WJ 709

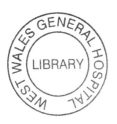

Standard Practice
in Sexual Medicine

ISSM STANDARDS COMMITTEE

Chairman: Hartmut Porst (*Germany*)
Co-Chairman: Jacques Buvat (*France*)

Sub-Committee: Preclinical Research and Animal Models in Sexual Medicine (Male and Female)
Chairman: François Giuliano (*France*)
Members: James G. Pfaus (*Canada*), Kevin McKenna (*USA*), Balasubramanian Srilatha (*Singapore*)

Sub-Committee: Psychobehavioral and Couple Aspects
Chairmen: Stanley E. Althof (*USA*), Raymond Rosen (*USA*)
Members: Eusebio Rubio-Aurioles (*Mexico*), Carolyn Earle (*Australia*), Marie Chevret-Measson (*France*)

Sub-Committee: Male Sexual Dysfunction
Medical Treatment in ED, Priapism and Peyronie's Disease
Chairmen: Hartmut Porst (*Germany*), Ajay Nehra (*USA*)
Members: Ganesan Adaikan (*Singapore*), Hussein Ghanem (*Egypt*), Sidney Glina (*Brazil*), Wayne Hellstrom (*USA*), Ira D. Sharlip (*USA*), Allen D. Seftel (*USA*)

Surgical Treatment of ED, Priapism and Peyronie's Disease
Chairmen: John P. Mulhall (*USA*) and Michael Sohn (*Germany*)
Members: Antonio Martin-Morales (*Spain*), Sudhakar Krishnamurti (*India*)

Ejaculatory Disorders
Chairmen: Chris G. McMahon (*Australia*), Marcel D. Waldinger (*The Netherlands*)
Members: David L. Rowland (*USA*), Pierre Assalian (*Canada*), Alan Riley (*UK*), Young Chan Kim (*South Korea*), Amado Bechara (*Argentina*)

Sub-Committee: Hormones, Metabolism, Aging, and Sexual Function
Chairmen: Jacques Buvat (*France*), Ridwan Shabsigh (*USA*)
Members: André Guay (*USA*), Louis Gooren (*The Netherlands*), Luiz Otavio-Torres (*Brazil*), Eric Meulemann (*The Netherlands*)

Sub-Committee: Female Sexual Disorders
Chairwoman: Alessandra Graziottin (*Italy*)
Members: Linda Banner (*USA*), Annamaria Giraldi (*Denmark*), Lorraine Dennerstein (*Australia*), Beverly Whipple (*USA*), Jeanne L. Alexander (*USA*)

Sub-Committee: Cardiovascular Issues in Sexual Medicine
Chairman: Graham Jackson (*UK*)
Member: Adolph Hutter (*USA*)

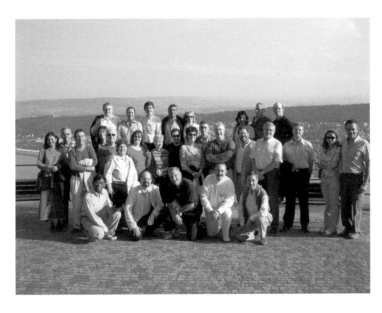

Members of the ISSM Standards Committee attending the preparatory meeting for *Standard Practice in Sexual Medicine* in Rüdesheim, Germany, 31st August–4th September, 2005.

Standard Practice in Sexual Medicine

EDITED BY

Hartmut Porst

Chairman, ISSM Standards Committee

Neuer Jungfernstieg 6a
20354 Hamburg
Germany

Jacques Buvat

Co-Chairman, ISSM Standards Committee

Centre ETPARP
3 Rue Carolus
59000 Lille
France

AND

The Standards Committee of the International Society for Sexual Medicine

Blackwell
Publishing

© 2006 International Society for Sexual Medicine
Published by Blackwell Publishing

Blackwell Publishing, Inc., 350 Main Street, Malden, Massachusetts 02148-5020, USA
Blackwell Publishing Ltd, 9600 Garsington Road, Oxford OX4 2DQ, UK
Blackwell Publishing Asia Pty Ltd, 550 Swanston Street, Carlton, Victoria 3053, Australia

First published 2006

1 2006

Library of Congress Cataloging-in-Publication Data

Standard practice in sexual medicine / edited by Hartmut Porst, Jacques Buvat.
     p.   ;   cm.
  Includes bibliographical references and index.
  ISBN-13: 978-1-4051-5719-3
  ISBN-10: 1-4051-5719-4
  1. Sexual disorders. I. Porst, Hartmut. II. Buvat, J. (Jacques)
  [DNLM: 1. Sexual Dysfunction, Physiological. 2. Genital Diseases, Female.
  3. Genital Diseases, Male. WJ 709 S785 2006]
  RC556. S73 2006
  616.6'9–dc22

2006018673

A catalogue record for this title is available from the British Library
ISBN-13: 978-1-4051-5719-3
ISBN-10: 1-4051-5719-4

Set in 9 on 12 pt Meridien by SNP Best-set Typesetter Ltd., Hong Kong
Printed and bound in the United Kingdom by TJ International Ltd, Padstow, Cornwall

Commissioning Editor: Stuart Taylor
Development Editor: Julie Elliott
Production Controller: Kate Charman

For further information on Blackwell Publishing, visit our website:
http://www.blackwellpublishing.com

Contents

List of Contributors

Ganesan Adaikan MD, PhD, DSc, ACS
President, ISSM
Department of Obstetrics and
    Gynaecology
National University Hospital
Yong Loo Lin School of Medicine
National University of Singapore
5 Lower Kent Ridge Road
Singapore 119074
Singapore

Jeanne L. Alexander MD, ABPN, FRCPC, FAPA, FACPsych
Director, Northern California Kaiser
    Permanente Medical Group
    Psychiatry Women's Health Program
Assistant Clinical Professor of Psychiatry,
    Stanford Medical School, PaloAlto,
    California
Founder, Alexander Foundation for
    Women's Health
1700 Shattuck Avenue, Suite 329
Berkely, CA 94709
USA

Stanley E. Althof PhD
Professor of Psychology
Case Western Reserve University School
    of Medicine
Executive Director, Center for Marital
    and Sexual Health of South Florida
1515 N. Flagler Drive
Suite 540
West Palm Beach, Florida 33401
USA

Pierre Assalian MD
Associate Professor, Department of
    Psychiatry, McGill University
Executive Director, Canadian Sex
    Research Forum
Director, Human Sexuality Unit,
    Montreal General Hospital
1650 Cedar
Montreal
Quebec H3G 1A4
Canada

Linda Banner PhD
Health Psychologist
Research Consultant, Stanford Medical
    Center
2516 Samaritan Drive D
San Jose, CA 95124
USA

Amado Bechara MD, PhD
Urologyst
Director, Instituto Médico Especializado
    (IME)
Av. Santa Fe 3312 6to D (1425)
Buenos Aires
Argentina

Jacques Buvat MD
Past President, SFMS and ISSM
Centre ETPARP
3 rue Carolus
59000 Lille
France

Marie Chevret-Measson MD
Psychiatrist and Sexologist
283, Rue de Créqui
69007 Lyon
France

Lorraine Dennerstein MBBS, PhD, FRANZCP, DPM
Director, Office for Gender and Health
Department of Psychiatry
The University of Melbourne
Level 1 North, Main Building Royal
    Melbourne Hospital Victoria 3050
Australia

Carolyn Earle
Manager / Sexologist
Keogh Institute for Medical Research
3rd Floor, A Block
Sir Charles Gairdner Hospital
2 Verdun Street
Nedlands
Western Australia
Australia

Hussein Ghanem MD
Professor of Andrology, Sexology and
    STDs
Cairo University
139(A) El Tahrir Street
Dokki, Cairo
Egypt

Annamaria Giraldi MD, PhD
President Elect, ISSWSH
Specialist Registrar and Lecturer in
    Sexology
Division of Sexological Research
Rigshospitalet 7111
Blegdamsvej 9
Copenhagen 2100
Denmark

François Giuliano MD, PhD
Professor of Therapeutics, Urology AP-
    HP, Neuro-Urology-Andrology Unit
Department of Physical Medicine and
    Rehabilitation
Raymond Poincaré Hospital
104 bd Raymond Poincaré
92380 Garches
France

Sidney Glina MD, PhD
Past President, ISSM
Director, Instituto H. Ellis
Rua Almirante Pereira Guimarães, 360
01250-000 São Paulo-SP
Brazil

Louis Gooren MD, PhD
Professor, Department of Endocrinology
Vrije Universiteit Medical Center
PO Box 7057
1007 MB Amsterdam
The Netherlands

Alessandra Graziottin MD
Director, Center of Gynecology and
    Medical Sexology
Consultant Professor of Sexual
    Medicine, University of Florence
    and Parma
H. San Raffaele Resnati
Via E. Panzacchi 6
20123 Milan
Italy

André Guay MD, FACP, FACE
Director, Center For Sexual
    Function/Endocrinology
Lahey Clinic Northshore
One Essex Center Drive
Peabody, MA 01960
USA

Wayne J.G. Hellstrom MD, FACS
Chief, Section of Andrology and Male
    Infertility
Tulane University School of Medicine
Department of Urology
1430 Tulane Avenue, SL 42
New Orleans, LA 70112
USA

Adolph Hutter MD
Professor of Medicine, Harvard Medical
    School
Yawkey 5B
Massachusetts General Hospital
55 Fruit Street
Boston, MA 02114
USA

**Graham Jackson MD, FRCP, FACC,
FESC**
Cardiothoracic Centre
St Thomas' Hospital
London SE1 7EH
UK

Young Chan Kim MD
Korean Sexual and Men's Health Center
3F. Han Central Bldg.
646-7 Yoksam-dong
Kangnam-ku 135-911
Seoul
Korea

Sudhakar Krishnamurti MD
Andromeda Andrology Center
1st Floor, Topaz
P.O. Box 1563
Greenlands Rd.
Hyderabad, 500 082 AP
India

**Chris G. McMahon MBBS,
FAChSHM**
Professor, Genitourinary Physician and
    Director, Australian Centre for Sexual
    Health
Suite 2-4
Berry Road Medical Centre
1a Berry Road
St Leonards NSW 2065
Australia

Kevin McKenna PhD
Professor, Departments of Physiology
    and Urology
Northwestern University Feinberg
    School of Medicine
Tarry Building 5-755 (M211)
303 East Chicago Avenue
Chicago, Il 60611-3008
USA

Antonio Martín-Morales MD
Unidad Andrología, Servicio Urología
Hospital Regional Universitario Carlos
    Haya
Plaza Hospital Civil s/n
Málaga, 29009
España

Eric Meuleman MD
Department of Urology
Free University Medical Center
PO Box 7057
1007 MB Amsterdam
The Netherlands

John Mulhall MD
Associate Professor
Department of Urology
Weill Medical College of Cornell
    University
Director, Sexual Medicine Programs
New York Presbyterian Hospital and
    Memorial Sloan Kettering Cancer
    Center
525 E 68th St
New York, NY 10021
USA

Ajay Nehra MD, FACS
Consultant, Department of Urology
Professor of Urology
Mayo Medical School
Mayo Clinic
Rochester
USA

James G. Pfaus PhD
Professor, Center for Studies in
    Behavioral Neurobiology
Department of Psychology
Concordia University
7141 Sherbrooke W.
Montreal, QC H4B IR6
Canada

Hartmut Porst MD
Professor of Urology
Urclogical Practice
Neuer Jungfernstieg 6a
20354 Hamburg
Germany

Alan Riley MSc, MBBS, MRCS, DRCOG, FFPM
Professor, Sexual Medicine
Lancashire School of Health and
  Postgraduate Medicine
University of Central Lancashire
Preston PR1 2HE
UK

Raymond Rosen PhD
UMDNJ-Robert Wood Johnson Medical
  School
671 Hoes Lane
Piscataway, NJ 08854
USA

David Rowland MD, PhD
Professor of Psychology
Office of Graduate Studies
Valparaiso University
Valparaiso, IN 46383
USA

Eusebio Rubio-Aurioles MD, PhD
Asociación Mexicana para la Salud
  Sexual, A.C. AMSSAC
Tezoquipa 26
Colonia La Joya
Delegación Tlalpan, México DF 14000
Mexico City
Mexico

Allen D. Seftel MD
Professor, Department of Urology
Case Western Reserve University
University Hospitals of Cleveland
11100 Euclid Ave
Cleveland, Ohio 44106-5046
USA

Ridwan Shabsigh MD
Associate Professor of Urology
Columbia University
Director, New York Center for Human
  Sexuality
161 Fort Washington Avenue
New York, NY 10032
USA

Ira D. Sharlip MD
President Elect, ISSM
Clinical Professor of Urology
University of California at San Francisco
2100 Webster St
Suite 222
San Francisco CA 94115
USA

Michael Sohn MD
Professor of Urology
Urologische Klinik
Frankfurter Diakonie Kliniken/Markus
  KH
Wilhelm-Epstein Str. 2
60431 Frankfurt
Germany

Balasubramanian Srilatha MD, PhD
Department of Obstetrics and
  Gynaecology
National University Hospital
Yong Loo Lin School of Medicine
National University of Singapore
5 Lower Kent Ridge Road
Singapore, 119074
Singapore

Luiz Otavio Torres MD
Past President, SLAMS
President, Brazilian Society of Urology,
  Section Minas Gerais
Director, Clinica de Urologia e
  Andrologia
Av. Afonso Pena 3111/204-205
CEP 30130-008 — Belo Horizonte
Minas Gerais
Brazil

Marcel Waldinger MD, PhD
Neuropsychiatrist
Department Psychiatry and
  Neurosexology
Haga Hospital Leyenburg
Leyweg 275
2545 CH The Hague
The Netherlands

Beverly Whipple PhD, RN, FAAN
Professor Emerita
Rutgers University
87 Matlack Drive
Voorhees, NJ 08043
USA

Preface

The modern era in sexual medicine started in the 1970s when a few devoted pioneers and visionaries began to revolutionize our thinking and understanding in this field.

Prior to that time, sexual dysfunctions in men, particularly erectile disorders, were thought to be purely psychogenic or in rare cases caused by testosterone deficiency. Treatment of sexual disorders was considered to be predominantly the business of sextherapists or rarely of endocrinologists. And at that time, knowledge about female sexual disorders was practically non-existent; female sexuality was little more than a blank spot in sexual medicine.

The introduction of completely new surgical procedures, such as corpus cavernosum revascularization and penile implants, for the treatment of impotence, and the invention of new and creative diagnostic procedures, such as penile angiography, dynamic cavernosometry and penile Doppler ultrasonography, expanded our knowledge in this field and contributed to the better understanding of the causes and treatments of sexual dysfunctions. Several exceptional medical scientists deserve to be considered the true pioneers of this novel thinking in sexual medicine. First, Vaclav Michal, a Czechoslovakian vascular surgeon, introduced the concept of passive erection for the diagnosis of vasculogenic erectile dysfunction and the technique of penile arterial revascularization for the treatment of vasculogenic impotence. Jean-Francois Ginestié and A. Romieu, the inventors of the radiologic exploration of impotence, introduced selective pudendal arteriography and dynamic cavernosography as key procedures in the diagnosis of vasculogenic impotence. M.P. Small and H.M. Carrion invented the first internationally marketed rigid penile implant and B. Scott invented the first hydraulic penile implant. Gorm Wagner focused his scientific investigations on the physiologic and pathophysiologic processes involved in sexual responses and how they contribute to the manifestation of sexual dysfunctions in both sexes. Dr Wagner later became the first President of the International Society for Impotence Research, later renamed the International Society for Sexual Medicine. In the late 1970s, Adrian W. Zorgniotti, of New York University, gave the new scientific field of sexual medicine an organizational framework by convening the first and second conferences on "Corpus Cavernosum Revascularization" in 1978 in New York and in 1980 in Monte Carlo. After 1980, these conferences were continued at two year intervals, becoming first the World Congresses of Impotence Research in the 1980s and 1990s and then the Congresses of the International Society for Sexual Medicine in the first decade of the new century. Gathering biennially up to 2000 physicians and researchers from around the world, the first several of these Congresses made it clear that considering sexual dysfunctions as purely psychogenic was inaccurate and a new era in the history of sexual medicine was launched.

Having attended all these Congresses since 1980, we learned in person of the rapid progress being made in the field of sexual medicine. This book, the work-product of the Standards Committee of the International Society for Sexual Medicine, classifies what has been accomplished so far and identifies where the main emphasis of future trends may be. This book updates current knowledge and present standards in the field of sexual medicine for both genders. It demonstrates as well the growing importance of female sexual medicine and psychology.

With this statement, we would like to express our thanks to all the members of the ISSM Standards Committee, especially to the Chairmen and Chairwomen of the respective sub-committees. Without their dedicated and untiring engagement, this work would never have happened in such a short time. Our deep gratitude extends also to the exceptional contribution of Astrid Brendt and the superb work of Helen Harvey and Blackwell Publishing without whose dedication and support this project could not have been completed.

By increasing knowledge in sexual medicine of many thousands of colleagues who deal with sexual dysfunctions across this globe, we hope that the work of the ISSM Standards Committee will provide even better health services in this medical discipline. It is our wish that this work will enhance sexual health and quality of life for the tens of million of couples world-wide who face the challenges of sexual dysfunction.

Hartmut Porst, MD
Chairman
Jacques Buvat, MD
Co-Chairman
ISSM Standards Committee
2006

Foreword

It is a mystifying paradox that among the most important functions of the human body, sexuality has drawn more public attention than any other, yet sexual function is one of the last areas to receive the careful attention of medical scientists.

Many studies have shown that sexual health is a very important element of overall health and quality of life. Yet in both the developed and the developing worlds, social taboos and religious restrictions surround human sexuality. In some places, ignorance about sexuality, illogical mores and/or irrational ritual practices impede medical research, interfere with medical education about sexual health, contribute to the propagation of sexually-transmitted diseases and/or prevent individuals from achieving a fully healthy and happy life.

Since its inception in 1982, the International Society for Sexual Medicine (ISSM) has strived to alter the paradox between the immense impact that sexuality has on human behavior and the limited state of scientific research and knowledge in human sexuality. The basic goal of the Society has been to introduce sound scientific knowledge to the experimental and clinical aspects of sexual medicine. In addition, ISSM aims to guide the field of sexual medicine into a position of prominence and prestige in the panoply of healthcare disciplines; to promote public education about sexual health; and to provide its members with a rich international environment for the exchange of scientific ideas and information.

In its global efforts to promote the highest standards of research, practice and treatment in sexual healthcare, ISSM conducts international scientific meetings in every continent, maintains an international registry of sexual health problems and promotes scientific publications in female and male sexual medicine. For example, the Society's official journal, *The Journal of Sexual Medicine*, has become widely acknowledged as the leading journal, by all standards, in this field.

Standard Practice in Sexual Medicine is another milestone in the history of the ISSM. As the Society addresses a multiplicity of challenges in sexual medicine, we are heartened at the focused consonance in this book between clinical problems and contemporary scientific literature. As its name states, this comprehensive volume proposes standards for current practice of both male and female sexual medicine and provides direction for future investigation. At the crossroads of our quest to enhance the quality of life for man and womankind, this book will be an invaluable source for many years to come, not only for the deeply inquiring young scientific mind but for the more seasoned practitioner as well.

We must be certain to recognize the Herculean efforts of the far-sighted Editors, Dr Hartmut Porst and Dr Jacques Buvat, and all of the individual chapter authors in making this book a reality. We are especially indebted to Dr Buvat who, during his term as President of ISSM, had the vision to create the ISSM Standards Committee. This scholarly book is the first work of that committee. The prodigious scientific contribution of Drs Porst and Buvat in compiling this book is an extraordinary legacy to the future of sexual medicine. On behalf of the ISSM, we place on record our sincere gratitude for their uncompromising and timely efforts.

P. Ganesan Adaikan
President
Ira D. Sharlip
President-Elect
International Society for Sexual Medicine
September 2006

CHAPTER 1

Preclinical Research and Animal Models in Sexual Medicine

François Giuliano, Kevin McKenna, Balasubramanian Srilatha, and James G. Pfaus

Introduction

Preclinical research typically involves the use of animal models of human sexual response, and is often conducted to investigate the effects of pharmacologic agents, instrumentation, new devices, or surgical procedures prior to clinical trials. This research may also examine certain side effects of such treatment; however, preclinical research may also include human tissue experiments or biochemical experiments with human products, e.g. native or recombinant enzymes. For the sake of simplicity, studies of toxicology, carcinogeniticity, fertility, and safety will not be included in the definition.

The key issue for clinicians is the ability to extrapolate the preclinical results to human clinical populations, and in particular to determine the likelihood that a treatment will be successful or will warrant subsequent human tests. Besides studies conducted in anesthetized animals that have been extremely useful in the study of sexual physiology, behavioral experiments are crucial to providing a more integrative approach to understanding the physiologic and pathophysiologic aspects of sexual function and dysfunction.

In all species, sexual behavior is directed by a complex interplay between steroid hormone actions in the brain that give rise to sexual arousability, and experience with sexual reward or pleasure that gives rise to expectations of competent sexual activity, including sexual arousal, desire, and performance. Sexual experience allows animals to form instrumental and Pavlovian associations that predict sexual outcome and thereby direct the strength of sexual responding. Although the study of animal sexual behavior by neuroendocrinologists has traditionally been concerned with mechanisms of copulatory responding; more recent use of conditioning and preference paradigms, and a focus on environmental circumstances and experience, has revealed behaviors and processes that resemble human sexual responses.

Accordingly, we have summarized behavioral paradigms used with rodents and other species that are analogous or homologous to human sexual arousal, desire, reward, and inhibition. At a superficial level, human copulatory behavior does not resemble copulatory behavior in animals. For example, there is no human counterpart to female rat lordosis (at least not as an unambiguous, estrogen-dependent postural display of sexual receptivity in females), and human sexual behavior is so shaped by experience and learning that it seems to defy hormone actions that are critical to the display of animal sexual behavior. However, insights into the human experience can indeed be derived from animals, and in ways that are far less difficult scientifically and ethically to obtain than from human populations.

We have not referenced any experimental techniques because this was far beyond the scope of this chapter. Instead, we have proposed a list of review papers that will provide the reader with more in-depth insight into different experimental models.

What is required for a good animal model?

Predictive validity is the most important requisite of an appropriate animal model. In addition to this,

Penile erection
Recording of intracavernous pressure increases in anesthetized or conscious
   animals
Penile reflex tests
Ex copula erections
In vitro studies of cavernosal strips / penile artery reactivity (organ baths)
Cavernosal smooth muscle cells culture
Biochemical studies of erectile tissue

Ejaculation
Mating test: latency to ejaculate
Urethrogenital reflex (anesthetized)
PCA-induced ejaculation (anesthetized or conscious)
Pudendal motoneuron reflex discharge (anesthetized)
Electrical stimulation of peripheral nerves (anesthetized)

La Peyronie's disease
TGF-β1-induced La Peyronie's like condition

Priapism
Rabbits exposed to corporal hypoxia, then penile erection elicited by neural
   stimulation and the base of the erect penis clamped
eNOS–/– and nNOS–/–, eNOS–/– mice

Female peripheral sexual arousal
Anesthetized dogs, rabbits and rats: vaginal vasculo-muscular response along
   with clitoral tumescence induced by peripheral electrical neural stimulation.

Table 1.1 Experimental paradigms that can be used as rodent models of human sexual functions. eNOS, endothelial nitric oxide synthase; nNOS, neural nitric oxide synthase; PCA, p-chloroamphetamine; TGF-β1, transforming growth factor beta 1.

animal models should be simple and practical enough to have "high throughput", meaning the ability to have experiments conducted relatively quickly. Issues of sample size and ease of testing and analysis are key factors. The validity of any homologous or analogous animal model can only be determined in situations that test whether a treatment that modifies behavior in the animal does so in humans.

Any animal "system" in which the homology or analogy has predictive validity to human responses or physiologic processes (and can be replicated) is a good model. If the model is practical from an experimental standpoint, then it will likely be used more than models that are cumbersome. In addition, the more information that is gathered from a particular model, the more the model will be used because it has a large literature associated with it. Rats continue to be the most frequently used animals in the study of sexual behavior. There are many reasons for this,

the most obvious being that they are practical (e.g. small, easy to handle, and quite social) and they have a large literature associated with them. Rats also resemble humans in many analogous and homologous ways. Certain tissues and neuroendocrine systems in rats are strikingly similar to our own (e.g. the physiologic control of erection, or uterine tissue growth following estrogen treatment).

Rectification of terms

In humans, sexual dysfunctions form around the categories of sexual arousal, desire, orgasm, and pain. Arousal may be separated into physiologic genital arousal (sometimes referred to as "potency") and subjective or psychologic arousal that denotes a conscious awareness of the genital sensations. However, this psychologic arousal may be an important component of sexual desire (sometimes referred to as "libido" or "motivation"). Sexual arousal and desire sum into behavioral responses of copulation

Table 1.2 Paradigms that can be used as rodent models of human sexual behavior (from Pfaus *et al.*, 2003).

Sexual arousal

Males

    Penile reflex tests (physiologic erectile function; responses to somatosensory stimulation)

    Noncontact erections ("psychogenic" erectile function; responses to primary or secondary conditioned sexual cues)

    Copulatory measures: latency to mount, intromit or ejaculate (shorter latency = greater arousal)

    Enforced interval effect (model of premature ejaculation)

    Coolidge effect (increased arousal by changing sexual stimuli)

Sexual desire

Females and males

    Excitement (motor responses in anticipation of sexual activity or in response to hormonal stimulation)

    Instrumental responding (desire to obtain a sex partner)

    Sexual preference paradigms (desire to obtain unconditioned or conditioned sexual incentive characteristics)

    Copulatory measures

Males

    Pursuit (desire to obtain sex partner)

Females

    Solicitation, hops and darts (desire to initiate sexual activity)

    Pacing (desire to regulate copulatory contact; increased pacing = decreased desire for copulatory contact)

    Lordosis (receptivity to vaginal penetration)

    Lateral tail displacement in hamsters (receptivity to vaginal penetration)

Sexual reward

Females and males (to examine what aspect of sexual responding is rewarding, e.g. copulatory stimulation vs. ejaculation in males, or the ability to control sexual interaction in females):

    Operant responding for primary or secondary sexual reinforcers

    Conditioned place preference

    Unconditioned or conditioned partner preference

    Conditioned copulatory behavior (e.g. copulatory responses in places paired with sexual or other rewards, or in the presence or absence of conditioned incentive cues)

Sexual inhibition

Females

    Copulatory behavior after several ejaculatory series

    Estrus termination

    Tests using ovariectomized females primed with estrogen alone

Males

    Primary sexual inhibition (using access to nonreceptive females)

    Second order sexual inhibition (using odors or other stimuli paired with access to nonreceptive females).

    Recovery from sexual exhaustion

(sometimes referred to as "performance"). The terms used in the animal literature often do not resemble those in the human literature, and a rectification of terms is necessary to translate between animal and human sexual functions. We propose the Incentive Sequence Model (Fig. 1.1) as a place to begin such a rethinking of nomenclature and to bridge the gap between animal research and the clinical practice.

Male Sexual Function

Peripheral sexual reflexes (erection and ejaculation), copulatory behaviour (mounts, intromissions,

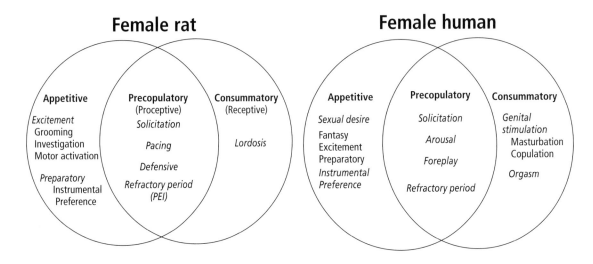

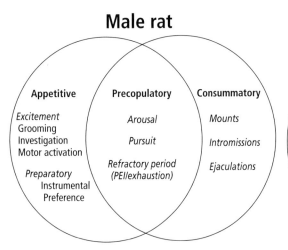

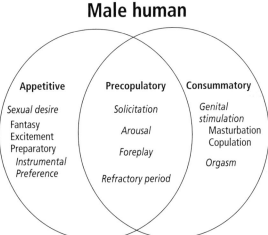

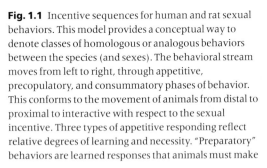

Fig. 1.1 Incentive sequences for human and rat sexual behaviors. This model provides a conceptual way to denote classes of homologous or analogous behaviors between the species (and sexes). The behavioral stream moves from left to right, through appetitive, precopulatory, and consummatory phases of behavior. This conforms to the movement of animals from distal to proximal to interactive with respect to the sexual incentive. Three types of appetitive responding reflect relative degrees of learning and necessity. "Preparatory" behaviors are learned responses that animals must make in order to acquire the incentive (e.g. operant behaviors, pursuit, etc.). "Anticipatory" behaviors are learned responses that occur in anticipation of an incentive, but are not necessary to obtain it (e.g. conditioned psychomotor stimulation that characterizes behavioral excitement). Unlearned appetitive responses also exist that are instinctual (e.g. unconditioned anogenital investigation). These aspects of behavior also occur once copulatory contact has been made, especially if copulation occurs in bouts (as it does in rats). From Pfaus, 1999.

and ejaculation), and appetitive conditioned sexual responses (e.g. conditioned arousal), have been examined in a variety of species. In most cases, sexual physiologic and behavioural responses are extremely similar between the species, making the generation of analogies and homologies, and their application to human male function and dysfunction, straightforward.

Penile erection

Experimental research on penile erection dates from at least the 19th century, with the work of pioneer physiologists such as Eckhardt, Langley and Anderson. Subsequently, during the 20th century significant advances were achieved thanks to the work of Semans and Langworthy in the 1930s, veterinary researchers performing experiments in conscious bulls and stallions in the 1970s, Sjöstrand using plethysmography to quantify penile erection in the rabbit, and then work by Lue's and Goldstein's groups in the 1980s, providing the scientific and medical community with experiments conducted in dogs, monkeys and rabbits that show the vascular component of penile erection and the crucial role of cavernosal smooth muscle fibers. Quinlan then introduced the first rat model to measure penile erection. More recently, investigations of penile erection have been performed in mice, opening the door to studies conducted with genetically modified animals.

From a physiologic perspective, it appears that there is a close similarity between local mechanisms of penile erection between non-human mammals and human males except for the role of striated muscles, which are less important in humans compared to various animal species.

Evaluation of erectile response in anesthetized animals

The gold standard for quantitative measurement of penile erection during experiments conducted in anesthetized and conscious animals is the recording of intracavernous pressure (ICP), also measurable in conscious animals by telemetry. It is noteworthy that ICP is closely dependant from arterial blood pressure. Penile erection can be elicited in anesthetized animals by electrical stimulation of peripheral nerves, i.e. pelvic or cavernous nerves (Fig. 1.2). It can also be elicited by electrical or chemical stimulation applied to brain structures. Drug delivery everywhere in the periphery (from intracavernosal injections to oral gavage) or within the central nervous system, including brain and spinal cord, is feasible in anesthetized animals to study their effect on penile erection.

Animal models have been widely used to establish the effects of phosphodiesterase-5 (PDE-5) inhibitors, and they have been predictive for the human situation for this class of compounds. There are crucial questions to be answered before extrapolating experimental data to humans, including: is the

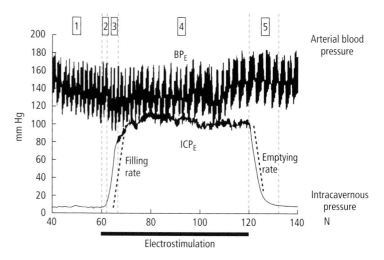

Fig. 1.2 Computer tracing of original recording of intracavernous and arterial blood pressures when stimulating cavernous nerve (6 volts, 10 Hz. 1 millisecond). 1: flaccid state; 2: latent phase; 3: tumescence phase; 4: maximal tumescence of the corpora cavernosa; 5: detumescence phase. ICP_E and BP_E were mean values of intracavernous and arterial blood pressures during full phase. Filling rate of corpora cavernosa is slope of increase of intracavernous pressure during tumescence phase. Slope of dramatic drop of intracavernous pressure after end of stimulation represents corpora cavernosa emptying rate.

receptor targeted by the compound under investigation the same in animals as compared to the human male and does it play the same role; e.g. intracavernosal prostaglandin E_1 (PGE_1) injections do not elicit penile erection in many animal species. When investigating the proerectile effect of pharmacologic compounds in animals, the following aspects must always be taken into account: dose used, route of administration, pharmacokinetics, half-life, metabolism of the studied compounds, etc.

In vitro reactivity studies of erectile tissue

These experiments are conducted in the investigation of the local cellular mechanisms of penile erection. Cavernosal strips from various animal species and humans have been studied in organ baths. These tissues are either pharmacologically precontracted, e.g. with phenylephrine, or electrically stimulated (electrical field stimulation) to elicit the release of neurotransmitters contained within the nerve terminals present in the tissue. Numerous compounds (e.g. prostanoids, α-adrenoceptor blockers, endothelin antagonists, PDE-5 inhibitors) have been found to be able to relax cavernosal strips by targeting various intracellular systems. Primary cell cultures derived from animal or human corpus cavernosum have also been used as *in vitro* models to define cellular mechanisms involved in erectile function.

Pathophysiologic models of erectile dysfunction

A wide variety of pathophysiologic models of erectile dysfunction (ED) have been proposed, aiming to mimic the numerous pathologic conditions responsible for ED in clinical practice. A non-exhaustive list of these models comprises: hypertensive rats, atherosclerotic rabbits, diabetic rats and rabbits, aged rats, castrated rats, cavernous nerve-injured rats, alcohol-treated, or nicotine-treated rats. The question of extrapolation to humans using these various experimental conditions must always be asked before drawing conclusions regarding applicability. It is noteworthy that there is no established standard in this domain, therefore we propose that the endpoints must be analogous or homologous (e.g. the restoration of erectile capability sufficient for copulation).

A special caution must be paid to castrated animals: many conclusions regarding the role of testosterone on penile erection have been drawn from experiments conducted in castrated rats; unfortunately this experimental paradigm is very different from the human situation, which is highly prevalent—i.e. the ageing male with partial androgen deficiency syndrome due to age in males (PADAM). So far no reliable model of PADAM has been proposed.

Due to advances in molecular biology, genetically engineered mice have now become available. Although the ultimate goal of these models is to develop gene therapy to rectify gene activity, transgenic or knockout mice have recently contributed to our understanding of the physiologic mechanisms of erectile function, as well as to various pathophysiologic processes occurring during ED.

Study of erection in conscious animals

In conscious rats, penile erections can be studied in isolation to obtain measures of physiologic arousal, or in response to different types of sexually arousing stimuli (e.g. noncontact erections in response to estrous odors) to obtain measures of psychogenic arousal.

Ex copula reflex erection is a commonly used unanesthetized rat model of erection. The rat is lightly restrained in a supine position and the penis is retracted from the sheath. Relatively predictable "spontaneous" penile erections are thus elicited. *Ex copula* reflex erections are generated by spinal reflex mechanisms and modulated by supraspinal control. The effects of drugs and various central neural lesions can be examined in this model. It has the advantage in that it does not involve social interaction with the female and it examines penile reactions directly.

Several pharmacologic agents acting at different central brain regions have been shown to elicit penile erection in conscious rats during *ex copula* penile erection tests, i.e. in isolation. Penile erection during these tests has been inferred from a series of motor acts like standing on the hind limbs, the head of the animal oriented towards the genital area, licking of the genital area, contractions of the hip muscles, and sometimes by direct observation of protrusion of the glans. It remains unknown whether or not the putative neural structures representing targets for these "proerectile drugs" are all activated during the penile erection that occurs in several natural contexts (sleep, copulation, psychogenic, reflex).

Male rats (but only pigmented strains) also show an analogy of "psychogenic erection" in response to the presence of estrous females, even when physical contact is prevented. A model of noncontact erections (NCEs) in rats was developed by Sachs and colleagues, and is studied in the presence of an inaccessible receptive female behind a mesh screen, or behind a series of walls with an air circulation system that brings the estrous odors to the male's compartment. Erections in response to these salient sexual cues are viewed as a model of psychogenic erection because they do not require direct somatosensory stimulation to be induced. The neurochemical and hormonal mechanisms that control their expression have been studied in detail. Analysis of NCEs following discrete brain lesions has demonstrated important distinctions in the neural control of copulatory performance and erectile capability. Drugs that enhance noncontact erections also induce a "penile erection and yawning syndrome" in rats in the absence of sexual stimulation. NCEs offer at least one advantage over the study of erection during copulation: they do not require complex motor responses or direct social interaction. This makes their study relatively less ambiguous as a measure of subjective sexual arousal. One concern is that the dependence of these responses on olfactory stimuli is unlike human sexual responses, which are more dependent on visual and auditory cues. However, olfaction is analogous to vision in this case, as the former is the dominant sense in rodents, whereas the latter is the dominant sense in humans.

Conclusions

Experimental research has been very productive regarding the physiology, pathophysiology and pharmacology of penile erection. There exist several rodent models of penile erection, from higher neural control down to molecular events within the erectile tissue. Although care must always be taken before extrapolating quickly from experimental data to the clinical situation, there is a high degree of predictability from rat models to men. Nature appears to have conserved mechanisms of erection in mammalian males.

Ejaculation and male orgasm

Most of the experimental work done so far for the investigation of ejaculation is based on behavioral experiments. Ejaculations in rats can be studied much the same way they are studied in humans, with the latency from first mount or intromission to ejaculation being the key variables (Fig. 1.3). Male rats typically ejaculate following several penile intromissions, and can ejaculate several times before becoming sexually exhausted, in which the male no longer responds to estrous odors or female solicitations. During successive ejaculatory series, the refractory period or post ejaculatory interval between each ejaculation and the subsequent resumption of copulation increases progressively. Penile intromission requires erection, and ejaculation typically requires sensory feedback from the penis that accumulates with multiple intromissions. The number of intromissions before ejaculation, the number of ejaculations achieved in a timed test, and the length of the post ejaculatory interval, are all dependent on autonomic arousal and can be enhanced or disrupted by drugs that have similar effects on copulatory performance in men. For example, drugs that delay or abolish orgasm in men (e.g. selective serotonin reuptake inhibitors such as fluoxetine, paroxetine), increase the ejaculation latencies and reduce the total number of ejaculations in rats. As in men, the reduced ability to ejaculate is more pronounced in rats following long-term daily administration. Acute alcohol intoxication also delays ejaculation in men and male rats.

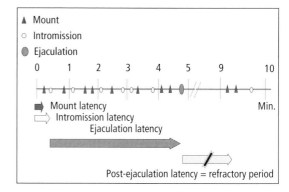

Fig. 1.3 Typical copulatory pattern in the male rat over a 10-min period.

Experimental investigation of ejaculation in anesthetized rats

Compared to penile erection much less research has been conducted in anesthetized animals in order to elucidate the physiology and the pharmacology of ejaculation. However, four interesting paradigms have been developed:

1 *Urethrogenital reflex:* the urethrogenital (UG) reflex is elicited by mechanical stimulation of the urethra in anesthetized and spinalized rat. Such a stimulation causes a spinal reflex to occur that consists of rhythmic contraction of the bulbospongiosus (BS) and the ischiocavernosus (IC) striated muscles associated with penile erection. It may be considered as mimicking the expulsion phase of ejaculation.

2 *PCA-induced ejaculation:* A model of pharmacologic induced ejaculation; p-chloroamphetamine (PCA) is an amphetamine derivative that liberates catecholamines and serotonin (5-hydroxytrptamine, 5-HT) from monoaminergic nerve terminals. Systemic administration of PCA has been reported to induce ejaculation in both conscious and anesthetized rats. Pharmacologic data indicate that the primary role in mediating the effect of PCA on ejaculation involves 5-HT, whereas noradrenaline (NA) appears to be of secondary importance.

3 *Electrical stimulation of peripheral nerves and ejaculation*: in anesthetized rats, electrical stimulation of the hypogastric nerve can partially reproduce the ejaculatory process, i.e. eliciting a rise in seminal vesicle and bladder neck pressures that correspond respectively to seminal vesicles contractions and closure of the bladder neck, but it fails to induce the expulsion reflex.

4 *Pudendal motoneuron reflex discharge*: the recording of electrical activity in the efferent branch of the ejaculatory reflex, i.e. the pudendal motor response discharge (PMRD) elicited by the electrical stimulation of the afferent branch of the expulsion reflex—the dorsal nerve of the penis, is thought to be an experimental model representing events that occur in humans during sexual intercourse and that culminate with the expulsion of sperm.

Orgasm and the consequences of ejaculation

Although it is not known whether male rats experi-ence orgasm during ejaculation, the peripheral reflexes appear very similar. Moreover, ejaculation is absolutely necessary for male rats to show subsequent evidence that sex was rewarding or "pleasurable". For example, ejaculation is required for the induction of conditioned place and partner preference in male rats. These preferences are not displayed if males are administered the opioid antagonist naloxone during conditioning, suggesting that ejaculation induces the activation of endogenous opioids in the brain that mediate the critical rewarding properties of sex.

Conclusions

This research is still in its infancy. Apart from behavioral studies, there is a need for standardization and more research is definitely mandatory in this area. There is no model available, for example, to investigate delayed or absent ejaculation or painful ejaculation, and the experimental equivalent of the male orgasm is lacking.

Sexual motivation and "desire"

Desire has always been difficult to define objectively. In the DSM-IV-TR, the diagnosis of hypoactive sexual desire disorder is given when "desire for and fantasy about sexual activity are chronically or recurrently deficient or absent." By converse logic, then sexual desire is the presence of desire for, and fantasy about, sexual activity. This definition appears coherent but is circular. How does desire manifest itself?

Like people, animals manifest sexual excitement behaviorally. They increase their motor output in anticipation of copulation and work for the opportunity to copulate or to obtain primary or secondary (conditioned) sexual rewards associated with copulation. Animals will also choose between two or more sexual incentives based on the strength of the incentive cues and the animal's own internal drive state. What characterizes these behaviors is that they occur before copulation: Courtship, operant responses, conditioned locomotion in anticipation of sex, time spent near a particular sexual incentive, or choices made between two or more incentives, can all be considered analogies of anticipatory sexual desire. The strength of the behavior can be observed as increases or decreases, or can be tested by increasing the criterion level of responding that animals must attain before they are given access to rewards. Simply put, animals with more "desire" will display more robust behavior than animals with less desire. Desire can also be inferred from certain appetitive responses that occur during copulation, such as solicitation in females or chasing behavior in males. A growing body of evidence indicates that these aspects of sexual behavior are altered in a relatively selective fashion by certain drugs that are known to alter desire in humans (e.g. by drugs that affect dopamine or melanocortin receptors).

Models of male sexual dysfunctions
Erectile dysfunction

Male rats that do not perform sexually are typically taken out of behavioral studies, so there is very little known about their actual erectile responsiveness. This proportion is generally low, especially if the males are pre-exposed to the test chambers prior to their initial sexual experiences. Some of these males do not display any interest in the female, and do not initiate any kind of sexual activity. However, other males display sexual interest and mount repeatedly, but do not achieve vaginal intromission. The lack of intromission may stem from an inability to achieve erection. Indeed, erectile responses in isolation and intromissions during copulation are both very sensitive to disruption by several classes of drug, including psychomotor stimulants, dopamine and noradrenergic antagonists, and opioid agonists. Acute or chronic treatment with selective serotonin reuptake inhibitors (SSRIs) does not appear to alter erectile responses or the number of intromissions prior to ejaculation. This profile of pharmacologic sensitivity is strikingly similar to clinical observations and anecdotes in men, thus male rats may be a useful model of drug-induced, if not also stress or vascular disease–related erectile dysfunction.

Premature ejaculation

In 1956, Knut Larsson published a series of studies that described many ways in which sexual reflexes and behaviors could be conditioned by experience. In one of these paradigms, called the "enforced interval effect", male rats were given repeated access to females that were removed physically from the testing chamber by the experimenter after every intromission. In this way, Larsson was able to vary the time between intromissions and found that male intromission intervals that lasted longer than normal resulted in males that learned to ejaculate with far fewer intromissions. One of the interpretations of this data was that the imposition of longer intromission intervals made males more sympathetically aroused, and led to either a faster ejaculation or one that required less tactile penile stimulation. This model of hyperstimulation of sympathetic outflow by either highly stimulating, unpredictable, or stressful sex, formed part of the basis of Masters and Johnson's model of premature ejaculation a decade later. Despite this, the model has not been developed further, nor has it been used widely to examine drug effects.

More recently it was reported that natural differences are found in the ejaculation latencies of male rats, which may indicate a more biological explanation of premature ejaculation that shares some of the characteristics of human premature ejaculation. In pooled populations of male albino Wistar rats during a 30 min standardized mating test, three categories of males were identified: (1) males that displayed a low number of ejaculations (0 to 1) and were considered as sexually "sluggish" or "hypo-sexual"; (2) a second category of rats that showed a range of two or three ejaculations and were considered as "normal" ejaculators; and (3) males who displayed four or five ejaculations and were considered as "rapid" ejaculators or "hypersexual" rats. The number of ejaculations across the various studies was distributed according to a Gaussian curve: on one side approximately 10% of rats display "hypo-sexual" behavior and on the other side 10% display "hyper-sexual" behavior after at least four successive weekly sexual tests of 30 min. Interesting differences were found between the "sluggish" and "rapid" groups of rats with regard to a variety of other parameters of sexual behavior, resembling clinical symptoms of men suffering from retarded and premature ejaculation, respectively.

The "hyper-sexual" animals have been further investigated in order to know whether they could be used as a model for human premature ejaculation. Compared to "normal" ejaculators, ejaculation latency was shorter in "rapid" ejaculators and longer in "sluggish" ejaculators. Intromission and mount frequencies, the latter being considered as a putative index of sexual motivation, did not differ between the three categories of ejaculators, suggesting no differences in appetitive components of sexual behavior. When investigating the effects of 8-hydroxy-2-di-n-propylamino-tetralin (8-OH-DPAT) in these three categories of males, this compound was shown to induce a statistically significant increase in the number of ejaculations displayed by "sluggish" and "normal" rats, and to decrease in a statistically significant way the ejaculation latency in the "sluggish", "normal" and "rapid" rats.

This experimental paradigm, despite the fact it has been recently reported and not yet confirmed by others, appears as extremely attractive. Indeed "hyper-sexual rats" likely represent a pathophysiologic model of premature ejaculation. It remains to be seen whether drugs that can counteract premature ejaculation in men can increase the latency of male rats to ejaculate in this condition. It also remains to be studied whether such males are uniquely susceptible to an "enforced interval effect".

Delayed ejaculation

Conversely, some male rats ejaculate infrequently, or take a long time to achieve ejaculation. As mentioned above, this can be induced pharmacologically with alcohol or chronic treatment with SSRIs, such as fluoxetine or paroxetine. It remains to be determined whether the subset of sexually "sluggish" male rats found in normal populations can be utilized as models of delayed ejaculation.

Hypoactive sexual desire

Some male rats do not copulate despite extreme attempts on the part of sexually receptive females to get them to do so (including repeated mounting of the male by the female). Some of these males can be stimulated to copulate with low levels of electric shock, tail pinch, or treatment with low doses of psychomotor stimulants, like amphetamine, suggesting that a more general hypoarousability mediates their lack of responsiveness. Stress may also induce hyposexual responsivity in male rats, especially if it is pre-

sent during their early sexual experience. For example, a sizable proportion (often nearly 50%) of male rats will not copulate during their first trial with sexually receptive females unless they are pre-exposed to the testing chamber. Indeed, a large proportion of these noncopulators will *never* copulate, despite repeated exposure to receptive females. Novel environments are stressful to male rats, and induce the activation of endogenous opioids. Treatment with the opioid antagonist naloxone can reverse this novelty-induced stress effect.

Another way to study hypoactive desire in male rats is to examine their sexual responsiveness following multiple ejaculations, a phenomenon known as "sexual exhaustion". Male rats are able to ejaculate several times before becoming unresponsive. During this period of sexual activity, there is a progressive increase in the post-ejaculatory refractory period consonant, with a decrease in the number of intromissions before each ejaculation and a lengthening of the interintromission interval (a state that suggests a progressive loss of erectile function as the number of ejaculations increases). After males become sexually exhausted, they remain unresponsive to female solicitations for up to 72 hrs. Rodriguez-Manzo and colleagues have examined the ability of several classes of drug to increase the responsiveness of these males, including the opioid antagonist naloxone, 8-OH-DPAT, and the α_2 presynaptic autoreceptor antagonist yohimbine. Only yohimbine increased the proportion of males that mounted, intromitted, and displayed an ejaculatory-like behavioral pattern (but without seminal emission), suggesting that a decline in adrenergic activity is an important component of inhibited sexual desire in males.

La Peyronie's disease

An experimental model of transforming growth factor beta 1 (TGF-β1)-induced La Peyronie's like condition in the rat has been proposed by Tom Lue's group. The fibrosis is induced by a single injection of TGF-β1 in the tunica albuginea of Sprague Dawley rats. Following TGF-β1 injection, a dramatic influx of inflammatory cells is observed in the tunica albuginea, whereas the normal architecture of the tissue remains preserved. At two weeks, the inflammation decreases and the tunica albuginea structure is disturbed, which leads to fibrosis development both in the tunica albuginea and the adjacent corpus cavernosum of the penis at six weeks. This fibrosis is considered as a La Peyronie's-like condition because it exhibits biochemical and structural features that are similar to the human La Peyronie's disease plaque. Therefore, this animal model appears as a relevant tool to test innovative La Peyronie's disease pharmacologic strategies.

Hypogonadism/agonadism

In male rats, castration or the administration of androgen synthesis inhibitors, like cyproterone acetate, disrupt and ultimately eliminate copulatory behaviors and penile reflexes progressively over time. They also shrink androgen sensitive peripheral tissues (e.g. penis and prostate). Although the degree of disruption depends on the amount of androgen synthesis inhibition that is induced (e.g. moderate following low doses of cyproterone acetate to total disruption following castration), the amount of time it takes to reach an asymptotic level of behavioral or reflexive performance depends on the level of sexual experience male rats have prior to treatment. In each case, subsequent exogenous administration of androgens or estrogens can restore sexual interest and copulatory behavior, with nonaromatizable androgens (such as dihydrotestosterone) restoring peripheral tissues, and aromatizable androgens (e.g. testosterone) restoring behavioural measures. As with hypogonadal men, restoration of copulatory responses in castrated rats requires a threshold dose of aromatizable androgen that can restore plasma levels lower than those found in gonadally intact, functional animals (higher circulating levels are required for additional anabolic effects on muscle). It is striking, however, that appetitive sexual responses are the least affected by castration and can be maintained for months following. This finding echoes observations that treatment of sex offenders with androgen synthesis inhibitors does not reduce certain appetitive patterns of abuse (e.g. fondling), despite the fact that these men do not achieve erection. There are currently no models of age–related hypogonadism, although a decline in the sexual responsiveness of older male rats (>one year) has been reported in a few studies. However, castrated males can be maintained on subthreshold doses of testosterone prior to behavioral tests, or on a threshold dose followed by a progressive lowering of the dose regimen to mimic a more progressive decline, such as might be seen clinically.

Female Sexual Function

Gonadally-intact female rats of reproductive age go into sexual "heat" every four to five days immediately after ovulation. This process is initiated by the sequential actions of estrogen and progesterone (and possibly also androgens) in the brain and periphery, so that sexual behaviour shows an "estrous cycle". Although women (and certain other primate females) can engage in sexual activity throughout their menstrual cycle, there is a peak rise in female-initiated sexual activity around the time of ovulation, suggesting that estrogen–induced neurochemical systems have been conserved throughout mammalian evolution.

Peripheral sexual reflexes (e.g. vaginal blood flow), copulatory behaviour (solicitations, pacing, lordosis), and appetitive conditioned sexual responses (e.g. conditioned arousal) have been examined in female rats (Fig. 1.4), rabbits, and primates such as macaques. The physiologic mechanisms that regulate vaginal blood flow are extremely similar between species, and more is known about the hormonal and neural regulation of the reflexive posture lordosis (the dorsiflexion of the back that denotes sexual "receptivity" in many species) than any other sexual reflex. Recent work has also begun to elucidate the hormonal and neural control of complex behaviors used by females to regulate the initiation and rate of copulation, offering a real potential to utilize female rats as models for human sexual function.

It is important to emphasize that compared to human males, in whom ability to achieve and maintain erections sufficient for sexual activity is also good for self-esteem related to competent sexual performance, in women there is no clear relationship between physiologic performance and sexual desire. The subjective feeling of sexual arousal

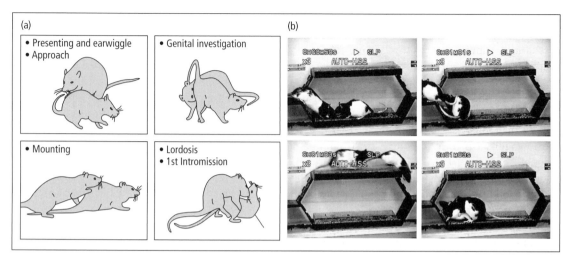

Fig. 1.4 Sexual behaviors displayed by male and female rats. (a) Line drawing of proceptive behaviors (presenting, ear wiggling and approach) and receptive behavior (lordosis) displayed by the female that evokes interest, investigation, chasing, and copulatory responses (mounts, intromissions, and ejaculation) in the male. (b) Female and male sexual behavior in a bilevel testing chamber. Top left: Female (right) makes a headwise orientation toward the male (left) characteristic of a solicitation. Top right: Female hops over the male to reveal her anogenital region, allowing the male to sniff and become aroused. Bottom left: Female runs away, forcing the male to chase her. Bottom right: Female holds a lordosis posture that allows the male to mount and gain vaginal penetration.

results more from cognitive processing of stimulus, meaning and content than from peripheral vasocongestive feedback. Indeed, there are well-identified discrepancies between physiologic and subjective measures of sexual arousal in women, and often no correlation between them (e.g. following treatment with PDE-5 inhibitors). It is not yet known how vaginal responses are integrated with behavioral responses. It remains questionable that increased vaginal blood flow could be perceived by females and participates in the stimulation of behavioral measures of sexual arousal. Accordingly, a more integrative approach is necessary to investigate female sexuality experimentally.

Genital sexual arousal

Upon sexual arousal, the blood supply to the vagina is rapidly increased and at the same time the venous drainage is reduced, thus creating vasocongestion and engorgement with blood. Such an increase in blood flow combined with an enhanced permeability of the capillary tufts induces a neurogenic transudate, which results in vaginal lubrication. From arousal to orgasm, there is also an increase of vaginal luminal pressure.

Reliable and standardized models to study the physiology/pharmacology of female vaginal sexual arousal have been described in dogs, rabbits and rats. In these models, vaginal sexual arousal along with clitoral tumescence is induced by peripheral electrical neural stimulation, while direct measurements of various vaginal physiologic variables are performed. These models have been useful to initiate the exploration of the peripheral physiology of female genital sexual response as well as the consequences of various experimental pathophysiologic conditions (e.g. atherosclerosis or hormonal deprivation).

Female orgasm, the urethra–genital reflex, and the consequences of paced copulation

It is not known whether female rats experience anything like orgasm during sex. However, like males, they display a genital reflex, called the "urethro–genital reflex" that is reminiscent of the orgasmic response in women. This reflex can be induced and studied in isolation by applying a mechanical stimulation to the urethra of anesthetized, spinalized female rats. The urethro–genital reflex includes rhythmic contractions of the vagina, uterus, and the anal sphincter, as well as the striated pelvic musculature. Stimulation of the urethra may mimic stimulation of the anterior wall of the vagina, which is the area with the highest "erotic" sensitivity. Indeed, the anterior wall of the vagina has a denser innervation than the posterior wall, and the distal area has more nerve fibers than the proximal.

During copulation, female rats typically control the initiation and rate of contact with males. In the same way that ejaculation is critical for conditioned sexual responses in males, the ability of female rats to pace their copulatory contact is critical for the induction of conditioned place or partner preferences. As in males, these consequences of sexual stimulation are blocked by administration of the opioid antagonist naloxone, suggesting that opioid activation is a critical feature of the sexual reward experienced during paced copulation. In addition, pacing imposes a delay between successive vaginal intromissions by the male. This delay distributes the vaginocervical stimulation that females receive over time, an effect that enhances reproductive capability and fertility in the female. Vaginocervical stimulation during orgasm in women may have a similar enhancing effect on reproductive capability.

Copulatory behavior and measures of female sexual motivation or "desire"

As in males, female sexual behavior can be divided into sequential appetitive and consummatory components (Fig. 1.1). In the female rat, these aspects of sexual behavior are also referred to as proceptive and receptive components, two different aspects of sexual behavior displayed by estrous females in the presence of sexually-active males. To solicit attention and approach of the male, the female displays a variety of active proceptive behavioral patterns, including solicitations, hops and darts, and ear-wiggles. As mentioned above, receptivity has been used to describe the behavioral postures assumed by

females to allow mounting by a male, with the lordosis reflex being the best known and most studied response. Unfortunately, there is no counterpart for lordosis in women. In contrast, psychologic arousal or desire in women is likely to be very close to proceptivity. For this reason, the study of proceptive behaviors is also relevant to any preclinical investigation of potential of compounds for the treatment of female sexual disorders or dysfunctions (FSD). Indeed, recently it has been reported that the melanocortin agonist, PT-141, increased rates of sexual solicitation and hops and darts in female rats selectively. This same drug increased female-initiated sexual activity in early Phase IIa clinical trials. These two observations were critically important to begin to establish solicitation as a valid model of female sexual desire.

Models of female sexual dysfunctions
Hypogonadism/agonadism and hypoactive sexual desire

Although there are currently no established models of female sexual dysfunction in rats, there are several reasons to believe that such models could exist. The most obvious would be the consequences of hypogonadism induced by ovariectomy followed by maintenance with different doses of estrogen alone, or estrogen and progesterone. Ovariectomized rats treated with estrogen and progesterone display a complete pattern of proceptive and receptive behaviors, whereas those treated with estrogen alone display no proceptive behaviors, low levels of lordosis, and high rates of rejection responses. Certain pharmacologic treatments (e.g. apomorphine, oxytocin, PT-141), are able to increase proceptive behaviors and reduce rejection responses in ovariectomized females treated or maintained on estrogen alone. This pattern of data suggests that such drugs may be useful in the treatment of hypoactive sexual desire disorder, with or without accompanying hypogonadism.

A similar loss of interest in sexual activity occurs during the phenomenon of "estrous termination". Estrous termination occurs progressively after the female receives a requisite number of intromissions and ejaculations during sex. It can also be induced by manual vaginocervical stimulation using a lubricated glass rod that approximates the size of a male rat penis, and that is inserted to mimic the stimulation received during intromission. The first behavioral set to disappear is solicitation, and this precedes a rise in rejection responses. Females given vaginocervical stimulation also show a faster loss of lordosis over the next 12 hrs, compared to females given sham stimulation. It would appear, then, that sexual stimulation in females, as in males, activates inhibitory systems that bring about refractoriness. It is not yet known how different pharmacologic treatments might delay the onset of estrous termination, and whether such effects might prove useful in treatment of low desire.

It will be important to consider how androgen administration may alter sexual behavior in ovariectomized females, with or without estrogen treatment. Currently, combined androgen—estrogen treatment is used in postmenopausal women to restore sexual desire and arousal. It should be straightforward to examine this combined hormone therapy in ovariectomized rats and categorize the effects, along with studying potential mechanisms (e.g. steroid receptor activation and interaction, role of peripheral sex hormone binding globulins).

It will also be critical to study the sexual behavior of older female rats. Female rats have a homologue of "menopause" in which ovarian function is disrupted then declines to a continuous state of vaginal diestrus (accompanied by a progressive atrophy of the vagina and clitoris). It is not known how these females would respond to sexual advances by a male, or to manually applied vaginocervical stimulation.

Hypoactive sexual arousal

Treatment of rats with the peripheral nitric oxide inhibitor nitro-L-arginine-methyl ester (L-NAME) reduces vaginal blood flow. It is not yet known if this treatment alters female sexual behavior.

Hypoactive sexual desire/conditioned inhibition

Female rats treated with the opioid antagonist naloxone during paced copulatory trials do not form conditioned place or partner preferences. Such preferences are typically examined on a final test, when the drug is not administered (thus revealing the necessity of opioid reward during paced copulation). However, during this final test without the drug, females previously treated with naloxone display a conditioned disruption of solicitation and lordosis relative to saline-treated females, despite being primed fully with estrogen and progesterone. As a result, males engage in fewer intromissions and achieve fewer ejaculations with those females. A pattern of diminished sexual solicitation and receptivity, which leads to more restricted sexual contact with males, is analogous in many ways to the pattern of sexual behavior displayed by women with hypoactive sexual desire disorder. It is not yet known if this pattern of disrupted appetitive sexual behavior can be restored by pharmacologic or experiential treatments that increase desire in women.

General Conclusion

Real progress has been made in understanding the neuroanatomical and neurochemical mechanisms of erection, ejaculation, solicitation, and other sexual responses, and in the design of rational pharmacologic treatments for certain sexual dysfunctions. We have begun to examine the mechanisms that underlie desire, and how sexual stimulation and reward impact on endpoints like sexual arousal, desire, attractiveness, and even mate choice. Progress in these areas could not have been made without the help of animal models. The evolution of sexual physiology and behaviour have been highly conserved, therefore animal models of human sexual response can be used successfully as preclinical tools so long as the functional endpoints are homologous or analogous, and carry predictive validity. When setting up testing paradigms to study preclinical models of human sexual function in laboratory animals, it is essential to ask the animals human questions that they can answer in their own species–specific manner. Although standardization of models (and of paradigms between laboratories) is critical, this should never limit the inspired intuition of researchers or clinicians to envision new models or paradigms.

Guidelines and Recommendations for Setting up a Preclinical Lab in Sexual Medicine

Research questions

The selection of a research topic is the most fundamental decision in establishing a preclinical laboratory in sexual medicine. This decision will control all subsequent considerations, such as research models and techniques, collaborative arrangements and funding needs. Clearly, the choice of a research program will be heavily influenced by one's interests and background. However, an often overlooked, but important, consideration is opportunity, such as the opportunity to achieve distinction, funding opportunities, or the opportunity to establish collaborative relationships with research groups that may have research techniques that can be usefully applied to questions in sexual medicine.

For the starting investigator, an important question to ask is what will be necessary to achieve both success and distinction? This can be difficult in an area which is already somewhat mature or has a number of well-established labs working in it. In a mature field, many of the bigger questions may have been answered. This may leave only opportunities to investigate details of previously-identified mechanisms, with reduced opportunities for recognition. Trying to compete against established labs can also lead to difficulty in achieving recognition. The new investigator with a small laboratory still developing techniques will be hard pressed to publish the first or the most comprehensive results compared to a larger established lab.

One approach is to identify research areas that are comparatively understudied. Some of the more fundamental questions may remain to be answered, with correspondingly higher recognition. The disadvantage to this approach is that understudied areas may lack well defined research models or they may be understudied precisely because they are too challenging. However, new investigators can often find a niche because they can see research fields with fresh eyes.

Selection of models

The selection of the appropriate model is crucial to progress. This chapter and others referenced here provide useful considerations on this topic. The new investigator should also seek advice from mentors and investigators in sexual medicine to help make these decisions about experimental models. Luckily, the field of sexual medicine is fairly new, with a relatively small, collegial community. Established investigators want to encourage growth of the field, and therefore are generally willing to help new investigators.

Experimental techniques

The choice of research models will dictate what research techniques will be needed. If these are new methods for the investigator, there are many approaches to acquiring the necessary technical skills. Some may be relatively straightforward to learn on one's own, using the literature. However, it may save considerable time to visit labs using the techniques to learn the little details and learn to troubleshoot problems. Other techniques may require more formal training. Many courses on scientific techniques are offered by professional societies and equipment/reagent manufacturers. Longer visits or mini-sabbaticals to other labs may also provide the necessary training.

Collaborations

Developing collaborative relationships can be extremely useful, or even essential for the new investigator, especially someone with a demanding clinical practice. Except in very large institutions, there are unlikely to be many other researchers in sexual medicine. Therefore, the most likely collaborators will be in related areas of cellular and molecular biology, physiology and pharmacology, endocrinology, or neuroscience, depending on the research topic. The collaborative arrangements can range from simply trading technical help to a complete sharing of labs. Typically, these relationships will begin with rather limited interactions and grow over time. It is probably unrealistic to expect that a potential collaborator will commit to an extensive interaction from the start. It is also likely that attempts at collaboration are not successful. Beyond the scientific interaction, the personal relationship is important.

In a successful collaboration, everyone must feel that they are benefiting. People often will be willing to provide limited help (such as teaching a technique) without expecting something in return. For a longer-term project, they will often need reasons to justify their expenditure of time and effort. The new investigator must identify the possible benefits of collaboration. These could be an entry into a young, interesting field with many opportunities, access to new sources of funding, or additional people, such as fellows, to work in their lab.

Further Reading

General reviews on animal models

Ågmo A, Ellingsen E. Relevance of nonhuman animal studies to the understanding of human sexuality. *Scand J Psychol* 2003;**44**:293–301.

Beach FA. Sexual behavior in animals and man. *The Harvey Lectures* 1950;**43**:259–279.

Bitran D, Hull EM. Pharmacological analysis of male rat sexual behavior. *Neurosci Biobehav Rev* 1987;**11**:365–389.

Dornan WA, Malsbury CW. Neuropeptides and male sexual behavior. *Neurosci Biobehav Rev* 1989;**13**:1–15.

Everitt BJ, Bancroft J. Of rats and men: The comparative approach to male sexuality. *Ann Rev Sex Res* 1991;**2**:77–118.

Larsson K. Conditioning of sexual behavior in the white laboratory rat. *Acta Psychologica Gothobourgensia* 1956;**1**:1–269.

McKenna KE, Adams MA, Baum M, Bivalacqua T, Coolen L, Gonzalez-Cadavid N, Hedlund P, Park K, Pescatori E, Rajfer J, Sato Y. Experimental models for the study of male sexual function. In: Lue TF, Basson R, Rosen R, Giuliano F, Khoury S, Montorsi F, eds. *Sexual Medicine.* Health Publications, 2004.

Meisel RD, Sachs BD. The physiology of male reproduction. In: Knobil E. Neil JD, eds. *The Physiology of Reproduction.* New York: Raven Press, 1994, vol. 2. pp. 3–105.

Pfaus JG, Kippin TE, Coria-Avila G. What can animal models tell us about human sexual response? *Ann Rev Sex Res* 2003;**14**:1–63.

Penile erection

Andersson, K-E, Wagner G. Physiology of penile erection. *Physiol Rev* 1995;**75**:191–236.

Bancroft J, Jannsen E. The dual control model of male sexual response: A theoretical approach to centrally mediated erectile dysfunction. *Neurosci Biobehav Rev* 2000;**24**: 571–579.

Burnett AL, Nelson RJ, Calvin DC, Liu JX, Demas GE, Klein SL, Kriegsfeld LJ, Dawson VL, Dawson TM, Snyder SH. Nitric oxide-dependent penile erection in mice lacking neuronal nitric oxide synthase. *Mol Med* 1996;**2**:288–296.

Christ GJ, Richards S, Winkler A. Integrative erectile biology: The role of signal transduction and cell-to-cell communication in coordinating corporal smooth muscle tone and penile erection. *Int J Impot Res* 1997;**9**: 69–84.

Ferrini M, Magee TR, Vernet D, Rajfer J, Gonzalez-Cadavid NF. Aging-related expression of inducible nitric oxide synthase and markers of tissue damage in the rat penis. *Biol Reprod* 2001;**64**:974–982.

Giuliano F, Rampin O, Mc Kenna K. Animal models used in the study of erectile dysfunction. In: Carson C, Kirby R, Goldstein I. eds. *Textbook of Erectile Dysfunction.* Oxford: ISIS Medical Media, 1999, pp 43–50.

Giuliano F. Rodents in impotence research: Functional and genetic aspects. *Int J Impot Res* 2001;**13**:1–3.

Heaton JP. Central neuropharmacological agents and mechanisms in erectile dysfunction: The role of dopamine. *Neurosci Biobehav Rev* 2000;**24**:561–569.

McKenna K. Central nervous system pathways involved in the control of penile erection. *Ann Rev Sex Res* 1999;**10**:157–183.

Sezen SF, Burnett AL. Intracavernosal pressure monitoring in mice: Responses to electrical stimulation of the cavernous nerve and to intracavernosal drug administration. *J Androl* 2000;**21**:311–315.

Rosen RC, Sachs BD. Central mechanisms in the control of penile erection: Current theory and research. *Neurosci Biobehav Rev* 2000;**24**:503–505.

Sachs BD. Placing erection in context: The reflexogenic-psychogenic dichotomy reconsidered. *Neurosci Biobehav Rev* 1995;**19**:211–224.

Saenz de Tejada I, Moroukian P, Tessier J, Kim JJ, Goldstein I, Frohrib D. Trabecular smooth muscle modulates the capacitor function of the penis. Studies on a rabbit model. *Am J Physiol* 1991;**260**(5 Pt 2):H1590–1595.

Saenz de Tejada I. Molecular mechanisms for the regulation of penile smooth muscle contractility. *Int J Impot Res* 2002;**14** Suppl 1:S6–10.

Ejaculation

Cantor JM, Binik YM, Pfaus JG. Chronic fluoxetine inhibits sexual behavior in the male rat: Reversal with oxytocin. *Psychopharmacol* 1999;**144**:355–362.

Coolen LM, Allard J, Truitt WA, McKenna KE. Central regulation of ejaculation. *Physiol Behav* 2004;**83**:203–215.

Johnson RD, Hubscher CH. Brainstem microstimulation differentially inhibits pudendal motoneuron reflex inputs. *Neuroreport* 1998;**9**:341–345.

McKenna KE. Ejaculation. In: Knobil E, Neill J.D, eds. *Encyclopedia of Reproduction*. Academic Press, 1998, pp.

Mos J, Mollet I, Tolboom JT, Waldinger MD, Olivier B. A comparison of the effects of different serotonin reuptake blockers on sexual behaviour of the male rat. *Eur Neuropsychopharmacol* 1999;**9**(1–2):123–135.

Olivier B, Chan JS, Pattij T, de Jong TR, Oosting RS, Veening JG, Waldinger MD. Psychopharmacology of male rat sexual behavior: Modeling human sexual dysfunctions? *Int J Impot Res* 2005 Apr 21; [Epub ahead of print].

Rènyi L. Ejaculations induced by p-chloroamphetamine in the rat. *Neuropharmacol* 1985;**24**:697–704.

Waldinger MD, Olivier B. Animal models of premature and retarded ejaculation. *World J Urol* 2005;**23**:115–118.

Bivalacqua TJ, Diner EK, Novak TE, Vohra Y, Sikka SC, Champion HC, Kadowitz PJ, Hellstrom WJ. A rat model of Peyronie's disease associated with a decrease in erectile activity and an increase in inducible nitric oxide synthase protein expression. *J Urol* 2000;**163**: 1992–1998.

El Sakka AI, Hassoba HM, Chui RM, Bhatnagar RS, Dahiya R, Lue TF. An animal model of Peyronie's-like condition associated with an increase of transforming growth factor beta mRNA and protein expression. *J Urol* 1997;**158**:2284–2289.

Vernet D, Ferrini MG, Valente EG, Magee TR, Bou-Gharios G, Rajfer J, Gonzalez-Cadavid NF. Effect of nitric oxide on the differentiation of fibroblasts into myofibroblasts in the Peyronie's fibrotic plaque and in its rat model. *Nitric Oxide* 2002;**7**:262–276.

Priapism

Munarriz R, Park K, Huang YH, Saenz de Tejada I, Moreland RB, Goldstein I, Traish AM. Reperfusion of ischemic corporal tissue: Physiologic and biochemical changes in an animal model of ischemic priapism. *Urology* 2003; **62**(4):760–764.

Champion HC, Bivalacqua TJ, Takimoto E, Kass DA, Burnett AL. Phosphodiesterase-5A dysregulation in penile erectile tissue is a mechanism of priapism. *Proc Natl Acad Sci* (USA) 2005;**102**(5):1661–1666.

Experimental investigation of female sexual function

Ågmo A, Soria P. GABAergic drugs and sexual motivation, receptivity and exploratory behaviors in the female rat. *Psychopharmacol* (Berl) 1997;**129**:372–381.

Giuliano F, Allard J, Compagnie S, Alexandre L, Droupy S, Bernabe J. Vaginal physiological changes in a model of sexual arousal in anesthetized rats. *Am J Physiol Regul Integr Comp Physiol* 2001;**281**:R140–149.

Erskine MS. Solicitation behavior in the estrous female rat: A review. *Horm Behav* 1989;**23**:437–502.

McKenna KE, Chung SK, McVary KT. A model for the study of sexual function in anesthetized male and female rats. *Am J Physiol* 1991;**261**:R1276–1285.

McKenna KE. The neurophysiology of female sexual function. *World J Urol* 2002;**20**:93–100.

Min K, O'Connell L, Munarriz R, Huang YH, Choi S, Kim N, Goldstein I, Traish A. Experimental models for the investigation of female sexual function and dysfunction. *Int J Impot Res* 2001;**13**:151–156.

Park K, Goldstein I, Andry C, Siroky MB, Krane RJ, Azadzoi KM. Vasculogenic female sexual dysfunction: The hemodynamic basis for vaginal engorgement insufficiency and clitoral erectile insufficiency. *Int J Impot Res* 1997;**9**: 27–37.

Pfaus JG, Shadiack A, Van Soest T, Tse M, Molinoff P. Selective facilitation of sexual solicitation in the female rat by a melanocortin receptor agonist. *Proc Nat Acad Sci* (USA) 2004;**101**(27):10201–10204.

Pfaus JG, Smith WJ, Coopersmith CB. Appetitive and consummatory behaviors of female rats in bilevel chambers: I. A correlational and factor analysis and the effect of ovarian hormones. *Horm Behav* 1999;**35**:224–240.

Pfaus JG, Smith WJ, Coopersmith CB. Appetitive and consummatory behaviors of female rats in bilevel chambers: II. Patterns of estrus termination following vaginocervical stimulation. *Horm Behav* 2000;**37**(1):96–107.

Shabsigh A, Buttyan R, Burchardt T, Buchardt M, Hayek OR, D'Agati V, Olsson C, Shabsigh R. The microvascular architecture of the rat vagina revealed by image analysis of vascular corrosion casts. *Int J Impot Res* 1999;**11**: S23–30.

Models of sexual desire

Ågmo A. Sexual motivation—An inquiry into events determining the occurrence of sexual behavior. *Behav Brain Res* 1999;**105**:129–150.

Everitt BJ. Sexual motivation: A neural and behavioral analysis of the mechanisms underlying appetitive and copulatory responses of male rats. *Neurosci Biobehav Rev* 1990;**14**:217–232.

Levine SB. The nature of sexual desire: A clinician's perspective. *Arch Sex Behav* 2003;**32**:279–285.

Pfaus JG. Revisiting the concept of sexual motivation. *Ann Rev Sex Res* 1999;**10**:120–157.

Pfaus JG, Kippin TE, Centeno S. Conditioning and sexual behavior: A review. *Horm Behav* 2001;**40**:291–321.

CHAPTER 2

Psychologic and Interpersonal Aspects and their Management

Stanley E. Althof, Raymond Rosen, Eusebio Rubio-Aurioles, Carolyn Earle, and Marie Chevret-Measson

Introduction

Psychologic and interpersonal factors play a major role in both the etiology and maintenance of sexual problems. However, especially in men, the importance of these factors has been downplayed due to the initial success of the novel phosphodiesterase type 5 inhibitors (PDE-5i) for the treatment of erectile dysfunction. More recently, as men discontinued treatment with PDE-5 inhibitors at higher than expected rates, the importance of the potential psychologic and interpersonal influences in the etiology, maintenance and course of treatment of male sexual dysfunction has regained prominence.

This chapter offers a holistic, patient-centered approach for the evaluation of male sexual dysfunction via clinical interviews and self-administered questionnaires. It highlights the salience of psychologic and interpersonal issues in the development and maintenance of sexual health, and presents a four-tiered paradigm for understanding the evolution and maintenance of sexual problems. Finally, this chapter will briefly review the rationale and efficacy of psychologic interventions for male sexual dysfunction, and the role of innovative, integrated treatment paradigms, and will offer recommendations for clinical management and future research.

Etiological Background of Sexual Dysfunction from a Psychologic/ Interpersonal Perspective

Sexual dysfunction is typically influenced by a variety of predisposing, precipitating, maintaining and contextual factors [1]. There are no current data available to suggest that any one factor is more important than another. Predisposing factors include both constitutional (e.g. congenital illness, anatomical deformities) and prior life experiences, such as problematic attachments, neglectful or critical parents, restrictive upbringing, sexual and physical abuse and violence. Predisposing factors are often associated with a greater prevalence of sexual dysfunction and emotional difficulties in adult life. While some individuals appear less vulnerable and more resilient in the face of stressors, others are more susceptible.

Precipitating factors are those that initiate or trigger sexual problems. For any one individual it is impossible to predict which factors, under what circumstances, will impair sexual desire or performance. Nonetheless, an individual's vulnerability to a particular set of circumstances can precipitate sexual dysfunction. For instance, traumatic events such as the discovery of a spouse's infidelity may cause one man to lose his sexual desire while another man's desire may increase. While initially a precipitating event may be problematic and distressing, it need not necessarily lead to a diagnosable dysfunction in the long term. Over time however, repetition of such events, especially those that damage self-confidence and self-esteem result in sexual dysfunction, even in reasonably resilient individuals. Examples of such precipitating events include conflictual separation or divorce, a sudden brush with death through an accident or disease process, or unsatisfying sexual experiences.

Finally, maintaining factors such as relationship conflict, performance anxiety, guilt, inadequate sexual information or stimulation, psychiatric disorders, loss of sexual chemistry, fear of intimacy, impaired self-image or self-esteem, restricted foreplay, poor communication and lack of privacy, may prolong and exacerbate problems, irrespective of the original predisposing or precipitating conditions. Maintaining factors also include contextual factors that can interfere or interrupt sexual activity, such as environmental constraints or anger/resentment towards a partner. Each of these four factors adversely contributes to, or diminishes, both the individual's and the couples' ability to sustain an active and satisfying sexual life. Often there is not a clear distinction between predisposing and precipitating and precipitating and maintaining factors. For instance, anxiety can increase an individual's vulnerability to sexual dysfunction as a common predisposing factor; it can also serve as a maintaining factor leading to sexual avoidance or arousal inhibition.

• *Recommendation 1. Clinical assessment should aim to identify the predisposing, precipitating, maintaining and contextual factors related to the individual's sexual dysfunction.*

Clinical Assessment

Sexual function assessment in the male

As recommended by the 2nd International Consultation on Sexual Dysfunction [2] the sexual, medical and psychosocial history are the essential elements in the basic evaluation and should be obtained in all male patients presenting with complaints of sexual dysfunction (A sexual function checklist to be filled out in general practice or specialty settings is provided in Table 2.1 on p. 26).

The essential components of sexual function assessment in the male always include erectile response (onset, duration, progression, severity of the problem, nocturnal/morning erections, self-stimulatory and visually erotic-induced erections), sexual desire, ejaculation, orgasm, sexually related genital pain disorders and partner sexual function, if available. Often, a dysfunction in one phase may precipitate a dysfunction in another. For instance, men with erectile dysfunction may report a loss of sexual desire or the onset of premature ejaculation.

Brief symptom scales or self-report questionnaires may assist the clinician in recognizing and diagnosing the sexual problem. These measures may also permit patients to acknowledge the problem and to initiate a clinical discussion with their health provider. Scales and questionnaires are also a valuable tool in clinical trials and outcomes research for male sexual dysfunctions.

Although valuable in recognizing and identifying sexual dysfunction, screening tools and questionnaires should not substitute for a thorough sexual, medical, and psychosocial history. For patients with multiple sexual dysfunction symptoms (e.g. erectile dysfunction (ED) and low libido), further evaluation of these symptoms is always recommended prior to initiating ED therapy. Whenever possible, the temporal association or causal relationship between the symptoms should be assessed.

Self-administered questionnaires

Sexual function symptom scales should be used routinely to assess functional level (e.g. ability to respond, level of interest) and to determine the impact of therapy. The most frequently used type of instrument is the self-administered questionnaire. As with all psychometric instruments, the fundamental requirements for psychometric validity include reliability and validity. Reliability refers to the consistency or replicability of data, while validity reflects the degree to which an instrument or scale measures what it intends or claims to measure. Two essential indicators of validity for measures of sexual function are: sensitivity to diagnostic status (e.g. functional versus dysfunctional); and sensitivity to treatment change. Both are crucial features of any scale that is designed to serve as a diagnostic and/or efficacy measure in either clinical or research settings. Validated symptom scales are available for the assessment of male sexual dysfunction, as well as couple and partner questionnaires, quality of life and well-being measures. Most of the scales described in the table are well established and widely used in research or clinical settings.

In Table 2.2 (on p. 27) we review measures of sexual function (in alphabetical order), that may be used in either men or women (e.g. CSFQ), or with men only (e.g. IIEF, IPE). Each measure is reviewed in terms of its psychometric properties, its clinical utility and an overall rating based on a five-point scale. Questionnaires still in development or older measures not meeting current psychometric standards were not included in the table.

Sexuality-related quality of life measures in men

Quality of life and treatment satisfaction measures are summarized in Table 2.3 (on p. 28). These measures have generally been developed for use in clinical trials and outcome studies. They have had limited use among clinicians. These measures vary greatly in the type and extent of validation that has been conducted. They are not recommended for primary care or widespread clinical use.

Clinical assessment of psychologic and interpersonal factors

The patient's psychologic state must be assessed in every case, with special attention to symptoms of anxiety or depression, past and present partner relationships, history of sexual trauma/abuse, occupational and social stressors, health issues in either partner, infertility, child-rearing difficulties, economic status, and educational level.

A critical aspect of assessment is the identification of patient needs and expectations, personal priorities and treatment preferences, which may be significantly influenced by cultural, social, ethnic and religious perspectives. Unfortunately, an in-depth discussion of the impact of culture is beyond the scope of this chapter.

Patient and partner education is also necessary in fostering a therapeutic relationship, facilitating patient–physician communication and enhancing treatment compliance. Although not always possible on the first visit, effort should be made to involve the patient's partner early in the process. However, it may not always be possible or practical for the partner to be present. At times it may be the couple's preference that the patient should be seen alone. When the partner participates in the evaluation, either with the patient or separately, it is important to corroborate the information that has been obtained and address any discrepancies that may arise. These discrepancies may be an indication of a troubled relationship, the man's denial, or the woman's hurt/anger.

Partner participation may be influenced by cultural and social expectations, as well as patient needs and preferences. When psychosocial assessment reveals the presence of significant psychologic distress or relationship difficulties, in-depth psychosocial evaluation and one-to-one counseling may be recommended.

How is psychogenic ED diagnosed?

Variability of erectile function is the hallmark of psychogenic ED. Take the example of the man who reports excellent morning erections, moderately good erections with fantasy or masturbation, and poor erections with foreplay and attempts at intercourse. This man, by history, has clear psychogenic ED. No physical scenario can explain the variability of erectile function. Note that in this example the patient's function worsens as he becomes involved with a partner, suggesting the role of performance anxiety or interpersonal anxiety.

However, most men do not present with psychogenic ED. The majority of men have mixed ED, that is a combination of biogenic and psychologic/interpersonal factors that contribute to the onset and maintenance of ED. Neglecting either the psychologic or physical does the man/couple a great disservice. Offering a prescription for a PDE-5 inhibitor with the simple statement such as, "Perhaps factors other than your diabetes are involved in your problem. It might be useful for you to consult with one of my colleagues who can help you with them".

Psychologic and relational variables can enhance or inhibit the physiologic aspects of sexual response. There is, however, great variability in men's vulnerability to sexual dysfunction and likewise ability to compensate for these factors. Psychologic factors can help men resist declining erectile function. For example, a man with good self-esteem, broad sexual experience, and a loving and arousing partner can partially compensate against organic factors for some length of time before the organic factors overwhelm his ability to maintain erections. Conversely, men with little self-confidence who are depressed and in poor relationships may have little resilience against organic factors, and report erectile function that is worse than expected with the organic factors alone.

The role of anxiety in sexual dysfunction

Anxiety played a significant role in early psychodynamic formulations of sexual dysfunction and later became the foundation for the etiologic concepts of sex therapy established by Masters and Johnson [3] and Kaplan [4]. Kaplan believed that sexually related anxiety became the "final" common pathway through which multiple negative influences led to sexual dysfunction.

More recent studies have suggested that it may not be the subjective role of anxiety, per se, that causes and maintains sexual dysfunction but rather the manner in which anxiety affects an individual's ability to focus on, and process sexual stimuli. Barlow [5] has offered a theoretical model explaining why anxiety may operate differentially in men with and without erectile dysfunction. His model emphasizes the role of cognitive interference in male arousal. In general, what appears to distinguish functional from dysfunctional responding is a difference in selective attention and distractibility. What sex therapists consider performance demand, fear of inadequacy or spectatoring are all forms of situation-specific, task-irrelevant, cognitive activities which distract dysfunctional individuals from task-relevant processing of stimuli in a sexual context [6].

Men with premature\rapid ejaculation try to distract themselves in an effort to prevent early ejaculation. They fear focusing on arousal, yet distraction does not effectively solve their problem. Counter intuitively, sex therapists teach men to focus on their arousal as a means of controlling ejaculation.

• *Recommendation 2. Ascertain the degree to which anxiety, distraction or the inability to maintain focus on sexual stimulation interferes with sexual response.*

Depression and Sexual Function

The relationship between depression and sexual functioning is of considerable interest to clinicians and researchers since both affective and sexual disorders are highly prevalent, are believed to be co-morbid, and may even share a common etiology [7,8]. It is generally agreed that the relationship between depressive mood and sexual dysfunction is bi-directional and further complicated by the sexual side effects of antidepressant medication [9].

The empirical evidence confirms a prominent role of depression in sexual dysfunction. While the exact direction of causality is difficult to ascertain, the data not only indicates a close correlational relationship between depression and sexual disorders but also supports a functional significance of mood disorders in causing and maintaining sexual dysfunction. Compared to functional controls, men and women with sexual dysfunction exhibit both higher levels of acute depressive symptoms and a markedly higher lifetime prevalence of affective disorders.

• *Recommendation 3. Inquire about depressive symptomotology (mood, sleep, appetite, libido, energy level, hopelessness, outlook regarding the future and suicidality). If present, inform the patient that depression can interfere with sexual response. Either begin treatment or refer.*

Interpersonal Dimensions of Sexual Function and Dysfunction

Clinically, it has been frequently observed that sexual problems may be either the cause of, or consequence of, dysfunctional or unsatisfactory relationships. Often, it is difficult to determine which is cause and effect: a non-intimate and non-loving relationship, or sexual desire and/or performance problems, leading to partner avoidance and antipathy. The research literature is contradictory on this topic, and often difficult to interpret since couples begin therapy with varying degrees of relationship satisfaction.

While the evidence is not conclusive, and most studies in the literature are not randomized controlled trials, the findings demonstrate a significant relationship between sexual and relationship functioning. While it is impossible to determine cause and effect with certainty, the literature suggests better long-term outcome when the relationship issues are treated and resolved. The relationship and sexual difficulties should be dealt with concurrently so that any unresolved relationship issues do not undermine the efficacy of the sexual dysfunction treatment. Clearly, randomized controlled trials need to be conducted in this area.

• *Recommendation 4. Inquire about the quality of the interpersonal relationship and identify potential relational factors that may precipitate, maintain and/or interfere with effective treatment.*

Psychologic Treatment of Male Sexual Dysfunction

Psychotherapy of erectile dysfunction

Men with lifelong and acquired erectile dysfunctions typically achieve significant gains initially and over the long term, following participation in sex therapy. Men with acquired disorders tend to fare better than those with lifelong problems. Masters and Johnson [3] reported initial failure rates of 41% and 26% for lifelong (primary) and acquired (secondary) erectile dysfunction, respectively. Their 2–5 year follow-up of this cohort indicated sustained gains.

Masters and Johnson's initial studies have been criticized for their methodological limitations. Their studies were not controlled and there were no placebo or waiting list controls used. Additionally, the treated group was a highly unusual, self selected group consisting of highly motivated patients who were required to attend Masters and Johnson's two-week residential program with no other activity (like work or children) interfering with their treatment. This is obviously a very unrepresentative group of patients. In all likelihood these highly motivated patients inflated the reported efficacy of treatment. The significance of Masters and Johnson's work lies in their innovative vision of treating couples and understanding the role of psychologic and interpersonal factors in the genesis of sexual problems. They were also the first to address the issue of performance anxiety.

In a review of the studies of treatment for erectile dysfunction, Mohr and Bentler [10] wrote, "The component parts of these treatments typically include behavioral, cognitive, systemic and interpersonal communication interventions. Averaging

across studies, it appears that approximately two-thirds of the men suffering from erectile failure will be satisfied with their improvement at follow-up ranging from six months to six years".

Sex therapy treatment of ED consists of a variety of interventions such as systematic desensitization, sensate focus, interpersonal therapy, behavioral assignments, psychodynamic interventions, sex education, communications and sexual skills training and masturbation exercises. It has not been possible to statistically analyze the precise contribution of any of these single interventions to overall success.

All studies with long-term follow-up indicate a tendency for men to relapse. To prevent relapse, McCarthy [11] has suggested that therapists schedule periodic "booster or maintenance" sessions following termination. Follow-up sessions have been recommended in order to resolve "glitches" that have interfered with progress.

While the studies on the efficacy of psychotherapy should ideally circumvent the "problem" of the "therapist factor"; the practical difficulties of designing such a clinical trial are difficult to surmount. However, psychotherapy is not different from other clinical interventions that rely on the mastering of specific techniques by the clinician making the intervention. Surgical techniques are perhaps the clearest example, but other techniques used in medicine also pose the same problem. With this reality being recognized, the dismissal of reports on the efficacy of psychotherapy on the sole ground of not controlling for the "psychotherapist factor" should be avoided.

Special issues

Honeymoon ED is a special circumstance that is common in non-western countries. The pain of this condition extends far beyond the sexual arena and involves extended families and their relationship to the newly-weds [12]. Most cases, particularly in sexually naïve men, may be related to poor understanding of human sexuality, inadequate sex education, and inhibition due to cultural and religious values, performance anxiety and other psychologic factors (gender identity concerns). Counseling, anxiety reduction, sexual education and PDE-5 inhibitors, may all be useful in the management of these patients. However, penile vascular abnormalities and neurogenic factors, as well as the more complex non-organic causes such as gender identity and gender preference, have to be excluded, especially if conventional treatment outcome is sub-optimal.

Psychotherapy with rapid ejaculation

Cognitive behavioral therapy, as well as multimodal, psychodynamic and behavioral treatment is described in review papers; however, there are no controlled outcome studies that examine the efficacy of these methods [13]. Masters and Johnson [3] utilizing multiple treatment techniques including the squeeze technique in combination with sensate focus and interpersonal therapy, reported failure rates of 2.2% immediately after treatment and 2.7% at the five-year follow-up. Other researchers have been unable to replicate Masters & Johnson's success rates. For instance, only 64% of men in Hawton's [14] study were characterized as successful in overcoming rapid ejaculation.

Hypoactive sexual desire disorder

There are no randomized clinical trials of psychologic intervention with hypoactive sexual desire disorder (HSDD). Clinical wisdom suggests that four dynamics are generally associated with psychologic HSDD. These include depression, anger, sexual arousal patterns that are not available within the present relationship (e.g. sexual arousal to a partner of another gender, sado-masochistic wishes), and relationship discord. By stabilizing mood, diminishing hostility and improving relationship satisfaction, interest in conventional sexual activities often improves. Unfortunately, men with unconventional sexual aspirations typically do not show much improvement in conventional sexual interest.

Role of sexual satisfaction of the female partner of sexually dysfunctional men

The role of the female partner in both treatment seeking behavior and treatment success has been recently highlighted. The female partner is an important agent in motivating the man to seek treatment for his ED [15]. ED also has an impact on female sexual response. Sexual desire, arousal, orgasm and satisfaction in the female are adversely effected prior to the man's developing ED [16]. Conversely, levels of sexual satisfaction in the female partner are significantly increased with successful ED treatment [17].

What follows are two vignettes that illustrate the role of the female partner first in facilitating treatment seeking behavior, and second in creating barriers for effective interventions.

Vignette A

Joseph, aged 50, developed ED three years ago. He has been married to Martha, aged 45, for 20 years. Over the past three years Martha has recognized that Joseph's erectile function is no longer reliable. Joseph has difficulty acknowledging that something was happening to his erections. He tells Martha that he is too tired or too stressed at work. She however insists that he consult his primary care physician. Routine testing revealed a previously undiagnosed diabetes mellitus that surprised both the doctor and Joseph. After initial control of the diabetes mellitus and treatment with PDE-5i, Martha and Joseph recovered the intensity of their sexual life. Joseph is thankful to Martha for insisting that he seek professional consultation for their problem.

Vignette B

Susan, aged 30 and John, aged 45 have been married for seven years. One year ago John developed ED, which had a tremendous impact on his relationship with Susan. For the last three months their sexual life has become almost non-existent. Susan is certain that John is involved with another woman and that this is the source of his ED. She is angry when he attempts to initiate lovemaking, believing that he is no longer attracted to her. John has no awareness of the foundation of Susan's extreme response. He seeks consultation from his physician who diagnoses hypercholesterolemia and prescribes a statin and a PDE-5i. The PDE-5i does not work on two consecutive attempts at lovemaking. Susan cannot accept that the cause of John's ED was hypercholesterolemia. Furthermore she tells John that she resents him using a pill to get turned on, rather than being turned on by her alone. After five unsuccessful attempts with a PDE-5i John returns to his physician stating, "This medication is not working, can you give me something stronger?"

The above examples illustrate how, in case A, the partner supports and motivates her husband to seek out consultation and treatment, while in case B the partner creates conflict because she believes her husband is no longer attracted to her.

Integrated treatment for sexual dysfunction

Medical treatments alone are often insufficient in helping couples resume a satisfying sexual life. The term integrated is used to denote concurrent or step-wise combinations of psychologic and medical interventions. Too often, medical treatments are directed narrowly at a specific sexual dysfunction and fail to address the larger biopsychosocial issues. While medical therapies, especially for ED, are generally efficacious (50–90%), approximately 50% of individuals fail to continue treatment. This may be due to the clinician's failure to address the relevant psychologic and interpersonal issues [18]. Examples of relevant biopsychosocial factors include: (1) patient variables such as performance anxiety and depression; (2) partner variables such as poor mental or physical health and partner disinterest; (3) interpersonal non-sexual variables such as quality of the overall relationship; (4) interpersonal sexual variables such as the interval of abstinence and sexual scripts; and (5) contextual variables such as current life stresses with money or children.

Ideally, the physician treating sexual concerns should be sensitive and able to recognize the need for more specialized psychologic intervention. The following list includes some of the clinical symptoms and features that make a referral to a mental health specialist desirable:

List of clinical features that make referral to a mental health practitioner of sexual medicine desirable:
• Primary erectile dysfunction, especially with no clear biogenic abnormality
• Failure of PDE-5i treatment when no clear biogenic abnormality is found
• Conflictual relationship, especially if conflict is not ameliorated with the prescription of erectile dysfunction treatment

• Antecedents of sexual assault or other traumatic sexual experience in the patient's or partner's sexual histories that interfere with sexual function or emotional intimacy
• Depressive symptoms, especially if they have not been treated
• Anxiety over sexual performance that is not ameliorated by initial treatment of the sexual dysfunction (with PDE-5i, or selective serotonin reuptake inhibitors (SSRIs))
• Hypoactive sexual desire in the man with no clear biogenic abnormality, which is not improved by the initial treatment
• Identification or suspicion of a psychiatric disorder both in the male or his partner

There is an emerging literature that demonstrates a synergistic benefit from the use of both psychologic interventions and pharmacologic treatments for a number of psychiatric conditions including depression, post-traumatic stress disorder and to a lesser degree, schizophrenia [19]. It is regrettable that there are so few well-designed randomized controlled studies focusing on integrated approaches to the treatment of sexual dysfunction. The studies that do exist focus on treatment for erectile dysfunction; there are only a few reports of combined therapies for female dysfunction.

Although to date there are no approved pharmacologic treatments for female sexual dysfunction (FSD), undoubtedly they will evolve. Psychosocial/contextual issues contribute to the etiology and maintenance of FSD and innovative integrated strategies will be necessary to treat these problems.

Conclusion

This chapter addresses the psychologic and interpersonal dimensions of male sexual dysfunction. These dimensions can be assessed by means of a clinical interview or self-administered questionnaires. Several validated questionnaire measures are reviewed in this chapter. Psychologic interventions and integrated treatment approaches are briefly described. Further research is needed to evaluate the short and long-term efficacy of these treatment approaches in randomized, controlled trials.

References

1 Hawton K, Catalan J. Prognostic factors in sex therapy. *Behavior Research & Therapy* 1986;**24**:377–385.

2 Lue TF, Basson R, Rosen R, Giuliano F, Khoury S, Montorsi F, eds. *Sexual Medicine: Sexual Dysfunction in Men and Women*. Paris, Editions 21, 2004.

3 Masters WH, Johnson VE. *Human Sexual Inadequacy*. Boston: Little Brown, 1970.

4 Kaplan HS. *The New Sex Therapy*. New York: Brunner/ Mazel, 1974.

5 Barlow DH. Causes of sexual dysfunction: The role of anxiety and cognitive interference. *Journal of Consulting and Clinical Psychology* 1986;**54**:140–148.

6 Cranston-Cuebas MA, Barlow DH. Cognitive and affective contributions to sexual functioning. *Annual Review of Sex Research* 1990;**1**:119–161.

7 Thase ME, Howland RH. Biological processes in depression: An updated review and integration. In: Edward E, Leber WR, eds. *Handbook of Depression*, 2nd edn. New York: Guilford Press, 1995.

8 Goldstein I. The mutually reinforcing triad of depressive symptoms, cardiovascular disease, and erectile dysfunction. *The American Journal of Cardiology* 2000;**86**:41F–44F.

9 Ferguson JM. The effects of antidepressants on sexual functioning in depressed patients: A review. *J Clin Psychiatry* 2001;**62**(suppl.3):22–34.

10 Mohr DC, Bentler LE. Erectile dysfunction: A review of diagnostic and treatment procedures. *Clinical Psychology Review* 1990;**10**:123–150.

11 McCarthy B. Cognitive–behavioral strategies and techniques in the treatment of early ejaculation. In: Leiblum SR, Rosen RC, eds. *Principles and Practice of Sex Therapy*, 3rd edn. New York: Guilford Press, 2000, pp. 141–167.

12 Usta MF, Erdogru T, Tefaki A, Koksal T, Yucel B, Kadioglu. A Honeymoon impotence: Psychogenic or organic in origin? *Urology* 2001;**57**(4):758–762.

13 Althof SE. Psychological treatment strategies for rapid ejaculation: Rationale, practical aspects and outcome. *World Journal of Urology* 2005;**23**(2):89–92.

14 Hawton K, Catalan J, Martin P, Fagg J. Long-term outcome of sex therapy. *Behavior Research & Therapy* 1986;**24**:665–675.

15 Fisher WA, Rosen RC, Eardley I, Niederberger C, Nadel A, Kaufman J, Sand M. The multinational men's attitudes to life events and sexuality (MALES) study phase II: Understanding PDE5 inhibitor treatment seeking patterns, among men with erectile dysfunction. *Journal of Sexual Medicine* 2004;**1**:150–160.

16 Fisher W, Rosen R, Goldstein I, Sand M. How are female sexual responses (desire, arousal, orgasm, and satisfaction) linked to male sexual responses? Results of the female experience of men's attitudes to sexuality and life events (F.E.M.A.L.E.S.) study. Presented at the International Society for Women's Sexual Health meeting, Las Vegas, 2005.

17 Goldstein I, Fisher WA, Sand M, Rosen RC, Mollen M, Brock G, Karlin G, Pommerville P, Bangerter K, Bandel TJ, Derogatis L. Women's sexual function improves when partners are administered Vardenafil for erectile dysfunction: A prospective, randomized, double-blind, placebo-controlled trial. *Journal of Sexual Medicine* 2005;**2**(6):819–832.

18 Althof S. When an erection alone is not enough: biopsychosocial obstacles to lovemaking. *International Journal of Impotence Research* 2002;**S1**:S99–104.

19 Nathan PE, Gorman JM, eds. *A guide to treatments that work*. New York: Oxford University Press, 1998.

20 Clayton AH, MacGarvey EL, Clavet GJ. The changes in sexual functioning questionnaire (CSFQ): Development, reliability, and validity. *Psychopharmacology Bulletin* 1997;**33**:731–745.

21 Clayton AH, MacGarvey EL, Clavet GJ, Piazza L. Comparison of sexual functioning in clinical and nonclinical populations using the changes in sexual functioning questionnaire (CSFQ). *Psychopharmacology Bulletin* 1997;**33**:747–753.

22 Bobes J, Gonzalez MP, Bascran MT, Clayton A, Garcia M, Rico-Villademoros F, Banus S. Evaluating changes in sexual functioning in depressed patients: Sensitivity to change of the CSFQ. *Journal of Sex and Marital Therapy* 2002;**28**(2):93–103.

23 Bobes J, Gonzalez MP, Rico-Villademoros F, Bascran MT, Sarasa P, Clayton A, Banus S. Validation of the Spanish version of the changes in sexual functioning questionnaire. *Journal of Sex and Marital Therapy* 2000;**26**:119–131.

24 Derogatis LR, Melisaratos N. The DSFI: A multidimensional measure of sexual functioning. *Journal of Sex and Marital Therapy* 1979;**5**(3):244–281.

25 Derogatis LR, Rust J, Golumbok S, Davis S, Bouchard N, Rodenberg C, *et al.* Validation of the profile of female sexual function (PFSF) in surgically and naturally menopausal women. *Journal of Sex and Marital Therapy* 2004;**30**(1):25–36.

26 Rust J, Golumbok S. The Golombok–Rust Inventory of Sexual Satisfaction (GRISS). *British Journal of Clinical Psychology* 1985;**24**:63–64.

27 Rosen RC, Riley A, Wagner G, Osterloh IH, Kirkpatrick J, Mishra A. The International Index of Erectile

Function (IIEF): A multidimensional scale for assessment of erectile dysfunction. *Urology* 1997;**49**:822–830.

28 Rosen RC, Cappelleri JC, Smith MD, Lipsky J, Pena BM. Development and evaluation of an abridged, 5-item version of the International Index of Erectile Function (IIEF-5) as a diagnostic tool for erectile dysfunction. *International Journal of Impotence Research* 1999; **11**:319–326.

29 Rosen RC, Cappelleri JC, Gendrano III N. The International Index of Erectile Function (IIEF): A state-of-the-science review. *International Journal of Impotence Research* 2002;**14**:226–244.

30 Rosen R, Catania J, Pollack L, Althof S, O'Leary M, Seftel A. The male sexual health questionnaire (MSHQ): Scale development and psychometric validation. *Urology* 2004;**64**(4):777–782

31 Althof S, Rosen R, Mundayat R, May K Symonds T. Index of premature ejaculation: A new questionnaire to assess changes in control over ejaculation and satisfaction with sex life. Presented to the World Congress of Sexology, Montreal, Canada, 2005.

32. Althof S. Quality of Life and Erectile Dysfunction. *Urology* 2002;**59**(6):803–810.

Table 2.1 Medical, psychosocial and sexual assessment questionnaire.

Please answer the following questions about your overall sexual function in the past 3 months:

Chronology
- When was the last time you had a satisfactory erection?
- Was the onset of your problem gradual or sudden?
- When was your last normal erection?

Quantify
- Do you have morning or night-time erections?
- On a scale of 1 to 5 rate your rigidity during sex?
  □ 1 2 3 4 5
- With sexual stimulation can you initiate an erection?
- With sexual stimulation can you maintain an erection?

Qualify
- Is your erectile dysfunction partner or situational specific?
- Do you lose erection before penetration, or before climax?
- Do you have to concentrate to maintain an erection?
- Is there a significant bend in your penis?
- Do you have pain with erection?
- Are there any sexual positions that are difficult for you?

Libido/interest
- Do you still look forward to sex?
- Do you still enjoy sexual activity?
- Do you fantasize about sex?
- Do you have sexual dreams?
- Are you easily sexually aroused (turned on)?
- Do you have a strong sex drive?

Ejaculation/orgasm/satisfaction
- Are you able to ejaculate when you have sex?
- Are you able to ejaculate when you masturbate?
- If you have a problem with ejaculating, is it:
  — You ejaculate before you want to?
  — You ejaculate before your partner wants you to?
  — You take too long to ejaculate?
  — You feel that nothing comes out?
- Do you have pain with ejaculation?
- Do you see blood in your ejaculation?
- Do you have difficulty reaching orgasm?
- Do you find your orgasm satisfying?
- What percentage of sexual attempts are satisfactory to your partner?

Are you satisfied with your sexual function?
Yes / No

If No, please continue:
- How long have you been dissatisfied with your sexual function?
  3 months, 6 months, 1 year, 2 years, more than 2 years?
- What effect, if any, has your sexual problem had on your partner relationship/s?
  Little or no effect, moderate effect, large effect?
- What is the most likely reason/s for your sexual problem?
  — Medical illness or surgery
  — Prescription medications
  — Stress or relationship problems
  — Don't know

Previous consultations
- Have you consulted a physician or counselor for your sexual problems?
- If yes, what type of physician or counselor have you consulted (check all that apply)
  — General practitioner
  — Urologist
  — Other specialist
  — Counselor or psychologist
- Are you taking any medication or receiving medical treatment for your sexual problem?
- If yes, what medical or other non-medical treatments are you using?

Table 2.1 *Continued*

How effective has the treatment been?
- Not at all effective
- Somewhat effective
- Very effective

What are your concerns about your sexual function?
(Check one or more)
- Problems with little or no interest in sex
- Problems with erection
- Problems ejaculating too early during sexual activity
- Problems taking too long, or not being able to ejaculate or have orgasm
- Problems with pain during sex
- Problems with penile curvature during erection
- Other

Which problem is most bothersome (circle) 1 2 3 4 5 6 7
What are your concerns in your personal life?
(Check for YES)
1. I have sexual fears or inhibitions

2. I have problems finding romantic/sexual partners
3. I am uncertain about my sexual identity
4. I have been subjected to emotional or sexual abuse
5. I have significant relationship problems with family members
6. I have been under considerable emotional or physical stress
7. I have a history of depression, anxiety, or emotional problems
8. I have had a recent change in employment or financial status

My sexual partner has problems with:
(Check for YES)
1. Health
2. Sexual interest
3. Sexual performance
4. Sexual fears or inhibitions
5. History of sexual abuse

Table 2.2 Questionnaire measures for male sexual dysfunction [20–31].

Questionnaire	Author/Date	Purpose	Psychometric Evaluation	Clinical Utility	Overall Rating (1–5)
Changes in Sexual Function Questionnaire (CSFQ)	Clayton *et al.*, 1997	Assess adverse effects of drugs on sexual function	Adequate reliability and validity. Lack of treatment sensitivity data	Limited usefulness in assessing adverse effects of drugs	3
Derogatis Interview for Sexual Functioning (DISF/DISF-SR)	Derogatis & Melisaratos, 1979	Multi-dimensional measure of five domains of sexual function	Adequate validity and reliability. Limited treatment sensitivity data	Limited use in clinical trials and patient screening	4
Golombek–Rust Inventory of Sexual Satisfaction (GRISS)	Rust & Golombek, 1985	Multi-dimensional measure of seven domains of sexual function	Adequate validity and reliability. Lack of treatment sensitivity data	Limited use in European trials. Evaluation of sex therapy outcomes	4
International Index of Erectile Function (IIEF)	Rosen *et al.*, 1997	Multi-dimensional measure of erectile function and related domains	Excellent reliability and validity. Robust treatment sensitivity	Widespread use of short form (IIEF-5) for ED screening	5
Male Sexual Health Questionnaire (MSHQ)	Rosen *et al.*, 2004	Multi-dimensional measure of four domains, including ejaculatory function	Adequate reliability and validity. Lack of treatment sensitivity data	New measure of ejaculatory function. Short form scale in development	4
Index of Premature Ejaculation (IPE)	Althof *et al.*, 2005	Multi-dimensional scale of premature ejaculation	Adequate reliability and validity. Treatment sensitivity under analysis	Potentially strong new self-report measure of PE	4

Table 2.3 Quality-of-life measures used in clinical trials and studies [1, 32].

QoL endpoint	No. of items	QoL construct	Item content	How scored
Questions 13 and 14 from the IIEF	2	QoL issues related to sexual dysfunction	Q13: How satisfied have you been with your overall sex life? Q14: How satisfied have you been with your sexual relationship with your partner?	Scored on a scale from 1 (very dissatisfied) to 5 (very satisfied)
EDITS	11	Treatment satisfaction	How satisfied with treatment overall; ease of use; time to onset; duration; continued use; naturalness; partner satisfaction	Scored on a scale from 1 (very satisfied) to 5 (very dissatisfied)
Erection Distress Scale	5	Disease-specific instrument	Were you frustrated about your erection problems? Did you feel weighed down by your erection problems? Were you discouraged by your erection problems? Did you feel despair over your erection problems? Were your erection problems a worry in your life?	Scored from 1 (none of the time) to 6 (all of the time)
Erectile Dysfunction Impact Scale	1	Disease-specific question	If you were to spend the rest of your life with your erectile condition the way it is now, how would you feel about that?	Scored on a scale from 1 (very satisfied) to 5 (very dissatisfied)
MOS Short Form 12: Mental Health	6	Summary of social, emotional functioning.	Energy, emotional problems affecting work or daily activities, interference with social activities, feeling low	The various items are scored anywhere from 1–4 to 1–12; higher scores indicate better health
Physical Health	6	Summary of perceived physical function and general health.	Ability to perform moderate activities, perceived general health, pain, limited in daily activities	
MOS Family Survey	7	Intrapersonal communication with partner.	Q1–Q6: Say anything wanted to say, trouble sharing personal feelings, feeling close to partner, partner supportive; Q7: How satisfied with partner relationship	

Instrument	Items	Domain	Description	Scoring
PGWBI:	5	Anxiety	Bothered by nervousness, tense, worried or upset, relaxed or agitated, under strain or stress	Each item is scored from 0–5, where 5 is the most positive response.
	4	Positive well-being	General spirits, satisfied with personal life, interesting daily life, cheerful, lighthearted	The total score for the 14 items is 0–70
	3	Emotional stability and self-control	Control of behavior, thoughts and emotions, losing control over speech, thoughts, feelings, emotionally stable	
	2	Depression	Feeling depressed, discouraged and hopeless	
Rosenberg Self-Esteem Scale	10	Self concept	I feel that I am a person of worth, have a number of good qualities, am a failure, am able to do things as well as others, do not have much to be proud of, believe in myself, am satisfied with myself, could have more respect for myself, am useless, am no good at all	From 1–4, with higher scores: better self-esteem
DUKE Health Profile	5	Generic instrument with 3 brief scales.	Physical Health: Ambulation and physical symptoms	Scored from 0–100, from worst to best
	5		Mental Health: Personal self-esteem, cognition	
	5		Social Health: Social self-esteem, social interaction	
MUSE questionnaire	11	3 domains of QoL	Personal wellness (contentment, self-esteem); relationship with partner; quality of erection; anxiety about erectile function; energy	
RAND-SF36	36	8 domains of QoL	Physical function, bodily pain, vitality, role-physical, general health, emotional well-being, social function, role-emotional	Each domain scored from 1–100, higher scores: Better QoL

Continued on p. 30

Table 2.3 *Continued*

QoL endpoint	No. of items	QoL construct	Item content	How scored
CARES-SF	8	Marital interaction scale	With partner: Difficulty talking about feelings, finances, taking care of me; not getting along well	From 0–4, lower scores: Better QoL
Litwin Survey	20	Prostate cancer-specific scale	Nine items on sexual bother, 6 items on urinary bother, and 5 items on bowel bother	Scored from 1–100, with higher scores representing better QoL
UCLA Prostate Cancer Index	8 1	Sexual function scale Sexual bother scale	Level of desire; ability to have an erection; ability to reach orgasm; quality of erections; frequency of erections; ability to function sexually	From 0–100, with higher scores: Better QoL
ICED		Medical comorbidity	Presence of 19 medical conditions and 11 physical impairments	
KDQoL (Kidney Disease Quality of Life)	36+	36-item health survey, supplemented with multi-item scales tailored to individuals with kidney disease	Symptoms/problems, effect on daily life, burden of kidney disease, cognitive function, work status, sexual function, social interaction, sleep	Scored from 1–100, with higher scores representing better QoL
QoL questionnaire, Denmark	317	5 questions on sexuality	Are you sexually active? How satisfied are you with your sex life now? Sexual orientation? Do you have a sexual problem now?	
QoL-MED	19	Disease-specific instrument	Items pertaining to masculinity, emotional responses, overall life satisfaction	Scored from 1 (not at all) to 4 (very much)
Life Satisfaction Checklist	8	Disease-specific instrument with 7 domains	Life as a whole, sexual life, partnership relation, family life, contacts, leisure, vocational situation, economy	Scored from 1 (very dissatisfying) to 6 (very satisfying)

IIEF, International Index of Erectile Function; MOS, Medical Outcomes Study; PGWBI, Psychologic General Well-Being Index; MUSE, Medicated Urethral System for Erection; RAND, a nonprofit organization (Santa Monica, CA); SF, short form; CARES, Cancer Rehabilitation Evaluation System; UCLA, University of California, Los Angeles; PCI, Prostate Cancer Index; KD = Kidney Disease; QoL-MED, QoL in Male Erectile Dysfunction; ICED, Index of Coexisting Disease.

CHAPTER 3

Anatomy and Physiology of Erection

Hartmut Porst and Ira D. Sharlip

Embryology of the Penis

The penis develops from the genital tubercles and the urethra from the genital folds (in the female: labia minora). The genetic sex (XY) induces testicular development, with the help of the sex-determining factor located on the Y chromosome [1]. Differentiation of the external genitals (male: phallus; female: clitoris) from the genital tubercles occurs when testosterone production begins in the Leydig cells in the 8th/9th embryonal week. The penis grows very rapidly and is fully developed along with the urethra at the 4th fetal month. Growth of the penis and the scrotum, as well as differentiation of the prostate from the urogenital sinus, are regulated by dihydrotestosterone (DHT), which is converted from testosterone by 5α-reductase in peripheral tissues. Androgen-induced genital development occurs via specific androgen receptors, which have increased affinity to DHT. The gene for the androgen receptor is located on the long arm of the X chromosome [2].

Development disorders of the internal and external genitals may be caused by chromosomal defects, disorders of testosterone and DHT synthesis, or disorders of androgen receptor functions (androgen resistance) and the Mullerian inhibiting hormone. Thus synchronous, combined action of testosterone, DHT and Mullerian inhibiting factor is essential for normal development of the internal and external genitals. In this regard fetal and pubertal development of the penis length first and foremost depends on sufficient testosterone and DHT tissue levels and, second, by the number of androgen receptors [3–5].

Anatomy of the Penis

The penis is composed of the paired corpora cavernosa and the single corpus spongiosum, which surrounds the urethra. In the mobile section, the corpora cavernosa communicate with each other through numerous pore-like junctions in the septum penis. The corpora cavernosa are characterized by a spongy tissue structure consisting of connective trabecular tissue surrounding the sinusoidal spaces. These spaces fill up with blood during erection and are lined with endothelial cells and the subjacent muscle cells. The vessels and nerves supplying the sinusoidal spaces run through the trabecular tissue. The corpora cavernosa are surrounded by the very firm tunica albuginea, which is between 1.7 and 3.3 mm thick and which is divided into two layers containing collagen and elastic fibers [6–7]. The corpora cavernosa diverge in the proximal section to insert as the crura penis on the periosteum of the respective inferior pubic ramus. In the proximal section the crura are surrounded by the striated ischiocavernous muscles.

The single or sometimes paired deep dorsal vein runs along the surface of the corpora cavernosa in a central groove. This vein is responsible for the drainage of the distal two thirds of the corpora cavernosa. The dorsal penile arteries and the dorsal penile nerve are situated lateral to the dorsal vein on both sides. These vessel/nerve structures are covered by Buck's fascia, which surrounds the corpora cavernosa and the corpus spongiosum. Buck's fascia merges with the tunica albuginea at the root of the penis and continues as the triangular suspensory ligament of penis. The strong suspensory ligament of penis anchors the penis base to the periosteum of the pubic bone and gives the penis the appropriate stability at its base to erect vertically and to not tilt to the side. A further, much weaker, suspensory apparatus is the fundiform ligament of penis, located distal to the suspensory ligament of the penis with mediolateral insertion into Colles' fascia. This is covered by the penile shaft skin, which is fused directly together with the tunica albuginea in the coronary sulcus without intermediate layers. It continues in the foreskin which consists of two sheets of epithelium and normally covering the glans penis completely.

Arterial/venous supply and microcirculation
Arteries

The ischiopudendal trunk originates on both sides from the internal iliac artery, giving off the obturator and inferior gluteal arteries and continuing as the internal pudendal artery. The internal pudendal artery is the main trunk for arterial penile blood supply and, in radio-anatomical terms, is divided into the pelvic segment (origin–obturator foramen), ischiorectal segment (corresponds to Alcock's canal in the obturator foramen) and the perineal segment (below obturator foramen). Their penile end branches are the bulbar artery and the urethral artery, which supply the corpus spongiosum, the dorsal penile artery, mainly responsible for the blood supply of the glans penis and the skin of the penile shaft, and the deep penile artery (syn: cavernous artery), which is mainly responsible for filling the cavernous bodies with blood during erection. The deep arteries run through the center of the corpora cavernosa near the septum and give off the corkscrew-shaped helicine arteries, whose end branches open either directly into the sinusoidal spaces or into subalbugineal venules via shunts. Shunts exist in a great individual variation between the deep penile and the dorsal penile artery, as well as between the deep penile artery and the urethral artery (corpus spongiosum).

Variations in the penile arterial supply are very common. Physiologically, they are not important for the erection mechanism. However, they may be important in cases of pelvic/perineal injuries such as external trauma or surgical interventions. The most important known variations are:

Accessory internal pudendal artery. It runs cranial to the obturator foramen and may be the main trunk for the penile arteries. Its incidence varies from between 5% and 14% [8].

Penile arteries originating from the obturator artery. The obturatory artery is the main anterior branch of the ischiopudendal trunk.

Unilateral arterialization. In this case all penile arteries, or only both dorsal or deep penile arteries, arise unilaterally from the internal pudendal artery and supply both halves of the penis.

Corpus cavernosum arterialization from the dorsal artery. In 20–30% of men, the dorsal artery gives off a thick branch to the corpus cavernosum, usually in the middle third of the penis. This branch either anastomoses with the deep penile artery or gives off an isolated distal deep penile artery [8].

Double penile arteries. Our own investigations using duplex ultrasound and angiography on several thousand patients showed unilateral or bilateral double penile arteries in approximately 10–15% of cases.

Numerous intracavernous and extracavernous shunts exist between the various penile arteries (e.g. deep artery – urethral artery), and between arteries and veins. These shunts are subject to neural regulation of blood circulation in the dorsal, cavernous and helicine arteries (Figs 3.1 and 3.2).

Veins

Blood drained off from the sinusoidal spaces or directly from arteriovenous shunts is collected in the distal two thirds of the corpora cavernosa via a direct subtunical venous plexus, and is then transported further via the oblique emissary veins that perforate the tunica albuginea. Several emissary veins open into a circumflex vein, which originates ventrally between the corpus spongiosum and the corpus cavernosum, and surrounds the corpus cavernosum like a hoop, finally opening into the central, deep dorsal vein (Fig. 3.1). The proximal third of the corpus cavernosum is drained by the deep veins, which originate as 3–5 veins directly from the crura penis and open into the pudendal plexus (Fig. 3.3). The deep dorsal vein opens into the periprostatic plexus (Santorini's plexus) beneath the arcuate ligament of pubis. The pudendal plexus and Santorini's plexus finally unite and drain into the internal iliac vein. Other penile veins are the comunicantes veins

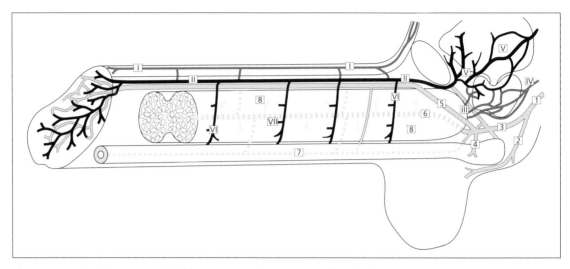

Fig. 3.1 Arterial and venous supply of the penis. Circulation: 1, internal pudendal artery; 2, superficial perineal artery; 3, penile artery; 4, bulbar artery; 5, dorsal penile artery; 6, deep penile artery; 7, urethral artery; 8, helicinearteries; I, superficial dorsal vein; II, deep dorsal vein; III, deep penile vein; IV, pudendal plexus; V, periprostatic plexus; VI, circumflex veins; VII, emissary veins.

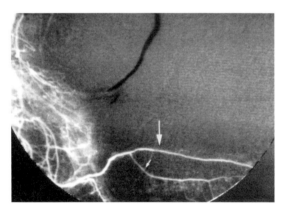

Fig. 3.2 Penile angiography — normal findings. Big arrow: dorsal penile artery. Small arrow: cavernous (deep) artery.

accompanying the dorsal arteries, and several superficial dorsal veins, which run between Colles' fascia and Buck's fascia. The superficial dorsal veins open into the great saphenous vein via the external pudendal veins, but also give off branches to the deep dorsal vein. Numerous venovenous anastomoses connect the different penile veins to each other.

Microcirculation

The difference between blood flow regulation in the flaccid state and the erect state is of particular importance. Nerve fibers containing vasoactive intestinal

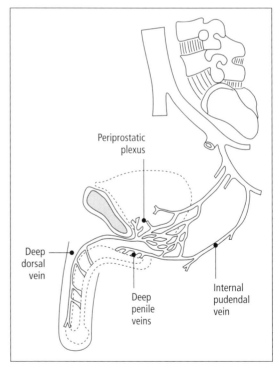

Fig. 3.3 The venous drainage of the penis.

polypeptide (VIP) and neuropeptide Y (NPY) in prominent longitudinal, subendothelial vascular wall cushions have been found at the sinusoidal opening sites of the helicine arteries. These nerve fibers are attributed regulatory functions in relation to blood flow into the sinusoidal spaces [9,10]. Blood flow to the sinusoidal spaces is regulated in particular via the sympathetic innervation of the corpus cavernosum tissue and penile vessels. Whereas α_1-adrenoceptors dominate in the cavernous smooth muscle cells, α_2-adrenoceptors prevail in the penile arteries, particularly in the cavernous arteries [11,12]. The blood flow is also regulated in the helicine arteries by β_2-adrenoceptors [13], which explains the negative effect that β-blockers may have on erection. Due to the fact that α_1- and α_2-adrenoceptors, and nerve endings containing neurotransmitters (e.g. NPY, VIP, calcitonin gene-related peptide (CGRP), substance P) have been described in the penile venous walls [14–16], active restriction of penile venous outflow by the autonomic nervous system seems likely.

Physiology of erection
Neurophysiology of erection

Parasympathetic nerve supply: Initiation of erection
Pro-erectile impulses are generated in the parasympathetic erection centers of the limbic system and the hypothalamus, in particular in the paraventricular nucleus and the medial preoptic area, which are the key regions for the central regulation of erection [17]. Perception of visual, auditory, imaginary, tactile or other erotic stimuli activate a variety of receptors which, in turn, stimulate via oxytocinergic, dopaminergic neurons the spinal parasympathetic reflexogenic erection center located at the level S_2–S_4. Parasympathetic nerve fibers, called nervi erigentes, leave the reflexogenic erection center and build along with the sympathetic nerve fibers, originating from the superior hypogastric plexus, the inferior hypogastric plexus that continues in the cavernous nerves. These cavernous nerves contain both sympathetic and parasympathetic fibers, and perforate the pelvic floor (urogenital diaphragma) to enter the cavernous bodies at the level where the cavernous crura diverge.

Erection-initiating neurotransmitters include, among others, dopamine (via D_2-receptors) and melanocortins. Five melanocortin receptors (MCR) have been identified. MC-4-R seems to have special importance for erection [18–20].

Oxytocin is an oligopeptide synthesized along with arginine vasopressin—another stimulatory neurotransmitter—in the paraventricular and supraoptic nuclei and stored in the posterior pituitary lobe. Serotonin may act as an erection stimulatory transmitter via 5-HT (1B/1C and 2A/2C) receptors; norepinephrine may have erection stimulatory action via α_1-adrenoceptors [11,21]; glutamate [22], EP peptides (hexarelin analogues) [23], and of course nitric oxide (NO) [24–25], also participate in the erection process. After entering the cavernous bodies the parasympathetic nerve fibers principally divide into two different types of nerve terminals: (1) cholinergic (acetylcholine, ACH) nerve terminals ending at the endothelial cells and stimulating NO-synthase, which catalyzes the production of NO from L-arginine and O_2; and (2) non-adrenergic, non-cholinergic (NANC-peptidergic) nerve terminals at the cavernous smooth muscle cells, from which NO and VIP are released into the smooth muscle cells. Within the smooth muscle cells NO activates guanylate cyclase, which catalyses the breakdown of guanosine triphosphate into 3′5′-cyclic guanosine monophosphate (cGMP) (Fig. 3.4).

cGMP is the most important second neurotransmitter of erection. It stimulates protein kinase G, which in turn initiates phosphorylation of membrane-bound proteins at the potassium channels (Fig. 3.5). This leads to potassium ion outflow into the extracellular space resulting in hyperpolarization. Hyperpolarization leads to closure of the L-type calcium channels subsequently resulting in a decrease in the intracellular Ca^{++} ion concentration. Physiologically, intracellular Ca^{++} along with calmodulin activate myosin light chain (MLC) kinase which catalyzes the phosphorylation of myosin light chains and induces actin–myosin interaction, finally resulting in contraction of the cavernous smooth musculature, thus preventing erection (Fig. 3.6). Phosphorylated myosin light chain is dephosphorylated by the active (dephosphorylated) form of MLC phosphatase, with the result being corpus cavernosum relaxation and erection. Phosphorylation

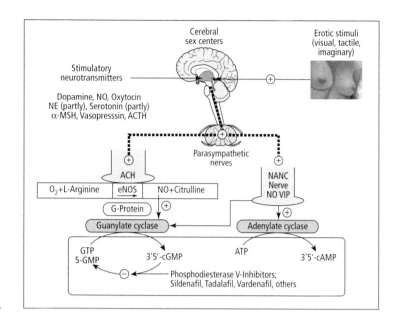

Fig. 3.4 Neurophysiology of erection.

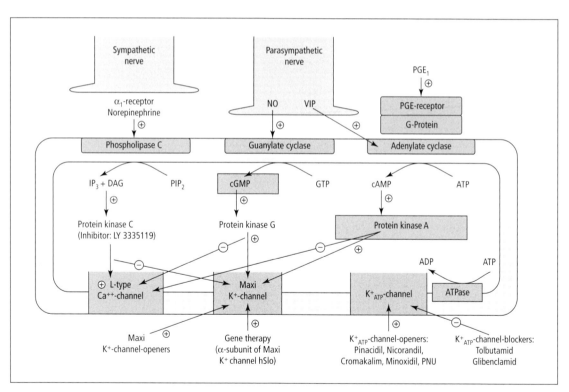

Fig. 3.5 The biochemical basics for the pharmacologic treatment of erectile dysfunction.

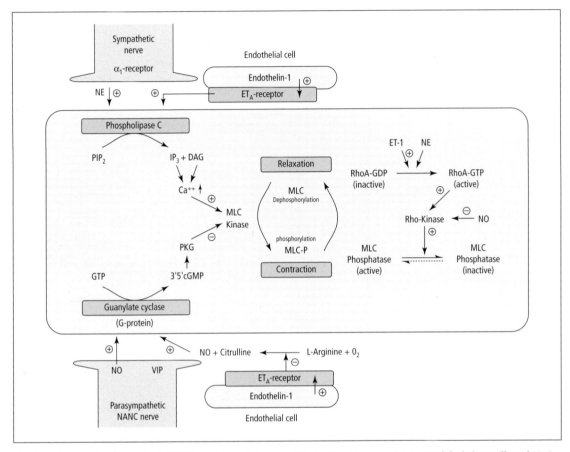

Fig. 3.6 The myosin light chain (MLC) kinase/phosphatase and RhoA/Rho-kinase pathway. Modified after Mills *et al.* [26].

that results in inactivation of MLC phosphatase is catalyzed by Rho-kinase A (RhoA) [26]. RhoA is a small GTPase which is inactive when GDP is bound but becomes active when GTP is bound. Activated RhoA stimulates the serine/threonine kinase named Rho-kinase. Rho-kinase itself phosphorylates MLC phosphatase at the myosin binding unit and thus inactivates this enzyme, resulting in smooth muscle contraction and flaccidity of the penis (Fig. 3.6). So-called Rho-kinase inhibitors, developed recently to assess their potential for the treatment of erectile dysfunction, activate MLC phosphatase and lead to relaxation and erection.

Sympathetic nerve supply: inhibition of erection
Erection inhibiting (anti-erectile) neurotransmitters are serotonin, which causes erection inhibition via 5-HT receptors (1A and 1B), γ-aminobutyric acid (GABA) [12], norepinephrine, which works via α_2-adrenoceptors, and opioids [12]. Erection-inhibiting impulses, originating in the cerebral centers, run along the spinal cord to an area at $Th_{11/12}–L_{2/3}$, which seems to function as a psychogenic erection center. Efferent nerve fibres leave the psychogenic erection center through the anterior root and then synapse in the sympathetic trunk ganglia, forming the superior hypogastric plexus. This plexus continues downwards as the inferior hypogastric plexus after joining the parasympathetic nervi erigentes. Along with these nerve fibers they become part of the cavernous nerves, which enter the cavernous bodies after penetrating the pelvic floor.

In the cavernous bodies the sympathetic nerve fibers innervate both the cavernous smooth muscle

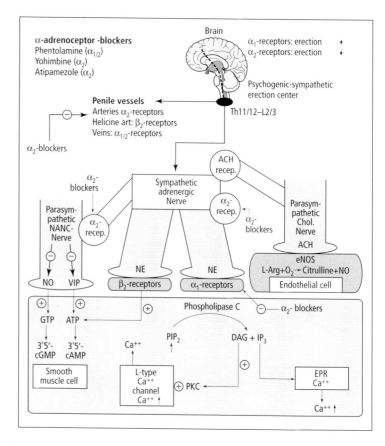

Fig. 3.7 The sympathetic innervation and its impact on erection.

cells as well as the cavernous vessels, i.e. arteries and veins. In the smooth muscle cells sympathetic nerve terminals end at α_1-adrenoceptors and at β_2-adrenoceptors. The ratio of α_1- to β_2-adenoceptors is 10 : 1 [27]. Among the α_1-adrenoceptors, the α_{1A}- and α_{1C}-subtypes dominate in the cavernous smooth musculature [12,28]. One research team found the following distribution pattern of α-adrenoceptors: $\alpha_{2A} > \alpha_{1A} > \alpha_{1B}$ [29]. The α_1-receptor density in the corpus cavernosum tissue is approximately the same as that of the prostate.

Alpha$_1$-adrenoceptors are stimulated either by direct release of norepinephrine from the sympathetic nerve terminals, or by epinephrine circulating in the plasma. Occupation of the α_1 receptors by norepinephrine or epinephrine respectively, leads to stimulation of the phospholipase C, which converts phosphatidylinositol biphosphate (PIP$_2$) to inositol triphosphate (IP$_3$) and diacylglycerol (DAG) (Fig. 3.7) [30,31]. DAG activates protein

kinase C, resulting in phosphorylation of membrane-bound proteins and activation of voltage-dependent L-type Ca^{++} channels. IP$_3$ causes release of Ca^{++} ions from intracellular sarcoplasmatic Ca^{++} stores. Activation of L-Type Ca^{++} ion channels and release of Ca^{++} ions from the endoplasmatic reticulum, results in an increase in intracellular Ca^{++} ion-concentrations, causing contraction of the cavernous smooth muscle cells and thus flaccidity, or prevention of erection. The contraction induced by norepinephrine is potentiated by endothelin 1 [21]. NPY has also been identified in some penile adrenergic nerve terminals.

Likewise norepinephrine or epinephrine stimulate α_1- and β_2-adrenoceptors. This results in activation of the adenylate cyclase which catalyzes the breakdown of ATP to 3′5′-cAMP, a second neurotransmitter in the physiology of erection. Cyclic AMP in turn stimulates protein kinase A leading to hyperpolarization and closure of L-type Ca^{++} ion channels (Fig. 3.7). Because β_2-adrenoceptors are in the minority as compared to the α_1-adrenoceptors, under physiologic conditions norepinephrine and epinephrine lead to contraction of smooth muscle cells and thus to detumescence and flaccidity.

Whereas α_1-adrenoceptors dominate within the cavernous bodies, α_2-adrenoceptors prevail in the penile arteries [12]. In addition, recent studies have shown that helicine arteries are rich in β_2-adrenoceptors, whose stimulation results in relaxation and increase of penile blood flow [13]. Both α_1- and α_2-adrenoceptors could be identified within the penile veins [16]. In addition, α_2-adrenoceptors are located presynaptically on sympathetic nerve terminals of α_1-adrenoceptors, inhibiting the sympathetic tone in these terminals [32]. A$_2$-adrenoceptors also have been detected presynaptically on parasympathetic NANC nerves, where they modulate parasympathetic activity (see also Fig. 3.7) [33].

In the aging male there is an increase in the density and sensitivity of α_1-adrenoceptors as well as a decrease in β_2-adrenoceptors. These changes in adrenoceptors are part of the reason why ED is an age-related phenomenon [34–36].

Somatic innervation

The somatic innervation of the penis occurs via the pudendal and dorsal nerves. The dorsal penile nerve innervates the glans penis, and the penile shaft and conveys sensory impulses to the reflexogenic erection center in the spinal cord at S_2–S_4.

At the spinal cord the sensory signals are processed either to the cerebral centers or to the somatic motoneurons of the pudendal nerve, which send motoric efferent branches to the pelvic floor. The pudendal nerve innervates the pelvic floor muscles and causes contraction of the bulbo and ischiocavernous muscles. This results in further blockade of the venous outflow from the cavernous bodies and increase of the intracavernous pressure, which ultimately leads to complete rigidity of the penis.

Endothelial factors

Angiotensin: The angiotensin I/II system and the angiotensin-converting enzyme play a role in the regulation of the cavernous smooth muscle tone [37,38].

Angiotensin II causes a dose-dependent contraction of the cavernous musculature, which can be blocked by specific AT$_1$-receptor antagonists such as losartan, but not by AT$_2$-antagonists. In patients with severe organic impotence in whom a penile implant was inserted, hypertrophied cells secreting angiotensin II have been detected in the corpus cavernosum [38]. This overproduction of angiotensin II may be one of the etiologic factors for ED in diabetes and hypertension [38]. Endothelial angiotensin II secretion has been shown to be significantly suppressed by PGE$_1$ and papaverine [38]. Angiotensin I also causes contraction, but only to a tenth of the extent of angiotensin II.

Endothelin: Of the three endothelins (ET$_{1-3}$) ET$_1$ is the most important in the cavernous bodies. The ET$_A$ receptor is relatively selective for ET$_1$ whereas the ET$_B$ receptor shows the same affinity for all three endothelins [39]. In in vitro trials on human corpus cavernosum muscle strips, the contraction strength of the three endothelins were classified as follows: ET$_1$ > ET$_2$ > ET$_3$ [40–41]. ET$_1$ activates phospholipase C after occupying the ET$_A$ receptor and causes the split off of IP$_3$ and DAG from PIP$_2$, resulting in an increase in intracellular Ca^{++} concentration. Increased Ca^{++} causes contraction and flaccidity of the corpora cavernosa (see Fig. 3.7). The contraction induced by ET$_1$ is eliminated by selective ET$_A$ receptor antagonists or blockers of the voltage-dependent L-type Ca^{++} ion channels [42]. It is argued that endothelin contributes to the manifestation of ischemic processes and arteriosclerotic changes, due to its contractile and proliferative properties [39]. Changes in the endothelin production or in endothelin receptors also appear to play a role in the manifestation of erectile dysfunction.

Prostanoids: A variety of prostanoids are synthesized and metabolized in the cavernous bodies. PGE$_1$ (alprostadil) causes strong relaxation, whereas PGE$_2$ at low concentrations causes weak relaxation. At high concentrations PGE$_2$ causes contraction of cavernous smooth muscle cells.

In contrast PGF$_{2\alpha}$, PGI$_2$, and most markedly thromboxan A$_2$ (TXA$_2$) lead to contraction. Prostacyclin (PGI$_2$) results in relaxation of the penile arteries, but contraction of the cavernous smooth muscle cells [43]. The release of the prostanoids is inhibited under hypoxemic conditions and increases with reoxygenation due to stimulation of prostaglandin H synthase (PGHS) [44]. Of the relaxing prostanoids, PGE_1 (alprostadil) has played a leading role in the management of ED. Alprostadil has been developed for intracavernous injection therapy, intraurethral therapy (Medicated Urethral System for Erection MUSE ®), and for topical therapy. PGE_1 stimulates adenylate cyclase via specific prostaglandin (EP) receptors [45], inhibits norepinephrine release at α_1-adrenoceptors, and hence acts as an anti-sympathetic drug. In addition, PGE_1 also causes reduction in angiotensin II secretion [38] and activates maxi K^+ channels, thus resulting in hyperpolarization and a decrease in intracellular Ca^{++} concentration.

Bradykinin has been reported to induce a dose-dependent relaxation of isolated human cavernous muscle strips due to an increase of the intracellular cAMP and cGMP concentrations.

The influence of hormones on erection

Testosterone (T)
Both fetal and later phallic growth are dependent on T and DHT tissue concentrations and androgen receptor density. At the cerebral level, testosterone stimulates the synthesis, storage and release of pro-erectile neurotransmitters such as dopamine, NO and oxytocin [14,24,46,47]. At the spinal level the somatic motoneurons of the bulbo- and ischiocavernous muscles are T dependent (Fig. 3.8).

At the corpus cavernosum level, NOS-containing parasympathetic nerves are T dependent [48]. Recent studies in animals have shown that T has a considerable effect on relaxation of cavernous smooth musculature and that T sites of action are also distal to the cGMP level [49]. Density and sensitivity of α-adrenoceptors are T dependent with an increase following T deprivation by castration [50]. Androgen (T) withdrawal is followed by programmed cell death (apoptosis) of the cavernous smooth musculature [51].

Dehydroepiandrosterone(sulfate) (DHEA(S))
DHEA(S) is an intermediate product of T biosynthesis. It is synthesized in significant amounts in the adrenal cortex. Although the serum concentrations of this androgen are a thousand-fold higher in primates than those of T, the importance of DHEA(S) is not yet well defined or understood. DHEA replacement therapy in men with proven DHEA deficiency resulted in increased vitality and

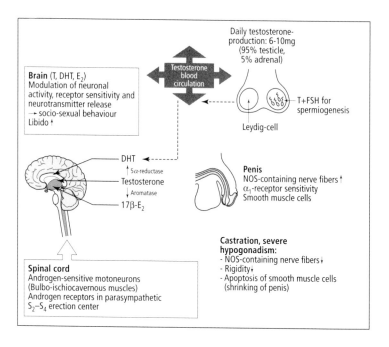

Fig. 3.8 Impact of testosterone on male sexual function.

well-being after oral administration of 50 mg DHEA/day [52], or in improvement of ED in impotent men [53].

Growth Hormone (GH) and insulin-like growth factor (IGF-1)

It has been proven that GH and IGF-1 affect penis growth and androgen production [54]. In cases with isolated GH deficiency and micropenis, continuous treatment with recombinant growth hormone normalizes the penile size [54]. Recently it has been suggested that GH also plays a role in erection [55]. Recombinant GH caused dose-dependent relaxation of cavernous smooth musculature by increasing intracellular cGMP levels. During erection a 90% increase in intracavernous GH concentration occurred in the tumescence stage.

References

1 Drews U. Geschlechtsdetermination und Entwicklung der Genitalorgane. *Urologe* 1997;**A37**:2–8.

2 Eberle J, Klocker H. Der Androgenrezeptor. *Urologe* 1993;**A32**:460–465.

3 Baskin LS, Sutherland RS, DiSandro MS, *et al.* The effect of testosterone on androgen receptors and human penile growth. *J Urol* 1997;**158**:1113–1118.

4 Neumann F. Endokrinologie der Geschlechtsentwicklung. *Urologe* 1997;**B37**:9–13.

5 Schweikert HU, Weidemann W, Romalo G. Intersexualität: Gonadendysgenesien und androgenresistenzsyndrome. *Urologe* 1997;**B37**:14–23.

6 Bitch M, Goldstein AMP, Melhan JP, *et al.* The fibrous skeleton of the corpora cavernosa and its possible function in the mechanism of erection. *Br J Urol* 1985;**57**:575.

7 Goldstein AMP, Padma-Nathan H. The microarchitecture of the intracavernosal smooth muscle on the cavernous fibrous skeleton. *J Urol* 1990;**144**:1144–1146.

8 Porst H. *Erektile Impotenz. Ätiologie, Diagnostik, Therapie.* Stuttgart: Enke-Verlag, 1987.

9 Fugleholm K, Schmalbruch H, Wagner G. The vascular anatomy of the cavernous body of green monkeys. *J Urol* 1989;**142**:181–188.

10 Fujita T, Shirai M. Mechanism of penile erection. *J Clin Exp Med* 1989;**148**:249–256.

11 Andersson KE, Holmquist F. Mechanisms for contraction and relaxation of human penile smooth muscle. *Int J Impotence Res* 1990;**2**:209–225.

12 Andersson KE, Wagner G. Physiology of penile erection. *Physiol Rev* 1995;**75**:191–236.

13 Saenz de Tejada I, Moncada J, Orte L, *et al.* β-Blockers potentiate the constrictor response of human helicine arteries to catecholamines. *Int J Impotence Res* 1996;**8**:No.3:D25.

14 Crowley WR, Zelman FP. The neurochemical control of mating behavior. In: Adler NT, ed. *Neuroendocrinology of reproduction, physiology and behavior.* New York: Plenum Press, 1981, p. 451.

15 Fontaine J, Schulman CC, Wespes E. Postjunctional alpha-1 and alpha-2 like activity in human isolated deep dorsal vein of the penis. *Br J Pharmacol* 1990;**101**:375–381.

16 Kirkeby HJ. Regulation of penile venous outflow. Experimental studies on endogenous control mechanisms. *Int J Impotence Res* 1994;**6,S2**:1–36.

17 Giuliano F, Allard J, Rampin U, *et al.* Proerectile effect of Apomorphine delivered at the spinal level in anaesthetized rat. *Int J Impotence Res* 2000;**12,S3**:S66:A22.

18 Gantert LT, Drisko JE, Nargund RP, *et al.* Melanocortin 4-receptor and 5 HT2C receptor modulation of erectogenesis in conscious rats as reported by telemetric measurement of intracavernous pressure. *Int J Impotence Res* 2001;**13,S5**:S53,Abstr.6.

19 Lindia JA, Nargund R, Sebhat J, *et al.* Erectogenic effects of a selective melanocortin-4 receptor (MC 4-R) agonist in a rat model of erectile activity. *Int J Impotence Res* 2001;**13,S5**:S55.

20 McGowan E, Cashen DE, Drisco JE, *et al.* Activation of melanocortin-4 receptor (MC 4-R) increases erectile activity in rats. *Int J Impotence Res* 2001;**13,S5**:S55Abstr.13.

21 Andersson KE. Classification, function and regulation of alpha adrenergic receptors in human penile tissue. *Vortrag Pre-Congress Session of ESIR:Erectile Dysfunction. XIVth Congress of EAU*, Stockholm, April 7, 1999.

22 Zahran AR, Vachon P, Courtois F, *et al.* Increases in intracavernous penile pressure following injections of excitatory amino acid receptor agonists in the hypothalamic paraventricular nucleus of anaesthetized rats. *J Urol* 2000;**164**:1793–1797.

23 Melis MR, Spano MS, Succu S, *et al.* EP 60761- and EP 50885- induced penile rection: structure-activitiy studies and comparison with apomorphine, oxytocin and N-metyl-D-aspartic acid. *Int J Impotence Res* 2000; **12**:255–262.

24 Horita H, Sato Y, Kurohata T, *et al.* Effect of testosterone replacement on nitric oxide synthase-containing cells in the rat brain. *Int J Impotence Res* 1998;**10,S3**: S12.

25 Sato Y, Horita H, Kurohata T, *et al.* Effect of testosterone replacement on extracellular nitric oxide in the PVN in aged rats. *J Urol* 1998;**159**:No.5 Suppl.99.

26 Mills TM, Chitaley K, Lewis RW. Vasoconstriction in erectile physiology. *Int J Impotence Res* 2001;**S5**: S29–S34.

27 Levin RM, Wein AJ. Adrenergic alpha-receptors outnumber beta-receptors in human penile corpus cavernosum. *Invest Urol* 1980;**18**:225–226.

28 Traish AM, Netsuwan N, Daley J, *et al.* A heterogeneous population of $alpha_1$ adrenergic receptors mediates contraction of human corpus cavernosum smooth muscle to norepinephrine. *J Urol* 1995;**153**:222–227.

29 Goepel M, Krege S, Price DT, *et al.* Characterization of alpha-adrenoceptor subtypes in the corpus cavernosum of patients undergoing sex change surgery. *J Urol* 1999;**162**:1793–1799.

30 Eckert RE, Bewermeier H, Utzt, *et al.* Role of phospholipase C in the $alpha_1$-adrenoceptor induced cavernous smooth muscle contraction. *J Urol* 1997;**157**:No.4, Suppl.356.

31 Holmquist F, Persson K, Garcia-Pascual A, *et al.* Phospholipase C activation by endothelin I and norepinephrine in isolated penile erectile tissue from rabbit. *J Urol* 1992;**147**:1632–1635.

32 Molderings GJ, Göthert M, van Ahlen H, *et al.* Modulation of noradrenaline release in human corpus cavernosum by presynaptic prostaglandin receptors. *Int J Impotence Res* 1992;**4**:19.

33 Saenz de Tejada I. Commentary on mechanisms for the regulation of penile smooth muscle contractility. *J Urol* 1995;**153**:1762.

34 Christ GJ, Maayani S, Valcic M, *et al.* Pharmacologic studies of human erectile tissue: Characteristics of spontaneous contractions and alterations in alpha-adrenoceptor responsiveness with age and disease in isolated tissues. *Br J Pharmacol* 1990;**101**:375–381.

35 Christ GJ, Stone B, Melman A. Age dependent alterations in the efficacy of phenylephrine-induced contractions in vascular smooth muscle isolated from corpus cavernosum of impotent men. *Can J Pharmacol* 1991;**69**:905–913.

36 Saenz de Tejada I, Moncada I. Pharmacology of penile smooth muscle. In: Porst H, ed., *Penile Disorders*. Berlin, Heidelberg, New York: Springer-Verlag, 1997, pp. 125–144.

37 Comiter CK, Sullivan MP, Kifor J. Effect of angiotensin II on corpus cavernosum smooth muscle in relation to nitric oxide environment: In vitro studies in canines. *Int J Impotence Res* 1997;**9**:135–140.

38 Kifor J, Williams GH, Vickers MA, *et al.* Tissue angiotensin II as a modulator of erectile function. I Angiotensin peptide content, secretion and effects in the corpus cavernosum. *J Urol* 1997;**157**:1920–1925.

39 Ferro CJ, Webb DJ. Endothelial dysfunction and hypertension. *Drugs* 1997;**53**:Suppl.1:30–41.

40 Christ GJ, Lerner SE, Kim DC, *et al.* Endothelin-1 as a putative modulator of erectile dysfunction: I characteristics of contraction of isolated corporal tissue stripes. *J Urol* 1995;**153**:1998–2003.

41 Traish AM, de los Morenas A, Goldstein I, *et al.* Biochemical and physiological studies of endothelin action in human corpus cavernosum. *J Urol* 1991;**145**: No.4,230.

42 Giraldi A, Serels S, Autieri M, *et al.* Endothelin-1 as a putative modulator of gene expression and cellular physiology in human corporal smooth muscle. *Int J Impotence Res* 1996;**8**:No.3,100.

43 Bosch RJLH, Benard F, Aboseif SR, *et al.* Changes in penile hemodynamics after intracavernous injection of prostaglandin E_1 and prostaglandin I_2 in pigtailed monkeys. *Int J Impotence Res* 1989;**1**:211–221.

44 Daley JT, Watkins MT, Brown ML, *et al.* Prostanoid production in rabbit corpus cavernosum II. Inhibition by oxidative stress. *J Urol* 1996;**156**:1169–1173.

45 Porst H. The rationale for prostaglandin E_1 in erectile failure: A survey of world-wide experience. *J Urol* 1996;**155**:802–815.

46 McEwen BS. Neural gonadal steroid actions. *Science* 1981;**211**:1303–1311.

47 Sato Y, Shibuya A, Adachi H, *et al.* Restoration of sexual behavior and dopaminergic neurotransmission by long term exogenous testosterone replacement in aged male rats. *J Urol* 1998;**160**:1572–1575.

48 Baba K, Yajima M, Carrier S, *et al.* Effect of testosterone on nitric oxide synthase-containing nerve fibres and intracavernous pressure in rat corpus cavernosum. *Int J Impotence Res* 1994;**6**:S1,D6.

49 Alcorn JF, Toepfer JR, Leipheimer RE. The effects of castration on relaxation of rat corpus cavernosum smooth muscle in vitro. *J Urol* 1999;**161**:686–689.

50 Mills TM, Stopper VS, Reilly CM. Androgens modulate the alpha-adrenergic responsiveness of vascular smooth muscle in the rat corpus cavernosum. *Int J Impotence Res* 1996;**8**,No.3,133.

51 Santarosa RP, Te A, Koo HP, *et al.* Androgen deprivation and apoptosis in rat erectile tissue. *J Urol* 1994;**151**: No.5,494A.

52 Morales A, Nolan JJ, Nelson JC, *et al.* Effects of replacement dose of dehydroepiandrosterone in men and

women of advancing age. *J Clin Endocrinol Metab* 1994; **78**:1360–1367.

53 Reiter WJ, Pycha A, Lodde M, *et al.* Dehydroepiandrosterone in the treatment of erectile dysfunction: a prospective, double-blind randomized, placebo-controlled study. *Int J Impotence Res* 1998;**10**,**S**3:S39, 1998

54 Levy JB, Husman DA. Micropenis secondary to growth hormone deficiency:does treatment with growth hormone alone result in adequate penile growth? *J Urol* 1996;**156**:214–216.

55 Becker AJ, Ückert S, Stief CG, *et al.* Possible role of human growth hormone in penile ereciton. *J Urol* 2000;**164**:2138–2142.

CHAPTER 4

History and Epidemiology of Male Sexual Dysfunction

Hartmut Porst and Ira D. Sharlip

It seems paradoxical that among the physiologic functions of the human body, sexual function has generated the greatest popular awareness and curiosity, but the least scientific inquiry. Despite the considerable human behavior, both virtuous and evil, that has been motivated by human sexuality, restrictive social attitudes and taboos have severely inhibited scientific investigation of human sexual function. Working within a restrictive social environment, a few irrepressible investigators and observers of human behavior have changed the course of modern social science and philosophy through their interests in sexual medicine and sexual psychology. Sigmund Freud brought new concepts of the importance of sexuality to the forefront of Western creative thinking at the end of the 19th century and beginning of the 20th century [1]. As early as 1896, the aphrodisiac effects of yohimbine were reported by Leopold Spiegel, who extracted this substance from the bark of the West African yohimbe tree [2]. Around that time reports on the successful treatment of "atonic impotence" by dorsal penile vein ligature procedures were also published in the literature [3,4]. Only a few years later in 1914, a patent for "a device for the artificial erection of the penis", the prototype of the vacuum devices, was awarded to Otto Lederer in Germany [5]. Decades later, Alfred Kinsey's epidemiologic studies of human sexual behavior, published in 1948 and 1953, profoundly liberalized popular attitudes about sexuality in American society [6]. In the 1960s, Masters and Johnson contributed groundbreaking studies of sexual anatomy and physiology as well as new concepts about sex therapy, further lessening societal barriers to open discussion of human sexuality [7,8]. At about the same time, research in sex steroid biochemistry led to the development of the birth control pill in the 1960s. The ability for women to control their own reproductive choices played a vital role in the rise of feminism in Western countries; and the rise of feminism was a crucial element in producing more liberal social attitudes about human sexuality and the resulting sexual revolution of the late 1960s and early 1970s.

Perhaps made possible by this sexual revolution, progress in male sexual medicine accelerated in the 1970s. Prior to this time, sexual dysfunction was considered to be an endocrine or a psychologic problem. The usual treatments were testosterone therapy for men with hypogonadism, and psychotherapy. In the early 1970s, Vaclav Michal, a vascular surgeon from Prague, began to investigate the role of penile revascularization techniques for the treatment of vasculogenic erectile dysfunction [9,10]. Interest in Michal's surgical techniques led Adrian Zorgniotti in 1978 to organize the First International Conference on Corpus Cavernosum Revascularization in New York. This conference evolved into biennial conferences, which expanded to cover the entire field of sexual medicine. By 1984, these conferences became the meetings of the International Society for Impotence Research (ISIR). ISIR has since been renamed the International Society for Sexual Medicine (ISSM).

Also in the early 1970s, Small, Carrion, Scott and others in the United States created a dramatic change in treatment options for erectile dysfunction with the introduction of the modern era of penile prostheses [11,12]. This resulted in new access to treatment for erectile dysfunction for tens of thousands of men worldwide, and created a new wave of popular and medical interest in sexual medicine.

Subsequently, in 1981 the serendipitous discovery in Paris by Ronald Virag of the erectogenic action of intracavernous injection of papaverine produced major advances in both the treatment of erectile dysfunction and the understanding of erectile physiology [13]. By the mid-1980s, intracavernous injection therapy with papaverine, the mixture of papaverine/pentolamine, and later with prostaglandin E_1, became a common and effective treatment for erectile dysfunction [14–17].

A particularly important development in sexual medicine occurred in 1992 when the National Institutes of Health in the United States called for a consensus development conference on impotence. The conference recommended using the term erectile dysfunction rather than impotence, and defined erectile dysfunction as the "consistent inability to attain or maintain a penile erection, or both, sufficient for adequate sexual relations." This effectively identified erectile dysfunction as a recognized disease state, thus helping to qualify it for governmental and private insurance medical benefits.

As scientists dedicated more and more effort in the 1990s to elucidating the molecular biology of sexual and erectile physiology, a major basic science breakthrough occurred in the mid-1990s with the discovery of the role of nitric oxide in smooth muscle relaxation of the corpus cavernosum. Only a few years later, the greatest clinical breakthrough event in the history of male sexual medicine occurred with the approval of sildenafil, the first effective oral therapy for erectile dysfunction, which was launched in March 1998 in the US [18]. The social impact of sildenafil may have been even greater than its medical impact. While some 25 million men have benefited from sildenafil, and another five million or more have benefited from the newer phosphodiesterase inhibitors, vardenafil and tadalafil; the commercialization of these drugs has brought the subject of sexual dysfunction into common parlance and social discussion for hundreds of millions of men and women throughout the world. The introduction of sildenafil may have been the most important event in medical history in destigmatizing sexual dysfunction and reducing taboos about discussing sexuality.

Proceeding into the beginning of the 21st century, new trends in sexual medicine promise to promote more popular interest and public discussion. A new and specific treatment for premature ejaculation, one of the most common forms of male sexual dysfunction, is in the final stages of clinical development and may be approved in 2007 [19]. And an entirely new method of treating erectile dysfunction using the cutting-edge technique of gene therapy has just entered the initial stages of clinical development [20]. Importantly, progress in both male and female sexual health has been aided by the World Health Organization (W.H.O.) which has designated the years 2004 to 2009 for worldwide public emphasis on sexual health using the campaign slogan, "Sexual Health: a new focus for W.H.O.". The recognition by W.H.O. of the importance of sexual health is another signal of the vital role that sexual medicine is likely to play in the future.

Epidemiology of Erectile Dysfunction

The scale and potential social impact of erectile dysfunction may be best understood by an appreciation of its international frequency. In 1995, it is estimated that there were 152 000 000 men worldwide suffering from erectile dysfunction. Because of the accelerating aging of the world population, coupled with the high prevalence of erectile dysfunction in men over 50, the world population of men with erectile dysfunction is expected to increase to 322 000 000 by the year 2025 [21]. With this high prevalence, erectile dysfunction will become a progressively more common and compelling public health problem throughout the world.

Many studies on the prevalence of erectile dysfunction have been published in recent years but their conclusions vary widely. The reasons for the varying results include differences in the design and methodology of the studies, the methods of selecting subjects for the study, the age and health of the cohort studied, the questions that are asked, how the questions are asked, cultural characteristics of the cohort under study, the prevailing attitudes about what constitutes a normal and an abnormal erection in the cohort under study, and prejudices of the investigators.

A review of 15 large-scale prevalence studies from

1994 to 2004, reporting men with erectile dysfunction as a percentage of the studied population shows that the prevalence of erectile dysfunction has varied from a low of 10.2% in Laumann's US study of men aged 18–59 years, to a high of 64% in Akkus' Turkish study of men over 40 (Table 4.1) [22–36]. Among all 15 studies, the Massachusetts Male Aging Study is the one that is most often referenced [22]. This study demonstrated an overall prevalence of erectile dysfunction of 52% in men aged 40–70. Of these 52%, 17.2% had minimal erectile dysfunction, 25.2% had

moderate erectile dysfunction and 9.6% had complete erectile dysfunction.

Prevalence studies have produced much practical information of clinical importance. Across all prevalence studies, when controlling for other factors, increasing age is a strong risk factor for erectile dysfunction. This effect becomes especially prominent after about age 50 years. For example, in 11 prevalence studies which report erectile dysfunction by decade of life, the prevalence of erectile dysfunction for men in their 30s is 2–15.9%, in their 40s is 9–

Table 4.1 Prevalence of erectile dysfunction.

Author	Year	Country	N	Age	Total (%)	Mild (%)	Moderate (%)	Complete (%)
Feldman [22]	1994	US	1.290	40–70 (⌀54)	52	17.2	25.2	9.6 (⌀54)
Dunn [23]	1998	UK	780	18–75 ⌀50	26			
Laumann [24]	1999	US	1.249	18–59	10.2			
Braun [25]	2000	Germany	4.489	30–80	19.2			
Chew [26]	2000	Australia	1.240	18–91 (⌀56)	39.4	9.6	8.9	18.6
Akkus [27]	2000	Turkey	1.982	>40	64.3	35.7	23	5.6
Vaaler [28]	2000	Norway	1.182	>40	33	NA	20	13
Meuleman [29]	2000	Netherlands	1.215	>40	13			
Mahmoud [30]	2000	Egypt	594	30–70 (⌀39)	54.9	32.3	20.4 (⌀39)	2.2
Koskimaki [31]	2000	Finland	2.128	50–70	48	22	14	12
Dogunro [32]	2000	Nigeria	917	35–70 (⌀43)	50.7	40.5	9.9	0.2
Kadiri [33]	2000	Morocco	646	>25 (⌀40)	53.6	37.5	15	1.1
M.-Morales [34]	2001	Spain	2.476	25–70	12.1	5.2	5	1.9
Rosen [35]	2004	Multinational	27.839	20–75	16			
Laumann [36]	2005	Multinational	13.618	40–80	12.9–28.1*			
deBoer [37]	2004	Netherlands	2.117	18–80	16.8	5.9	3.6	6.9
Ponholzer [38]	2005	Austria	2.869	20–80	32.3	23.7	7.2	1.3

* Variation of prevalence depends on the region under investigation.

39%, in their 50s is 16–67%, in their 60s is 27–76%, and in their 70s is 37–83% [22–26,29–31,33,34, 36–38] (Table 4.2). Other major risk factors for erectile dysfunction include hypertension, hyperlipidemia, diabetes, cardiovascular disease, and probably smoking. The common element, which links these risk factors and erectile dysfunction, is endothelial dysfunction. Epidemiologic studies are producing the very important new concepts that erectile dysfunction may be an early manifestation of endothelial dysfunction, that erectile dysfunction may be a harbinger of generalized endothelial dysfunction, and that erectile dysfunction may be a precursor for various forms of cardiovascular disease [40]. These concepts, if true, will have powerful implications for strategies to promote cardiovascular health and to prevent catastrophic cardiovascular diseases such as stroke and coronary thrombosis.

Many of the erectile dysfunction prevalence studies have been done in populations from specific nations. While there are large variations among these studies, the variances in study design, methodology and subject recruitment prevent the conclusion that the prevalence of erectile dysfunction is discernibly more or less common in any one country.

Even though erectile dysfunction increases significantly with increasing age, there is evidence of continued sexual activity in men over 70, and even beyond age 80. For men in the age range 70 to 79, a study conducted in Germany [25] reported that 71% of men were sexually active, and a study in Japan [41] reported that 55% to 70% of men were sexually active [41]. The Japanese study also reported that 44% of men over age 80 were sexually active. Another study showed that, for men aged 50 to 80 in the United States and six European countries, the number of sexual activities per month was consistently between 5.4 and 6.5 (Fig. 4.1) [42]. These epidemiologic studies strongly suggest that a large percentage of men remain sexually active into their 70s and beyond.

Another important concept in epidemiologic studies of erectile dysfunction is that the overall preva-

Table 4.2 Prevalence of erectile dysfunction by decade of life.

Author			Country	N (total)	Decade of Life				
					30–39	40–49	50–59	60–69	70–80
Feldman [22]	1998		USA	1.790	?	39%	48%	57%	67%
Laumann [24]	1999		USA	1.249	9%	11%	18%	NA	
Braun [25]	2000		Germany	4.489	2.3%	9.5%	15.7%	34.4%	53.4%
Chew [26]	2000		Australia	1.240	8.4%	13.1%	33.5%	51.5%	69.2%
Kadiri [33]	2000		Morocco	646	5%	?	?	56.7%	?
Mahmoud [30]	2000		Egypt	594	15.9%	?	?	35.7%	?
Koskimaki [31]	2000		Finland	2.178	?	?	67%	76%	83%
Glina [39]	2000		Brazil	825	2%	9%	16%	27%	49%
Meuleman [29]	2000		Netherlands	1.779	10%				78%
M.-Morales [34]	2001		Spain	2.476	1%	1.7%	4.5%	11.7%	—
Rosen [35]	2004		Multinational	27.839	11%	15%	22%	30%	37%
DeBoer [37]	2004		Netherlands	2.117	5.6%	13.7%	23.7%	40%	41.9%
Ponholzer [38]	2005		Austria	2.869		28.9%	37.5%		71.2%

NA, not available.

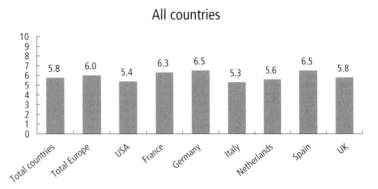

Fig. 4.1 Sexual activities per month in age groups 50 to 80 years. From Rosen R. *et al.* [42].

lence of concern in men with erectile dysfunction is only about one half of the overall number of men with erectile dysfunction. Prevalence studies and pharmaceutical sales data show that only a fraction of men with erectile dysfunction seek and use treatment chronically. In the multinational MALES study of 27 839 men between the ages of 20 and 75 years, 16% or about 4450 men, self-reported erectile dysfunction. Of these men with self-reported erectile dysfunction, 58% acknowledged that they had discussed erectile dysfunction with a doctor but only 22% had used sildenafil more than once and only 15.7% used sildenafil continuously [35]. Another study published in 2000 showed that of 4483 German men aged 30 to 80 who responded to a postal questionnaire, 19.2% reported having erectile dysfunction, but only 6.8% had urologic treatment for erectile dysfunction [25]. This suggests that only about one third of these men with erectile dysfunction were bothered enough to want medical treatment for erectile dysfunction. Although another report from The Netherlands showed that two thirds of men with ED were bothered by this disease. Interpreting all of these studies broadly, it seems reasonable to conclude that about one half of men with erectile dysfunction are bothered by it and one half are not.

References

1 Freud S. Über die allgemeinste Erniedrigung des Liebeslebens. *Jahrbuch für Psychoanalytische und Psychopathologische Forschungen* 1912;**4**(1):40–50.
2 Spiegel L. Untersuchungen einiger neuer Drogen(I. Yohimbeherinde). *Chemiker-Zeitung* 1886;**97**:970–971.
3 Wooten JS. Ligation of the dorsal vein of the penis as a cure for atonic impotence. *Tex Med J* 1902;**16**:325–328.
4 Lydston GF. The surgical treatment of impotency: further observations on the resection of the vena dorsalis penis in appropriate cases of impotence in the male with a record of experiences. *Am J Clin Med* 1908;**15**:1571–1573.
5 Lederer O. Vorrichtung zur künstlichen Erektion des Penis.Patentschrift Nr. 268874, Klasse 30d, Gruppe 15. Kaiserliches Patentamt 1914. (Available from European patent office, Den Haag, The Netherlands, 1914.)
6 Kinsey AC, Pomeroy WB, Martin CE, eds. *Sexual behavior in the human male*. Philadelphia: W Saunders Co., 1948.
7 Masters WH, Johnson VE, eds. *Human sexual response*. Boston: Little Brown and Co., 1966.
8 Masters WH, Johnson VE, eds. *Human sexual inadequacy*. Boston: Little Brown and Co., 1970.
9 Michal V, Kramar R, Pospichal J. Direct arterial anastomosis to the cavernous body in the treatment of erectile impotence. *Rozhal Chir* 1973;**52**:587–591.
10 Michal V, Kramar R, Pospichal J, *et al.* Arterial epigastricocavernous anastomosis for the treatment of sexual impotence. *World J Surg* 1977;**1**:515–520.
11 Scott FB, Bradley WE, Timm GW. Management of erectile impotence. Use of implantable inflatable prosthesis. *Urology* 1973;**2**:80–82.
12 Small MP, Carrion HM, Gordon JA. Small Carrion penile prosthesis. *Urology* 1975;**5**:479–486.
13 Virag R. Intracavernous injection of papaverine for erectile failure. *Lancet* 1982;**2**:938.
14 Zorgniotti AW, Lefleur RS. Autoinjection of the corpus cavernosum with a vasoactive drug combination for vasculogenic impotence. *J Urol* 1985;**133**:39–41.
15 Adaikan PG, Kottegoda SR, Ratnam SS. A possible role for prostaglandin E_1 in human penile erection. In: *Abstract Book Second World Meeting on Impotence*. Abstr.2.6, Prague, 1986.

16 Porst H. Stellenwert von Prostaglandin E_1 (PGE) in der Diagnostik der erektilen dysfunktion (ED) im Vergleich zu Papaverin und Papaverin/Phentolamin bei 61 Patienten mit ED. *Urologe A* 1988;**27**:22–26.

17 Stackl W, Hasun R, Marberger M. Intracavernous injection of prostaglandin E_1 in impotent men. *J Urol* 1988;**140**:66.

18 Boolell M, Allen MJ, Ballard SA, *et al.* Sildenafil: an orally active type 5 cyclic GMP-specific phosphodiesterase inhibitor for the treatment of penile erectile dysfunction. *Int J Impotence Res* 1996;**8**:47–52.

19 Pryor JL, Althof SE, Steidle C, *et al.* Efficacy and tolerability of Dapoxetine in the treatment of premature ejaculation. *J Urol* 2005;**173**:Suppl. 201,740.

20 Melman A, Bar-Chama N, Christ G. The first phase I human gene transfer trial: Ion channel therapy for the treatment of ED-preliminary results. *J Sex Med* 2004;**1**:Suppl.1, 141, Abstr. UP 153.

21 Aytac IA, McKinlay JB, Krane RJ. The likely worldwide increase in erectile dysfunction between 1995 and 2025 and some possible policy consequences. *BJU Int* 1999;**84**:50–56.

22 Feldman HA, Goldstein I, Hatzichristou DG, *et al.* Impotence and first medical and psychosocial correlates: Results of the Massachusetts Male Aging Study. *J Urol* 1994;**151**:54–61.

23 Dunn KM, Croft PR, Hackett GI. Sexual problems: a study of the prevalence and need for health care in the general population. *Fam Pract* 1998;**15**:519–524.

24 Laumann EO, Paik A, Rosen RC. Sexual dysfunction in the United States. Prevalence and Predictors. *JAMA* 1999;**281**:537–544.

25 Braun M, Klotz T, Reifenrath B, *et al.* Die Prävalenz von männlichen Erektionsstörungen in Deutschland heute und in der Zukunft. *Akt Urol* 2000;**31**:302–307.

26 Chew KK, Earle CM, Stuckey BGA, *et al.* Erectile dysfunction in general medicine practice: prevalence and clinical correlates. *Int J Impotence Res* 2000;**12**:41–45.

27 Akkus E, Kadioglu A, Esen A, *et al.* The prevalence and correlates of erectile dysfunction in Turkey. *Int J Impotence Res* 12, 9th World Meeting on Impotence Research, Perth, 2000, M 64, p. 57.

28 Vaaler S, Lövkist H, Svendsen KOB, *et al.* Prevalence of erectile dysfunction in men over 40 years seeing general practitioners. *Int J Impotence Res* 2000;**12**:Suppl.5, S.8:29.

29 Meuleman E, Kolman D, Donkers L, *et al.* Male erectile dysfunction: Prevalence and quality of life in the Netherlands: The UREPIC-study. *Int J Impotence Res* 2000;**12**:Suppl.5, S8:28.

30 Mahmoud KZ, Azim SA, Gadallah M, *et al.* A patient based epidemiology study to find the prevalence and correlates of erectile dysfunction (ED) in Egypt. *Int J Impotence Res* 2000;**12**:Suppl.5, S24:P46.

31 Koskimaki J, Hakama M, Tammela TLJ. Prevalence of erectile dysfunction in Finland. *Int J Impotence Res* 2000;**12**:Suppl.5, S25:P47.

32 Dogunro S, Osegbe D, Jaguste VS, *et al.* Epidemiology of erectile dysfunction (ED) and its correlates: a patient based study in Nigerian population. *Int J Impotence Res* 2000;**12**:Suppl.5, S25:P47.

33 Kadiri N, Berrada S, Tahiri S, *et al.* Prevalence of erectile dysfunction (ED) and its correlates in Morocco: A population based epidemiology study. *Int J Impotence Res* 2000;**12**:Suppl.5, S25:P48.

34 Martin-Morales A, Sanchez-Cruz JJ, Saenz de Tejada I, *et al.* Prevalence and independent risk factors for erectile dysfunction in Spain.Results of the Epidemiologia de la Disfuncion Erectil Masculina Study. *J Urol* 2001;**166**:569–574.

35 Rosen RC, Fisher WA, Eardley I, *et al.* The multinational Men's Attitudes to Life Events and Sexuality (MALES) study: I. Prevalence of erectile dysfunction and related health concerns in the general population. *Curr Med Res Opin* 2004;**20**:607–617.

36 Laumann EO, Nicolosi A, Glasser DB, *et al.* Sexual problems among women and men aged 40–80y: prevalence and correlates identified in the global study of sexual attitudes and behaviour. *Int J Impotence Res* 2005;**17**:39–57.

37 de Boer BJ, Bots ML, Lycklama a Nijeholt AAB, *et al.* Erectile dysfunction in primary care: relevance and patient characteristics. The ENIGMA study. *Int J Impotence Res* 2004;**16**:358–364.

38 Ponholzer A, Temml C, Mock K, *et al.* Prevalence and risk factors for erectile dysfunction in 2869 men using a validated questionnaire. *Eur Urol* 2005;**47**:80–86.

39 Glina S, Melo LF, Martins FG, *et al.* Brazilian survey on aging and sexual performance. 9th World Meeting on Impotence Research, Perth. *Int J Impotence Res* 2000;**12**:p. 55:M58.

40 Billups K, Bank AJ, Padma-Nathan H, *et al.* Erectile dysfunction is a marker for cardiovascular disease: Results of the minority health institute expert advisory panel. *J Sex Med* 2005;**2**:40–52.

41 Kumamoto Y, Tsukamoto T, Satoh T, *et al.* Epidemiological study on aging changes of sexual activity in Japanese men and women. *The Aging Male* 2000;**3**:Suppl.1,9 Abstr. 0–18.

42 Rosen R, Altwein J, Boyle P, *et al.* Lower urinary tract symptoms and male sexual dysfunction: The multinational survey of the aging male (MSAM-7). *EurUrol* 2003;**44**:637–649.

CHAPTER 5

Etiology and Risk Factors of Erectile Dysfunction

Hussein Ghanem and Hartmut Porst

Introduction

Our understanding of the etiology and risk factors for erectile dysfunction (ED) has grown immensely over the past twenty years. Masters and Johnson [1] (1970) suggested that most cases of impotence were psychogenic, while Helen Kaplan (1974) estimated that erectile failure was psychogenic in 90% of cases and organic in 10% of cases [2]. However, the introduction of modern diagnostic tools in the area of sexual medicine revealed that vascular, neurologic, endocrinal, and other factors, contribute significantly to the development of ED [3]. The current consensus is that in most patients ED is of mixed etiology that may be either predominantly psychogenic or predominantly organic. The main etiologies and risk factors for ED are presented in Table 5.1.

Psychogenic Factors

Several predisposing, precipitating, maintaining, and contextual factors influence the development and maintenance of ED. Please refer to Chapter 2 (Psychologic and Interpersonal Aspects and their Management).

Lifestyle

Lifestyle factors frequently reported to be associated with ED include a sedentary lifestyle, smoking, alcohol or drug abuse, and obesity. Sleep deprivation has recently been suggested to inhibit nocturnal erections [4]. An increase in body mass index by 1 kg/m^2 reduced the Sexual Health Inventory for Men

(SHIM), also known as IIEF-5 (5-item version of the International Index of Erectile Function), by 0.141, independent of age ($P = 0.005$) [5]. In a study of 593 men 30 to 70 years old, midlife lifestyle modification appeared to be too late to reverse the adverse effects of nicotine, obesity, and alcohol consumption on sexual function, while physical activity appeared to be effective in reducing the risk of ED even if initiated in midlife [6]. A controlled study in obese men (BMI > 30) revealed that increase of physical activity from 48 to 195 min/week, and a decrease in BMI from 36.9 to 31.2 over two years, resulted in an increase of the International Index of Erectile Function (IIEF) score from 13.9 to 17 ($P < 0.001$) [7].

Age

Although many men continue to function sexually into later age, epidemiologic studies confirm that the prevalence of ED increases significantly with age (see also Chapter 4). In the Massachusetts Male Aging Study (MMAS), 39% of men had some degree of ED at the age of 40 [8]. The prevalence gradually increased to reach 67% at the age of 70. A strong relationship of patient age with both prevalence and severity of ED was also recently confirmed by a large-scale study of 2476 Spanish men [9]. In this regard it is obvious that the strong age-related increase of the prevalence of ED is predominantly due to the increasing risk factors with age.

Poor Physical and Psychological Health

In a recently published report involving 447 men

Table 5.1 Etiology and risk factors of ED.

Psychogenic factors (see Chapter 2)
• Lifestyle factors and individual health conditions
• Sedentary life-style
• Nicotine
• Alcohol abuse
• Drug addictions
• Possible factors: obesity, sleep deprivation, general poor health
• Age

Cardiovascular risk factors
• Hypertension
• Dyslipidemia
• Coronary artery disease (CAD)
• Peripheral arterial occlusive disease (PAOD)

Cavernous factors
• Cavernous veno-occlusive dysfunction
• Cavernous myopathy
• Cavernous fibrosis after priapism
• Peyronie's disease
• Penile fracture

Diabetes mellitus
• Diabetes type 1
• Diabetes type 2

Endocrine factors (see Chapter 18)
• Hypogonadism
• Hypoprolactinemia and prolactinoma
• Thyroid disorders

Iatrogenic ED
• Drug induced (see Table 5.3)
• Post-operative
• Post-radiation

LUTS (lower urinary tract symptoms) and BPH
Other medical disorders
• Hepatic insufficiency
• Respiratory disorders and sleep apnea
• Renal insufficiency
• Neurogenic disorders (MS, Parkinson's disease, stroke)

Post-traumatic ED
• Neural and vascular lesions

attending general practice clinics in London, it was found that men with sexual dysfunctions were in poorer physical and psychologic health (Nazareth and Boynton, 2003). The diagnosis of sexual dys-

function was according to ICD-10 (International Classification of Diseases, 10th revision).

Nicotine abuse

Smoking has been shown to be an important risk factor for ED, whether in the long or short term. The detrimental effects of smoking on sexual function have been shown to be independent of other nicotine related health problems. Long-term cigarette smoking has been shown to be an independent risk factor for arteriogenic impotence [29]. Juenemann *et al.* suggested that smoking could significantly interfere with the cavernous veno-occlusive mechanism [30]. Smoking cigarettes directly before an intracavernous injection of papaverine significantly reduced the erectile response to the medication [31].

Cardiovascular Risk Factors

More than 20 years ago the vascular surgeon Vaclav Michal from Prague recognized that chronic arterial disease, compromising the blood flow in the cavernous arteries, can be a significant cause of ED [11]. Atherosclerosis appears to be the most common cause of vasculogenic erectile dysfunction. Smoking, hypertension, diabetes mellitus and dyslipidemias have been shown to initiate the cascade of events resulting in atherosclerosis. These include endothelial injury, cellular migration, and smooth-muscle proliferation [12].

These same risk factors leading to the manifestation of ED are shared with coronary artery disease (CAD). Studies suggest ED as a strong predictive factor for CAD [13,14]. Vasculogenic impotence has been reported to be the first sign of a generalized arteriopathy suggesting that physicians should check ED patients for ischemic heart disease, which can be diagnosed by stress ECG or other investigations prior to starting treatment for ED [15,16]. The presence of silent co-existing myocardial ischemia should be considered in men who present with ED, particularly when they have other cardiovascular risk factors [17].

Hypertension

Hypertension is a major risk factor for the development of vascular ED. Muller *et al.* reported a very high incidence (85%) of cavernous artery insufficiency in a group of 117 hypertensive patients [18]. Oaks and Moyer reported that 8–10% of hypertensive patients suffered ED at their initial diagnosis with hypertension [19]. In a more recent study Burchardt *et al.* reported a 68% ED incidence rate in treated hypertensive patients with 7.6% suffering from mild, 15.4% from moderate, and 45.2% from severe ED, according to the IIEF [20].

Dyslipidemia

In animal experiments, acute and chronic hypercholesterolemia resulted in impairment of neural and endothelial-mediated relaxation of the cavernous smooth muscle cells through inhibition of NO-synthesis [21–23].

A high level of total cholesterol or a low level of high density lipoproteins (HDL) were reported as important risk factors for ED [8,24].

In clinical studies pathologic HDL and LDL (low density lipoprotein) values were associated with vascular ED and veno-occlusive dysfunction [25,26]. Lowering elevated total, and especially LDL, cholesterol levels, either by dietary measures or by administration of cholesterol lowering drugs (statins), resulted in a significant improvement of erectile function in both animals and humans [27,28].

Diabetes Mellitus (Table 5.2)

Several studies confirmed the etiologic role of diabetes in ED. ED develops in 35–75% of diabetics [32]. In the MMAS complete ED has been shown to occur three times more frequently in diabetics than in non-diabetics [8].

Diabetes mellitus may be involved in the pathogenesis of ED through several mechanisms, including sensory neuropathy, autonomic neuropathy, or vascular insufficiency (macro- or microangiopathy). Psychogenic or mixed factors may be also involved in ED in diabetic patients.

Based on animal models and human *in vitro* trials, a variety of cellular, biochemical and molecular changes in the cavernous tissue have been reported in the literature over the past 20 years (see Table 5.2).

ED in diabetics has been reported to be more common than retinopathy or nephropathy [33]. It occurs earlier in type I diabetes and may be the first sign of diabetes mellitus in 12% of patients [34]. Peak systolic velocity in the cavernous artery was found to be lower in diabetics in a study of 105 patients [35]. Endothelium-dependent and nerve-mediated corporal smooth muscle relaxation were also impaired with diabetes [36].

Medical Disorders

Several systemic diseases are associated with ED, including neurologic disorders, respiratory diseases, renal and hepatic disorders.

Neurologic diseases

ED can occur as a result of various neurologic diseases or lesions. The hippocampus and paraventricular nucleus and medial preoptic area are considered as the main centers regulating sexual drive and behavior [37,38]. Lesions at these areas may result in ED, depending on their severity. Central neurologic disorders frequently associated with ED include disorders at the level of the brain (e.g. multiple sclerosis, temporal lobe epilepsy, Parkinson's disease, stroke or Alzheimer's disease), or at the level of spinal cord (e.g. spinal cord injury) [39,40,41]. Peripheral neurologic disorders related to ED include afferent (sensory) neuropathies, such as dorsal penile nerve affections (e.g. diabetic neuropathy), or efferent (autonomic) lesions, such as autonomic neuropathy or lesions of the cavernous nerves after radical pelvic surgery [42].

Respiratory diseases

Chronic obstructive pulmonary disease has been associated with ED in up to 30% of cases despite intact penile vasculature, suggesting pulmonary disease as a primary etiologic factor [43]. Hypoxia may be a possible mechanism for this. An association between obstructive sleep syndrome, as well as sleep apnea, and ED was suggested by several other authors [44,45].

Hepatic insufficiency

ED has been reported in up to 50% of patients with

Table 5.2 Pathogenesis of ED in diabetes mellitus.

Angiopathy	
Macroangiopathy (rarely):	Iliac arteries
Microangiopathy (frequently):	Penile arteries and microcirculation
Polyneuropathy	
Somatic nervous system:	Pudendal and dorsal penile nerve
Autonomic nervous system:	Parasympathetic $\rightarrow$ pelvic and cavernous nerves (Impairment of erection)
	Sympathetic $\rightarrow$ pelvic and cavernous nerves (Loss of emission and ejaculation)
Impairment of neurotransmitter synthesis/release	
Cerebral/spinal level:	NO$\downarrow$
Peripheral level (penis):	NO$\downarrow$, VIP$\downarrow$, ACH$\downarrow$

Endothelial and smooth muscle cell dysfunction
Upregulation of ET_B-receptors
Impairment of eNOS (NO$\downarrow$)
Impairment of prostanoid synthesis (Prostacyclin: $PGI_2\downarrow$, $PGE_1\downarrow$)
Upregulation of arginase (NO$\downarrow$)
Upregulation of protein kinase C (PKC) β II
Impairment of KATP-channels (additionally enhanced by sulfonylurea antidiabetics)
Upregulation of insulin-like growth factor binding protein 3 (IGFBP-3) precursor
Downregulation of estrogen β-receptor expression
Upregulation of α_1-adrenoceptors
Glycosylated hemoglobin C-induced decrease of NO-release

Impairment of cavernous tissue architecture
Enhanced apoptosis of smooth muscle cells and endothelium
Enhanced collagen synthesis (TGF $\beta1\uparrow$) and fibrosis

NO, nitric oxide; VIP, vasoactive intestinal polypeptide; ACH, acetylcholine; eNOS, endothelial derived nitric oxide synthase; ET_B-receptors, endothelin type B receptors; PGI_2, prostacyclin; PGE_1, prostaglandin E1; TGF, transforming growth factor.

chronic liver dysfunctions, and may reach up to 75% in alcoholic liver cirrhosis [46]. Suggested mechanisms for ED in hepatic failure include hyperprolactinemia, increased sex hormone binding globulin synthesis resulting in decreased bioavailable testosterone, and elevated levels of estrogens [47].

Renal insufficiency

Renal failure may result in ED in up to 50% of patients. Possible mechanisms for ED in patients with renal disease include vascular insufficiency, autonomic or sensory neuropathy, endocrine factors with decreased testosterone and elevated prolactin levels, significant anemia, zinc deficiency, associated diabetes, psychologic stress, and anti-erectile medications such as antihypertensives [48,49]. In pa-

tients requiring dialysis, occlusions of the cavernous arteries was found in 78%, and veno-occlusive dysfunction in 90% of patients [50].

Iatrogenic Disorders

Iatrogenic disorders include post-operative, post-radiation, and drug-induced ED.

Post-operative ED

Surgery may lead to ED, either by compromising the vascular or nerve supply, or by hormonal deprivation (e.g. post castration, due to advanced prostate cancer or post pituitary surgery). Transurethral and open prostate adenomectomy may result in ED in between 5 and 40% of patients depending on the series reported [51–53]. Procedures frequently resulting in the manifestation of ED include radical pelvic surgery, such as radical prostatectomy (non nerve sparing), or cystectomy, abdominoperineal resection of the rectum and aorto–iliac bypass surgery. With knowledge of the anatomical course and identification of the cavernous nerves from the spinal center to the erectile tissue, and with the possible aid of intraoperative neurostimulation, the cavernous nerves may be identified and preserved, thereby preventing iatrogenic impotence [54,55].

Radiogenic impotence

Studies have shown that 20 to 75% of patients who received radiation for malignant disease suffered from ED, with an onset of as early as one month up to four years. In particular, vascular (arterial) factors were discussed [56].

Drug induced ED

Several classes of medications and recreational drugs have been linked to the manifestation of ED (Table 5.3). This list is not meant to be inclusive of all medications that could cause ED. Drugs exhibit their adverse effects either through central inhibitory neuroendocrine mechanisms and/or local neurovascular actions, or they have an impact on the hormonal milieu (testosterone, prolactin). Psychotropic medications may exert their inhibitory effects through their effect on central neurotransmitter pathways (serotonergic, adrenergic or dopaminergic). Beta-adrenergic blockers may exhibit central inhibitory effects or allow predominance of peripheral α-mediated vasoconstrictive effects [57]. Antiandrogens may suppress libido. Almost all recreational drugs have been reported to be associated with sexual dysfunctions, including Marijuana, opiates and cocaine [58,59]. In addition to the central nervous system (CNS) inhibitory effect, opiates have demonstrated an acute suppression of luteinizing hormone (LH) release from the pituitary gland, followed by a secondary drop in plasma testosterone levels [60].

Post-traumatic ED

Patients with a history of pelvic fracture with associ-

Table 5.3 Selection of medications and recreational drugs commonly associated with ED.

Antihypertensives
Thiazide diuretics
Beta blockers
Calcium channel blockers

Antidepressants/Neuroleptics
Tricyclic antidepressants
Selective serotonin reuptake inhibitors
Phenothiazines
Butyrophenones

Antiarrhythmics
Digoxin
Amiodarone
Disopyramide

Medications impacting on hormone milieu
Anti-androgens
GnRH agonists (leuprolide, goserelin, others)
Flutamide
Ketoconazole
Spironolactone
H2 blockers
Cimetidine
Estrogens

Recreational substances
Marijuana
Opiates
Cocaine
Nicotine
Alcohol

GnRH, gonadotophin releasing hormone; H2 blockers, histamine-2 receptor blockers.

ated urethral trauma could suffer from ED due to disruption of the neurovascular pathway [61]. Spinal cord injuries also often result in ED, depending on the level of the lesion. Patients with incomplete lesions have a higher likelihood of preservation of sexual function. Ejaculation and orgasm may also adversely be affected in spinal cord injury patients [62]. According to Chapelle *et al.*, three different erection patterns may be distinguished in patients with spinal cord injuries [63].

Psychogenic erections

Originating in the sympathetic psychogenic spinal erection center (Th$_{10}$–L$_2$), these are especially observed in lower motor lesions. Psychogenic erections are mostly partially rigid, frequently not allowing satisfactory intercourse.

Reflexogenic erections

Originating in the preserved parasympathetic reflexogenic spinal erection center (S$_2$–S$_4$), these are present in the event of upper motor lesions. Reflexogenic erections quite often result in rigid erections, allowing satisfactory intercourse.

Mixed erections

They contain patterns from both psychogenic and reflexogenic erections.

Penetrating or blunt penile trauma may result in corporeal or tunical rupture (so called fracture of penis) or scarring. Penile fracture is not that rare an event and may either result in acute severe hematoma of the penis, with or without simultaneous rupture of the urethra, requiring immediate surgical intervention, or more often may result in a cracking noise without apparent hematoma, but subsequent manifestation of a Peyronie's-like plaque with penile deviation, with or without simultaneous ED. A review of the literature comprising 25 references with a total of 393 cases, reported the following causes of penile fractures [64]:

- Vigorous masturbatory activities: 43%
- Sexual intercourse: 28%
- Fall, blow or bending (erect penis): 16%
- Rolling over asleep: 11%
- Fall, blow or bending (flaccid penis): 2%

Acute perineal (straddle) trauma may disrupt the neurovascular bundle with or without accompanying urethral rupture, and may result in ED [65].

Chronic perineal trauma in the sense of a chronic compression syndrome, which is occasionally observed in cyclists who spend a long time in the saddle, may lead to impairment of the penile blood supply with effects on the pudendal nerve (numbness of penis), and subsequent manifestation of ED [66–68].

Significant testicular injury resulting in testicular atrophy or hypogonadism could potentially lead to ED.

Endocrine Factors

Endocrine diseases that are significantly related to sexual function include diabetes mellitus, hyperprolactinemia and hypogonadism. Testosterone affects various physiologic actions, and plays an important role in the function of many organs and the development of male secondary sex characters. See Chapters 3 and 18).

Lower Urinary Tract Symptoms (LUTS)

There has been a recent increased interest in the association between LUTS and ED, both conditions being prevalent among older men. Recent epidemiologic data support such a link. El Sakka recently studied 476 male patients with ED and reported that 77% suffer from LUTS; of those, 22.8% had mild, 42% had moderate, and 35.2% had severe grades of ED. Significant associations between LUTS and both the longer duration and the increased severity of ED, were also observed [69]. Suggested mechanisms for the postulated LUTS–ED association include: (1) decreased or altered NOS/NO levels in the prostate and penile smooth muscle; (2) increased adrenergic tone effects on LUTS, prostate growth and ED; (3) alternate pathway/mechanism: Rho kinase activation/endothelin activity; and (4) pelvic atherosclerosis [70].

Etiologies and Co-morbidities in Relation to Prevalence of ED

Vascular disease and diabetes mellitus are the most commonly associated etiologic factors for organic ED. Neurogenic disorders, drugs and endocrine factors are also prevalent [71–74] (Fig. 5.1). Anxiety and depression are the most common psychogenic co-morbid conditions, while hypertension, hypercholesterolemia, diabetes mellitus and cardiovascular disease remain the most common physical disorders associated with ED [72] (Fig. 5.2).

Conclusion

The understanding of the various etiologies and

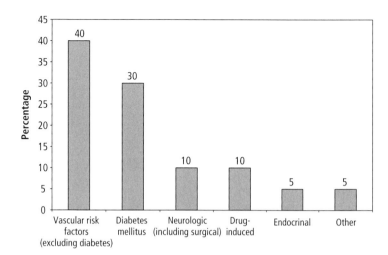

Fig. 5.1 Commonly reported physical etiologies for ED.

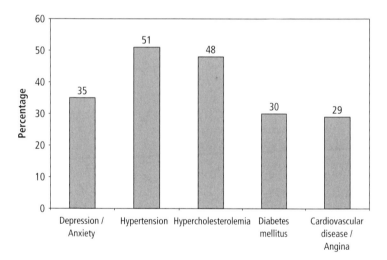

Fig. 5.2 The most prevalent co-morbid conditions associated with ED.

risk factors for ED is imperative to guide the management plan. Expertise can assist us in tailoring the history-taking and physical examination to identify reversible risk and lifestyle factors, as well as to select the appropriate laboratory tests and investigations, as needed. Unnecessary, expensive, and potentially invasive investigations are dispensable in the majority of ED patients, so costs can be saved. Such knowledge would also allow us to educate our patients and their partners and to assist them in modifying reversible causes of erectile dysfunction, thus enhancing the treatment outcome.

References

1 Masters WH, Johnson VE, eds. *Human Sexual Inadequacy.* Boston: Little Brown, 1970.

2 Kaplan HS, ed. *The New Sex Therapy.* New York: Brunner/Mazel, 1974.

3 Melman A, Tiefer L, Pederson R. Evaluation of the first 406 patients in urology department-based service center for male sexual dysfunction. *Urology* 1988; **32**:6–10.

4 Kamp S, Ott R, Knoll T, *et al.* REM-sleep deprivation leads to a decrease of nocturnal penile tumescence (NPT) in young healthy males: The significance of NPT-

measurements. (611.13) *XVII World Congress of Sexology*, July 10–15, Montreal, Canada, 2005.

5 Kratzik CW, Schatzl G, Lunglmayr G, *et al*. The impact of age, body mass index and testosterone on erectile dysfunction. *J Urol* 2005;**174**:240–243.

6 Derby CA, Mohr BA, Goldstein I, Feldman HA, Johannes CB, McKinlay JB. Modifiable risk factors and erectile dysfunction: can lifestyle changes modify risk? *Urology* 2000;**56**(2):302–306.

7 Esposito K, Giugliano F, Di Palo C, *et al*. Effect of lifestyle changes on erectile dysfunction in obese men. *JAMA* 2004;**291**:2978–2984.

8 Feldman HA, Goldstein I, Hatzichristou DG, Krane RJ, Mckinaly JB. Impotence and its medical and psychosocial correlates: results of the massachusetts male aging study. *J Urol* 1994;**151**:54–61.

9 Martin-Morales A, Sanchez-Cruz JJ, Saenz de Tejada I, Rodriguez-Vela L, Jimenez-Cruz JF, Burgos-Rodriguez R. Prevalence and independent risk factors for erectile dysfunction in Spain: results of the Epidemiologia de la Disfuncion Erectil Masculina Study. *J Urol* 2001;**166**:569–574.

10 Nazareth I, Boynton P. Problems with sexual function in people attending London general practitioners: cross sectional study. *BMJ* 2003;**327**:423–428.

11 Michal V. Arterial disease as a cause of impotence. *Clin Endocrinol Metab* 1982;**11**:725–748.

12 Sullivan ME, Keoghane SR, Miller MA. Vascular risk factors and erectile dysfunction. *BJU Int* 2002;**87**(9):838–45.

13 Shamloul R, Ghanem H, Salem A, Elnashaar A, Elnaggar W, Darwish H, Mousa A. Correlation between penile duplex findings and stress electrocardiography in men with erectile dysfunction. *Int J Impot Res* 2004;**16**:235–237.

14 Billups KL, Bank AJ, Padma-Nathan H, *et al*. Erectile dysfunction is a marker for cardiovascular disease: results of the minority health institute expert advisory panel. *J Sex Med* 2005;**2**:40–52.

15 Lochman A, Gallmetzer J. Erectile dysfunction of arterial origin as possible manifestation of atherosclerosis. *Minerva Cardioangiol* 1996;**44**(5):243–246.

16 Mittleman MA, Siscovick DS. Physical exertion as a trigger of myocardial infarction and sudden cardiac death. *Cardiol Clin* 1996;**14**:263–270.

17 O'Kane PD, Jackson G. Erectile dysfunction, is there silent obstructive coronary artery disease? *Int J Clin Prac* 2001;**55**(3):219–220.

18 Muller SC, El Damanhoury H, Ruth J, Lue TF. Hypertension and Impotence. *Eur Urol* 1991;**19**:29–34.

19 Oaks WW, Moyer JH. Sex and Hypertension. *Med Aspects Hum Sexual* 1972;**6**:128–137.

20 Burchardt M, Burchardt T, Baer L, *et al*. Hypertension is associated with severe erectile dysfunction. *J Urol* 2000;**164**:1188–1191.

21 Ahn TY, Saenz de Tejada I. Effects of hypercholesterolemia and nitric oxide synthesis inhibition on rabbit corpus cavernosum tissue. *Int J Impotence Res* 1992;**4**:Suppl.2,A5.

22 Chen JH, Lee KR. Lipid composition of human corpus cavernosum analyzed by high resolution 1H and 13C-nuclear magnetic resonance spectroscopy. *J Urol* 1997;**157**:No.4,Suppl.360.

23 Seftel AD, Azadzoi K, Krane RJ, *et al*. Hypercholesterolemia impairs neurogenic and endothelium-dependent responses in rabbit cavernosal arteries. *J Urol* 1993;**149**:No.4,Suppl.247.

24 Wei M, Macera C, Davis D, Hornung Ca, Nankin H, Blair S. Total cholesterol and high density lipoprotein cholesterol as important predictors of erectile dysfunction. *Am J Epidemiol* 1994;**140**:930–937.

25 Juenemann KP, Muth S, Rohr G, *et al*. Does lipid metabolism influence the pathogenesis of vascular impotence? – Part 1. *Int J Impotence Res* 1990;**2**:Suppl.2,33.

26 Manning M, Schmidt P, Juenemann KP, *et al*. The role of blood lipids in erectile failure. *Int J Impotence Res* 1996;**8**:No.3, D179.

27 Kim JH, Klyachkin MC, Svendsen E, *et al*. Experimental hypercholesterolemia in rabbits induces cavernosal atherosclerosis. *J Urol* 1993;**149**:No.4,Suppl.246.

28 Saltzman EA, Guay AT, Jacobson J. Improvement in erectile function in men with organic erectile dysfunction by correction of elevated cholesterol levels: a clinical observation. *J Urol* 2004;**172**:255–258.

29 Rosen MP, Greenfield AJ, Walker TG, Grant P, Dubrow J, Bettman MA, Fried LE, Goldstein I. Cigarette smoking: an independent risk factor for atherosclerosis in the hypogastric–cavernous arterial bed of men with arteriogenic impotence. *J Urol* 1991;**145**:759–763.

30 Juenemann KP, Lue TF, Luo JA, Benowitz NL, Abozeid M, Tanagho EA. The effect of cigarette smoking on penile erection. *J Urol* 1987;**138**(2):438–441.

31 Glina S, Reichet AC, Leao PP, Dos-Reis JM. Impact of cigarette smoking on papaverine-induced erection. *J Urol* 1988;**140**(3):523–524.

32 Hatzichristou DG, Seftel A, Saenz De Tejada I. Sexual dysfunction in diabetes and other autonomic neuropathies. In: Singer C, Weiner WJ, eds. *Sexual Dysfunction: A Neuro-Medical Approach* Armonk: Futura Publishing Company, 1994, pp. 167–198.

33 Lehman TP, Jacobs JA. Etiology of diabetic impotence. *J Urol* 1983;**129**:291–294.

34 Koncz L, Balodimos MC. Impotence in diabetes mellitus. *Med Times* 1970;**98**:159–170.

35 Jonler M, Moon T, Brannan W, Stone N, Heisey D, Bruskewitz RC. The Effect of age, ethnicity and geographical location on impotence and quality of life. *Brit J Urol* 1995;**75**:651–655.

36 Metro MJ, Broderick GA. Diabetes and vascular impotence: Does insulin dependence decrease the relative severity? *Int J Impotence Res* 1999;**11**:87–89.

37 Saenz De Tejada I, Goldstein I, Azadoi K, Krane RJ, Cohen RA. Impaired neurogenic and endothelium-medicated relations of penile smooth muscle from diabetic men with impotence. *New Eng J Med* 1989;**320**:1025–1030.

38 Sachs BD, Meisel RL. The physiology of male sexual behavior. In: Knobil E, Neill J, eds. *The Physiology of Reproduction*. New York: Raven, 1988, pp. 1393–1485.

39 Giuliano, F. Key issues in CNS regulation of penile erection. *Int J Impotence Res* 12, 9th World Meeting on Impotence Research, Perth, 2000, p. 7:S1.

40 Sáenz de Tejada I, Angulo J, Cellek S. Pathophysiology of erectile dysfunction. *J Sex Med* 2005;**2**(1):26–39.

41 Goldstein I, Siroky MB, Sax DS, Krane RJ. Neurologic abnormalities in multiple sclerosis. *J Urol* 1982;**128**:541–545.

42 Eardly I, Kirby RS. Neurogenic impotence. In: Kirby RS, Carson CC, Webster GD, eds. Impotence: *Diagnosis and management of male erectile dysfunction*. Butterworth-Heinmann, 1991, pp. 227–231.

43 Fletcher EC, Martin RJ. Sexual dysfunction and erectile impotence in chronic obstructive pulmonary disease. *Chest* 1982; **81**:413–421.

44 Seftel A, Kingman P, Strohl P, *et al.* Sleep disorders and erectile dysfunction. *Int J Impotence Res* 2000;**12**:Suppl.3,S73.

45 Moreland B, Simopoulos DN, Nehra A. What is the underlying pathology of sleep apnea associated erectile dysfunction? *Int J Impotence Res* 1999;**11**: Suppl.1,S78.

46 Cornely CM, Schade RR, van Thiel DH, Gavaler JS. Chronic liver disease and impotence: Cause and effect. *Hepatology* 1984;**4**:1227–30.

47 Zonszein J. Diagnosis and management of endocrine disorders of erectile dysfunction. *Urol Clin North Am* 1995;**22**(4):789–802.

48 Carson CC. Impotence and chronic renal failure. In: Bennet AH, ed. *Impotence, Diagnosis and Management of Erectile dysfunction*. Philadelphia: WB Saunders, 1980, pp. 124–134.

49 Nogues MA, Starkstein S, Davalos M, Berthier M, Leiguarda R, Garcia H. Cardiovascular reflexes and pudendal evoked responses in chronic hemodialysis patients. *Funct Neurol* 1991;**9**:359–365.

50 Kaufman JM, Hatzichristou DG, Mulhall JP, Fitch WP, Goldstein I. Impotence and chronic renal failure: a study of the hemodynamic pathophysiology. *J Urol* 1994;**151**:612–618.

51 Altwein JE, Keuler FU. Benign prostatic hyperplasia and erectile dysfunction: A review. *Urol Int* 1992;**48**:53–57.

52 Lotti T, Mirone V, Imbimbo C, *et al.* Benign prostatic hyperplasia (BPH) and sexuality. *J d'Urologie* 1995; **101**:13–15.

53 Tscholl R, Largo M, Poppinghaus E, *et al.* Incidence of erectile impotence secondary to transurethral resection of benign prostatic hyperplasia, assessed by preoperative and postoperative snap gauge test. *J Urol* 1995;**153**:1491–1493.

54 Lue TF, Zeineh SJ, Schmidt RA, Tanagho EA. Neuroanatomy of penile erection: Its relevance to iatrogenic impotence. *J Urol* 1984;**131**:273–280.

55 Quinlan DM, Epstein JI, Carter BS, Walsh PC. Sexual function following radical prostatectomy: Influence of preservation of neurovascular bundles. *J Urol* 1991;**145**:998–1002.

56 Goldstein I, Feldman MI, Deckers PJ, Babayan RK, Krane RJ. Radiation-associated impotence: A clinical study of its mechanism. *JAMA* 1984;**251**: 903–910.

57 Sáenz de Tejada I, Angulo J, Cellek S. Pathophysiology of erectile dysfunction. *J Sex Med* 2005;**2**(1): 26–39.

58 Horowitz JD, Goble AJ. Drugs and impaired male sexual function. *Drugs* 1979;**18**(3):206–217.

59 Mirin SM, Meyer RE, Mendelson JH, Ellingboe J. Opiate use and sexual function. *Am J Psychiatry* 1980;**137**(8):909–915.

60 Millar JG. Drug-induced impotence. *Practitioner* 1979;**223**(1337):634–639.

61 Van Arsdalen K, Wein AJ, Hanno PM, *et al.* Erectile failure following pelvic trauma: A review of pathophysiology, evaluation and management, with particular reference to penile prosthesis. *J Trauma* 1984;**24**: 579–583.

62 Bors E, Comarr A. Neurological disturbances of sexual function with special reference to 529 patients with spinal cord injury. *Urol Surv* 1960;**10**:191–220.

63 Chapelle PA, Durand J, Lacert P. Penile erection following complete spinal cord injury in man. *Brit J Urol* 52;**216**:1980.

64 Porst H. Congenital and acquired penile deviations and penile fractures. In Porst, H, ed. *Penile Disorders*. Berlin-Heidelberg, New York: Springer-Verlag, 1997, pp. 37–56.

65 Munarriz RM, Yan RQ, Nehra, Udelson D, Goldstein I. Blunt Trauma: The pathophysiology of hemodynamic injury leading to erectile dysfunction. *J Urol* 1995;**153**:1831–1840.

66 Mulhall JP, Garcia-Reboll L, Salimpour P, *et al.* The effects of bicycle seat compression on cavernosal artery hemodynamics. *Int J Impotence Res* 1996;**8**:No. 3, 130.

67 Anderson KV, Bovim G. Impotence and nerve entrapment in long distance amateur cyclists. *Acta Neurol Scand* 1997;**9**:233–240.

68 Schwarzer U, Wiegand W, Bin-Saleh A, *et al.* Genital numbness and impotence rate in long-distance cyclists. *J Urol* 1999;**161**:Suppl. No.4, 178.

69 El-Sakka A. Lower urinary tract symptoms in patients with erectile dysfunction: Analysis of risk factors. *J Sex Med* 2006;**3**:144–149.

70 McVary K. The relationship between erectile dysfunction and lower urinary tract symptoms. *J Sex Med* 2004;**S1**:11–14.

71 Brotons F, Campos J, Gonzalez R, *et al.* Core document on erectile dysfunction: key aspects in the care of a patient with erectile dysfunction. *Int J Impotence Res* 2004;**16**:S26–S39.

72 Eardley I, Neiderberger C, Fisher C, *et al.* Prevalence of comorbidity among men with ED in the M.A.L.E.S. 2004 longitudinal cohort. *J Sexual Med* 2005;**S1**:18 (Abstract).

73 Lue TF. Drug therapy: erectile dysfunction. *New Engl J Med* 2000;**342**:1802–13.

74 Miller TA. Diagnostic evaluation of erectile dysfunction. *Am Fam Phys* 2000;**61**:95–104, 109–110.

CHAPTER 6

Diagnosis of Erectile Dysfunction

Allen D. Seftel

Male sexual dysfunction encompasses many areas. These include desire or libido disorders, erectile dysfunction and ejaculatory dysfunction. This chapter focuses specifically upon the standards for the diagnosis of male erectile dysfunction (ED).

The patient-oriented approach to the evaluation and treatment of male ED is the preferred and accepted approach for the majority of men with ED, and serves as the basis for this chapter [1]. This implies that the history and physical exam are the paramount factors contributing toward the successful diagnosis of ED. The American Urological Association ED guidelines panel also accepts this scheme [2]. The treatment of male ED is based upon the patients' personal goals, and is covered elsewhere in this textbook.

Questionnaires

Physicians who are not facile with the specifics of the ED office evaluation may turn to questionnaires to aid in the diagnosis. Questionnaires are not mandatory in the evaluation of male ED, but often serve as an important adjunct to the proper diagnosis. Prior to, or in addition to, being seen by the physician (and as a significant part of the history), it is advised that the patient fill out a questionnaire to delineate the extent of the erection problem. There are several questionnaires available. One of the simpler questionnaires in use is the Sexual Health Inventory for Men (SHIM), which has five questions, detailed in Table 6.1, and appended in full at the end of this chapter (Appendix A), which deal specifically with erectile activity using a five-point Likert-type scale [3]. The SHIM asks about erectile function over

a six-month time frame, which may be too long a period for some men. Nonetheless, the SHIM is an extremely worthwhile instrument for the diagnosis of male ED. The five questions are simple, straightforward, yet comprehensive.

A normal healthy male will have a score of 22 or more (scoring is detailed in Table 6.2), while the middle-aged man with garden variety ED will have score of 12–16. There are a variety of other more general questionnaires available that contain ED questions, such as the International Index of Erectile Function (IIEF), and the Male Sexual Health Questionnaire (MHSQ) [4,5]. The SHIM is validated and has been well studied, making it an ideal, simple instrument for use. While the IIEF has been used for many clinical studies, it can be used for routine office practice as well. The length of the IIEF questionnaire may be a barrier to its routine clinical use.

Diagnostic Evaluation Setting

The initial evaluation of male ED should include a complete medical, social and sexual history. This evaluation should be performed in a non-judgmental fashion, in a friendly environment, without undue interruption. Ideally, this encounter should not be a hurried, exit-type interview, but a thorough review of the sexual problem. The prime goal should be to understand the specific sexual dysfunction. In as much as many couples do not use vaginal intercourse as the barometer for a successful sexual encounter, this issue should be explored at the outset. What does the couple define as sexual dysfunction? What does the couple define as erectile dysfunction? The definition of male ED is "the

Table 6.1 Sexual Health Inventory for Men (SHIM).

1. How do you rate your confidence that you could get and keep an erection?

2. When you had erections with sexual stimulation, how often were your erections hard enough for penetration?

3. During sexual intercourse, how often were you able to maintain your erection after you had penetrated (entered) your partner?

4. During sexual intercourse, how difficult was it to maintain your erection to completion of intercourse?

5. When you attempted sexual intercourse, how often was it satisfactory for you?

Total score ranges from 5 to 25 and is based on five questions.
Each rated on a Likert scale of 1 = least functional to 5 = most functional.
With permission from Rosen RC, et al. Int J Impot Res 1999;11:319–326

Table 6.2 Sexual Health Inventory for Men (SHIM) scoring. The score characterizes ED severity.

22–25 Normal erectile function
17–21 Mild ED
12–16 Mild to moderate ED
8–11 Moderate ED
<7 Severe ED

consistent or recurrent inability of a man to attain and/or maintain a penile erection sufficient for sexual performance" [6]. The definition emphasizes and verifies the movement away from intercourse as the end point for the definition of male ED.

The onset of the sexual problem is a pivotal question. Did the onset of the ED occur suddenly, implying a possible psychogenic erectile dysfunction? The gradual onset of ED is most consistent with an organic etiology. Delineating the situation under which it occurs is also a crucial question. Does the ED occur under all circumstances? Does the ED occur with the partner only? Does the ED occur with masturbation? Does the ED occur with fantasy or watching an erotic video? If the ED occurs only with the partner, then the ED is most likely psychogenic. If the ED occurs under all circumstances, such as with an erotic video, masturbation and with the partner, then it is more likely organic.

The quality of erection should be explored, as well as the duration of the erection. These two items are of high importance in the diagnosis of male ED, as many men with ED will still be able to have intercourse but will be thought of as having ED due to the lack of satisfaction with the quality of the erection. As noted in the definition of ED, this is a function of sexual satisfaction. Thus, a young man with an erection that is less hard as compared to his earlier, historical erections, assuming that the decrease in the hardness of erections is bothersome to him, may be considered as having ED, in spite of the fact that his erections may be of sufficient rigidity for intercourse. This is a major departure from the earlier definitions that used intercourse as the end point definition of ED.

The frequency and quality of the nocturnal erections, the frequency and quality of the morning erections, the ability to successfully engage in vaginal intercourse; heterosexuality vs. homosexuality; the extent of concern about the problem, ejaculatory success, ejaculatory volume, ejaculatory pain, orgasmic function, are all additional important items for discussion.

The degree of sexual desire or libido, may signal hypogonadism or reactive or fulminant depression. The Androgen Deficiency in the Aging Male (ADAM) questionnaire [7] (Table 6.3) has been touted as a useful instrument to ascertain hypogonadism. In my experience, this questionnaire has some degree of sensitivity for hypogonadism, but is not specific. Meaning, the ADAM questionnaire can also detect other conditions as well.

The level of partner sexual interest should be ascertained as it has been shown that the partner of men with ED suffers with sexual dysfunction as well [8].

The partner may have a medical disease that precludes sexual relations, such as urinary incontinence [9], or hip arthritis that precludes abduction of the thighs. Partner issues and partner satisfaction are among the other areas that should be explored. Table

Table 6.3 Androgen deficiency in aging men (ADAM) questionnaire.

1. Do you have a decrease in libido (sex drive)?
2. Do you have a lack of energy?
3. Do you have a decrease in strength, endurance or both?
4. Have you lost height?
5. Have you noticed a decreased enjoyment of life?
6. Are you sad, grumpy, or both?
7. Are your erections strong?
8. Have you noted a recent deterioration in your ability to play sports?
9. Are you falling asleep after dinner?
10. Has there been a recent deterioration in your work performance?

Table 6.4 Brief checklist of questions for male erectile dysfunction.

What is the problem you are experiencing?
When did it start; was it at some exact time point, or has the problem developed gradually over time?
When was the last time you had sexual intercourse?
Are the erections hard enough for vaginal penetration?
How often are the erections not hard enough for intercourse?
Are you satisfied with the hardness of the erection?
Are you satisfied with the duration of the erection?
Is the erection curved?
Is the erection painful?
Does the erection problem occur with your partner?
Does the erection problem occur when you awake in the morning, or watch an erotic video?
Does the erection problem occur with masturbation?
Are you heterosexual, homosexual or bisexual?
If heterosexual, is your partner concerned or unhappy with your sexual activity?
Does your partner have any problems that preclude sexual activity?
How is your sex drive?
Are you still attracted to your partner?
Are you able to ejaculate?
Is the ejaculation too quick or too rapid?
Is the ejaculation painful?
Is the ejaculation volume less?
Is the force of the ejaculation a problem?
Is there burning or pain with the ejaculation?

6.4 outlines the most germane questions to ask of the man with erectile dysfunction.

Physical Examination

The physical examination remains an essential component of sexual dysfunction evaluation. In most cases, the physical examination will not identify the specific etiology or cause of sexual dysfunction, but will help in formulation of the diagnosis. The physical examination should include a general screening for medical risk factors or comorbidities that are associated with sexual dysfunction, such as body habitus (secondary sexual characteristics), assessment of the cardiovascular, neurologic and genital system, with particular focus on the genitalia and secondary sex characteristics. The physical examination is used to corroborate aspects of the medical history and may sometimes reveal unsuspected physical findings (e.g. decreased peripheral pulses, atrophic testes, penile plaque). Every effort should be made to ensure the patient's privacy, confidentiality and personal comfort while conducting the physical examination.

The physical examination (Table 6.5) should include specific attention to the genitalia. The examination starts preferably in a standing position as possible gynecomastia, abnormal pubic fat-deposition with shortening of the penis and varicocele, are best visible and palpable in the upright position. On occasion, pathologic conditions may be encountered. Carbone *et al.* [10] found the following pathology in 207 patients (average age 60 years, range 17 to 88 years) who consulted a physician exclusively because of erectile dysfunction. These men had undergone a complete urologic status, including urinalysis, rectal examination, PSA and ultrasound, before initiating specific ED diagnostic methods.

The results of the general urologic examination were amazing: 31 (15%) of the 207 ED patients showed malignancies on a thorough diagnostic screening:
• 16 patients (7.7%) had prostate cancer with prostate-specific antigen (PSA) values between 4.1 and 14.5
• 12 patients (5.8%) had superficial bladder cancer

Table 6.5 Brief points to cover in the physical examination of the male with ED.

check for gynecomastia
check for body hair distribution
check the penis size and suprapubic fat pad
check the femoral pulses
check for inguinal hernia
check for sexually-transmitted disease
check the penis for foreskin
check the foreskin, if present for ability to retract, warts, cancer and other lesions.
check the glans for balanitis and other similar conditions, warts and cancer.
check position of the urethra
check the tunica for plaques
check the urethra for warts, and strictures
check the penile skin for lesions
check the testis size and consistency
check the testis lie
check for varicocele
check for the presence of two testis
check the spermatic cord for the vas and any pathology
check the rectum for prostate size, volume, lesions, tenderness
check the rectum for hemorrhoids, anal cancer, anal stenosis, anal tone

- 2 patients (1%) had small renal cell cancer
- 1 patient (0.5%) had penile cancer

Although the 15% incidence of urologic malignancies is unusually high in this study with only ED patients, it highlights the importance of the general urologic physical examination in men with ED. Other pathologic findings may include Peyronie's plaques, testicular atrophy, varicocele, inguinal hernia, femoral arterial occlusive disease, sexually transmitted disease, prostatitis, and anal pathology, such as hemorrhoids, anal stenosis, anal fissure, rectal cancer and weak anal tone (seen in diabetes and neurologic disease).

Overlapping Diseases and Points of Confusion

Shabsigh *et al.* demonstrated that ED and depression coexist and are quite common [11]. One hundred and twenty men with ED or benign prostatic hyperplasia (BPH) were divided into three groups. Group 1 had ED only, group 2 had BPH only, and group 3 had both ED and BPH. Patients were screened for depressive symptoms using Primary Care Evaluation of Mental Disorders (PRIME-MD) and the Beck Depression Inventory (BDI). They were also surveyed for comorbidity, marital status, severity of ED, levels of libido, prior ED treatment choice (if any), success of treatment, and others. Depressive symptoms were reported by 26 (54%) of 48 men with ED alone, 10 (56%) of 18 men with ED and BPH, and 7 (21%) of 34 men with BPH alone. Patients with ED were 2.6 times more likely to report depressive symptoms than men with BPH alone ($P < 0.005$). Patients with depressive symptoms reported lower libido than other patients ($P < 0.0001$). Severity of comorbidities did not differ among the three groups. The conclusion is that ED is associated with high incidence of depressive symptoms, regardless of age, marital status, or comorbidities.

In as much as depression is often seen in men with ED, a screening questionnaire to elicit depressive symptoms may be quite useful. The Centers for the Epidemiologic Survey – Depression (CES-D) (Table 6.6) [12] is a public domain, useful instrument for such purposes. Other instruments include the Hamilton depression scale (HDS) and the BDI. It is incumbent upon the clinician to be aware of this relationship and to ask pointed questions, or use a questionnaire to elicit or exclude the diagnosis of depression.

Many men also confuse ejaculatory dysfunction (EjD), such as rapid or delayed ejaculation, with ED. Thus, the clinician must be keen and tease out the specific male sexual dysfunction. Indeed, EjD and ED may overlap, as depicted by Rosen *et al.* (Table 6.1) in the Multinational Study of the Aging Male [13]. This survey, which included postal questionnaires to men aged 50–80 in seven countries, demonstrated that EjD and ED were both highly prevalent and highly bothersome (Figs 6.1 and 6.2).

Misconceptions

Many clinicians have misconceptions about many aspects of ED, rendering ED a low priority item on

Table 6.6 The Centers for the Epidemiologic Survey-Depression (CES-D) questionnaire to evaluate depressive symptoms, used by urologists at the University Hospitals of Cleveland.

Below is a list of ways you might have felt or behaved. Please tell me how often you have felt this way during the past week. Please CIRCLE ONE number for each item.

	Rarely or none of the time (Less than 1 day)	Some or a little of the time (1–2 days)	Occasionally or a moderate amount of the time (3–4 days)	Most or all of the time (5–7 days)
1 I was bothered by things that usually don't bother me	0	1	2	3
2 I did not feel like eating: my appetite was poor	0	1	2	3
3 I felt that I could not shake off the blues even with help from my family or friends	0	1	2	3
4 I felt that I was just as good as other people	0	1	2	3
5 I had trouble keeping my mind on what I was doing	0	1	2	3
6 I felt depressed	0	1	2	3
7 I felt that everything I did was an effort	0	1	2	3
8 I felt hopeful about the future	0	1	2	3
9 I thought my life had been a failure	0	1	2	3
10 I felt fearful	0	1	2	3
11 My sleep was restless	0	1	2	3
12 I was happy	0	1	2	3
13 I talked less than usual	0	1	2	3
14 I felt lonely	0	1	2	3
15 People were unfriendly	0	1	2	3
16 I enjoyed life	0	1	2	3
17 I had crying spells	0	1	2	3
18 I felt sad	0	1	2	3
19 I felt that people dislike me	0	1	2	3
20 I could not get going	0	1	2	3

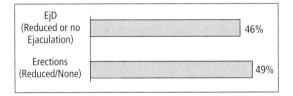

Fig. 6.1 ED and EjD are highly prevalent in a cohort of men in the MSAM-7.

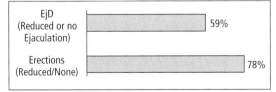

Fig. 6.2 ED and EjD are highly bothersome to the men in the MSAM-7 survey.

Table 6.7 Obstacles for clinician evaluation of ED.

Misconceptions
    Low prevalence
    ED primarily managed by urologists
    Perceived time constraints
    Only a quality-of-life issue
    High CV risk with sexual activity
Reimbursement issues
Unfamiliarity with topic can cause embarrassment

CV, cardiovascular.

the problem list. Several of these misconceptions are listed below (Table 6.7). Thus, a major barrier toward the accurate treatment and diagnosis of ED is to raise the level of awareness of this significant medical problem.

Medical Aspects of the ED Evaluation

The epidemiology of male ED, which is discussed in another chapter, provides guidance to the clinician faced with the ED patient. In as much as many men with ED will have a variety of medical problems, the astute clinician should recognize that ED is a significant part of these medical diseases. Indeed, recent epidemiologic data provides guidance to the clinician regarding the prevalence of ED in men with four medical diseases [16]. These diseases are hypertension, hyperlipidemia, diabetes and depression. Thus, it is incumbent upon the physician to delineate the extent of these four diseases in men with ED. As can be seen in the table, these four diseases were clearly noted to be present in men identified with ED in a large, managed-care database (Table 6.8).

In this study of a managed-care database, 272 325 men with a diagnostic code for ED were identified. Four specific diseases were then cross-referenced, including diabetes, depression, hypertension and hyperlipidemia. Thus, the man with hypertension or diabetes has a significant chance of having ED. Clinicians who treat these patients on a daily basis should ask about ED as a routine part of the medical history. Other studies provide guidance regarding this issue as well, as is readily discerned from Table 6.9.

Several chronic medical diseases impact negatively on male erectile function, again highlighting the need to ask about ED in men with these conditions. Newer areas of study include associations between ED and obesity, as well as ED, as the metabolic syndrome (Figure 6.3) [19]. Thus, those men with the metabolic syndrome may deserve an evaluation for male ED. The ATP-III guideline suggests a working definition of the metabolic syndrome that includes the presence of at least three of the following characteristics: abdominal obesity, elevated triglycerides, reduced levels of high density lipoprotein (HDL) cholesterol, high blood pressure, and high fasting glucose. In particular, the cut off values are the following: waist circumference greater than 102 cm in men and greater than 88 cm in women; triglycerides >150 mg/L (1.69 mmol/L); HDL cholesterol less than 40 mg/L (1.04 mmol/L) in men and less than 50 mg/L (1.29 mmol/L) in women; blood pressure greater than 130/85 mmHg; fasting glucose greater than 110 mg/L (6.1 mmol/L) [20].

Partner evaluation

The partners of men with ED are affected, to a lesser or greater degree by the ED, as is the male. As alluded to by Dr Wagner and colleagues [21], quality of life (QoL) has become one of the important parameters in the evaluation of treatment and assessment of medical conditions, and it may be an important tool in determining the urgency of the need for therapeutic intervention for ED. It is important to evaluate the QoL of the couple, because men and women alike will suffer as a result of male erectile disability.

Involvement of the partner in the diagnosis and treatment of ED has been shown to better delineate the nature of the female sexual dysfunction as well as the extent of the couples' problem. Partner involvement may enhance the outcome [22]. These authors used the Index of Sexual Life (ISL) questionnaire, specifically designed to measure the impact of ED on female partners' sexuality. They demonstrated that ED has a negative impact on the sexual life of female partners, specifically on their sexual satisfaction and sexual drive. Further analyses showed lower sexual satisfaction and sex drive for women reporting a disturbance or change in their own sex lives, than for women who did not. Older women had lower scores

Table 6.8 Prevalence of medical diseases in men with a diagnosis of ED.

Crude population prevalence rates (%)	Disease
41.6	Hypertension
42.4	Hyperlipidemia
20.2	Diabetes mellitus
11.1	Depression
29.3	Hypertension and hyperlipidemia
12.8	Hypertension and diabetes mellitus
11.5	Hyperlipidemia and depression

n = 272 325. Only 32% (87 163) had no comorbid diagnosis of hypertension, hyperlipidemia, diabetes mellitus or depression. From Seftel, Sun, Swindle. J Urol 2004;171: 2341–5.

Table 6.9 Medical diseases as a risk factor for ED.

Chronic disease	ED risk multiplied*
Diabetes	4.1
Prostate disease	2.9
Peripheral vascular disease	2.6
Cardiac problems	1.8
Hyperlipidemia	1.7
Hypertension	1.6

* Age-adjusted odds ratio.

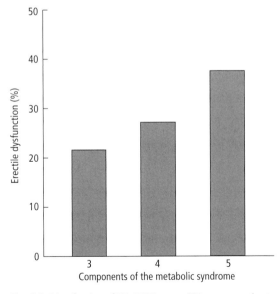

Fig. 6.3 Distribution of ED (IIEF score <21) among patients by the presence of 3 (n = 62), 4 (n = 25), and 5 (n = 13) components of the metabolic syndrome. The differences between bars are significant ($P < 0.05$)

compared to younger women, independent of whether their partner had ED or not.

As discussed by Dunn [23], the new modes of pharmacologic therapy give health care practitioners an unprecedented opportunity to treat patients with erectile dysfunction. Yet even with a portfolio of effective treatment modalities, such as phosphodiesterase type 5 (PDE-5) inhibitors, nonpharmacologic interventions should be considered as a means to support and augment the effects of these agents. Of equal value and necessity is the involvement of the man's partner in both the assessment and treatment processes. Because men see the primary care physician's office as a natural and expected place in which to address issues of sexual health, those healthcare professionals who are prepared to initiate discussion of ED can offer patients and their partners the possibility of effective and enduring treatment success, and the restoration of a satisfying relationship.

Summary

The patient (and partner) histories are the key toward the successful diagnosis of male ED. ED is highly prevalent in men with a variety of medical diseases, including depression, and is often confused with ejaculatory disorders. The clinician should have a high index of suspicion when evaluating men with these medical diseases for ED. The clinician must also be aware of the psychologic aspects of male ED, with a referral to a sex or marital therapist indicated as necessary. Finally, there is an evolving paradigm that ED may be a predictor/

marker of cardiovascular disease. This topic is covered elsewhere in this textbook.

Laboratory Tests

Most experts believe that certain laboratory tests are obligatory before treating ED. In as much as the epidemiology suggests that men with ED may have diabetes or dyslipidemia, laboratory testing should follow that path.

Routine laboratory tests

These should include a blood sugar and a fasting lipid profile in all men with ED without a diagnosis of diabetes mellitus or dyslipidemia, respectively. A PSA should be determined in the case of abnormal findings during palpation of the prostate, or as per the physicians' PSA screening protocol. A urinalysis is also helpful to look for glucose, ketones and proteinuria, as well as blood and white blood cells.

Blood pressure, weight and waist circumference should be measured as a part of the ED evaluation, as ED has been linked to the metabolic syndrome.

Free testosterone, testosterone, prolactin and dehydroepiandrosterone sulfate (DHEAS) are the specific hormones that may be part of the ED evaluation. These hormones have been associated with sexual desire. Luteinizing hormone (LH), follicle-stimulating hormone (FSH) and sex hormone-binding globulin (SHBG) are determined for further differential diagnosis in the case of low testosterone values, to ascertain primary or secondary hypogonadism. Estradiol, growth hormone or, better, insulin-like growth factor 1 (IGF-1) and thyroid parameters are determined in individual cases to diagnose further hormonal deficits.

It is recognized that serum testosterone levels decrease below the eugonadal range in some men with advancing age. Restoration of testosterone levels to the eugonadal range (300–1000 ng/dL) appear to correct many of the clinical abnormalities (impaired sexual function, negative changes in body composition, etc.) commonly associated with hypogonadism [24]. With respect to hypogonadal males, a number of studies have demonstrated that testosterone replacement therapy can significantly affect a number of the fundamental indicators of apposite sexual functioning, including intensity of libido, frequency of nocturnal erections, and frequency of sexual activity [25,26]. Furthermore, additional research in which an acute hypogonadal state was induced (in experimental animals and eugonadal males), not only confirmed the importance of physiologic levels of testosterone in maintaining normal sexual behavior, but also highlighted the dose–response relationships between testosterone levels and the various androgen-dependent processes, including sexual function.

Other data suggests that hypogonadism may affect the ability of the erectogenic agents to fully restore erectile function. Shabisgh *et al.* [27] have shown that the addition of testosterone to hypogonadal men with testosterone deficiency, who additionally have had a suboptimal response to PDE-5 inhibitors, was highly beneficial. Thus, a total and or free morning serum testosterone level may be indicated as a blood test for men with ED.

Confirmatory testing for a more comprehensive understanding of the etiology of the ED is optional, but should be available to the patient when appropriate. Such testing may include nocturnal penile tumescence (NPT) testing, penile duplex ultrasonography with color Doppler, cavernosometry, cavernosography, neurophysiologic testing, office intracavernosal injection of a vasoactive agent, such as prostaglandin E1 (PGE_1). All or some of these tests should be available to the patient as directed by the physician. Controversy exists as to the usefulness, relative value, and the indications for these tests. In general, the tests are relegated to the domain of the urologist, who will offer a variety of tests as per specific patient indications.

Invasive Testing

Intracavernous injection test combined with Doppler/duplex ultrasound

This specific diagnostic test in the hands of the urologist (or perhaps radiologist) should be thought of as an optional part of the evaluation. It is the optimal method of reliably diagnosing relevant disturbed arterial blood supply to the penis, and of obtaining an approximate idea of the relaxation capacity and thus cavernous function in practice. In addition, the drug-induced erection reveals possible cavernous deformations in Peyronie's disease such as cavernous notches, or deviations that could themselves impair sexual intercourse [28,29]. These anatomic changes of the corpus cavernosum or tunica albuginea, could be relevant in certain cases. Many clinicians find the expense of the Doppler/ duplex ultrasound cost prohibitive, and thus move to less costly devices. The Knoll/MIDUS Ultrasound System serves to evaluate the penile blood flow after injection of a vasoactive agent such as PGE_1 [30]. While the type of ultrasound used may be left to the discretion of the clinician, it is clear that the ultrasound combined with the injection of a vasoactive agent provides a clear evaluation of the cavernosal arterial supply to the penis.

Vasoactive substances used in the intracavernous injection test

In practice, PGE_1 (alprostadil) is the substance of choice for diagnostic purposes. It is available worldwide in 10 or 20 µg ampoules under the names of Caverject® (manufactured by Pharmacia) or Viridal®/Edex® (manufactured by Schwarz Pharma). The crucial advantage of PGE_1 is that it causes priapism requiring treatment in only approximately 0.5–1% of cases, as compared to other, older substances such as papaverine or papaverine/phentolamine, which cause priapism requiring treatment in up to 10% of cases in the diagnostic titration phase [31].

A PGE_1 dosing regimen for diagnostic tests depends on patient history and underlying diseases. The following dosing schedule has proven useful [33]:

• Neurologic underlying disease (multiple sclerosis (MS), spinal cord injury, pelvic surgery) — 5 µg PGE_1
• Standard dose with normal history — 10 µg PGE_1
• Severe organic underlying disease (e.g. diabetes) — 20 µg PGE_1

Goldstein *et al.* have proposed the concept of redosing, whereupon an additional dose of PGE_1 is given during the Doppler ultrasound in an attempt to induce greater vasodilation and cavernosal smooth muscle relaxation. Further, Goldstein *et al.*, as well as others, have proposed a variety of drug combina-

tions for use during the diagnostic Doppler ultrasound, as well as in clinical practice [32].

A combination of papaverine/phentolamine or papaverine/phentolamine/PGE_1 continues to be used by some colleagues as an alternative to PGE_1 alone [33]. As is the case for PGE_1, the dose used for diagnostic tests depends on the patient's history and underlying diseases, and should be adjusted accordingly. As already mentioned, the main risk of the papaverine/phentolamine combination is that it induces priapism that requires intervention in up to 10% of cases [31].

After the injection site has been cleansed with an alcohol swab, a 27–30 g needle is used to inject the vasoactive substance into the corpora cavernosa as a bolus from one side. Doppler or duplex ultrasound is performed when marked tumescence has occurred. The patient then has to remain in the waiting room for one hour, the extent of erection being checked after 10, 20, 30 and 60 min. It is prudent to monitor blood pressure during this procedure. Normal values for the post-injection cavernosal arterial flow, range from 25–35 cm/sec, while the normal value for end diastolic flow ranges from 0–8 cm/sec [34,35].

Office PGE_1 test

Clinicians inject PGE_1 in the office setting in an attempt to identify vascular disease of the penis, without the aid of an ultrasound device [36]. Sometimes the opinion is supported that a positive PGE_1 test (20–40 µg) excludes a vascular cause of ED, and that it could dispense with the need for Doppler/duplex ultrasound of the penile arteries. This does not correspond at all to the personal experiences, which showed that many patients with a positive injection test had severely arteriogenic ED in duplex ultrasound. A positive intracavernous injection test only demonstrates the integrity of the veno-occlusive mechanism, i.e. it excludes a so-called venous leak.

Visual Sexual Stimulation (VSS)

Visual sexual or erotic stimulation is an investigation method that has been used for many years in the diagnosis of ED. It is usually combined with intracavernous injection of vaso-active substances, say during Doppler/duplex ultrasound, to achieve a maximum erection response and thus to be able to draw conclusions on the maximum relaxation ability of the corpora cavernosa. VSS facilitates relaxation of the cavernosal tissue and overcomes potential psychogenic barriers toward the creation of an erection during vascular testing [37].

Cavernosometry and Cavernosography

Prior to 1998, cavernosometry and cavernosography [38,39] were widely used for the diagnosis of male erectile dysfunction. However, with the launch of a new oral drug treatment—sildenafil (Viagra®), [40], the need to diagnose cavernous insufficiency has changed greatly. What was the reason for this? Quite simply stated, the treatment of ED was no longer a function of any testing. Rather, the introduction of the oral phosphodiesterase type 5 inhibitors (PDE-5i) changed the diagnostic and treatment paradigm. Invasive diagnostic testing was no longer required for the introduction of treatment of ED. Essentially, if a man complained of ED, then he was offered a PDE-5i for his ED. The distinction between organic and psychogenic ED became blurred and the etiology of the ED, be it arteriogenic, neurogenic or venogenic was no longer a prerequisite for treatment.

Historically, animal experiments and clinical observations in humans have demonstrated that a chronic, disturbed arterial blood supply to the cavernous tissue with subsequent hypoxemic/ischemic conditions, impaired the veno-occlusive mechanism in the long term and resulted in the symptoms of cavernous insufficiency [41,42]. The severity of arteriosclerosis correlated with the severity of the veno-occlusive dysfunction. These observations led to the implementation of cavernosography and cavernosometry.

Cavernosometry

The technique, involving use of a 27–30 g needle, is used to inject varying μg (microgram) doses of PGE_1 (Caverject®), or a triple drug mixture, approximately 5–15 min before the actual investigation. The penile shaft is then draped with a sterile,

perforated drape. Patients who are sensitive to pain receive 1–2 cm³ of a 1% local anesthetic containing lidocaine, which is infiltrated prior to insertion of the 19 g butterfly needle. The butterfly needles should be applied vertically to the penis axis to avoid needle dislocation during erection and subsequent edema. The cavernosography pump is then used to infuse pre-heated physiologic saline in 20–40 mL/min steps until an erection considered firm enough for intercourse is achieved. The infusion is then stopped at a cavernous pressure of 150 mm Hg, and the fall in pressure within 30–60 sec is measured. The infusion is then restarted. When an erection considered firm enough for intercourse is achieved again (i.c. pressure > 90–100 mm Hg), the maintenance flow that is necessary to maintain a stable erection is measured.

Cavernsography

Non-ionic contrast agent is then added via a three-way stopcock, and after 50–100 mL of contrast agent, X-ray is performed in four different planes. This includes two anterior/posterior projections with the penis bent upwards and downwards, as well as two lateral/oblique projections using the urethrogram technique. Infusion is then stopped and 300–500 μg of phenylephrine is injected intracavernosally to achieve detumescence. The butterfly cannula are removed after detumescence has occurred and the puncture sites are compressed with a sterile swab for 2–3 min. An elastic compression dressing is applied at the end of the investigation for 1–2 h.

Gravity cavernosometry, first described by Puech Leao in 1990 [43] is a simplified method of cavernosometry/cavernosography. A pump is not required for this method. Cavernous pressure is continuously measured using a manometer via one butterfly needle, and saline at body temperature is infused via the other butterfly needle. The infusion solution is placed at a gravity pressure of 112 mm Hg. Following injection of the vasoactive substance, intracavernous pressure is measured continuously until a plateau has been achieved (equilibrium pressure). The infusion tube is then completely opened and the maximum cavernous pressure is measured using a manometer. However, gravity cavernosometry could never establish itself against pump cavernosometry as a routine method.

Penile Angiography

Until the mid 1980s, penile angiography was regarded as the gold standard in the diagnosis of arteriogenic impotence. This technique was mainly developed at the end of the 1970s by Ginestié and Romieu, whose standard work on this topic remains valid today [44]. As a result of standardization of vascular diagnostic in erectile dysfunction, using non-invasive Doppler and duplex ultrasound, penile angiography is no longer a standard diagnostic test (45). The only remaining indications for penile angiography is in younger men under 50 years of age in whom an isolated vascular occlusion with the absence of further risk factors makes the option of penile revascularization appear logical. Penile angiography is used for arterial embolization in cases of high-flow priapism [46].

Bulbocavernous Reflex Latency Times (BCR) and Somatosensory Evoked Potentials (SSEP)

This method is used to prove the integrity of somatic penile innervation, which is transmitted via the pudendal nerve and its motor terminal branches to the pelvic floor muscles or their sensory branch—the dorsal nerve of penis. Measuring the reflex latency times of the BCR checks the peripheral reflex arch (S_2–S_4), and measuring central latency times (SSEP) checks central (spinal) nerve transmission.

A ring electrode on the distal shaft of the penis is used to apply rectangular impulses lasting 0.2 msec via a constant current stimulator, and the reflex latency time is measured via the needle electrodes placed in the bulbocavernous muscles. Stimulus thresholds are chosen which permit constant reflex responses. These are generally six to eight times the sensory stimulus threshold, which varies individually between 7 and 12 mA. The interval between the stimuli is 40–60 sec, 10 consecutive responses being recorded.

The pudendal, somatosensory-evoked potentials and their latency times are also recorded via two electrodes located on the scalp at reference points C_{Z-2} and F_{pZ} [47].

The latency times of the pudendal, somatosensory evoked potentials depend on how tall the individual is. The latency time until the first positive amplitude P_1 of SSEP is calculated according to the following formula [48].

$$P_1 \text{ latency (SSEP)} = 5.41 + 0.207 \times \text{height of individual}$$

If the latency times of the BCR of the two control groups listed in Table 6.3 are compared to the results cited in the literature, mean BCR latency times $> 40 - 42$ msec must be generally considered as pathologic [48].

Based on the normal values mentioned for BCR latency times and SSEP, Porst [49] showed that 65 (50%) of 130 patients with ED had pathologic BCR findings. Of 116 patients with ED, in whom SSEP was also measured, 31% (36) had pathologic findings. In total, 76 (66%) of 130 patients with ED showed abnormalities in neurophysiologic investigations [49]. In the group investigated by Bemelmans, 58 (47%) of 123 impotent patients had pathologic findings in the various neurophysiologic investigations [48].

Nocturnal Penile Tumescence (NPT) Testing

This method is useful for select individuals. NPT testing takes advantage of the fact that men with normal erectile function have 4–6 episodes of involuntary, nocturnal erections lasting 20–50 minutes during a 6–8 hour sleep cycle. These erections occur mostly during REM (rapid eye movement) sleep. NPT testing in the diagnosis of ED has been described and is known worldwide [50]. NPT is best used to distinguish between organic and psychogenic ED.

Other simple and inexpensive methods such as the stamp test [51], the snap gauge band [52], and the erectiometer [53], were developed originally to record nocturnal erections. The common drawback of all these methods was that they could only record one nocturnal event. Thus no information could be obtained on the duration and frequency of nocturnal erections, and the degree of erection could not be sufficiently quantified.

The introduction of a computerized system called Rigiscan® made it possible to measure both tumescence and rigidity during an 8-h sleep cycle. Interpretation of Rigiscan® results has been simplified by new, more extensive software (Rigiscan®-plus), which includes four new parameters. In the Rigiscan®, which is the most commonly-used device to measure NPT worldwide, two loops at the penile base and tip (coronary sulcus) are contracted every 20 sec to constantly record and store circumference and rigidity changes, i.e. the erection status. A personal computer can then be used to print out the data [54].

Corpus Cavernosum Electromyography (CCEMG)

This procedure is used in the measurement of the reflex latency time of the BCR and pudendal, somatosensory-evoked potentials. This method has a considerable shortcoming in that it only checks the integrity of the somatic penile nervous system and does not allow any statement in terms of autonomic penile innervation, the system that is mainly responsible for the induction of erection (parasympathetic nervous system) and detumescence (sympathetic nervous system).

The greatest obstacle to evaluation of autonomic penile innervation, and in particular of the parasympathetic nervous system, is the fact that the cavernous muscle is the target organ of autonomic innervation of the penis, and that this is smooth muscle. No standard clinical procedure has been established to date to measure the electrical activity of smooth muscle, unlike the case for striated muscle, which has been measured by a standard procedure for decades.

More than ten years ago, the research efforts of Wagner and Gerstenberg led to the first published results for measuring the electrical activity of the cavernous muscle [55]. The Hanover team led by Stief *et al.* took up this method and refined it under the term "single potential analysis of cavernous electrical activity" (SPACE). In their first publication on this topic, they came to the conclusion that

SPACE could be useful in the diagnosis of autonomic neuropathy of the cavernous and/or myopathy of the cavernous muscles [56]. Based on the results obtained in 214 patients with ED, and 39 normally-potent patients, they observed that 52% of all impotent patients had pathologic results in SPACE. Further refinement of this method showed that surface electrodes as well as conventional concentric needle electrodes could be used to measure the electrical activity of the cavernous nerves.

With respect to the present status of CCEMG, it may be concluded that this method can detect abnormalities in cavernous muscle to a certain extent, although these pathologic alterations can be attributed to both damage to autonomic penile innervation and to degenerative processes of the cavernous smooth muscle. There are indications that CCEMG amplitudes correlate with the density of the cavernous smooth muscle. To date, there are no generally accepted standard criteria that would enable exact differentiation between normal and pathologic, and etiologic classification of the various ED forms is not possible. Thus, despite the fact that CCEMG has been around for 10–20 years, it is still considered experimental. It is far from becoming a routine procedure in the evaluation of ED etiology, especially in terms of autonomic neuropathy.

Sympathetic Skin Response (SSR)

Measurement of heart beat variation and the sympathetic skin response are generally accepted and now standardized investigation methods to demonstrate involvement of the autonomic nervous system, e.g. in diabetes, although the SSR method evaluates the sympathetic nervous system. SSR is infrequently used in the diagnostic evaluation of male ED, or in planning treatment for male ED.

The method makes use of a somatic afferent/sympathetic reflex, via which the activation of sweat gland secretion in certain skin domains is transmitted, which in turn is accompanied by a change in electrical potential. The method can in principle be used on different skin domains, although the palms and the soles are the most common domains.

Various authors have described SSR measurement

on the penis [57]. Penile sympathetic skin responses could be provoked in 85% of normal individuals with latency times of 1100–1600 msec [58]. Daffertshofer *et al.* showed that the SSR can be the only neurophysiologic test with a pathologic result in some patients, although other neurophysiologic tests were normal [57].

Summary

While many tests are available for the diagnosis of male ED, the history, physical and partner discussions have surmounted the minimally invasive or more rigorous testing schema used for the evaluation of male ED in the 1980s and early 1990s. This evolution was predicated on the introduction of oral therapies for male ED (PDE-5i), which supplanted and obviated the need for these tests.

References

1 Lue TF. A patient's goal-directed approach to erectile dysfunction and Peyronie's disease. *Can J Urol* 1995;**2**(Suppl):13–17.

2 Montague DK, Jarow JP, Broderick GA, Dmochowski RR, Heaton JP, Lue TF, Milbank AJ, Nehra A, Sharlip ID. Chapter 1: The management of erectile dysfunction: an AUA update. *J Urol* 2005;**174**(1):230–239.

3 Cappelleri JC, Rosen RC. The Sexual Health Inventory for Men (SHIM): a 5-year review of research and clinical experience. *Int J Impot Res* 2005;**17**(4):307–319.

4 Rosen RC, Riley A, Wagner G, Osterloh IH, Kirkpatrick J, Mishra A. The international index of erectile function (IIEF): a multidimensional scale for assessment of erectile dysfunction. *Urology* 1997;**49**(6):822–830.

5 Rosen RC, Catania J, Pollack L, Althof S, O'Leary M, Seftel AD. Male Sexual Health Questionnaire (MSHQ): scale development and psychometric validation. *Urology* 2004;**64**(4):777–782.

6 Recommendations of the 1st International Consultation on Erectile Dysfunction. In: Jardin A, *et al.* eds. *Erectile Dysfunction*. Plymouth, UK, Health Publication Ltd, 2000.

7 Morley JE, Perry HM 3rd, Kevorkian RT, Patrick P. Comparison of screening questionnaires for the diagnosis of hypogonadism. *Maturitas* 2006, Mar 20;**53**(4):424–9, Epub 2005, Sept 2.

8 Fisher WA, Rosen RC, Eardley I, Sand M, Goldstein I. Sexual experience of female partners of men with erectile dysfunction: the female experience of men's attitudes to life events and sexuality (FEMALES) study. *J Sex Med* 2005;**2**(5):675–684.

9 Aslan G, Koseoglu H, Sadik O, Gimen S, Cihan A, Esen A. Sexual function in women with urinary incontinence. *Int J Impot Res* 2005;**17**(3):248–251.

10 Carbone JR, DJ, Harrison LH, McCullough DL. Incidence of previously undiagnosed urologic malignancies in a population presenting solely with the complaint of erectile dysfunction. *J Urol* 1999;**161**, No 4, Suppl, 180.

11 Shabsigh R, Klein LT, Seidman S, Kaplan SA, Lehrhoff BJ, Ritter JS. Increased incidence of depressive symptoms in men with erectile dysfunction. *Urology* 1998;**52**(5):848–852.

12 Sheehan TJ, Fifield J, Reisine S, Tennen H. The measurement structure of the Center for Epidemiologic Studies Depression Scale. *J Pers Assess* 1995;**64**(3):507–521.

13 Rosen R, Altwein J, Boyle P, Kirby RS, Lukacs B, Meuleman E, O'Leary MP, Puppo P, Robertson C, Giuliano F. Lower urinary tract symptoms and male sexual dysfunction: the multinational survey of the aging male (MSAM-7). *Eur Urol* 2003;**44**(6):637–649.

14 Eid JF, *et al.* eds. *Cliniguide® to Erectile Dysfunction*. New York: Lawrence DellaCorte Publications Inc, 2001.

15 Muller JE, Mittleman MA, Maclure M, Sherwood JB, Tofler GH. Triggering myocardial infarction by sexual activity. Low absolute risk and prevention by regular physical exertion. Determinants of myocardial infarction onset study investigators. *JAMA* 1996;**275**(18):1405–1409.

16 Seftel AD, Sun P, Swindle R. The prevalence of hypertension, hyperlipidemia, diabetes mellitus and depression in men with erectile dysfunction. *J Urol* 2004;**171**(6 Pt 1):2341–2345.

17 Martin-Morales A, Sanchez-Cruz JJ, Saenz de Tejada I, Rodriguez-Vela L, Jimenez-Cruz JF, Burgos-Rodriguez R. Prevalence and independent risk factors for erectile dysfunction in Spain: results of the Epidemiologia de la Disfuncion Erectil Masculina Study. *J Urol* 2001;**166**(2):569–574.

18 Braun M, Wassmer G, Klotz T, Reifenrath B, Mathers M, Engelmann U. Epidemiology of erectile dysfunction: results of the "Cologne Male Survey". *Int J Impot Res* 2000;**12**(6):305–311.

19 Esposito K, Giugliano D. Obesity, the metabolic syndrome, and sexual dysfunction. *Int J Impot Res* 2005;**17**(5):391–398.

20 Executive Summary of the Third Report of the National Cholesterol Education Program (NCEP). Expert Panel

on Detection, Evaluation, and Treatment of High Blood Cholesterol in Adults (Adult Treatment Panel III). *JAMA* 2001;**285**:2486–2497.

21 Wagner G, Fugl-Meyer KS, Fugl-Meyer AR. Impact of erectile dysfunction on quality of life: patient and partner perspectives. *Int J Impot Res* 2000;**4**: S1.44–46.

22 Chevret M, Jaudinot E, Sullivan K, Marrel A, De Gendre AS. Impact of erectile dysfunction (ED) on sexual life of female partners: assessment with the Index of Sexual Life (ISL) questionnaire. *J Sex Marital Ther* 2004;**30**(3):157–172.

23 Dunn ME. Restoration of couple's intimacy and relationship vital to reestablishing erectile function. *J Am Osteopath Assoc* 2004;**104**(Sl- 4):S6–10.

24 Steidle C, Schwartz S, Jacoby K, Sebree T, Smith T, Bachand R. North American AA2500 T Gel Study Group. AA2500 testosterone gel normalizes androgen levels in aging males with improvements in body composition and sexual function. *J Clin Endocrinol Metab* 2003; **88**(6):2673–2681.

25 Burris AS, Banks SM, Carter CS, Davidson JM, Sherins RJ. A long-term, prospective study of the physiologic and behavioral effects of hormone replacement in untreated hypogonadal men. *J Androl* 1992;**13**(4): 297–304.

26 Arver S, Dobs AS, Meikle AW, Allen RP, Sanders SW, Mazer NA. Improvement of sexual function in testosterone deficient men treated for 1 year with a permeation enhanced testosterone transdermal system. *J Urol* 1996;**155**(5):1604–1608.

27 Shabsigh R, Kaufman JM, Steidle C, Padma-Nathan H. Randomized study of testosterone gel as adjunctive therapy to sildenafil in hypogonadal men with erectile dysfunction who do not respond to sildenafil alone. *J Urol* 2004;**172**(2):658–663.

28 Caretta N, Palego P, Roverato A, Selice R, Ferlin A, Foresta C. Age-matched cavernous peak systolic velocity: a highly sensitive parameter in the diagnosis of arteriogenic erectile dysfunction. *Int J Impot Res* 2006;**18**(3):306–10.

29 Schaeffer EM, Jarow JP Jr, Vrablic J, Jarow JP. Duplex ultrasonography detects clinically significant anomalies of penile arterial vasculature affecting surgical approach to penile straightening. *Urology* 2006;**67**(1): 166–169.

30 Wylie KR, Davies-South D, Steward D, Walters S, Iqbal M, Ryles S. A comparison between portable ultrasound (MIDUS) and nocturnal RigiScan when confirming the diagnosis of vascular organic erectile disorder. *Int J Impot Res* 2005 in press.

31 Porst H, Derouet H, Idzikowski, *et al.* Oral phentolamine (Vasomax®) in erectile dysfunction — Results of a German Multicenter-Study in 177 patients. *Int J Impotence Res* 1996;**8 No.3**:117.

32 Mulhall JP, Daller M, Traish AM, Gupta S, Park K, Salimpour P, Payton TR, Krane RJ, Goldstein I. Intracavernosal forskolin: role in management of vasculogenic impotence resistant to standard 3-agent pharmacotherapy. *J Urol* 1997;**158**(5):1752–1758.

33 Seyam R, Mohamed K, Akhras AA, Rashwan H. A prospective randomized study to optimize the dosage of trimix ingredients and compare its efficacy and safety with prostaglandin E1 *Int J Impot Res* 2005;**17**(4): 346–353.

34 Connolly JA, Borirakchanyavat S, Lue TF. Ultrasound evaluation of the penis for assessment of impotence. *J Clin Ultrasound* 1996;**24**(8):481–486.

35 Altinkilic B, Hauck EW, Weidner W. Evaluation of penile perfusion by color-coded duplex sonography in the management of erectile dysfunction. *World J Urol* 2004;**22**(5):361–364.

36 Elhanbly S, Schoor R, Elmogy M, Ross L, Hegazy A, Niederberger C. What nonresponse to intracavernous injection really indicates: a determination by quantitative analysis. *J Urol* 2002;**167**(1):192–196.

37 Pescatori ES, Silingardi V, Galeazzi GM, Rigatelli M, Ranzi A, Artibani W Audiovisual sexual stimulation by virtual glasses is effective in inducing complete cavernosal smooth muscle relaxation: a pharmacocavernosometric study. *Int J Impot Res* 2000;**12**(2).

38 Stief CG, Diederichs W, Benard F, Bosch R, Lue TF, Tanagho EA. The diagnosis of venogenic impotence: dynamic or pharmacologic cavernosometry? *J Urol* 1988;**140**(6):1561–1563.

39 Meuleman EJ, Wijkstra H, Doesburg WH, Debruyne FM. Comparison of the diagnostic value of pump and gravity cavernosometry in the evaluation of the cavernous veno-occlusive mechanism. *J Urol* 1991; **146**(5):1266–1270.

40 Goldstein I, Lue TF, Padma-Nathan H, Rosen RC, Steers WD, Wicker PA. Oral sildenafil in the treatment of erectile dysfunction. Sildenafil Study Group. *N Engl J Med* 1998;**338**(20):1397–1404.

41 Persson-Juenemann C, Diederichs W, Lue TF, *et al.* Correlation of impaired penile ultrastructure to quantified clinical impotence. *Proc. 3rd Biennial World Meeting on Impotence* Boston 1988, Abstr.15.

42 Azadzoi KM, Siroky MB, Goldstein I. Study of etiologic relationship of arterial atherosclerosis to corporal veno-occlusive dysfunction in the rabbit. *J Urol* 1996;**155**: 1795–1800.

43 Puech-Leao P, Chao S, Glina S. Gravity cavernosometry — simple diagnostic test for cavernosal incompetence. *Brit J Urol* 1990;**65**:391.

44 Ginestié IF, Romieu A, eds. *Radiologic exploration of impotence*. The Hague, Boston, London: Martinus Nijhoff Medical Division, 1978.

45 McMahon CG. Correlation of penile duplex ultrasonography, PBI, DICC and angiography in the diagnosis of impotence. *Int J Impot Res* 1998;**10**(3):153–158.

46 Ciampalini S, Savoca G, Buttazzi L, Gattuccio I, Mucelli FP, Bertolotto M, De Stefani S, Belgrano E. High-flow priapism: treatment and long-term follow-up. *Urology* 2002;**59**(1):110–113.

47 Porst H, Tackmann W, van Ahlen H. Bulbokavernosus-reflex -Latenzzeitmessung (BCR) und somatosensorisch evozierte Potentiale (SSEP) in der Diagnostik der erektilen Dysfunktion. *Akt Urol* 1987;**18**:198–202.

48 Bemelmans BLH, Meuleman EJH, Anten BWM, *et al.* Penile sensory disorders in erectile dysfunction. Results of a comprehensive neuro-urophysiological diagnostic workup in 123 patients. In: Meuleman, EJH, ed. *Recent progress in the diagnosis of erectile dysfunction*. Benda, Nijemegen, 1991, pp. 81–94.

49 Porst H, Tackmann W, van Ahlen H. Neurophysiological investigations in potent and impotent men. *Brit J Urol* 1998;**61**:445–450.

50 Karacan J, Salis PJ, Thornby JI, *et al.* The ontogeny of nocturnal penile tumescence. *Waking and Sleeping* 1976;**1**:27–44.

51 Marshall P, Morales A, Phillips P, *et al.* Nocturnal penile tumescence with stamps: A comparative study under sleep laboratory conditions. *J Urol* 1983;**129**:288–290.

52 Ek A, Bradley WE, Krane RJ. Nocturnal penile rigidity measured by snapgauge band. *J Urol* 1983;**129**: 964–967.

53 Jonas U. Erektiometer: Ein einfacher und sicherer test in der diagnostik der erektilen impotenz. *Akt Urol* 1982;**13**:324–327.

54 Levine LA, Lenting EL. Use of nocturnal penile tumescence and rigidity in the evaluation of male erectile dysfunction. *Urol Clin North Am* 1995;**22**(4):775–788.

55 Wagner G, Gerstenberg T. Human in-vivo studies of electrical activity of corpus cavernosum. *J Urol* 1988;**139**:Part 2, 327 A.

56 Stief CG, Bosch R, Diederichs W, *et al.* Cavernous smooth muscle changes during penile erection and sympathetic stimulation. *Int J Impotence Res* 1991; **3**:15–20.

57 Daffertshofer M, Linden D, Syren M, *et al.* Assessment of local sympathetic function in patients with erectile dysfunction. *Int J Impotence Res* 1994;**6**:213–225.

58 Jost WH, Derouet H, Osterhage J, *et al.* Elektrophysiologische diagnostik bei der erektilen dysfunktion. *Urologe* 1996;**A35**:120–126.

Appendix A The abridged 5-item version (ED intensity scale) of the International Index of Erectile Dysfunction (IIEF-5).

Over the past six months:					
1. How do you rate your **confidence** that you could get and keep an erection?	Very low	Low	Moderate	High	Very high
	1	2	3	4	5
2. When you had erections with sexual stimulation, **how often** were your erections hard enough for penetration?	Almost never/never	A few times (much less than half the time)	Sometimes (about half the time)	Most times (much more than half the time)	Almost always/always
	1	2	3	4	5
3. During sexual intercourse, **how often** were you able to maintain your erection after you had penetrated (entered) your partner?	Almost never/never	A few times (much less than half the time)	Sometimes (about half the time)	Most times (much more than half the time)	Almost always/always
	1	2	3	4	5
4. During sexual intercourse, **how difficult** was it to maintain your erection to completion of intercourse?	Extremely difficult	Very difficult	Difficult	Slightly difficult	Not difficult
	1	2	3	4	5
5. When you attempted sexual intercourse, **how often** was it satisfactory for you?	Almost never/never	A few times (much less than half the time)	Sometimes (about half the time)	Most times (much more than half the time)	Almost always/always
	1	2	3	4	5

The IIEF-5 score is the sum of the ordinal responses to the five items. Thus, the score can range from 5 to 25. Severity categorization of ED: Score 5–10, severe ED; Score 11–15, moderate ED; Score 16–20, mild ED; Score 21–25, normal (no ED).

CHAPTER 7

Oral Pharmacotherapy of Erectile Dysfunction

Hartmut Porst

Introduction

Up until a few years ago, pharmacologic treatment of erectile dysfunction (ED) was limited to a few substances, most of which had to be injected directly into the corpora cavernosa. The oral substances available to treat ED included drugs containing yohimbine, and in some special cases the serotonin re-uptake inhibitor trazodone, officially approved for the indication of depression, and occasionally administered in an off-label use for ED. There was also a plethora of aphrodisiacs or sexual tonics available, which usually contained a mixture of various substances, such as testis sicca, testosterone, yohimbine, ginseng, caffeine, barbituric acid, saw palmetto, cayenne fruit, and many others, in one preparation. Meanwhile many of these preparations disappeared from the market; some, however, are still available, in particular via the internet.

These include a range of drugs which contain yohimbine, vitamins (in particular vitamin E and vitamin B complex), dried extracts of muira-puama, gingseng and other herbal and plant extracts, or bamethan sulfate and benzyl nicotinate, respectively.

Common to all these aphrodisiacs, offered mostly by mail order sex companies or in sex shops, is the fact that their efficacy was never proven in well-designed placebo-controlled and double-blind clinical trials, and that only the belief in them may contribute to their promised efficacy, but not the usual homeopathic doses of the various compounds contained in these aphrodisiacs.

This chapter on pharmacologic treatment deals with all those substances, which have been clinically tested in a variety of ED studies and/or were finally approved in the indication of ED, at least in some countries of the world. In addition to drugs officially approved by the health authorities, this chapter also touches briefly on those medications/substances with which clinical studies in the indication of ED were conducted and reported in the literature, and which may be available in some countries, although not officially be approved for ED treatment.

Yohimbine

Yohimbine is the main alkaloid from the bark of the tree called *Coryanthe johimbe* K. Schum (yohimbehe tree), found particularly in central Africa. This tree belongs to the Rubiaceae family. The alkaloid was first isolated from the bark of the yohimbehe tree (hence the name) by L. Spiegel in 1896. The bark of this tree is still used today as the raw material for the various yohimbine preparations. Information on its use combined with papaverine in the treatment of ED was published as early as in 1923 [1]. Until the launch of sildenafil and the other phosphodiesterase-5 (PDE-5) inhibitors, yohimbine was the most prescribed substance worldwide for the treatment of ED.

Pharmacologic profile

Yohimbine is in particular a central α_2-adrenoceptor blocker, its activity being 50–100 times higher on presynaptic receptors than on postsynaptic ones [2]. A peripheral site of action is also presumed because yohimbine acts on the α_2-receptors of the penile arteries and on presynaptic α_2-adrenoceptors, which are localized on α_1-adrenoceptors of sympathetic nerve endings [3] (see also Fig. 3.7, p. 37). At these presynaptic α_2-adrenoceptors, α_2-blockers inhibit erection-suppressing impulses mediated by sympathetic α_1-adrenoceptors, which facilitates initiation of erection. Yohimbine at higher doses is also reported to act on cholinergic, vasoactive intestinal peptidergic (VIPergic) and dopaminergic receptors [2], and to exert antagonistic or inhibitory properties on serotonin receptors, monoamino-oxidase and the rapid sodium channels [4]. Based on these multiple, partly complex pharmacologic properties, yohimbine has three principal mechanisms of action in the treatment of erectile dysfunction.

Central

Unlike α_1-adrenoceptors, cerebral α_2-adrenoceptors mediate erection-inhibiting impulses. Thus yohimbine facilitates erection at a central level.

Peripheral

Yohimbine directly blocks α_2-adrenoceptors, which dominate in the penile arteries. Thus it counteracts the vasoconstriction induced by norepinephrine/epinephrine release, and in turn the reduction in blood flow.

By presynaptically inhibiting α_1-adrenoceptor activity in the cavernous smooth muscle cells, yohimbine facilitates their relaxation.

Pharmacokinetics and dosage

Yohimbine hydrochloride is orally well absorbed and has a plasma half-life of between 0.25 and 2.5 h [5,6]. However, the effects triggered by yohimbine, which can be traced back to an increase in plasma norepinephrine, may last for more than 13 h [6]. Only about 1% of yohimbine appears in the urine, indicating a predominantly hepatic clearance [6]. Doses described in the literature range from 5 to 15 mg three times a day, and may be a single daily administration of up to 100 mg (2,4,7,8). Doses of 5–15 mg three times daily for 6–8 weeks are the most commonly used regimen in the studies [2,8,9].

Efficacy

The efficacy and safety of yohimbine have been analyzed in numerous studies, some of which include a placebo-controlled, double blind, prospective design [2]. The efficacy rates range from no effect as compared to placebo, even at high doses, to efficacy rates of 71%, as compared to 40% for placebo, in non-organic impotence [7,8,10]. A meta-analysis of seven large yohimbine studies, which met the strict quality criteria, showed a superiority of yohimbine vs. placebo. Based on these data the authors concluded that there is a rationale for the use of yohimbine in suitable ED patients [2]. The Clinical Guidelines Panel on Erectile Dysfunction of the American Urologic Association (AUA) came to the conclusion that the data currently available on yohimbine do not allow it to be recommended as standard treatment in ED, particularly not in organic etiologies; this statement of the AUA ED Guideline Panel was not changed in the 2005 update[11,12].

Apart from its use in ED, yohimbine has also been reported effective in orgasmic disorders, i.e. delayed ejaculation or orgasm [13].

Side effects and contraindications

The side effects commonly observed with yohimbine can mostly be traced back to the partially increased sympathetic activity: anxiety, nausea, restlessness, agitation, sleeplessness tachycardia, palpitations, rarely diarrhea, manic symptoms [4,7,9]. In addition, after yohimbine, either increases or more infrequently decreases in blood pressure were reported, which may become of clinical relevance if hypertensive patients are taking this medication.

In 25 hypertensive patients who had not been treated with drugs, Grossmann *et al.* demonstrated that a mean increase in blood pressure of 5 mmHg (p < 0.01) occurred 1 h after taking 20 mg yohimbine, and that plasma norepinephrine levels measured in the cubital vein increased by an average of 66% (p < 0.001) [14]. Rate and severity of side effects is clearly dose-dependent, i.e. the occurrence of side effects particularly with higher doses (10–15 mg three times) leads to requests for the discontinuation of treatment significantly more often. It should also be noted that yohimbine may potentiate the effect of tricyclic antidepressants and antagonize the effects of clonidine treatment [4]. Severe cardiovascular diseases such as unstable angina or recent myocardial infarction, difficult to treat hypertension, severe psychiatric diseases, as well as severe hepatic impairment, are considered to be contraindicated for yohimbine use.

Conclusions and recommendations.

If yohimbine has any potential in ED then it is only in patients with non-organic ED. In those patients yohimbine may be used for a maximum of two months, either on a regular regimen (3×10 mg/day), or on an as-needed regimen, taking 10–15 mg, 30–60 min prior to sexual activities.

Apomorphine SL

The history of apomorphine dates back to 1869 when its first synthesis from morphine was reported by Mathiessen [15]. The dopaminergic activities of apomorphine were first published in the mid 1960s when it was successfully administered in Parkinson's disease to suppress refractory motor oscillations [16]. Apomorphine was formerly used as an emetic in the treatment of poisoning to prevent absorption of orally ingested poisons. The erection-inducing effect of apomorphine in humans was first described by Lal *et al.* [17]. In 1995 Heaton *et al.* reported positive results for orally administered apomorphine in seven out of 10 patients with psychogenic impotence [18].

Pharmacologic profile

Apomorphine is a central dopamine receptor agonist with effects on D_1 and D_2 receptors (dominantly on D_2). Predominant sites of action are located in the paraventricular nucleus, stria terminalis, medial preoptic area, and amygdaloid nucleus [19,20]. Apomorphine-induced erections are both testosterone and NO dependent [21,22], i.e. the erection-triggering effects of apomorphine diminish or may even be absent in the case of a clinically-relevant NO or testosterone deficiency/withdrawal. Following stimulation of the cerebral dopamine receptors the apomorphine-induced erections are mainly transmitted via parasympathetic oxytocinergic nerve fibers, and lead to an increase of arterial blood supply in the penis [23] as well as in the clitoris and vaginal wall [24]. In addition to its known cerebral

mechanisms of action, apomorphine also exerts pro-erectile properties at a spinal level [25].

Pharmacokinetics

As apomorphine has shown no efficacy via the gastrointestinal tract after oral intake (first-pass effect), a sublingual preparation was developed, which is absorbed via the oral mucosa. The sublingual apomorphine tablet is rapidly absorbed, with measurable plasma concentrations within 10 min after application and a T_{max} of 40–60 min [26]. The $T_{1/2}$ ranged in a dose-dependent manner between $2.7 \, h \pm 1.4 \, SD$ for the 2 mg, and $4.2 \, mg \pm 2.9 \, SD$ for the 4 mg dose.

Efficacy

Although apomorphine SL has shown statistically significant efficacy vs. placebo in the phase II/III clinical program, the net benefit ratio (active efficacy minus placebo efficacy) with figures between only 11 and 13%, were not convincing at all [27,28]. This limited efficacy of apomorphine SL, especially in organic ED, was recently confirmed in 130 diabetic ED patients in whom apomorphine SL 3 mg resulted in response rates of 22.9% vs. 17.3% for placebo [29]. Meanwhile several prospective studies between apomorphine SL and sildenafil were reported in the literature, with all of them resulting in a highly statistically significant superiority of sildenafil, and preference rates of 94–95% in favour of sildenafil [30–32]. Due to that overwhelming superiority of PDE-5 inhibitors, apomorphine SL never reached noteworthy acceptance or reasonable market shares in those countries where it was approved; meanwhile the drug marketed as Uprima® was withdrawn from nearly all markets in Europe, except in the UK where it is still marketed as 3 mg tablets.

Side effects

A summary of the side effects of the 3 mg apomorphine SL dose, as reported in several phase three trials shows the following outcome [33]: nausea 4.7%, headache 2.9%, dizziness 2.6%, yawning 1.9%, somnolence 1.5%, sweating 1.2%, vasodilation 0.9%, vomiting 0.2%, hypotension 0.2%, syncope 0.2%.

In apomorphine SL/alcohol interaction studies,

ingestion of 0.6 g/kg ethanol before administration of 6 mg apomorphine SL resulted in significant drop of blood pressure in some patients [26]. Therefore patients should be counselled to reduce alcohol intake together when prescribed apomorphine SL.

Conclusions and recommendations

As previously mentioned, due to its inferior efficacy apomorphine SL is withdrawn from most of the markets for which it was approved in 2001/2002. In those countries where it is still available it should only, if ever, be used in those patients with proven non-organic ED.

Phosphodiesterase-5 Inhibitors: Sildenafil (Viagra®), Tadalafil (Cialis®) and Vardenafil (Levitra®)

The physiological basis of erection (Fig. 7.1)
Pro-erectile impulses are generated in the parasympathetic erection centers of the limbic system and the hypothalamus, in particular in the paraventricular nucleus and the medial preoptic area, which are the key regions for the central regulation of erection [25]. Perception of sexual (erotic) stimuli, such as visual, imaginary or tactile stimuli, activate a variety

of receptors processing the stimulatory signals, which in turn are running via oxytocinergic/dopaminergic neurons to the spinal parasympathetic reflexogenic erection center, located at the level S_2–S_4. Parasympathetic nerve fibers, the so-called nervi erigentes, leave the reflexogenic erection center and build along with the sympathetic nerve fibers originating from the superior hypogastric plexus—the inferior hypogastric plexus—which continues in the cavernous nerves. These cavernous nerves contain both sympathetic and parasympathetic fibers and perforate the pelvic floor (urogenital diaphragma) to enter the cavernous bodies at the level where the cavernous crura are diverging.

Erection-initiating neurotransmitters are dopamine (via D_2-receptors) and melanocortins, for which five melanocortin receptors (MCR) have been identified, of which the MC-4-R seems of special importance for erection. After entering the cavernous bodies the parasympathetic nerve fibers principally divide into two different nerve terminals: cholinergic (acetylcholine, ACH) nerve terminals ending at the endothelial cells and stimulating nitric oxide (NO)-synthase, which catalyzes the production of NO from L-arginine and O_2, and non-adrenergic,

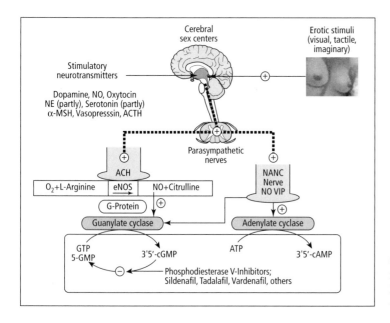

Fig. 7.1 Physiology of erection and the impact of PDE-5 inhibitors on erection. Please see text above for an explanation of this figure.

non-cholinergic (NANC-peptidergic) nerve terminals at the cavernous smooth muscle cells, from which NO and VIP (vasoactive intestinal polypeptide) are released into the smooth muscle cell. There, NO activates guanylate cyclase, which catalyses the breakdown of guanosine triphosphate into 3'5'-cyclic guanosine monophosphate (cGMP),the key second messenger for erection.

The Phosphodiesterase (PDE) System

Currently the PDE system includes 11 families, with a total of more than 50 splice variants (isoforms) [34–40]. The distribution and density of PDEs varies among the different tissues. The PDEs catalyze the breakdown of either cGMP or cyclic adenosine monophosphate (cAMP), which are both second messengers with specific physiologic functions. By hydrolyzing the phosphodiesterase bond of cAMP or cGMP, these second messengers are converted to the biologically-inactive monophosphates, resulting in termination of their physiologic functions.

In addition to PDE-5, which is the most abundant one in the corpus cavernosum, to date at least 13 other PDEs have been identified in the cavernous bodies: PDE-1A, PDE-1B, PDE-1C, PDE-2A, PDE-3A, PDE-4A, PDE-4B, PDE-4C, PDE-4D, PDE-7A, PDE-8A, PDE-9A, PDE-10A [39,40].

Apart from their direct impact on cavernous function, PDE-4 and -5 inhibitors also inhibit proliferation and migration of smooth muscle cells [37]. PDE-3 and PDE-4 inhibition can reduce restenosis after angioplasty procedures, individually, or by acting synergistically, and are therefore under investigation for their potential on angiogenesis [37].

General considerations for the three PDE-5 Inhibitors

For a better understanding of differences among, and comparisons between the three PDE-5 inhibitors, some terms frequently used in publications have to be explained.

IC_{50} is defined as the concentration of a PDE-5 inhibitor required to reduce the activity of PDE-5 by 50%. The IC_{50} values provide an overview of the clinical efficacy of a PDE-5 inhibitor. Generally speaking the lower the IC_{50} values the more potent

and therefore more effective a compound is for this enzyme.

Clinical efficacy

Regarding the clinical efficacy of a PDE-5 inhibitor several tools are used in clinical trials.

Regarding the general assessment question (GAQ): "Has the treatment you have been taking improved your erections?" This efficacy tool does not really tell whether the patient is able to attain an erection sufficient for sexual intercourse or not. This relatively weak efficacy measure is widely used, especially by pharmaceutical companies, because usually it yields the highest success rates.

International index of erectile function (IIEF) [48]

The IIEF was originally developed to evaluate the clinical efficacy of sildenafil (Viagra®) and became the most accepted and used efficacy tool for drugs assigned to treat ED world wide. It comprises 15 questions in five domains, addressing erectile and orgasmic function, sexual desire, sexual satisfaction and overall satisfaction. Each question has six response options scoring between zero (worst) and five (best result). For evaluation of the erectile efficacy of a drug the IIEF erectile function (EF) domain, comprising questions 1–5 and 15, represents the strongest efficacy tool, with a score >25 indicating a normal erectile function.

Sexual encounter profile (SEP)

The sexual encounter profile relies on the recordings of the patients in the patient diaries distributed to the patients with the study medication and collected at each study visit. The SEP comprises the following five questions:

1 Were you able to achieve at least some erection (some enlargement of the penis?)
2 Were you able to insert your penis into your partner's vagina?
3 Did your erection last long enough for you to have successful intercourse?
4 Were you satisfied with the hardness of your erection?
5 Were you satisfied overall with this sexual experience?

SEP question 3 (ability to complete sexual intercourse) turned out to be the most rigorous and most frequently-used efficacy measure in clinical ED trials.

Selectivity

The selectivity of a drug such as a PDE-5 inhibitor provides data on how selective a compound is with regard to the enzyme in question (here PDE-5), on which the efficacy is desired compared to other enzymes (PDE 1–4 and 6–11), and on which an efficacy has to be regarded undesirable.

Therefore the selectivity of a PDE inhibitor is assessed by comparing its potency (IC_{50}) to inhibit a PDE in question (here PDE 1–4 and 6–11), and its potency to inhibit the PDE desired (here PDE-5).

$$\text{Selectivity Ratio: } \frac{IC_{50} \text{ for a PDE in question}}{IC_{50} \text{ for PDE-5}}$$

The selectivity ratio is used for all three PDE-5 inhibitors to show how selective they are for PDE-5, as compared to anyone of the other ten PDEs. The higher this selectivity ratio is for PDE-5 compared to the PDE investigated, the more specific the PDE-5 inhibitor can be considered. In the clinical use all three PDE-5 inhibitors show, at the highest doses, a sufficiently high safety margin to all the other PDEs, except for sildenafil which shows only a 11-fold higher selectivity ratio for PDE-5, and for vardenafil which shows a 25-fold higher selectivity profile for PDE-5 as compared to PDE-6—an enzyme exclusively located in the retina that is responsible for our color and brightness discrimination abilities. In terms of PDE-11, an enzyme just recently isolated in several tissues (Table 7.1), without knowing in detail its physiologic function, the selectivity ratio of tadalafil turned out to be only five-fold higher for PDE-5.

Pharmacokinetic issues of the three PDE-5 inhibitors—onset and duration of clinical efficacy

The pharmacokinetic profile of a drug comprises all the different steps between its entry into the body and its elimination. In this regard of special interest is the speed of absorption, which is best defined by the T_{max} (time needed to reach the maximum plasma concentrations—C_{max}) and $T_{1/2}$ (half-life), defined as the time it takes for the fall of the plasma-concentrations of a drug to half of its C_{max} values. In the clinical setting the T_{max} corresponds quite well with the speed of clinical efficacy (onset of erection) and the $T_{1/2}$ (half-life), with the period of clinical -efficacy.

As illustrated in Table 7.2, all three drugs show similar earliest onset of action times, with vardenafil being a bit ahead. In this context it must taken into consideration that both with sildenafil and vardenafil, the pharmacokinetic parameters T_{max}, onset of action and C_{max} are clearly dependent on food intake; that means that after intake of a high fat (59% fat) meal a delay in T_{max} of 60 min and a reduction in C_{max} of 29% was observed with sildenafil [56]; similar data are valid for vardenafil [58,59]. On the other hand, with tadalafil, no food interaction was reported even with high fat meal [65].

Regarding the duration of efficacy, both with tadalafil and vardenafil, large placebo-controlled, double-blind trials were dedicated to figure out the real window of responsiveness, which is not the case for sildenafil [54,55,60]; although two studies with a very limited and thus not representative number of patients were able to show responsiveness of up to 12 hours for sildenafil [62,63]. Tadalafil steady-state plasma concentrations of 1.6-fold of the applied single dose are attained within five days if given once daily. Less than 0.0005% of the administered tadalafil dose appear in the semen.

Pharmacodynamics

The term pharmacodynamics covers all actions of a drug on the different body organs, and in turn on their functions (for example blood pressure, heart rate, vision). The pharmacodynamic interactions of any drug are influenced by the number of receptors available in the target organ and the affinity of the compound for the receptors in question. So for example it was just recently reported that vardenafil has, with 85%, a clearly higher proportion of high-affinity components to the PDE-5 catalytic site than sildenafil (with 50%) and tadalafil (with 60%) [61]. Given the fact that the high affinity components of a PDE-5 inhibitor show a considerably

Table 7.1 Current knowledge of the phosphodiestrase system and tissue distribution pattern [37,40,44,47].

Family	Substrate	Special Issues	Tissue Distribution Pattern
PDE 1	cGMP > cAMP	Ca^{++}/Calmodulin-dependent	Heart, brain, liver, kidney, skeletal muscle, vascular and visceral smooth musculature
PDE 2	cGMP = cAMP	Stimulated by cGMP	Brain, heart, adrenal cortex, kidney, liver, skeletal muscle, olfactory neurons, visceral smooth musculature, corpus cavernosum
PDE 3	cAMP	Inhibited by cGMP	Heart, vascular and visceral smooth musculature platelets, liver, kidney, fat, corpus cavernosum
PDE 4	cAMP		Lung and bronchus, brain, heart, liver, kidney, skeletal muscle, vascular and visceral smooth musculature, lymphocytes, mast cells, thyroid, testis, corpus cavernosum
PDE-5	cGMP		Corpus cavernosum, platelets, vascular and visceral smooth musculature, urogenital system (prostate, ureter, bladder)
PDE 6	cGMP > cAMP		Retina (rod and cone cells)
PDE 7	cAMP >> cGMP		Skeletal muscle, heart, brain, liver, lymphocytes, pancreas, thyroid, epididymis, tye
PDE 8	cAMP >> cGMP		Testis, ovary, small intestine, colon, liver, eye
PDE 9	cGMP >> cAMP		Small intestine, spleen, brain, kidney
PDE 10	cGMP > cAMP		Brain (putamen, caudate nucleus), testis
PDE 11	cGMP > cAMP		Testis, pituitary, heart, prostate, liver, kidney, salivary glands, skeletal muscle, corpus cavernosum

Table 7.2 Pharmacokinetics of the three PDE-5 inhibitors.

Drug (Authors)	T_{max} (min)	Onset of Action (min) earliest and >50% pt.response		$T_{1/2}$ (h)	Duration of Efficacy (h) (% succesful coitus)	C_{max} ng/ml
Sildenafil 100 mg [56,59]	70 (30–120)	14	20	3.82 ± 0.84	4 (81%)	327 ± 236
Tadalafil 20 mg [52–55,57,59]	120 (30–720)	16	30	17.5	36 (59 and 62%)	378
Vardenafil 20 mg [51,58,60]	40 (15–180)	11	25	3.94 ± 1.31	8 ± 2 (69%)	20.9 ± 1.83

pt, patient.

longer dissociation time, this explains why varde-nafil showed in clinical use a clearly longer duration of efficacy than could be inferred from its half-life time [60].

Intrinsic and extrinsic factors, drug-interactions

In patients with renal and hepatic insufficiency special dose adjustments have to be considered in

dependence of the severity of organ failure and the applied PDE-5 inhibitor (see Table 7.3)

Bleeding time
Both with aspirin 150 mg and warfarin, no increase in bleeding time was observed with the PDE-5 in-hibitors. After heparin, sildenafil showed an additive effect on bleeding time in rabbits, but this interaction trial was not conducted in humans.

Table 7.3 Pharmacodynamic issues with the three PDE-5 inhibitors (Source: Last Us-Label as of July 2005).

Parameter/Condition	Sildenafil	Tadalafil	Vardenafil
CYP 3A4 inhibitors[1]	Start dose 25 mg	Max.dose 10 mg/72 h	Max.2.5 mg/day
CYP 3A4 inhibitors[2]	Start dose 25 mg Max.dose 25 mg/day	Max.dose 10 mg/72 h	Max.dose 2.5 mg/72 h
Age >65 years	Start dose 25 mg	No dose adjustment	Start dose 5 mg
Severe renal failure (Creatinine clearance <30 ml/min.)	Start dose 25 mg	Max.dose 5 mg	No dose adjustment
Mild/mod.hepatic failure (Child Pugh A/B)	Start dose 25 mg	Max.dose 10 mg	Start dose 5 mg Max.dose 10 mg
Blood pressure drop systolic/diastolic	8.4/5.5 mmHg	1.6/0.8 mmHg	7/8 mmHg
α-blockers	Interval of 4 h recommended	Stable α-blocker therapy recommend. Start dose 5 mg	Stable α-blocker therapy recommend. Start dose 10 mg
Antihypertensives (all drug classes)	No interactions of clinical relevance	No interactions of clinical relevance	No interactions of clinical relevance
Alcohol intake (0.5–0.6 g/Kg)	No additional hypotensive effect	No additional hypotensive effect	No additional hypotensive effect
Contraindications	Nitrates and NO donors[3]	Nitrates and NO donors	Nitrates and NO donors
Safe interval for nitrate medication in emergencies	Not defined (presumably 24 h)	48 hours	24 hours

[1]CYP 3A4 inhibitors: erythromycin, ketoconacole, itraconacole: up to 3–10 fold increases in the plasma concentrations of the respective PDE-5 inhibitors. Cimetidine: 56% increase in sildenafil plasma concentrations; not valid for vardenafil; tadalafil not reported.
[2]CYP 3A4 inhibitors: protease inhibitors ritonavir, indinavir, saquinavir: increase in plasma concentrations of the respective PDE-5 inhibitors between 1.5-fold (tadalafil) and 16-fold (vardenafil). CYP 3A4 inducers: Rifampin: decrease of PDE-5 inhibitor plasma levels up to 88% (reported for tadalafil)
[3]Nitrates and NO donors: all short and long-acting nitrate-containing drugs, including recreational drugs such as "poppers" as well as molsidomine and nitroprussid-natrium containing medications

Cardiovascular risk patients

Those with left ventricular outflow obstruction (aortic and subaortic stenosis), recent (<6 months) myocardial infarction, and stroke or life threatening arrhythmias, as well as hypotensive (RR < 90/50) and hypertensive (RR > 170/110) patients, can be particularly sensitive to the systemic actions of PDE-5 inhibitors.

In conditions/drugs with a known risk of priapism, such as sickle cell disease, leukemia and multiple myeloma, PDE-5 inhibitors must be used with special precautions.

α blockers

Sildenafil 25 mg simultaneously applied with doxazosin 4 mg resulted in symptomatic postural hypotension, which was also the case with tadalafil 20 mg [56,57]. After tamsulosin 0.4 mg, both tadalafil 20 mg and vardenafil 5 mg did not exert any clinically relevant influence on blood pressure, whereas vardenafil 5 mg, if simultaneously applied with terazosin 10 mg, resulted in symptomatic hypotension, which could not be observed if both drugs were taken six hours apart [57, 58]. Tadalafil 20 mg applied with alfuzosin 10 mg did not result in clinically significant hemodynamic interaction [66].

Nitrate-/NO donor interactions

All three PDE-5 inhibitors showed clinically relevant interactions with nitrates in the sense of symptomatic blood pressure decays if given simultaneously [56–58,68–69]. Therefore all three PDE-5 inhibitors are contraindicated for patients with nitrate medications. The time interval considered to be safe between the administration of a PDE-5 inhibitor and a nitrate medication is 24 hours for the short-acting sildenafil and vardenafil, and 48 hours for tadalafil [56–58,68].

Efficacy

The efficacy of the three PDE-5 inhibitors was investigated world wide in large-scale trials, both in mixed ED populations as well as in subpopulations, like patients with diabetes, and after nerve-sparing radical prostatectomy (Table 7.4). To interpret Table 7.4 correctly it has to be mentioned that SEP 2 and SEP 3 diary data were available in all the tadalafil and vardenafil trials, whereas in the early sildenafil trials SEP 2 and 3 were not available, the tool "successful intercourse" was used instead.

All three PDE-5 inhibitors were remarkably successful in a variety of ED subpopulations including patients with diabetes, patients with neurologic disorders such as spinal cord injuries and multiple sclerosis, patients after radical prostatectomy—provided they have undergone a nerve sparing procedure, patients with hypertension or coronary artery disease, as well as patients with renal insufficiency or after kidney transplant.

Table 7.4 Efficacy of the three PDE-5 inhibitors in various ED populations.

ED Population	Sildenafil/Placebo (50/100 mg)		Tadalafil/Placebo (10/20 mg)			Vardenafil/Placebo (10/20 mg)		
	GAQ(%)	SEP/2/3(%)	GAQ(%)	SEP 2(%)	SEP 3(%)	GAQ(%)	SEP 2(%)	SEP 3(%)
Mixed	82/24	66/20	81/35	Not rep.	75/32	80/30	Not rep.	75/39
	(n = 1600–1787) [56]			(n = 1112) [70]			(n = 601) [71]	
						85/28	81/52	67/33
							(n = 804) [72]	
Diabetes	56/10	48/12	64/25	57/30	48/20	72/13	64/36	54/23
	(n = 268) [56,73]			(n = 216) [74]			(n = 452) [75]	
BNSP RRP	No controlled multicenter studies		62/23	54/32	41/19	65/13	48/22	37/10
				(n = 303) [76]			(n = 427) [77]	

Having said that, it has to be stated that all three PDE-5 inhibitors yielded very similar success rates, with only minor differences in the efficacy endpoints (Table 7.4).

Long-term efficacy

Long-term studies (two years) were able to prove that, in general there is no loss of efficacy among the three PDE-5 inhibitors. In recent experimental research studies no upregulation of PDE-5 in the penis was observed with the long-acting PDE-5 inhibitor tadalafil [78–81]. Apart from improvement in ED, improvements in other sexual domains such as orgasmic function, overall satisfaction with the sexual experience, and the quality of life [82] along with improvement of depressive symptoms [83], and increases in partner satisfaction with the sexual life [84,85], were regularly reported with the use of PDE-5 inhibitors.

First-dose-success

Large cohort studies were able to show that even with the very first dose of a PDE-5 inhibitor, the overwhelming majority of patients with 87% SEP 2 rates (successful vaginal penetration) for vardenafil 10 mg [86], and with 79% SEP 2 rates for tadalfil 20 mg [88], could successfully be treated.

Safety

As shown in Table 7.5, the side effects observed with the use of PDE-5 inhibitors are principally the same, except for color and brightness visual disturbances, which almost exclusively occurred after sildenafil, and back/muscle pain being ob-

served in a small portion of patients after tadalafil. In the overwhelming majority, these drug-related adverse events were mild to moderate and resulted in only 1–2% of early drop-outs in the clinical trials.

Cardiovascular safety

As shown in Table 7.6, in all trials the risk for myocardial infarction and death per 100 patient-years with PDE-5 inhibitors was not greater than with placebo. In addition, several trials in patients with coronary artery disease were able to confirm that PDE-5 inhibitors do not have any detrimental effect on the cardiovascular safety, which is also valid for patients taking antihypertensives, regardless of the number of antihypertensives currently administered in the same patient [90–97]. Moreover, many patients currently taking nitrates can be withdrawn from this treatment without facing disadvantages, and can then be successfully treated with a PDE-5 inhibitor [98].

Occular safety

Just recently reports in the mass media that PDE-5 inhibitors may induce blindness due to so-called non-arteric anterior ischemic optic neuropathy (NAION), made patients unsure about the safety of these medications. Although at the moment the FDA could not see the proof for a causal connection between the cases reported and the use of PDE-5 inhibitors, the PDE-5 manufacturers were requested to include in their new label warnings about NAION. Conditions with a higher likelihood for NAION are: age > 50 years, heart disease, diabetes, hypertension, high cholesterol, nicotine use, certain eye problems.

Side effect	Sildenafil[88] (n = 5.918)	Vardenafil[89] (n = 2.203)	Tadalafi[70] (n = 804)
Headache	14.6%	14.5%	14%
Flush	14.1%	11.1%	4%
Dyspepsia	6.2%	3.7%	10%
Rhinitis	2.6%	9.2%	5%
Back pain	0%	0%	6%
Visual disturbances	5.2%	0%	0%

Table 7.5 Drug-related adverse events with the three PDE-5 inhibitors. Integrated analysis of pooled data from phase III trials.

Table 7.6 Cardiovascular safety of PDE-5 inhibitors in clinical trials.

Demographics	Sildenafil[90]		Vardenafil[91]		Tadalafil[92] (controlled trials)		Tadalafil treated[92] patients in all trials
Study drug	Placebo	Active	Placebo	Active	Placebo	Active	Active
Number patients	3.627	5.148	793	1.812	2.118	5.228	10.480
Mean age (years)	54	54	57	57	55	55	Not reported
Hypertension	28%	26%	35%		26%	27%	Not reported
Diabetes	26%	22%	30%		20%	20%	Not reported
CAD	10%	11%	7%		Not reported		Not reported
Dyslipidemia	12%	13%	24%		16%	15%	Not reported
MI/insult rate per 100 patient-years	0.84	0.80	0.4	0.05	0.41	0.26	0.33
Cardiac death per 100 patient-years	0.19	0.23	0%		Not reported		0.12

Overdose [56,57]

Sildenafil: doses of up to 800 mg increased dose–dependently the well-known drug-related adverse events, without occurrence of new side effects currently not seen under therapeutic doses. Tadalafil: single doses of up to 500 mg and daily dosing of 100 mg for three weeks (in this study design patients reached tadalafil plasma levels equivalent to 160 mg single dose), resulted in a dose-dependent increase in drug-related adverse events already observed under therapeutic doses, but no new unknown side effects occurred.

Non-responders to PDE-5 inhibitors

Of course there are real non-responders to PDE-5 inhibitors. Real non-responders mostly have a severe end-organ failure, which means that the cavernosal tissue has lost a considerable portion of its functional smooth musculature [99]. In the clinical setting these PDE-5 inhibitor non-responders show severe veno-occlusive dysfunction, with many of them also non-responding to intracavernosal injection of vasoactive drugs such as alprostadil or the trimix combination. Quite frequently this veno-occlusive dysfunction (syn: venous leak or cavernous insufficiency) is associated with severe impairment of the penile arterial blood supply in the penile color Doppler findings. But many so-called non-responders may be rescued by appropriate counseling, by treatment of concomitant diseases or change in medication use. The definition of a real non-responder is justified if no success is seen under the following conditions: use of at least four tablets with the highest dose of the respective PDE-5 inhibitor, at four different occasions, under optimal conditions (appropriate sexual stimulation, appropriate interval between tablet intake and sexual activity, with sildenafil and vardenafil—fasting conditions for two hours, and with tadalafil—keeping an interval of at least two hours between intake and sexual activity) (personal experience).

In the literature the following measures resulted in convincing salvage rates from previously defined PDE-5 non-responders:

1 Re-counseling of the patients/couples in the proper use of PDE-5 inhibitors, including especially

the use of the highest doses, with salvage rates of up to 60% depending on the study population under investigation [100–103].

2 Optimal treatment of concomitant diseases, such as optimal diabetes control (elevated gycosylated hemoglobin can directly impair the relaxant capacity of the cavernosal smooth musculature [104]) or hypertension control. In addition, treatment of hypercholesterolemia with statins such as atorvastatin were able to improve erectile function per se, due to the fact that statins decrease low density lipoprotein (LDL) levels and subsequently the negative effect of oxidized LDL on endothelial function [105].

3 Treatment of concomitant hypogonadism. As it is proven that testosterone regulates the expression of PDE-5 and the responsiveness to PDE-5 inhibitors in the corpus cavernosum [106], and that androgens per se improve the cavernous vasodilation [107], hypogonadal men with ED show principally a poorer responsiveness to PDE-5 inhibitors and also other erectogenic drugs. In this regard many authors have provided evidence that hypogonadal ED patients, originally unresponsive to PDE-5 inhibitors, may be rescued by testosterone replacement therapy [108–110].

4 "High dose" (overdosing) PDE-5 inhibitor therapy i.e. doubling the maximum dose, resulted in a 24% salvage rate of ED patients (n = 54) previously unresponsive to 100 mg sildenafil [111]. According to personal experience, this concept may also apply for vardenafil and tadalafil in suitable patients—especially in unresponsive diabetics.

5 Shifting patients to another PDE-5 inhibitor: Shifting of real non-responders from sildenafil to vardenafil resulted in a rescue success rate of 12% [112]. According to personal experience with more than 7000 patients on PDE-5 inhibitors, only a small minority (5–8%) of real non-responders (vaginal penetration not possible after four attempts with the highest dose) to one PDE-5 may be rescued by another one.

6 Daily dosing with PDE-5 inhibitors for several months in patients, previously unresponsive, is able to rescue more than 50% of failures [113,114]. Although this was proven for sildenafil and tadalafil, it can be assumed that this also holds true for all PDE-5

inhibitors, in particular in patients with severe organic ED.

Chronic daily dosing of PDE-5 inhibitors

Although all three PDE-5 inhibitors were developed and approved for as-needed use, many experts in this field moved to daily dosing, provided the patients could afford it. Daily dosing of PDE-5 inhibitors at bed time became a successful treatment option in early sexual rehabilitation of patients after nerve-sparing radical prostatectomy [116–118]. But beyond this indication, daily dosing with PDE-5 inhibitors turned out to be very successful in non-responders to on-demand treatment [113], supported by personal observations and also increased nocturnal erection events in healthy men [119–120]. According to personal experience with more than 100 patients currently on daily dosing with tadalafil 5–10 mg, this concept is very promising for organic ED patients with several cardiovascular risk factors, and relieves the patients from scheduling sexual activities. This is especially welcomed by their partners. In addition, chronic dosing with PDE-5 inhibitors, either short-acting (here sildenafil) or long-acting (tadalafil), resulted in improvement of endothelial dysfunction. This holds true not only for the cavernous bodies, but also for the endothelium in the whole vascular system [121–123]. In this regard it may be speculated that daily dosing with PDE-5 inhibitors may have long-term beneficial effects on the whole vascular system, and perhaps also on voiding difficulties related with benign prostate hyperplasia, as PDE-5 is widely distributed within the prostate [124].

Conclusions on PDE-5 inhibitors

As described in the extension to this chapter, all three PDE-5 inhibitors are very effective and safe and can be applied to nearly all ED patients, with the exception of those under nitrate or NO donor medications and those suffering from very severe eye diseases (retinitis pigmentosa and NAION). In terms of efficacy they are not really distinguishable, although it might quite often happen in the daily routine use of these drugs that one PDE-5 inhibitor produces better erections in an individual than the other one, or one PDE-5 inhibitor might be better tolerated than the other. In this regard it seems to be wise and reasonable to offer the patients the option to try all three drugs in order to choose the optimal one for long-term use. Daily dosing with PDE-5 inhibitors seems to be a very promising new option, especially in difficult to treat patients—provided they can afford it.

Other Oral Drugs Used but not Approved for ED

Trazodone

Trazodone, approved for the treatment of depression, is a centrally-acting, selective serotonin re-uptake inhibitor**,** which inhibits cerebral serotonin turnover. Trazodone's α-adrenoceptor blocking properties are a further important function of trazodone in relation to its erection-inducing effect. Both Saenz de Tejada *et al.* and Azadzoi *et al.* demonstrated that trazodone inhibits contraction of the cavernous smooth muscle, i.e. it facilitates relaxation. [125,126].

It is still unclear which of the two effects (serotonin re-uptake inhibition or blocking of α-adrenoceptors) is more important with respect to the erection-inducing properties of trazodone. The success rates of trazodone in placebo-controlled trials were up to 67% vs. 39% for placebo [127–129].

Side effects occur relatively often during trazodone treatment and may be attributed to its cerebral effects, via interference with serotonin metabolism, and to its peripheral, anti-adrenergic properties. The most common side effects described so far are marked fatigue and sleepiness, headache, dizziness, fall in blood pressure and nausea. Patients find the marked fatigue and dizziness particularly troublesome and they are the mostly the cause for premature discontinuation rates in 20–30% of cases (130, personal experience).

Conclusions

In the era of very successful PDE-5 inhibitors the only indication for an attempt with trazodone appears to be the constellation of psychogenic ED and concomitant depression. In this regard it has to be mentioned that the literature contains reports of more than 200 cases of priapism associated with trazodone therapy.

Phentolamine (Vasomax®)

Phentolamine is a competitive, non-selective α_1- and α_2-adrenoceptor antagonist, which blocks both presynaptic and postsynaptic α-adrenoceptors. This explains its general cardiovascular effects, such as lowering of blood pressure. Its proerectile effects, when injected directly into the cavernous bodies, were described by several authors [131,132]. The real breakthrough for phentolamine came when it was successfully used along with papaverine for intracavernous self-injection therapy, which is still in place to date [133]. The same author [134] described successes in 21 out of 69 cases (30%), with a new buccally-administered preparation of phentolamine (20 mg).

Phentolamine mesylate in tablet form for oral administration was developed by Zonagen, and has been tested for efficacy and safety between 1995 and 1997 in three large multicenter studies in Germany, Mexico and the USA [135,136].

Oral phentolamine was temporarily approved in some countries of South America in 40 mg tablets, but was withdrawn early from the market due both to its very limited efficacy, and to the fact that the FDA refused its approval in the US because it was said to induce brownish discoloration of the fat tissue in rats.

L-arginine

L-arginine is the precursor of NO synthesis (Fig. 7.1). Zorgniotti *et al.* conducted a placebo-controlled study with 2800 mg L-arginine per day in 20 impotent men for two weeks. Of the 15 men who completed the study, six reported an improvement in the ability to achieve an erection, nine experienced no improvement [137].

In a placebo-controlled, crossover study on 21 patients with ED of different etiology, the efficacy of 500 mg L-arginine applied three times daily, was tested over a period of twice 17 days without showing a superiority over the placebo [138].

A high-dose, prospective, randomized, double-blind and placebo-controlled study with 5g L-arginine per day for six weeks was conducted in 50 patients (aged 55–75 years) with organic, complete ED (unable to perform coitus), for at least six months [139]. This study resulted in success rates (sexual intercourse possible) of 31% in the L-arginine group, compared to 12% in the placebo group. It was interesting to note that significantly higher urine concentrations of the stable NO metabolites, NO_2 and NO_3, were measured in the arginine responders than in the non-responders, although the responders had lower urine concentrations of NO_3 prior to treatment. Thus the question arises as to whether supraphysiologic doses of L-arginine given over a long period of time can lead to a permanent improvement in cavernous function in some of the ED patients. No side effects were observed, except a fall in blood pressure of maximum 10% in some patients, which did not result in clinical symptoms.

Gingko biloba extract

In a prospective, double-blind and placebo-controlled study in 32 patients, the efficacy of gingko biloba was evaluated over a period of 24 weeks [140]. Gingko biloba did not result in a subjective, or a statistically significant objective (NPT testing)—improvement of erection.

Korean red ginseng

In a three arm, placebo-controlled study with trazodone, placebo or ginseng in 90 patients (30 in each arm), global efficacy rates of 60% (p < 0.05) were reported for ginseng and 30% for both placebo and trazodone [140]. The erection-promoting effect of ginseng is attributed to its saponin content, although its exact mechanism of action is unclear.

References

1 Fleischer K, Hirsch-Tabor O. Zur Potenzierung der Yohimbine-Wirkung. *Münchner Med Wochenschrift* 1923;**51**:1506–1508.

2 Ernst E, Pittler MH. Yohimbine for erectile dysfunction: A systematic review and meta-analysis of randomized clinical trials. *J Urol* 1998;**159**:433–436.

3 Saenz de Tejada I. Commentary on mechanisms for the regulation of penile smooth muscle contractility. *J Urol* 1995;**153**:1762.

4 Köhler LD, Borelli S, Vogt HJ. Yohimbin-HCL in der Behandlung von Erektionsstörungen. *Sexuologie* 1995;**3**:209–217.

5 Owen JA, Nakatsu SL, Fenemore J, *et al*. The pharmacokinetics of yohimbine in man. *Eur J Clin Pharmacol* 1987;**32**:577–582.

6 Hedner T, Edgar B, Edvinsson L, *et al*. Yohimbine pharmacokinetics and interaction with the sympathetic nervous system in normal volunteers. *Eur J Clin Pharmacol* 1992;**43**:651–656.

7 Telöken C, Rhoden EL, Sogari P, *et al*. Therapeutic effects of high dose yohimbine hydrochloride on organic erectile dysfunction. *J Urol* 1998;**159**:122–124.

8 Vogt HJ, Brandl P, Kockott G. Double-blind, placebo-controlled safety and efficacy trial with yohimbine hydrochloride in the treatment of non-organic erectile dysfunction. *Int J Impotence Res* 1997;**9**:155–161.

9 Hartmann U, Stief CG, Djamilian M, *et al*. Therapieversuch der erektilen dysfunktion mit oraler. Medikation bei selktionierten patienten. *Urologe B* 1991;**31**:204–206.

10 Kunelius P, Häkkinen J, Lukkarinen O. Is high-dose yohimbine hydrochloride effective in the treatment of mixed-type impotence? A prospective, randomized, placebo controlled double-blind cross-over study. *Urology* 1997;**49**:441–444.

11 Montague DK, Barada JH, Belker AM, *et al*. Clinical guidelines panel on erectile dysfunction: summary report on the treatment of organic erectile dysfunction. *J Urol* 1996;**156**:2007–2011.

12 Montague D, Jarow JJ, Broderick GA, *et al*. Chapter 1: The management of erectile dysfunction: An AUA Update. *J Urol* 2005;**174**:230–239.

13 Adeniyi AA, Andrews HD, Helal MA, *et al*. Yohimbine in orgasmic dysfunction. *Int J Impotence Res* 2000;**12**:(Suppl.5),S7:26.

14 Grossman E, Rosenthal T, Peleg E, *et al*. Oral yohimbine increases blood pressure and sympathetic nervous outflow in hypertensive patients. *J Cardiovascul Pharmacol* 1993;**22**:22–26.

15 Mathiesen A, Wright CRA. Researches into the chemical constitution of the opium bases. Part I. On the action of hydrochloric acid on morphine. *Proc R Soc London B Biol Sci* 1869;**17**:455–462.

16 Cotzias GC, van Woert MH, Schiffer LM. Aromatic amino acids and modification of parkinsonism. *N Engl J Med* 1967;**276**:374–379.

17 Lal S, Laryea E, Thavundayil JX, *et al*. Apomorphine-induced penile tumescence in impotent patients. *Prog Neuopsychopharmacol Biol Psychiatry* 1987;**11**:235–242.

18 Heaton JPW, Morales A, Adams MA, *et al.* Recovery of erectile function by the oral administration of apomorphine. *Urology* 1995;**45**:200–206.

19 Andersson KE, Steers WD. The pharmacologic basis of sexual therapeutics. In Morales, A, ed. *Erectile Dysfunction. Issues in Current Pharmacotherapy*. London: Martin Dunitz Ltd, 1998, pp. 97–124.

20 Chen KK, Chan JYH, Chan SHH, *et al.* Elicitation of penile erection after administration of apomorphine to paraventricular nucleus of hypothalamus in the rat. *Int J Impotence Res* 1996;**8**:No.3,105.

21 Chen KK, Chan JYH, Chan SHH, *et al.* Testes-dependent elicitation of penile erection after administration of apomorphine into paraventricular nucleus of hypothalamus in the rat. *J Urol* 1997;**157**:No.4,35.

22 Melis MR, Argiolas A. Nitric oxide synthase inhibitors prevent apomorphine- and oxytocin-induced penile erection and yawning in male rats. *Brain Research Bulletin* 1993;**32**:71–74.

23 Paick JS, Lee SW. The neural mechanism of apomorphine-induced erection: an experimental study by comparison with electrostimulation-induced erection in the rat model. *J Urol* 1994;**152**:2125–2128.

24 Tarcan T, Goldstein I, Park K, *et al.* Systemic administration of apomorphine increases clitoral and vaginal arterial inflow in the rabbit. *Int J Impotence Res* 1998;**10**:(Suppl.3),S58.

25 Giuliano F, Allard J, Rampin U, *et al.* Proerectile effect of apomorphine delivered at the spinal level in anaesthetized rat. *Int J Impotence Res* 2000;**12**:(Suppl.3),S66:A22.

26 Argiolas A, Hedlund H. The pharmacology and clinical pharmacokinetics of apomorphine SL. *BJU International* 2001;**88**:(Suppl.3),18–21.

27 Stief C, Padley RJ, Perdok RJ, Sleep DJ. Cross-study review of the clinical efficacy of apomorphine SL 2 and 3 mg: Pooled data from three placebo-controlled, fixed-dose cross-over studies. *Eur Urol* 2002;(Suppl.1):12–36.

28 Heaton J, Sleep D, Perdok R, *et al.* Efficacy and safety of Uprima (apomorphine SL) in patients with documented comorbidities of hypertension, coronary artery disease (CAD) or diabetes. *Int J Impotence Res* 2001;**13**:(Suppl.4),S32,Abstr.87.

29 Gontero P, Antonio RD, Pretti G, *et al.* Clinical efficacy of apomorphine SL in erectile dysfunction of diabetic men. *Int J Impotence Res* 2005;**17**:80–85.

30 Pavone C, Curto F, Anello G, *et al.* Prospective, randomized, cross-over comparison of sublingual apomorphine (3 mg) with oral sildenafil (50 mg) for male erectile dysfunction. *J Urol* 2004;**172**:2347–2349.

31 Eardley I, Wright P, MacDonagh R, *et al.* An open-label, randomised, flexible-dose, crossoverstudy to assess the comparative efficacy and safety of sildenafil citrate and apomorphine hydrochloride in men with erectile dysfunction. *BJU Int* 2004;**93**:1271–1275.

32 Porst H, Jacob G, Albrecht S. Sildenafil (Viagra®) versus apomorphin in der behandlung der erektilen dysfunktion (ED): Multizentrische, offene, randomisierte,cross-over studie. *Urologe* 2004;(Suppl.1), S65.

33 Ralph DJ, Sleep DJ, Perdok RJ, Padley RJ. Adverse events and patient tolerability of apomorphine SL 2 and 3 mg: a cross-study analysis of phase II and II studies. *Eur Urol* 2002;(Suppl.1):21–27.

34 Beavo JA. Cyclic nucleotide phosphodiesterases: functional implications of multiple isoforms. *Physiol Reviews* 1995;**75**:No.4:725–748.

35 Corbin JD, Francis SH, Webb D. Phosphodiesterase type 5 as a pharmacologic target in erectile dysfunction. *Urology* 2002;**60**:Suppl:SB,4–11.

36 Corbin JD, Francis SH. Pharmacology of phosphodiesterase 5 inhibitors. *IJCP* 2002;**56**(6):453–459.

37 Maurice DH. Phsophodiesteraes and sexual function and dysfunction. Presented at the ISSIR Symposium, Molecular Mechanisms of Erectile Function at the 4th Biennal Congress of ESSIR, Rome, 29 September 2001.

38 Rybalkin SD, Beavo JA. Multiplicity within cyclic nucleotide phosphodiesterases. *Biochemical Society Transactions* 1997;**24**:1005–1009.

39 Küthe A, Wiedenroth A, Mägert HJ, *et al.* Expression of different phosphodiesterase genes in human cavernosum smooth muscle. *J Urol* 2001;**165**:280–283.

40 Corbin JD. Mechanism of action of PDE-5 inhibition in erectile dysfunction. *Int J Impotence Res* 2004; **16**:(Suppl.1),S4–S7.

41 Gantert LT, Drisko JE, Nargund RP, *et al.* Melanocortin 4-receptor and 5 HT2C receptor modulation of erectogenesis in conscious rats as reported by telemetric measurement of intracavernous pressure. *Int J Impotence Res*. 2001;**13**:(Suppl.5),S53,Abstr.6.

42 Lindia JA, Nargund R, Sebhat J, *et al.* Erectogenic effects of a selective melanocortin-4 receptor (MC 4-R) agonist in a rat model of erectile activity. *Int J Impotence Res* 2001;**13**:(Suppl.5),S55,2001.

43 McGowan E, Cashen DE, Drisco JE, *et al.* Activation of melanocortin-4 receptor (MC 4-R) increases erectile activity in rats. *Int J Impotence Res* 2001;**13**:(Suppl.5), S55,Abstr.13.

44 Francis SH, Turko IV, Corbin JD. Cyclic nucleotide phosphodiesterases: relating structure and function. *Prog Nucleic Acid Res Mol Biol* 2001;**65**:1–52.

45 Hetman JM, Soderling SH, Glavas NA, *et al*. Cloning and characterization of PDE 7B a cAMP-specific phosphodiesterase. *PNAS* 2000;**97**:472–476.

46 Fawcett L, Baxendale R, Stacey P, *et al*. Molecular cloning and characterization of a distinct human phosphodiesterase gene family: PDE 11 A. *Proc Natl Acad Sci* 2000;**97**:3702–3707.

47 Üeckert S, Kuethe A, Stief CG, *et al*. Phosphodiesterase isoenzymes as pharmacological targets in the treatment of male erectile dysfunction. *World J Urol* 2001; **19**:14–22.

48 Rosen RC, Riley A, Wagner G, *et al*. The international index of erectile function (IIEF): A multidimensional scale for assessment of erectile dysfunction. *Urology* 1997;**49**:822–830.

49 Gbekor E, Bethell S, Fawcett L, *et al*. Phosphodiesterase 5 inhibitor profiles against all human phosphodiesterase families: Implications for use as pharmacological tools. *J Urol* 2002;**167**:No.4 Suppl, p. 246 Abstr.967.

50 Padma-Nathan H, Stecher VJ, Sweeny J, *et al*. Minimal time to successful intercourse after sildenafil citrate: Results of a randomized, double-blind, placebo-controlled trial. *Urology* 2003;**62**:400–403.

51 Montorsi F, Padma-Nathan H, Buvat J, *et al*. Earliest time of action leading to successful intercourse with Vardenafil determined in an at-home setting: a randomized, double-blind, placebo-controlled trial. *J Sex Med* 2004;**1**:168–178.

52 Rosen R, Padma-Nathan H, Shabsigh R, *et al*. Determining the earliest time within 30 minutes to erectogenic effect after Tadalafil 10 and 20 mg: a multicenter, randomized, double-blind, placebo-controlled, at-home study. *J Sex Med* 2004;**1**: 193–200.

53 Patterson B, Bedding A, Hayley J, Chris P, Male M. Dose normalized pharmacokinetics of tadalafil administered as single dose to healthy volunteers. *Eur Urol* 2002;(Suppl.1), pp. 152.

54 Porst H, Padma-Nathan H, Giuliano F, *et al*. Efficacy of tadalafil for the treatment of erectile dysfunction at 24 and 36 hours after dosing: A randomized controlled trial. *Urology* 2003;**62**:121–125.

55 Young JM, Feldman RA, Auerbach SM, *et al*. Tadalafil improved function at twenty-four and thirty-six hours after dosing in men with erectile dysfunction: US trial. *J Androl* 2005;**26**:310–318.

56 Viagra (sildenafil citrate) US Labe (LAB-0221–2.4, July 2005).

57 Cialis (tadalafil) US Label, July 2005.

58 Levitra (vardenafil HCL) US-Label, July 2005.

59 Bischoff E. Vardenafil preclinical trial data: potency, pharmacodynamics, pharmacokinetics, and adverse events. *Int J Impotence Res* 2004;**16**:S34–S37.

60 Porst H, Sharlip ID, Hatzichristou D, *et al*. Extended duration of efficacy when taken 8 hours before intercourse: a randomized, double-blind placebo-controlled study. *Eur Urol* 2006, *in* press.

61 Blount MA, Beasley A, Zoraghi R, *et al*. Binding of tritiated sildenafil, tadlafil, or vardenafil to the phosphodiesterase-5 catalytic site displays potency, specifity, heterogenity, and cGMP stimulation. *Molecular Pharmacology* 2004;**66**:144–152.

62 Gingel C, Sultana SR, Wulff MB, *et al*. Duration of action of sildenafil citrate in men with erectile dysfunction. *J Sex Med* 2004;**1**:179–184.

63 Moncada I, Jara J, Subira D, *et al*. Efficacy of sildenafil citrate at 12 hours after dosing: Reexploring the therapeutic window. *Eur Urol* 2004;**46**:357–361.

64 Rajagopalan P, Mazzu A, Xia C, *et al*. Pharmacokinetics of the PDE-5 inhibitor vardenafil following a high-fat breakfast and a moderate-fat evening meal. *Int J Impotence Res* 2002;**14**:(Suppl.4),S64.

65 Patterson B, Bedding A, Jewell H, *et al*. The effect of intrinsic and extrinsic factors on the pharmacokinetic properties of tadalafil (IC351). *Int J Impotence Res* 2001;**13**:(Suppl.4),S43,Abstr.120.

66 Giuliano F, Kaplan S, Fournier P, *et al*. Tadalafil shows no clinically significant hemodynamic interaction with alfuzosin. *Eur Urol* 2005;(Suppl.4), pp. 137.

67 Kloner R, Jackson G, Emmick JT, *et al*. Interaction between the phosphodiesterase 5 inhibitor tadalafil and two alpha-blockers doxazosin and tamsulosin. *J Urol* 2004;**171**:(Suppl.315).

68 Kloner RA, Hutter AM, Emmick JT, *et al*. Time course of the interaction between tadalafil and nitrates. *J Am Coll Cardiol* 2003;**42**:1855–1860.

69 Webb DJ, Freestone S, Allen MJ, *et al*. Sildenafil citrate and blood pressure lowering drugs: results of drug interaction studies with an organic nitrate and a calcium antagonist. *Am J Cardiol* 1999;**83**:21C–28C.

70 Brock GB, McMahon CG, Chen KK, *et al*. Efficacy and safety of tadalafil for the treatment of erectile dysfunction: Results of integrated analyses. *J Urol* 2002;**168**:1332–1336.

71 Porst H, Rosen R, Padma-Nathan H, *et al*. The efficacy and tolerability of vardenafil, a new, oral, selective phosphodiesterase type 5 inhibitor, in patients with erectile dysfunction: the first at-home clinical trial. *Int J Impotence Res* 2001;**13**:192–199.

72 Hellstrom WJG, Gittelman M, Karling G, *et al*. Vardenafil for treatment of men with erectile dysfunction:

Efficacy and safety in a randomized,double-blind, placebo-controlled trial. *J Andrology* 2002;**23**: 763–771.

73 Rendell MS, Rajfer J, Wicker PA, *et al.* Sildenafil for treatment of erectile dysfunction in men with diabetes. *JAMA* 1999;**281**:421–426.

74 Saenz de Tejada I, Anglin G, Knight JR, *et al.* Effects of tadalafil on erectile dysfunction in men with diabetes. *Diabetes Care* 2002;**25**:2159–2164.

75 Goldstein I, Young JM, Fischer J, *et al.* Vardenafil, a new phosphodiesterase type 5 inhibitor, in the treatment of erectile dysfunction in men with diabetes. *Diabetes Care* 2003;**26**:1–7.

76 Montorsi F, Padma-Nathan H, McCullough AM, *et al.* Tadalafil in the treatment of erectile dysfunction following bilateral nerve sparing radical retropubic prostatectomy: A randomized, double-blind, placebo-controlled trial. *J Urol* 2004;**172**:1036–1041.

77 Brock G, Mehra A, Lipschultz LL, *et al.* Safety and efficacy of tadalafil for the treatment of men with erectile dysfunction after radical retropubic prostatectomy. *J Urol* 2003;**170**:1278–1283.

78 Fink HA, McDonald R, Rutks IR, *et al.* Sildenafil for male erectile dysfunction. A systematic review and metaanalysis. *Arch Intern Med* 2002;**162**: 1349–1360.

79 Montorsi F, Verheyden B, Meuleman E, *et al.* Long-term safety and tolerability of tadalafil in the treatment of erectile dysfunction. *Eur Urol* 2004;**45**:339–345.

80 Stief C, Porst H, Saenz de Tejada I, *et al.* Sustained efficacy and tolerability with vardenafil over 2 years of treatment in men with erectile dysfunction. *Int J Clin Pract* 2004;**58**:230–239.

81 Vernet D, Magee TR, Qian A, *et al.* Tadalafil does not upregulate the expression and activity of phosphodiesterase 5 (PDE-5) in the penis. *J Urol* 2005;**173**: (Suppl.287).

82 Donatucci C, Taylor T, Thibonnier M, *et al.* Vardenafil improves patient satisfaction with erection hardness, orgasmic function, and overall sexual experience, while improving quality of life in men with erectile dysfunction. *J Sex Med* 2004;**1**:185–192.

83 Hatzichristou D, Cuzin B, Martin-Morales A, *et al.* Vardenafil improves satisfaction rates, depressive symptomatology, and self confidence in a broad population of men with erectile dysfunction. *J Sex Med* 2005; **2**:109–116.

84 Montorsi F, Althof SE. Partner responses to sildenafil citrate (Viagra) treatment of erectile dysfunction *Urology* 2004;**63**:762–767.

85 Althof SE, Eid JF, Talley DR, *et al.* Tadalafil is an effective treatment for men with erectile dysfunction as confirmed by their partners. *J Sex Med* 2004; (Suppl.1),41 Abstr.O39.

86 Valiquette LB, Young J, Porst H, *et al.* Reliability and safety of vardenafil 10 mg for the treatment of erectile dysfunction; the reliability-vardenafil for erectile dysfunction (RELY I) trial. *J Sex Med* 2004;(Suppl.1),78 Abstr.MP57.

87 Schulman CC, Shen W, Stothard DR, *et al.* Integrated analysis examining first-dose success, success by dose , and maintenance of success among men taking tadlafil for erectile dysfunction. *Urology* 2004;**64**:783–788.

88 Padma-Nathan H, Eardley I, Kloner RA, Laties AM, Montorsi F. 4 year update on the safety of sildenafil citrate (Viagra®). *Urology* 2002;**60**:(Suppl.2B):67–90.

89 Kloner R, Porst H, Mohan P, Norenberg C, Pomerantz K, Segerson T, Glasser S. Cardiovascular safety of the selective PDE-5 inihibitor vardenafil in patients with erectile dysfunction; an analysis of five placebo-controlled clinical trials. *Int J Impotence Res* 2002;**14**: (Suppl.4),S22.

90 Mittelman MA, Glasser DB, Orezam J. Clinical trials of sildenafil citrate (Viagra®) demonstrate no increase in risk of myocardial infarction and cardiovascular death. *Int J Clin Pract* 2003;**57**:597–600.

91 Porst H, Kloner RA, Mohan P, *et al.* Cardiovascular safety of the selective PDE-5 inhibitor vardenafil in patients with erectile dysfunction;an analysis of five placebo-controlled clinical trials. *Int J Impotence Res* 2002;**14**:S22,Abstr.P-O92.

92 Jackson G, Kloner RA, Costigan T, *et al.* Update on clinical trials of tadalafil demonstrates no increased risk of cardiovascular adverse events. *J Sex Med* 2004;**1**:161–167.

93 Boshier A, Wilton LV, Shakir SA. Evaluation of the safety of sildenafil for male erectile experience gained in general practice use in England. *BJU International* 2004;**93**:796–801.

94 Wysowski DK, Farinas E, Swartz L. Comparison of reported and expected deaths in sildenafil (Viagra) users. *Am J Cardiol* 2002;**89**:1331–1334.

95 Rosano GMC, Leonardo F, Pagotta F, *et al.* Effects of phosphodiesterase-5 inhibition on myocardial ischemia in patients with chronic stable angina in therapy with β-blockers. *Eur Heart J* 1999;**20**:(Suppl.541), Abstr.P2846.

96 Chen YJ, Du R, Traverse JH, *et al.* Effect of sildenafil on coronary active and reactive hyperemia. *Circulation* 1999;**100**:(Suppl.1),Abstr.3772.

97 White WB, Hellstrom W, Norenberg C, *et al.* Cardio-vascular safety of vardenafil in patients on antihy-pertensives and/or α-blockers: analysis of 17 placebo-controlled trials. Presented at the World-Congress on Sexology, Montreal, 2005.

98 Jackosn G, Martin E, McGing E, *et al.* Successful with-drawal of oral long-acting nitrates to facilitate phos-phodiesterase type 5 inhibitor use in stable coronary disease patients with erectile dysfunction. *J Sex Med* 2005;**2**:513–516.

99 Wespes E, Rammal A, Garbar C. Sildenafil non-repon-ders: hemodynamic and morphometric studies. *Eur Urology* 2005;**48**:136–139.

100 Atiemo HO, Szostak MJ, Sklar GN. Salvage of silde-nafil failures referred from primary care physicians. *J Urol* 2003;**170**:2356–2358.

101 Jiann B-P, Yu C-C, Huang J-K. Rechallenge prior silde-nafil non-responders. *Int J Impotence Res* 2004; **16**:64–68.

102 Vardi Y, Chen Y, Sheinfield O, *et al.* A multi-center study, evaluating the effect of instruction and redosing of sildenafil failures. *Int J Impotence Res* 2002;**14**: (Suppl.4),S15,Abstr.PS-4–4.

103 Hatzimouratidis K, Hatzichristou G. Treatment options for erectile dysfunction in patients failing oral drug therapy. *EAU Update Series* 2004;**2**:75–83.

104 Cartledge J, Eardley J, Orchard C, *et al.* Impairment of corpus cavernosal smooth muscle relaxation by glycosylated haemoglobin. *Eur Urol* 1999;**35**: (Suppl.2), 100,Abstr.399.

105 Saltzman EA, Guay AT, Jacobson J: Improvement in erectile function in men with organic erectile dysfunc-tion by correction of elevated cholesterol levels: a clin-ical observation. *J Urol* 2004;**172**:255–258.

106 Zhang X-H, Morelli A, Luconi M, *et al.* Testosterone regulates PDE-5 expression and in vivo responsive-ness to tadalafil in rat corpus cavernosum. *Eur Urol* 2005;**47**:409–416.

107 Aversa A, Isidori AM, Spera G, *et al.* Androgens improve cavernous vasodilation and response to silde-nafil in patients with erectile dysfunction. *Clin Endocrinol* 2003;**58**:632–638.

108 Shabsigh R, Kaufman JM, Steidle C, Padma-Nathan H. Randomized study of testosterone gel as adjunctive therapy to sildenafil in hypogonadal men with erectile dysfunction who do not respond to sildenafil alone. *J Urol* 2004;**172**:658–663.

109 Kalinchenko SY, Kozlov GL, Gontcharov NP, Katsiya GV. Oral testosterone undecanoate reverses erectile dysfunction associated with diabetes mellitus in patients failing sildenafil citrate alone. *Aging Male* 2003;**6**:94–99.

110 Schulman C, Destraix R, Roumeguere T. Testosterone and PDE-5 inhibitors non responders. *J Sex Med* 2004;**1**:(Suppl.1),57 Abstr.O89.

111 McMahon C. High dose Sildenafil citrate as a salvage therapy for erectile dysfunction. *Int J Impotence Res* 2002;**14**:(Suppl.3),S89,Abstr,P5.11.

112 Brisson TE, Broderick GA, Pinkstaff DM. Can patients failing a PDE-5 inhibitor be rescued by another tablet?: An objective assessment of 351 patients with erectile dysfunction. *J Urol* 2005;**173**:(Suppl.236), Abstr.871.

113 McMahon C. Efficacy and safety of daily tadalafil in men with erectile dysfunction previously unrespon-sive to on demand tadalafil. *J Sex Med* 2004;**1**:292–300.

114 Porst H. Salvagetherapie mit täglicher dosierung von sildenafil bei non-respondern auf on-demand therapie mit 100 mg sildenafil. *Urologe A* 2003;**42**: (Suppl.1),S93.

115 McMahon C. Comparison of efficacy, safety and toler-ability of on-demand tadalafil and daily dosed tadalafil for the treatment of erectile dysfunction. *J Sex Med* 2005;**2**:415–427.

116 Montorsi F, Maga T, Strambi LF, *et al.* Sildenafil at bed-time significantly increases nocturnal erections: results of a placebo-controlled study. *Urology* 200;**56**:906–911.

117 Padma-Nathan H, McCullough A, Guiliano F, *et al.* Postoperative nightly administration of sildenafil cit-rate significantly improves the return of normal spon-taneous erectile function after bilateral nerve-sparing radical prostatectomy. *J Urol* 2003;**169**:375 Abstr.1402.

118 Schwartz EJ, Wong P, Graydon RJ. Sildenafil preserves intracorporeal smooth muscle after radical l retropu-bic prostatectomy. *J Urol* 2004;**171**:771–774.

119 Yaman Ö, Tokath Z, Inal T, *et al.* Effect of sildenafil on nocturnal erections of potent men. *Int J Impotence Res* 2003;**15**:117–121.

120 Chen J, Piero M, Greenstein A, *et al.* Effects of sildenafil on quality of erection in healthy volunteers-NPT Rigiscan. *Int J Impotence Res* 2003;**15**:(Suppl.6),S58, Abstr.P-O29.

121 Ahn GJ, Kim JM, Choi SM, *et al.* Effects of chronic treatment with a phosphodiesterase type inhibitor on erectile function in spontaneously hypertensive rats. *J Sex Med* 2004;**1**:(Suppl.1),63 Abstr.MP7.

122 Behr-Roussel D, Gorny D, Mevel K, *et al.* Chronic sildenafil improves erectile function and endothelium-dependent cavernosal relaxations in rats: Lack of tachyphylaxis. *Eur Urol* 2005;**47**:87–91.

123 Rosano GMC, Aversa A, Vitale C, *et al.* Chronic treatment with tadalafil improves endothelial function in men with increased cardiovascular risk. *Eur Urol* 2005;**47**:214–222.

124 Montorsi F, Corbin J, Pillips S. Review of phosphodiesterases in the urogenital system: New directions for therapeutic intervention. *J Sex Med* 2004;**1**: 322–336.

125 Azadzoi KM, Payton T, Krane RJ, *et al.* Effects of intracavernosal trazodone hydrochloride: animal and human studies. *J Urol* 1990;**144**:1277–1282.

126 Saenz de Tejada I, Ware JC, Blanco R, *et al.* Pathophysiology of prolonged penile erection associated with trazodone use. *J Urol* 1991;**145**:60–64.

127 Aydin S, Odabas O, Ercan M, *et al.* Efficacy of testosterone, trazodone and hypnotic suggestion in the treatment of non-organic male sexual dysfunction. *Brit J Urol* 1996;**77**:256–260.

128 Kurt Ü, Özkardes H, Altug U, *et al.* The efficacy of antiserotoninergic agents in the treatment of erectile dysfunction. *J Urol* 1994;**152**:407–409.

129 Lance R, Costabile RA, Albo M, *et al.* Oral trazodone for erectile dysfunction. *J Urol* 1995;**153**:(Suppl.473).

130 Meinhardt W, Schmitz PJM, Kropman RF, *et al.* Trazodone, a double blind trial for treatment of erectile dysfunction. *Int J Impotence Res* 1997;**9**:163–165.

131 Brindley GS. Cavernosal alpha-blockade: A new treatment for investigating and treating erectile impotence. *Br J Psychiatry* 1983;**143**:332–337.

132 Blum MD, Bahnson RR, Porter TN, *et al.* Effect of local alpha-adrenergic blockade on human penile erection. *J Urol* 1985;**134**:479–481.

133 Zorgniotti AW, Lefleur RS. Autoinjection of the corpus cavernosum with a vasoactive drug combination for vasculogenic impotence. *J Urol* 1985;**133**:39–41.

134 Zorgniotti AW: Experience with buccal phentolamine mesylate for impotence. *Int J Impotence Res* 1994;**6**:37–41.

135 Goldstein I, Ferguson D. Vasomax study group: Efficacy and safety of oral phentolamine (Vasomax™) for the treatment of erectile dysfunction using a crossover study design. *Int J Impotence Res* 1998;**10**: (Suppl.3),S61.

136 Porst H, Derouet H, Idzikowski, *et al.* Oral phentolamine (Vasomax®) in erectile dysfunction—Results of a german multicenter-study in 177 patients. *Int J Impotence Res* 1996;**8**:No.3,117.

137 Zorgniotti AW, Lizza EF. Effect of large doses of the nitric oxide precursor L-arginine on erectile dysfunction. *Int J Impotence Res* 1994;**6**:33–36.

138 Mathers M, Klotz T, Bloch W, *et al.* Effectiveness of oral L-arginine in the treatment of impotence in a prospective, randomized cross-over study. *Eur Urol* 1999;**35**(Suppl. 2), 67.

139 Chen J, Wollman Y, Chernichovsky T, *et al.* Effect of administration of high-dose nitric oxide donor L-arginine in men with organic erectile dysfunction: results of a double-blind, randomized, placebo- controlled study. *BJU International* 1999;**83**:269–273.

140 Sikora R, Sohn MH, Engelke B, *et al.* Randomized placebo-controlled study on the effects of oral treatment with gingko biloba extract in patients with erectile dysfunction. *J Urol* 1998;**159**:No.5,(Suppl.240).

141 Choi HK, Seong DH, Rha KH. Clinical efficacy of Korean red ginseng for erectile dysfunction. *Int J Impotence Res* 1995;**7**:181–186.

CHAPTER 8

Self-Injection, Trans-Urethral and Topical Therapy in Erectile Dysfunction

Hartmut Porst and Ganesan Adaikan

Self-Injection Therapy

The demonstration by Virag in 1982 that intracavernous (IC) injection of papaverine produced a fully-rigid erection in normal males, introduced a new route of administration in the clinical management of pharmacologic agents for the treatment of erectile failure [1,2]. Intracavernous injection of a vasoactive agent that readily produces erection has greatly simplified the multidisciplinary diagnostic investigations and management of erectile dysfunction (ED). Three groups of drugs are presently used for self-injection therapy worldwide, or at least in some parts of the world. These include papaverine, α-adrenoceptor blocking agents such as phentolamine or moxisylyte, and prostaglandin E1 (PGE_1). These compounds have proven to be effective in all etiologies of erectile failure such as psychogenic, neurogenic or vasculogenic impotence.

Other agents that have been investigated for their suitability in self-injection therapy, but never reached the stage of official approval or even off-label use, comprise calcium channel blocking agents, vasoactive intestinal polypeptide, ketanserin, histamine, β-adrenergic agonists, nitric oxide donors (linsidomine or sodium nitroprusside) etc. Generally speaking, compounds that were able to relax the smooth muscle cells of both the penile arteries and the cavernous tissue, subsequently resulting in blood engorgement of the cavernous sinusoidal spaces, with activation of the veno-occlusive mechanism through compression of the subtunical veins, may be principally considered for self-injection therapy in ED.

Up to 1998, self-injection therapy was the only effective pharmacologic treatment in ED and was considered a first-line option in this indication. But with the launch of sildenafil (Viagra®) IC self-injection therapy became generally a second-line option for the majority of ED patients, with the exception of those men in whom phosphodiesterase-5 (PDE-5) inhibitors were contraindicated, or turned out to be ineffective. In the following, the essential features of those compounds are described, which are either approved and/or mostly used, even in off-label use, for self-injection therapy.

Alprostadil (PGE_1—Caverject®, Edex®, Viridal®)

The effect of PGE_1 on the human corpus cavernosum (CC) was first described in 1975 by Karim & Adaikan [3]. Of more than 30 prostaglandins tested in vitro on the human CC, PGE_1 is the only compound that produced relaxation conducive for erection [4]. All other prostaglandins produced either a dual effect (contraction and relaxation) or contraction only. The relaxant effect of PGE_1 on the human CC has been further demonstrated in vitro [5,6]. Initial studies on the effectiveness and mechanism by which IC administration of PGE_1 produced erection were very encouraging [7–10]. Several investigators have assessed, in large groups of patients, the effectiveness of PGE_1 for the treatment of erectile failure in man.

PGE$_1$-induced relaxation of CC muscle is mediated through the activation of EP prostaglandin receptors and subsequent activation of the membrane bound adenylate cyclase, resulting in an increase in intracellular concentrations of cAMP in the cavernous tissue [11]. Further consequences of the PGE$_1$-mediated relaxation of human CC are the activation of maxi K channels, resulting in hyperpolarization and changes in transmembrane Ca^{2+} flux [12]. These effects are complimented by the ability of PGE$_1$ to inhibit the release of noradrenaline from sympathetic nerve endings and to suppress angiotensin II secretion in the cavernosal tissues [13,14] (Fig. 8.1).

Intracavernous injection of PGE$_1$ has definite advantages over the use of other drugs, such as the mixture of papaverine/phentolamine. PGE$_1$ is readily metabolized in the body by 15-hydroxyprostaglandin dehydrogenase, an enzyme that was identified in the human CC ([6]. The enzymic degradation of PGE$_1$ within the human CC probably contributes to the remarkably low incidence of undesirable side effects, such as prolonged erection and priapism.

PGE$_1$ was also shown to suppress the collagen synthesis by TGF-beta 1 in cultured human CC, suggesting that PGE$_1$ may play a key role in modulation/prevention of collagen synthesis with subsequent fibrosis of the CC [17]. This suppressive effect correlates well with the low incidence of local fibrotic lesions reported in PGE$_1$-injected primates and ED patients [15,18,19] (Table 8.2) and the unaltered intracavernous structures in patients with biopsies performed after intracavernous PGE$_1$ injection [20].

In the meta-analysis involving literature review and personal experience in 4577 patients with erectile failure, PGE$_1$ showed a response rate of more than 70% (Table 8.1) and compared to the mixture of papaverine and phentolamine, a considerably lower risk of priapism (0.35% versus 6%, respectively) as well as of local fibrotic complications such as penile nodules, indurations, or fibrosis during long-term injection therapy [15]. Intra-penile pain or tension following intracavernosal injection of PGE$_1$ is the other most frequently reported complaint in 7.2% of patients (Table 8.2). Except for rare cases of blood pressure decrease, no systemic side effects were observed after intracavernous injection of PGE$_1$ [15].

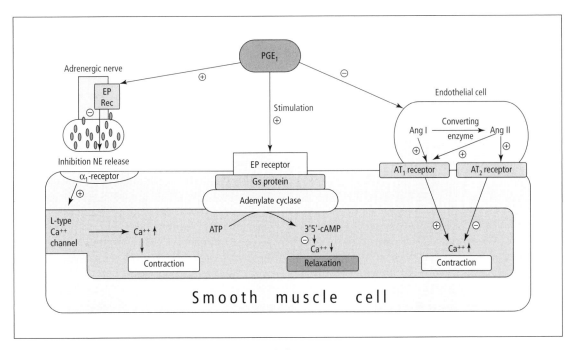

Fig. 8.1 Physiologic actions of alprostadil (PGE$_1$) on erectile function.

Table 8.1 Efficacy of vasoactive substances in the diagnosis of ED. Literature review of evaluable publications. From Porst [15].

Substance	Dose (Min/Max)	Publications	No. of patients	Responders
Papaverine	30/110 mg	19	2161	61% (987 out of 1,616)
Papaverine/ phentolamine	15 mg/1.25 mg 60 mg/2 mg	13	3016	68.5% (2065 out of 3,016)
PGE$_1$ (alprostadil)	5 μg/40 μg	27	10353	72.6% (7519 out of 10,353)

Table 8.2 Side effects of vasoactive substances in intracavernous injection treatment. Literature review of evaluable publications. From Porst [15].

Substance	N	No. Publications	Priapism >6 h	Fibrosis	Pain	Elevated liver enzyme
Papaverine	1527	15	7.1% (92 out of 1300)	5.7% (60 out of 1056)	4% (18 out of 452)	1.6% (5 out of 314)
Papaverine/ phentolamine	2263	22	7.8% (122 out of 1561)	12.4% (288 out of 1843)	11.6% (141 out of 1215)	5.4% (43 out of 799)
PGE$_1$ (alprostadil)	2745	10	0.36% (10 out of 2745)	0.8% (18 out of 2180)	7.2% (40 out of 558)	0%

There are data indicating that intracavernosal PGE$_1$ therapy may also promote transient, partial or complete restoration of spontaneous erections. Although the mechanism of this effect is not clear, both psychogenic factors and local effects on penile arterial and cavernous smooth muscle function have been implicated [21–23]. The recent observation that PGE$_1$ is not cytotoxic on cultured endothelial cells of human CC, may be considered as the beneficial effect of long-term self-injection PGE$_1$, as the endothelium of the corpus cavernosum plays an important role in the cascade of signal transduction of penile erection [24].

Alprostadil (PGE$_1$) is approved for self-injection therapy in ED as Caverject® (Pfizer/Pharmacia, USA) in 10 and 20 μg dual chamber syringes, and as Edex®/Viridal® (Schwarz Pharma, Germany) in 10, 20 and 40 μg dual chamber syringes.

Papaverine

Papaverine is a non-opiate derivative from *Papaver*

somniferum (poppy plant) and was the first clinically effective pharmacologic therapy for ED tried as an IC injection.

As a good smooth muscle relaxant, papaverine has shown to evoke relaxation of isolated CC strips, penile arteries, cavernous sinusoids, and penile veins in vitro; papaverine caused marked vasodilation of the penile arteries and decreased venous outflow, as recorded by Doppler [2]. Furthermore, papaverine also attenuated contractions induced by stimulation of adrenergic nerves and exogenous noradrenaline [25,26]. An IC injection of 80 mg papaverine in normal volunteers and patients with psychogenic impotence produced rigid erections.

At the cellular level, papaverine is a nonspecific phosphodiesterase inhibitor that causes increases in intracellular cAMP and cGMP, resulting in corporal smooth muscle relaxation and penile erection. It may also modulate cavernosal smooth muscle tone through inhibition of voltage-dependent L-type Ca^{2+} channels independent of cAMP, as reported in tracheal smooth muscle, and also leads to suppression of angiotensin II secretion in cavernosal tissue [14,27].

It is well established that IC injection of papaverine may cause cavernosal fibrosis. In a meta-analysis of the literature, including 15 retrospective studies, fibrotic changes were observed in 5.7% and 12.4% of patients after papaverine, and the mixture of papaverine/ phentolamine, respectively [15] (Table 8.2). Compared with PGE_1, an increased risk of prolonged erection and penile fibrosis was associated with long-term IC papaverine given weekly for eight months in primates [18].

Increased damage to cavernosal endothelial cells by papaverine had been reported within the human CC after injection of papaverine and papaverine/ phentolamine, but not after injection of PGE_1 [28,29]. Using cultured endothelial cells of human CC, Schultheiss *et al.* clearly demonstrated that papaverine produced cytotoxic effects as measured by increased release of lactate dehydrogenase, a marker of cytotoxicity and a significant decrease in the viable cell count and metabolic activity of the cultures [24]. The acidity (pH < 5) of papaverine or papaverine/ phentolamine solutions probably contributes to both the cytotoxic and fibrotic effects of papaverine. To avoid incurring permanent damage to endothelial cells, these findings encourage the use of alprostadil-containing preparations instead of papaverine-containing formulations for intracavernous injection therapy. Papaverine is extensively metabolized in the liver and papaverine-induced hepatotoxicity has also been reported (see Table 8.2).

Papaverine hydrochloride is marketed in many countries under a variety of trade names, mostly in 1–2 ml ampoules containing 30 mg papaverine per 1 ml. The most commonly used doses in ED were 30–60 mg; the dose range described in the literature varies between 10 and 110 mg [15].

Alpha-adrenoceptor blockers
Phentolamine
Phentolamine is a competitive, non-selective α_1- and α_2-adrenoceptor blocker that acts both on presynaptic and postsynaptic α-adrenoceptors. In addition its actvities are also attributed to potassium channel opening and endothelin-antagonist proper-

ties, as well as to NO synthase (NOS) stimulatory effects [30,31]. In the dog model intracavernously injected phentolamine resulted in a 50–100% increase in arterial blood flow without showing any impact on the veno-occlusive mechanism [32]. In contrast, in the same animal experiment papaverine resulted in a 300–700% increase in blood circulation and simultaneous blockade of venous drainage. The intracavernous injection of phentolamine 5 mg only resulted in penile tumescence but not rigidity [33], whereas a combination of phentolamine and papaverine showed additive efficacy resulting in long-standing rigid erections sufficient for sexual intercourse [34].

Moxisylyte
Moxisylyte is an α-adrenoceptor blocker with predominance of α_1-adrenoceptors [35]. Moxisylyte was developed for self-injection therapy in France and marketed in several European countries as Icavex®. Although its sucess rates were reported to range between 40% and 61%, regarding the induction of rigid erections sufficient for successful vaginal penetration, its efficacy was clearly inferior to alprostadil in a direct head to head comparative trial [36]. This may be the reason why this drug was not widely used for self-injection therapy despite its low side-effect profile. Just recently in the spring 2005 the manufacturer of Icavex® decided to withdraw this drug from the European market, presumably due to its low market shares. In experienced hands moxisylyte was especially helpful in the treatment of patients with ED after RRP, in whom PDE-5 inhibitors have failed and PGE_1 injections resulted in painful erections.

Vasoactive intestinal polypeptide
Vasoactive intestinal polypeptide (VIP) was considered to be one of the strong candidates for penile erection in the 1980s. The reasons for that is the fact that it is one of the naturally occurring neurotransmitters present in considerable amounts in the male genital tract. VIPergic nerves are densely distributed in the penis supplying the pudendal arteries and the cavernous smooth muscle cells. VIP is said to mediate facilitatory effects on blood flow, secretion and

muscle tone, suggesting that this peptide neuro-transmitter may play an important role in the neural control of male erectile function [37].

Interestingly, VIP was found in co-localization with NOS within the perivascular and trabecular nerve fibres of the penile erectile tissue [38]. In view of the findings that these nerve fibers contain vesicular acetylcholine transporter, a specific marker for cholinergic neurons, the NO and VIP-containing nerves were also considered to be cholinergic [39]. Furthermore, VIP-related peptides such as PHM, PACAP and helospectin (Hel-1), also coexist with VIP in nerve structures within the human cavernous tissue [40,41].

Whereas VIP is a potent relaxant of the CC and penile vascular smooth musculature in vitro, the ineffectiveness of VIP antiserum to inhibit the neurogenic relaxation in CC strips suggested that VIP was not released from the nitrergic (NANC) nerves during field stimulation [42]. This significant study made it unlikely that VIP is the erectile neurotransmitter and set off further research for potential neurotransmitters involved in the erection process. Another finding from this study was that intracavernous injection of VIP in man produced tumescence and not erection. Therefore, the finding that VIP was not able to induce penile rigidity adequate for coitus, when injected intracavernosally in normal volunteers and impotent men, made a potential role as a primary neurotransmitter for penile erection unlikely [42,43]. This is in line with the results obtained in healthy adult male volunteers in whom no significant changes were detected in systemic and cavernous plasma levels of VIP once the flaccid penis became rigid [44]. However, VIP may play a significant role in the mechanism of male sexual arousal as cavernosal VIP levels were elevated during penile detumescence and following ejaculation [44]. It was recently shown that chemical castration in patients who underwent radical prostatectomy does not influence VIP immunostaining of human CC, suggesting that VIP is not an androgen–dependent neuromediator of penile erection and that it may be responsible for sexually-induced erections in these castrated patients [45].

Similar to PGE_1, the effects of VIP are mediated by a specific membrane-bound receptor linked to adenylate cyclase via a stimulatory G-protein. VIP has been shown to elevate cAMP concentrations in cavernosal tissues without affecting cGMP [41–46].

Drug combinations for self-injection therapy
General considerations

PGE_1 is still the first line option for patients who either do not respond or show contraindications for oral phosphodiesterase-5 inhibitors. Besides PGE_1 mono therapy, several potentially useful combinations have been used for self-injection therapy as second line options. The vasoactive agents most commonly used in combination therapy, were phentolamine, papaverine, PGE_1, and VIP. Potential advantages of the use of combination therapies over mono therapy may depend on the number of drugs/strength of the mixtures used, an increase of efficacy by targeting different sites of action in the erection process, reduction of side effects such as priapism or fibrosis, and reduction of costs per application.

For instance, in vitro studies on human and rabbit cavernosal strips demonstrated that phentolamine significantly potentiated relaxation induced by sildenafil, VIP and PGE_1. These vasodilators also significantly enhanced relaxation induced by phentolamine in the cavernosal tissue strips. The enhancement of VIP and PGE_1-induced relaxation (cAMP-mediated) by phentolamine suggests a synergistic interaction, while the interaction between phentolamine and sildenafil (cGMP-mediated) appears to be additive [47]. The same investigators were also able to show that sildenafil and PGE_1 has additive and synergistic effects, respectively, with phentolamine-induced relaxation. Therefore, in combination therapy using phentolamine as an adjunct, the efficacy of vasodilators that initiate erection via independent relaxant pathways is increased due to a reduction in adrenergic tone, through the α-adrenoceptor blockade.

Combination of papaverine and phentolamine (Androskat®)

The combination of papaverine/phentolamine has become popular since the publication of Adrian

Zorgniotti 1985, and has competed with alprostadil mono therapy for a long time [34]. The mixture of papaverine/phentolamine is commercially available and approved as Androskat® in several countries worldwide, especially in Europe. Androskat® is marketed in 2 ml ampoules containing 15 mg papaverine and 0.5 mg phentolamine per 1 ml, i.e. a total content of 30 mg papaverine +1 mg phentolamine per ampoule. As a rule of thumb, the efficacy of one ampoule Androskat® is comparable to 10 μg alprostadil, and two ampoules Androskat® to 20 μg alprostadil [15] (Table 8.1). The major disadvantages of papaverine/phentolamine is its relatively high risk of priapism >6 hours ranging between 2 and >10% (mean 7.8%) depending on the concentration of the first dose used [15], (Table 8.2).

The main indication for using the mixture of papaverine/phentolamine are patients with ED in whom PGE_1-induced erections were felt intolerably painful, which is relatively often the case after major pelvic surgery (RRP, cystectomy, rectum amputation), or this minority of patients in whom PGE_1 mono therapy turned out to be inferior to papaverine/phentolamine. Long-term use of the mixture of papaverine/phentolamine was marked with a considerably higher risk of cavernous fibrosis compared to alprostadil monotherapy [15].

Combination of papaverine/phentolamine/PGE_1 (Triple drug, syn. Trimix)

The use of the triple drug combination of papaverine/phentolamine/PGE_1 was reported for the first time in 1990 by Goldstein [48]. Since this publication a variety of reports on the usefulness of this drug combination was published in the literature, with wide range of dose recommendations (see Table 8.3). A direct comparative study investigated the equivalent doses of alprostadil monotherapy to the triple-drug combination in terms of efficacy [56] (Tables 8.4 and 8.5).

Table 8.3 Triple drug compositions: intracavernous injection of Trimix, a mixture of papaverine, phentolamine and PGE_1, is indicated for patients unsuitable for PGE_1 injection due to poor response, pain or cost. Various dose combinations have been reported with the range of ratio (based on mass) for papaverine [12–30]: PGE_1 (0.006–0.02): phentolamine (taken as 1).

Reference	Trimix Stock Solution			Ratio (equimass basis)			Injection volume (ml)
	Papaverine	PGE_1	Phentolamine	Papaverine	PGE_1	Phentolamine	
Bennett et al [49]	17.6 mg/ml	5.9 μg/ml	0.59 mg/ml	30	0.01	1	0.25
Govier et al [50]	22.5 mg/ml	8.3 μg/ml	0.83 mg/ml	27	0.01	1	0.36
Israilov et al [51]	19.4 mg	16.4	1.6	12.1	0.01	1	NA
Marshall et al [52]	12 mg	9 μg	1 mg	12	0.009	1	0.1–0.8
Shenfield et al [53]	4.5 mg/0.5 ml	5 μg/0.5 ml	0.25 mg/0.5 ml	18	0.02	1	0.5
Mulhall et al [54]	30 mg	10 μg	1 mg	30	0.01	1	NA
	30 mg	25 μg	2 mg	15	0.0125	1	NA
Montorsi et al [55]	150 mg	30 μg	5 mg	30	0.006	1	0.18–0.21
	300 mg	100 μg	10 mg	30	0.01	1	0.18–0.21
	300 mg	200 μg	20 mg	15	0.01	1	0.18–0.21

The Trimix stock solution of Montorsi et al. [55] is in 3 ml.

There is no question that at present the triple drug combination represents the most effective regimen in self-injection therapy, which was also preferred over alprostadil in the cited trial [56]. The major disadvantage of this powerful drug-combination is the fact that up to now, no commercially available preparation exists worldwide, i.e. the patients or the pharmacists have to reconstitute this combination individually, which is relatively complicated and cumbersome for many patients.

Combination of VIP and Phentolamine (Invicorp®)

The use of the combination of VIP and phentolamine in a larger series of patients with ED was published for the first time in 1992 [57]. After a couple of studies [58,59], the mixture of VIP/phentolamine in doses of 25 μg/1 mg or 25 μg/

2 mg was introduced commercially as Invicorp®, available with a very user-friendly automatic injection device for single use (Senetek-CA, USA), and approved in some countries (Denmark, UK, New Zealand). Although the VIP/phentolamine combination was very promising, especially due to its self-injection device and relatively high efficacy, it was never marketed worldwide. This is presumably due to the considerable decrease of the market for injectables in ED. To the knowledge of the authors, at present the VIP/phentolamine combination is not officially available in any country.

Other drug combinations for self-injection therapy

There are a variety of other drug combinations, mostly with PGE_1 (alprostadil), such as triple drug with PGE_1/papaverine/chlorpromazine (0.5 mg/ml) instead of phentolamine, or triple drug + atropine, PGE_1 + ketanserin, PGE_1 + CGRP (calcitonin gene-related peptide), PGE_1 + forskolin (activates the enzyme adenylate cyclase and increases intracellular cAMP), or triple drug and forskolin, but none of these combinations were able to achieve any market acceptance or official approval [60].

Combination of self-injection therapy and oral drug therapy

The successful conversion of non-responders either to high dose alprostadil mono-therapy (40 μg) or to the triple drug combination (40 μg PGE_1/48 mg papaverine/3.2 mg phentolamine) by combining

Table 8.4 Equivalent efficacy doses of alprostadil powder (Caverject®) and papaverine/phentolamine/PGE_1 combination (triple drug solution) in 68 patients. From Kulaksizoglu *et al.*[56].

Alprostadil powder (PGE_1 (μg))	Papaverine(mg)/ phentolamine (mg)/PGE_1 (μg)
4	1.47/0.05/0.49
8	3.2/0.1/1.1
12	4.6/0.15/1.55
16	6.8/0.22/2.27
20	7.6/0.25/2.5

Table 8.5 Intra-individual comparative study of alprostadil powder (Caverject®) and papaverine/phentolamine/PGE_1 (triple drug solution). From Kulaksizoglu *et al.* [56].

	Alprostadil powder (PGE_1 Caverject)	Papaverine/phentolamine/PGE_1 (triple drug solution)	No preference (both the same)
Overall assessment better	23%	46%	31%
Improved rigidity	22%	37%	41%
Erection maintenance better	19%	37%	44%
Reproducibility better	15%	35%	50%
Orgasm/ejaculation better	0	0	100%

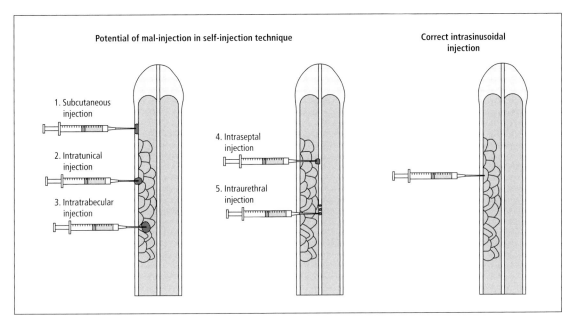

Fig. 8.2 Technique of self-injection therapy. From Porst [60].

self-injection therapy with 100 mg sildenafil, was reported in 34% [32] of 93 patients treated in this way [61]. In another prospective, placebo (against sildenafil) controlled study with 40 patients experiencing unsatisfactory erections at both the 50 and 100 mg dose of sildenafil, the combined treatment with 20 µg IC-PGE$_1$ resulted in a statistically significant improvement of the erectile response as assessed by the IIEF-EF in 65% of the patients [62].

Technique and complications of self-injection therapy

In order to overcome the reservations and to increase the acceptance of patients on the one hand, but to decrease at the same time the complications of self-injection therapy on the other hand, a thorough instruction of the patients in a proper technique and use of ultra-thin needles is mandatory. According to the experiences of the authors it takes, in many patients, at least two teaching sessions before the patient is sure that he has mastered this technique correctly and avoids potential mal-injection risks (see Fig. 8.2).

The most frequent side effects encountered with self-injection therapy are:

Prolonged erections/priapism: the frequency of which has been shown to be drug- and dose–dependent (see Table 8.2). Priapisms lasting longer than six hours must be interrupted by injecting IC a sympathomimetically acting antidote (see Chapter 15 on conservative management of priapism), and/or evacuation of the entrapped blood through a butterfly cannula. The six hour time limit has absolutely to be considered in order to avoid irreversible ischemic damage to the cavernous tissue.

Fibrosis of the cavernous tissue: the occurrence of which has also shown a clear drug dependency (see Table 8.2). The follow up of fibrotic changes occurring both in the European multicenter 4-year study with alprostadil (Viridal®/Edex®), or in the US 5 year trial (Caverject®), showed that between 33–47% of these nodules/plaques healed spontaneously [63,64]. In a recently published study on the outcome of fibrotic changes due to self-injection therapy in 44 patients, 52% (n = 23) of the patients showed spontaneous improvement despite most of

Author	No. of patients	MUSE®	IC alprostadil
Ghazi 1998[71]	125	48% (61)	79% (98)
Werthman 1997[72]	100	37%	89%
Porst 1997[73]	103	43% (44)	70% (72)
Shabsigh 1998[74]	106	27%	66% (buckling test)
Shabsigh 200[75]	68	53%	83% (at home use)
Flynn 1998[76]	Literature review	45%	>70%

Table 8.6 Efficacy rates of transurethral alprostadil (MUS®) vs. self-injection therapy with alprostadil (Caverject®, Viridal®, Edex®).

them (91%) continuing self-injection therapy [65]. The tendency for spontaneous disappearance of the fibrotic changes may be supported by temporary discontinuation of self-injection therapy for two to four months, followed by a re-education of the patient in the correct self-injection technique (see Fig. 8.2). In roughly half of the patients, fibrotic changes are followed by the development of penile deviations frequently requiring surgical intervention.

Penile hematoma/bruising is the most often encountered side effect observed with self-injection therapy, and occurred between 33% and 47% in the European four years long-term trial (63). Hematoma occurred more frequently in those patients who developed fibrotic changes in the further course, pointing to the potential role of mal-injection technique in this regard. In some patients repeated occurrence of hematoma may be followed by dark coloring of the penile skin due to hemosiderin deposits.

Rare complications with self-injection therapy are the occurrence of infections/abscesses, needle breakages requiring surgical removal, or even the development of cavernous thrombosis with involvement of the pelvic veins and subsequent lethal pulmonary embolism [66].

Special populations/features with self-injection therapy
Patients on anticoagulants
According to the literature and my own experience, self-injection therapy can be performed even in men on warfarin or phenprocoumon-containing anticoagulants, without increasing the risk of bleeding/ecchymosis [67].

Transplant patients
The literature does not show any increased risk with self-injection therapy in patients who have received kidney or heart transplants [68].

Diabetics
Both in the literature and in own patient populations, ED patients with diabetes are revealed at increased risk of fibrosis and painful sensations with self-injection therapy [69].

Trans(intra)urethral Therapy
Transurethral alprostadil (PGE₁) with MUSE® (Medicated Urethral System for Erection)
A new alprostadil preparation using transurethral application with a small single-use applicator was introduced in 1994, and later on developed as MUSE® (Medicated Urethral System for Erection) for market approval in US, 1996 (VIVUS, USA) followed by many other countries worldwide [70]. Although the transurethral application route seemed at first glance to be preferable to self-injection therapy the outcome and especially direct comparative trials to intracavernously-applied alprostadil (Caverject®, Edex®, Viridal®), revealed a distinct inferiority of MUSE® [71–76] (Table 8.6).

Typical frequent side effects of MUSE® are penile/urethral pain between 25 and 43%, and urethral bleeding (around 5%). Infrequently reported adverse events are dizziness with fall in blood pressure (1–5%), and even the occurrence of syncope between 0.4 and 3% [70–76].

Of importance for achieving the best efficacy with MUSE® and avoidance of bleeding is a correct technical application, i.e. to insert MUSE® directly upon micturition with the urethra still being moist. The efficacy of MUSE® may be enhanced by simultaneous application of a constriction bandage on the base of the penis to avoid quick drainage of the medication through the penile veins. Successful salvage of non-responders to mono therapy either with sildenafil or MUSE® using a combination of both methods was reported by several authors [77,78]. At present transurethral alprostadil therapy with MUSE® must be considered a niche therapy in ED. The main indications of MUSE® are patients, non-responsive to PDE-5 inhibitors due to damage of the autonomic penile nerve supply after pelvic surgery or trauma (RRP, cystectomy).

Transurethral route used with other compounds

Transurethral application with other compounds such as lyophilized liposomal PGE_1 (LLPGE) [79,80] or PGE_2 [81,82] was investigated several times, but then abandoned, and never reached the stage of market approval.

Topical Therapies

Provided topical application can be as effective as oral or injection therapy, it would certainly have a greater popularity and acceptance, particularly for those patients with needle phobia fearing injection therapy, or those with contraindications for the use of PDE-5 inhibitors. Ideally, topical applications are considered to be non-invasive and have minimal systemic side effects that are commonly associated with oral pharmacotherapies. Currently, the application sites for topical therapy for ED are the skin of the penile shaft and the glans penis. Unlike certain skin areas such as the impermeable back or palms, the stratum corneum of the penile skin is more easily permeable to agents applied topically [83]. However, to reach the level of the corpora cavernosa, the agents applied on penile skin have to permeate fascial layers and the tunica albuginea with its thick layers of collagen. In view of the proven existence of venous communications between corpora cavernosa and glans penis [84], some studies have also investigated the efficacy of topical application on the glans penis to reach the CC. This approach is expected to minimize the venous return of the agents into systemic circulation thereby prolonging the local action. However, in spite of the advantages, i.e. ease of administration and patients' preference for topical therapy, the high concentration of an agent needed for topical application as against the direct intracavernous route may increase the likelihood of local and even systemic effects, and also could not be considered cost effective. For instance, 1000 μg of PGE_1 is required for an intraurethral application (MUSE®) compared to an equipotent dose of 20 μg to 40 μg of PGE_1 by the IC route. As for topical application on the glans penis, the dose of 2.5 mg (2500 μg: Topiglan®) PGE_1 used (0.25 ml of 1% alprostadil), which was effective in 38.9% of the ED patients under investigation), is more than 125 times that of the average 20 μg dose of PGE_1 used for IC injection [85].

Minoxidil is a potent vasodilator–antihypertensive agent used in patients refractory to a standard antihypertensive regimen. It is also used topically for alopecia. In view of its ability to relax vascular and other smooth muscle cells, it was also tested topically on the glans penis for the treatment of ED. One ml of 2% minoxidil solution, applied on the glans penis 20 minutes before attempted intercourse, was investigated in a total of 21 patients (age ranging from 29–65 years) [86]. One patient with psychogenic impotence and another patient who became impotent after excision of Peyronie's plaque, reported rigid erections adequate for intercourse. The latter one could subsequently achieve erection without minoxidil. The remaining 19 patients had no improvement of erectile rigidity. Similarly, Chancellor *et al.* [87]. who compared papaverine injection and vacuum constriction device (VCD) against topical minoxidil in the treatment of ED due to spinal cord injury, noted that both subjective and objective erectile responses to minoxidil were poor as compared to 77% success rates with papaverine and 57% with VCD [87]. However, in another study it was reported that three out of four paraplegic men have had a positive erectile response [88]. It may be suggested that the lack of erectile effect by minoxidil could be due to the fact that hepatic biotransformation is needed for the formation of the active metabolite, minoxidil *O*-sulfate [89]. However, in another prospective, double-blind controlled study, where transcutaneous application of minoxidil on the glans penis was tested against nitroglycerin (2.5 g, 10% ointment) and placebo, involving 116 patients, Cavallini *et al.* reported that minoxidil proved to be significantly superior to nitroglycerin, which was, in turn, more effective than the placebo [90].

Nitroglycerine: Nunez and Anderson [91] reported three cases of successful treatment of impotence using topical nitroglycerin ointment. In another placebo-controlled, double-blind study, using 2% nitroglycerin paste, the authors observed an improvement of blood flow in the cavernous arteries and tumescence after erotic stimulation in 18 of 26 patients [92].

Studies on the use of topical *papaverine gel* are rare. In a phase I, placebo-controlled, non-blinded study, Kim *et al.* investigated the efficacy of 15% and 20% papaverine base gels applied to the scrotum, perineum and penis [93]. The authors claimed a significant increase in cavernous arterial diameter (36%) and concluded that topical papaverine augmented reflex erections in their spinal cord injury patients. However, Chiang *et al.*, using a combination of 20% papaverine base gel with an enhancer against 500 µg PGE$_1$ were not able to yield a satisfactory erectile response after these combined vasoactive agents [94].

Whereas there have been several sporadic reports/personal observations on locally applied agents for the treatment of ED, the paucity of well controlled trials indicates poor success and acceptance rates of these drugs and precludes their widespread use in ED. Currently, there is no worldwide approved topical therapy for the treatment of ED on the horizon, although topical agents have been widely investigated in clinical studies and trials.

References

1 Virag R. Intracavernous injection of papaverine for erectile failure *Lancet* 1982;**2**(8304):938

2 Virag R, Frydman D, Legman M, Virag H. Intracavernous injection of papaverine as a diagnostic and therapeutic method in erectile failure. *Angiology* 1984;**35**(2):79–87.

3 Karim SMM, Hillier K. Physiological roles and pharmacological actions of prostaglandins in relation to human reproduction. In Karim SMM, ed. *Prostaglandins and Reproduction*. Lancaster: MTP Press Ltd, 1975, pp. 23–75.

4 Adaikan PG. Pharmacology of human penis. MSc Thesis. University of Singapore 1979, pp. 1–213.

5 Adaikan PG, Karim SM, Kottegoda SR, Ratnam SS. Cholinoreceptors in the corpus cavernosum muscle of the human penis. *J Auton Pharmacol* 1983;**3**(2):107–11.

6 Hedlund H, Andersson KE. Contraction and relaxation induced by some prostanoids in isolated human penile erectile tissue and cavernous artery. *J Urol* 1985;**134**(6):1245–1250.

7 Adaikan PG, Kottegoda SR, Ratnam SS. A possible role for prostaglandin E$_1$ in human penile erection. In: Abstracts of the 2nd World Meeting on Impotence, Prague, 1986;**2**:6.

8 Ishii N, Watanabe H, Irisawa C, Kikuchi Y, Kawamura S, Suzuki K, Chiba R, Tokiwa M, Shirai M. Studies on male sexual impotence. Report 18. Therapeutic trial with prostaglandin E1 for organic impotence. *Nippon Hinyokika Gakkai Zasshi* 1986;**77**(6):954–962.

9 Adaikan PG. Investigations and management of male impotence. In Proceedings of the XXI Malaysia-Singapore Congress of Medicine. Academy of Medicine, Malaysia, 1987, pp. 103–109.

10 Virag R, Adaikan PG. Effects of prostaglandin E1 on penile erection and erectile failure. *J Urol* 1987;**139**:1010.

11 Lin JS, Lin YM, Jou YC, Cheng JT. Role of cyclic adenosine monophosphate in prostaglandin E1-induced penile erection in rabbits. *Eur Urol* 1995;**28**(3):259–265.

12 Lee SW, Wang HZ, Zhao W, Ney P, Brink PR, Christ GJ. Prostaglandin E1 activates the large-conductance K$_{Ca}$ channel in human corporal smooth muscle cells. *Int J Impot Res* 1999;**11**(4):189–199.

13 Molderings GJ, van Ahlen H, Gothert M. Modulation of noradrenaline release in human corpus cavernosum by presynaptic prostaglandin receptors. *Int J Impot Res* 1992;**4**:19–25.

14 Kifor I, Williams GH, Vickers MA, Sullivan MP, Jodbert P, Dluhy RG. Tissue angiotensin II as a modulator of erectile function. I. Angiotensin peptide content, secre-

tion and effects in the corpus cavernosum. *J Urol* 1997;**157**(5):1920–1925.

15 Porst H. The rationale for prostaglandin E1 in erectile failure: a survey of worldwide experience. *J Urol* 1996;**155**(3):802–815.

16 Roy AC, Adaikan PG, Sen DK, Ratnam SS. Prostaglandin 15-hydroxydehydrogenase activity in human penile corpora cavernosa and its significance in prostaglandin-mediated penile erection. *Br J Urol* 1989;**64**(2):180–182.

17 Moreland RB, Traish A, McMillin MA, Smith B, Goldstein I, Saenz de Tejada I. PGE1 suppresses the induction of collagen synthesis by transforming growth factor-beta 1 in human corpus cavernosum smooth muscle. *J Urol* 1995;**153**:826–834.

18 Adaikan PG, LC Lau, Singh G, Susheela K, Vasatha Kumari K, Ratnam SS. Long-term intracavernous injection of papaverine and saline are detrimental to the primate cavernosum as compared to PGE₁. *Int J Impot Res* 1990;**2**(2):237–238.

19 Moemen MN, Hamed HA, Kamel II, Shamloul RM, Ghanem HM. Clinical and sonographic assessment of the side effects of intracavernous injection of vasoactive substances. *Int J Impot Res* 2004;**16**(2):143–145.

20 Wespes E, Sattar AA, Noel JC, Schulman CC. Does prostaglandin E1 therapy modify the intracavernous musculature? *J Urol* 2000;**163**(2):464–466.

21 Brock G, Tu LM, Linet OI. Return of spontaneous erection during long-term intracavernosal alprostadil (Caverject) treatment. *Urology* 2001;**57**:536–541.

22 Marshall GA, Breza J, Lue TF. Improved hemodynamic response after long-term intracavernous injection for impotence. *Urology* 1994;**43**(6):844–848.

23 Thiounn N, Flam T, Zerbib M, Debre B. Does prostaglandin El (PGE1) help restoration of spontaneous erections? *J Urol* (Paris) 1993;**99**(3):136–138.

24 Schultheiss A, Pilatz A, Gabouev N, Schlote J, Wefer H, Mertsching M, Sohn U, Jonas C. Stief. Cytotoxicity of different intracavernous vasoactive drugs on cultured endothelial cells of human corpus cavernosum penis. *Urology* 2004;**64**(3):598–602.

25 Adaikan PG, Ratnam SS. Pharmacological considera- tion of intracavernous drug injection in the treatment of impotence. *Acta Urol Belg* 1988;**56**(2):149–153.

26 Kirkeby HJ, Forman A, Andersson KE. Comparison of the papaverine effects on isolated human penile cir- cumflex veins and corpus cavernosum. *Int J Impot Res* 1990;**2**:49–54.

27 Iguchi M, Nakajima T, Hisada T, Sugimoto T, Kurachi Y. On the mechanism of papaverine inhibition of the

voltage-dependent Ca++ current in isolated smooth muscle cells from the guinea pig trachea. *J Pharmacol Exp Ther* 1992;**263**(1):194–200.

28 van Ahlen H, Piechota H-J, Hermanns M, Kruger E. Metabolic changes in the human corpus cavernosum under vasoactive substances. *Int J Imp Res* 1990;**2**(suppl 2):244.

29 Stackl W, Loupal G, Holzmann A. Intracavernous injection of vasoactive drugs in the rabbit. *Urol Res* 1988;**16**:455–458.

30 Gupta S, Gallant C, Traish A, *et al.* Relaxation of corpus cavernosum smooth muscle by phentolamine via a non-adrenergic mechanism. *Int J Impotence Res* 1998;**10**:Suppl 3, S27.

31 Traish AM, Gupta S, Gallant C, *et al.* Phentolamine me- sylate relaxes penile corpus cavernosum by adrenergic and non-adrenergic mechanisms. *Int J Impotence Res* 1998;**10**:215–223.

32 Juenemann KP, Lue TF, Fournier JR, GR, *et al.* Hemody- namics of papaverine- and phentolamine-induced pe- nile erection. *J Urol* 1986;**136**:158–161.

33 Blum MD, Bahnson RR, Porter TN, *et al.* Effect of local alpha-adrenergic blockade on human penile erection. *J Urol* 1985;**134**:479–481.

34 Zorgniotti AW, Lefleur RS. Autoinjection of the corpus cavernosum with a vasoactive drug combination for vasculogenic impotence. *J Urol* 1985;**133**:39–41.

35 Buvat J, Lemaire A, Buvat-Herbaut M, *et al.* Safety of in- tracavernous injections using an alpha-blocking agent. *J Urol* 1989;**141**:1364–1367.

36 Buvat J, Costa P, Morlier D, *et al.* Double-blind multi- center study comparing alprostadil alpha cyclodextrin with moxisylyte chlorhydrate in patients with chronic erectile dysfunction. *J Urol* 1998;**159**:116–119.

37 Polak JM, Gu J, Mina S, Bloom SR. Vipergic nerves in the penis. *Lancet* 1981;**2**(8240):217–219.

38 Ehmke H, Juenemann KP, Mayer B, Kummer W. Nitric oxide synthase and vasoactive intestinal poly- peptide colocalization in neurons innervating the human penile circulation. *Int J Impot Res* 1995;**7**(3): 147–156.

39 Hedlund P, Ny L, Alm P, Andersson KE. Cholinergic nerves in human corpus cavernosum and spongiosum contain nitric oxide synthase and heme oxygenase. *J Urol* 2000;**164**(3 Pt 1):868–875.

40 Kirkeby HJ, Fahrenkrug J, Holmquist F, Ottesen B. Vasoactive intestinal polypeptide (VIP) and peptide histidine methionine (PHM) in human penile corpus cavernosum tissue and circumflex veins: localization and in vitro effects. *Eur J Clin Invest* 1992;**22**(1):24–30.

41 Hedlund P, Alm P, Ekstrom P, Fahrenkrug J, Hannibal J, Hedlund H, Larsson B, Andersson KE. Pituitary adenylate cyclase-activating polypeptide, helospectin, and vasoactive intestinal polypeptide in human corpus cavernosum. *Br J Pharmacol* 1995;**116**(4):2258–2266.

42 Adaikan PG, Kottegoda SR, Ratnam SS. Is vasoactive intestinal polypeptide the principal transmitter involved in human penile erection? *J Urol* 1986;**135**(3): 638–640.

43 Roy JB, Petrone RL, Said SI. A clinical trial of intracavernous vasoactive intestinal peptide to induce penile erection. *J Urol* 1990;**143**(2):302–304.

44 Becker AJ, Uckert S, Stief CG, Scheller F, Knapp WH, Machtens SA, Kuczyk MA, Jonas U. Systemic and cavernous plasma levels of vasoactive intestinal polypeptide during sexual arousal in healthy males. *World J Urol* 2002;**20**(1):59–63.

45 Cormio L, Gesualdo L, Maiorano E, Bettocchi C, Palumbo F, Traficante A, Schenaand FP, Selvaggi FP. Vasoactive intestinal polypeptide (VIP) is not an androgen-dependent neuromediator of penile erection. *Int J Impot Res* 2005;**17**:23–26.

46 Miller MA, Morgan RJ, Thompson CS, Mikhailidis DP, Jeremy JY. Effects of papaverine and vasointestinal polypeptide on penile and vascular cAMP and cGMP in control and diabetic animals: an in vitro study. *Int J Impot Res* 1995;**7**(2):91–100.

47 Kim NN, Goldstein I, Moreland RB, Traish AM. Alpha-adrenergic receptor blockade by phentolamine increases the efficacy of vasodilators in penile corpus cavernosum. *Int J Impot Res* 2000;**12**(Suppl 1):S26–36.

48 Goldstein I, Borges FD, Fitch WP, *et al.* Rescuing the failed papaverine/phentolamine erection: A proposed synergistic action of papaverine, phentolamine and prostaglandin E₁. *J Urol* 1990;**143**:4 Suppl, 304A.

49 Bennett AH, Carpenter AJ, Barada JH. An improved vasoactive drug combination for a pharmacological erection program. *J Urol* 1991;**146**(6):1564–1565.

50 Govier FE, McClure RD, Weissman RM, *et al.* Experience with triple-drug therapy in a pharmacological erection program. *J Urol* 1993;**150**:1822–1824.

51 Israilov S, Niv E, Livne PM, *et al.* Intracavernous injections for erectile dysfunction in patients with cardiovascular diseases and failure or contraindications for sildenafil citrate. *Int J Impot Res* 2002;**14**(1):38–43.

52 Marshall GA, Breza J, Lue TF. Improved hemodynamic response after long-term intracavernous injection for impotence. *Urology* 1994;**43**(6):844–848.

53 Shenfeld O, Hanani J, Shalhav A, *et al.* Papaverine-phentolamine and prostaglandin E1 versus papaverine-phentolamine alone for intracorporeal injection therapy: a clinical double-blind study. *J Urol* 1995;**154**(3):1017–1019.

54 Mulhall JP, Jahoda AE, Cairney M, *et al.* The causes of patient dropout from penile self-injection therapy for impotence. *J Urol* 1999;**162**(4):1291–1294.

55 Montorsi F, Salonia A, Zanoni M, *et al.* Current status of local penile therapy. *Int J Impot Res* 2002;**14**(Suppl): S70–81.

56 Kulaksizoglu H, Hakim LS, Nehra A, *et al.* Comparison of alprostadil sterile powder (Caverject™) with trimix Nomogram and patient satisfaction. *J Urol* 1997;**157**: No. 4 Suppl, 180.

57 Gerstenberg TC, Metz P, Ottesen B, *et al.* Intracavernous self-injection with vasoactive intestinal polypeptide and phentolamine in the management of erectile failure. *J Urol l* 1992;**47**:1277–1279.

58 Hackett G, and the UK-group of investigators. A 12-month multicenter placebo-controlled study of Invicorp™ in the treatment of non-psychogenic erectile dysfunction. *Int J Impotence Res* 1998;**10**:Suppl. 3, S21.

59 Sandhu D, Curless E, Dean J, *et al.* A double blind, placebo-controlled study of intracavernosal vasoactive intestinal polypeptide and phentolamine mesylate in a novel autoinjector for the treatment of non-psychogenic erectile dysfunction. *Int J Impotence Res* 1999;**11**:91–97.

60 Porst, H. Manual der Impotenz, Uni-Med Verlag, 2000, Bremen, Germany.

61 McMahon CG, Samali R, Johnson H. Treatment of intracorporeal injection nonresponse with sildenafil alone or in combination with triple agent intracorporeal injection therapy. *J Urol* 1999;**162**:1992–1998.

62 Gutierrez P, Hernadez P, Mas M. Combining programmed intracavernous PGE1 injections and sildenafil on demand to salvage sildenafil nonresponders. *Int J Impot Res* 2005;**17**:354–358.

63 Porst H, Buvat J, Meuleman E, *et al.* Intracavernous alprostadil alfadex—an effective and well tolerated treatment for erectile dysfunction. Results of a long-term European study. *Int J Impotence Res* 1998;**10**: 225–231.

64 Linet OJ. Long-term safety of Caverject™ (alprostadil S.PO, PGE) in erectile dysfunction (ED). *Int J Impotence Res* 1998;**10**:Suppl.3, S37.

65 Chew KK, Stuckey BGA. Clinical course of penile fibrosis in intracavernosal prostaglandin E1 injection therapy: a follow-up of 44 patients. *Int J Impotence Res* 2003;**15**:94–98.

66 Hashmat AJ, Abrahams J, Fani K, *et al.* A lethal complication of papaverine-induced priapism. *J Urol* 1991; **145**:146–147.

67 Limoge JP, Olins E, Henderson D, *et al.* Minimally invasive therapies in the treatment of erectile dysfuction in anticoagulated cases: A study of satisfaction and safety. *J Urol* 1996;**155**:1277–1279.

68 Mansi MF, Ackhudair WK, Huraib S. Treatment of erectile dysfunction after kidney transplantation with intracavernosal self-injection of prostaglandin E$_1$. *J Urol* 1998;**159**:1927–1930.

69 Plekhanov AY, Zhivovo AV, Goryachew LA. Comparative complications rate after alprostadil intracavernous pharmacotherapy for erectile dysfunction in diabetes mellitus vs. non-diabetic patients. *Int J Impotence Res* 1998;**10**:Suppl 3, S50

70 Padma-Nathan H, Keller T, Poppiti R, *et al.* Hemodynamic effects of intraurethral alprostadil: The Medicated Urethral System for Erection (MUSE®). *J Urol* 1994;**151**:No. 5, 345.

71 Ghazi SA, AlMeligy A. Transurethral alprostadil and the prostaglandin E1 intra corporal injection in treatment of erectile dysfunction: A comparative study. *Int J Impotence Res* 1998;**10**:Suppl.3, S13.

72 Werthman P, Rajfer J. MUSE-therapy: preliminary clinical observations. Urology 1997;**50**:809–811.

73 Porst H. Transurethral alprostadil with MUSE™ (Medicated Urethral System for Erection) vs. intracavernous alprostadil—a comparative study in 103 patients with erectile dysfunction. *Int J Impotence Res* 1997;**9**:187–192.

74 Shabsigh R, Padma-Nathan H, Gittelman M, *et al.* and the EDEX®/VIRIDAL® Study Group: Comparative results of efficacy and safety of intracavernous alprostadil alfadex (EDEX®/VIRIDAL®) and intraurethral alprostadil (MUSE®) plus ACTIS®. *Int J Impotence Res* 1998;**10**:Suppl., S51.

75 Shabsigh R, Padma-Nathan H, Gitteman M, *et al.* Intracavernous alprostadil alfadex is more efficacious, better tolerated and preferred over intraurethral alprostadil plus optional actis: a comparative, randomized, crossover, multicenter study. *Urology* 2000;**55**: 109–113.

76 Flynn TN, Guest JF. Intracorporeal and transurethral application of alprostadil: A review of the literature. *Int J Impotence Res* 1998;**10**:Suppl.3, S47.

77 Mydlo JH, Volpe, MA, Maccia RJ. Inital results utilizing combination therapy for patients with a suboptimal response to either alprostadil or sildenafil monotherapy. *Eur Urol* 2000;**38**:30–34.

78 Nehra A, Hakim L, Barrett DM, *et al.* Effectiveness of combination therapy of MUSE and Viagra in the salvage of erectile dysfunction patients desiring non-invasive therapy: 18-month follow-up. Int J Impotence Res. 12, 9th World Meeting on Impotence Research, Perth, 2000;p.**23**:P23

79 See RJ, Williams J, Sparkuhl A, *et al.* Lyophilized Liposomal Prostaglandin E$_1$ released by a dilute detergent for intrameatal delivery to treat erectile failure. *J Urol* 1997;**157**: No.4, Suppl.201

80 Engelhardt PF, Plas E, Hübner WA, *et al.* Comparison of intraurethral liposomal and intracavernosal prostaglandin E1 in the management of erectile dysfunction. *Br J Urol* 1998;**81**:441–444.

81 Schmidt AC. Prostaglandin E$_2$ gel: an alternative treatment for erectile dysfunction. *Int J Impotence Res* 1994;**6**:Suppl.1, A43.

82 Wolfson B, Pickett S, Scott NE, *et al.* Intraurethral prostaglandin E$_2$ cream: a possible alternative treatment for erectile dysfunction. Urology 1993;**42**:73–75.

83 Maibach HI, Feldman RJ, Milby TH, Serat WF. Regional variation in percutaneous penetration in man. *Arch Environ Health* 1971;**23**(3):208–211.

84 McVary KT, Polepalle S, Riggi S, Pelham RW. Topical prostaglandin E1 SEPA gel for the treatment of erectile dysfunction. *J Urol* 1999;**162**(3 Pt 1):726–730.

85 Goldstein I, Payton TR, Schechter PJ. A double-blind, placebo-controlled, efficacy and safety study of topical gel formulation of 1% alprostadil (Topiglan) for the in-office treatment of erectile dysfunction. Urology 2001;**57**(2):301–305.

86 Radomski SB, Herschorn S, Rangaswamy S. Topical minoxidil in the treatment of male erectile dysfunction. *J Urol* 1994;**151**(5):1225–1226.

87 Chancellor MB, Rivas DA, Panzer DE, Freedman MK, Staas WE Jr. Prospective comparison of topical minoxidil to vacuum constriction device and intracorporeal papaverine injection in treatment of erectile dysfunction due to spinal cord injury. *Urology* 1994;**43**(3): 365–369.

88 Beretta G, Saltarelli O, Marzotto M, Zanollo A, Re B. Transcutaneous minoxidil in the treatment of erectile dysfunctions in spinal cord injured men. *Acta Eur Fertil* 1993;**24**(1):27–30.

89 Johnson GA, Barsuhn KJ, McCall JM. Minoxidil sulfate, a metabolite of minoxidil. *Drug Metab Dispos* 1983; **11**(5): 507–508.

90 Cavallini G. Minoxidil versus nitroglycerine: a prospective, double-blind, controlled trial in transcutaneous therapy for organic impotence. *Int J Impot Res* 1994;**6**(4):205–212.

91 Nunez BD, Anderson DC Jr. Nitroglycerin ointment in

the treatment of impotence. *J Urol* 1993;**150**(4): 1241–1243.

92 Owen JA, Saunders F, Harris C, Fenemore J, Reid K, Surridge D, Condra M, Morales A. Topical nitroglycerin: a potential treatment for impotence. *J Urol* 1989;**141**(3):546–548.

93 Kim ED, el-Rashidy R, McVary KT. Papaverine topical gel for treatment of erectile dysfunction. *J Urol* 1995;**153**(2):361–365.

94 Chiang HS, Kao YH, Sheu MT. Papaverine and prostaglandin E1 gel applications for impotence. *Ann Acad Med Singapore* 1995;**24**(5):767–769.

CHAPTER 9

Future Aspects of Pharmacotherapy in Erectile Dysfunction

Hartmut Porst

The overwhelming success of sildenafil in the management of male erectile dysfunction (ED) encouraged both researchers and the pharmaceutical industry to enforce their endeavors in this special field of medicine. Meanwhile two further PDE-5 inhibitors tadalafil and vardenafil have joined sildenafil. Because they are not really distinguishable from sildenafil in terms of efficacy and side effects, but only from the pharmacokinetic profile, they are now directly competing with this very first protagonist. The ED market continues to be very attractive for pharmaceutical companies and independent researchers, in particular due to the fact that at present only between 15 and 20% of all men suffering from ED are treated. The purpose of the following chapter is to provide a brief overview of the main sites of the current research dedicated to the pharmacologic treatment of ED.

Centrally Acting Drugs Under Clinical Investigation

After apomorphin SL, a dopamine $D_{1/2}$ receptor agonist with dominant action on D_2, has failed on the European market, due to lack of efficacy and clear inferiority to the phosphodiesterase-5 (PDE-5) inhibitors. The main focus in drug development is now directed to other central neurotransmitters known to be involved in processing erection.

Melanocortin receptor (MCR) agonists

Presently there are five MCRs identified and all five are activated by adrenocorticotropin hormone (ACTH) and four out of five, except MC2R, by alpha-melanocyte stimulating hormone (α-MSH) [1]. Of the five MCRs only two (MC3R and MC4R) are expressed in cerebral regions known to be involved in the modulation of erectile function. The origin of both α-MSH and ACTH is the pro-opiomelanocortin (POMC) gene, and the biologic effects of these two hormones are mediated via activation of one or more of the five MCRs. All five MCRs use cAMP as the second neurotransmitter mediating the final biologic (physiologic) effects upon their activation.

Melanotan II and its active metabolite *PT-141* (Bremelanotide), are cyclic peptide analogues of α-MSH, targeting four of the five MCRs (not MC2R), which have been under investigation for nearly 10 years for their usefulness in the management of ED [2]. Following the first research studies Melanotan II was investigated both as subcutaneous injection and as intranasal spray [3,5].

Recently the results with the intranasal melanocortin receptor agonist PT-141 in an at home, multi-center, double-blind, placebo-controlled parallel-arm study in 271 sildenafil-responsive patients were reported, with improved erections in 66–67% with the 10–20 mg dose [5]. As shown in Fig. 9.1 there was no dose-dependent efficacy between 10 and 20 mg. In two further Rigiscan studies with a subcutaneous (s.c.) application of PT-141 in doses between four and 10 mg, efficacy was reported even in a small group of patients (n = 25) with a history of inadequate response to 100 mg sildenafil and an IIEF-EF-score <17 [4]. A first response was seen approximately 37 min after the 10 mg dose. Mean duration of efficacy (definition: ≥60% penile base rigidity) was 41 min for the 6 mg s.c. dose [4], whereas in another study the mean duration of efficacy after intranasal PT-141 was 26

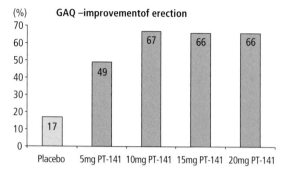

Fig. 9.1 At home efficacy of PT-141, an intranasal MCR-agonist, in 271 sildenafil-responsive patients [5].

min (6 mg dose) and 54 min (20 mg dose), respectively, compared to 18.5 min in patients receiving placebo [3]. Co-administration of low doses of intranasal PT-141 (7.5 mg) and sildenafil (25 mg) in men suffering from ED resulted in an enhanced erectile response [6].

A major problem with this new MCR agonist may be its side effect profile, with nausea rates up to 36% after 6 mg s.c and 17% after intranasal application [3,4]. Further drug related side effects >5% were headache (up to 27%), flushing (up to 17%) vomiting (up to 9%), back-pain (up to 9%), muscle cramps (up tp 9%), and fatigue (up to 8%).

There is no doubt that this completely new approach with MCR agonists seems to be promising in terms of efficacy, but at present there are some uncertainties regarding their side effect profile.

Centrally Acting Compounds with the Potential for Pharmacotherapy in ED

Positive effects on the erectile mechanism were reported from the following centrally-acting compounds.

Oxytocin

In the rat model oxytocin micro-injections into the nucleus paraventricularis and the medial septum of the hippocampus induced erections [7], which is not the case if these regions were injured through trauma [8]. In small clinical trials, conducted about 30 years and 10 years ago, oxytocin was able to im-

prove ED in patients with psychogenic etiology [9–11]. As the patent for oxytocin (syntocinon) was revoked long ago, no pharmaceutical company seems to be interested in investigating the potential of this hormone in psychogenic ED.

Serotonin receptor agonists

Generally speaking, serotonin (5-hydroxytryptamine, 5-HT) receptors are attributed inhibitory effects in the erectile mechanism, but the serotonin receptor subtypes $5\text{-HT}_{1C/2A}$ and $_C$ are suggested to facilitate both erection in male and female sexual proprioceptive behaviour [12–14]. There were two 5-HT_{2C} agonists in preclinical or clinical phase I/IIA investigations named RSD 992 and YM 348, with no results being reported so far. The pro-erectile effects of RSD 992 were blocked by the $5\text{-HT}_{2A/C}$ antagonist ritanserin but not by the 5-HT_{2A} antagonist ketanserin, indicating that the 5-HT_{2C} receptor is the more important one in facilitating an erectile response [14].

Glutamate

In the rat model it was shown that hippocampal glutamate receptors are involved in the erectile response [15]. The injection of glutamate subtype receptor agonists such as NMDA, ACPD and AMPA, resulted in multiple episodes of erectile responses [15].

Hexarelin analogues

Hexarelin, a growth hormone (GH)-releasing hexapeptide, induced erections upon intra-paraventricular injection [16]. In the rat model several hexarelin analogues were able to induce erections after injection into the paraventricular nucleus, which resembled the erections caused by apomorphine [16,17].

Peripherally-Acting Drugs Under Clinical Investigation

New PDE-5 inhibitors

DA 8159 is a new PDE-5 inhibitor from a South Korean pharmaceutical company with a selectivity that is similar to sildenafil with a T_{max} of 1.0–1.5 h and a $T_{1/2}$ of 11–13 h. This new PDE-5 inhibitor was recently investigated in a large multicenter, double-blind placebo-controlled home trial for 12 weeks, in doses of 100 and 200 mg, in 319 men with ED [18].

As shown in Fig. 9.2, the SEP 3 rates reached nearly 70%, against only 17% at baseline. Side effects >5% were flushing and headache.

TA-1790 (avanafil) is also a new PDE-5 inhibitor developed for the treatment of ED. Its pharmacokinetic profile shows a T_{max} < 1 h and a $T_{1/2}$ of about 1 hour. In a phase II A Rigiscan study, doses of 50/100/200 mg TA 1790 were compared to sildenafil 50 mg and placebo. Whereas the efficacy (rigidity >60% at penile base) of TA 1790 was superior to sildenafil in a time frame of 20–40 min after application, it was inferior to sildenafil after a time frame of 100–120 min [19]. The most commonly observed adverse event was flushing in between four and 11% of patients. The future will show whether these two PDE-5 inhibitors will be developed up to market approval, and whether these two PDE-5 will have the potential to compete with the three marketed PDE-5 inhibitors.

Topical alprostadil (Alprox®)

Topical alprostadil (Alprox®-TD) in doses of 100, 200 and 300 μg was investigated against a placebo in two multicenter pivotal phase 3 trials involving 1732 patients with mild to severe ED [20]. The demographics of the study population showed diabetes in 21%, hypertension in 44%, RRP in 12%, CAD in 21%, and nitrate or α-blocker medication in 16%. The SEP 3 data obtained after 12 weeks of treatment as shown in Fig. 9.3, indicate a clearly inferior efficacy if compared to PDE-5 inhibitors, whose SEP 3 data ranged in the literature between 65 and 75%. It may be presumed that topical alprostadil may play a role in the future combination treatment strategies if PDE-5 inhibitors only are not able to induce satisfactory responses.

Peripherally-Acting Drugs with the Potential for Pharmacotherapy in ED

S-Nitrosylated α-blockers

Nitrosylation of α-blockers has been reported both with yohimbine and moxisylyte [21]. The additional nitrosylation has no negative impact on the α-

adrenoceptor blocking properties but enhances their erectile-inducing efficacy by the additional NO-donor activities. Although this concept was introduced nearly 10 years ago, no results of clinical studies are reported to date.

Nitric oxide-releasing PDE-5 inhibitors

NCX-911 a novel nitric oxide-releasing PDE-5 inhibitor, turned out to be superior to sildenafil in the rabbit model if there was a lack of endogenous NO [22]. To date no data on clinical trials have been reported.

Guanylate cyclase (GC) activators

Several research groups were focusing in the past couple of years on guanylate cyclase, on the GC-B, a membrane bound enzyme in particular involved in the physiologic process of erection by promoting the cleavage of cGMP from GTP [23,24]. At least two GC activators, i.e. YC-1 and BAY 41-2272,

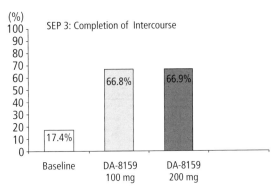

Fig. 9.2 Results (SEP 3) of the multicenter trial with the PDE-5 inhibitor DA 8159 (udenafil [18]); N=319.

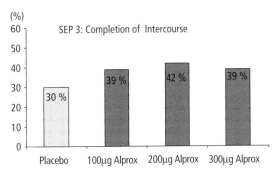

Fig. 9.3 Results of the two pivotal trials with topical alprostadil (Alprox® TD) [19].

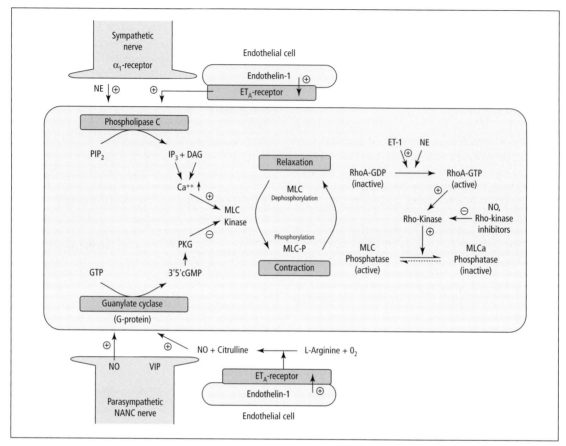

Fig. 9.4 The role of Rho A and Rho-kinase in the erectile process. Modified after Mills *et al.* [34].

have shown potential efficacy both in animal models and in vitro experiments with human corpus cavernosum muscle strips [25–28]. At present no data are available on clinical trials, but based on findings in experiments with diabetic rats it is speculated that GC activators may be more effective in diabetic ED than the common PDE-5 inhibitors. This speculation relies on the observation that endogenous NO release is significantly decreased in diabetes, and that NO-independent GC activators as well as NO-releasing PDE-5 inhibitors may be more useful in diabetic ED [28].

Rho-kinase inhibitors

A variety of research findings emphasize the role of Rho-kinase in the regulation of the corpus cavernosum smooth muscle tone, i.e. maintaining con-

traction and thereby preventing erection [29,30] (Fig. 9.4, see also Chapter 3, p.36). It has been shown that Rho-kinase expression and activity is clearly up-regulated, both in diabetes and hypertension and in hypoxemic conditions [31,32,33]. In the animal model Rho-kinase inhibitors were able to ameliorate ED [34,35]. Recent studies performed in hypertensive rats have provided evidence that the combination of PDE-5 inhibitors and Rho kinase inhibitors are superior to the respective mono-therapies [35]. Finally the topical application of the Rho-kinase inhibitor Y-27632 to the rat tunica albuginea resulted in an erectile response [36].

Conclusions

As briefly described in this chapter, there are a

variety of targets worthy of being considered for the development of pharmaceutical drugs in the indication of male ED, both on the central and the peripheral level. Without any doubt the following couple of years will be exciting in this field.

References

1 Martin WJ, MacIntyre DE. Melanocortin receptors and erectile function. *Eur Urol* 2004;**45**:706–713.

2 Wessells H, Fusciarelli K, Hansen J, *et al.* Melanotropic peptide for the treatment of psychogenic erectile dysfunction: double-blind cross over vehicle controlled study. *Int J Impotence Res* 1996;**8**:147.

3 Diamond LE, Earle DC, Rosen RC, *et al.* Double-blind, placebo-controlled evaluation of the safety, pharmacokinetic properties and pharmacodynamic effects of intranasal PT-141, a melanocortin receptor agonist, in healthy males and patients with mild to moderate erectile dysfunction. *Int J Impotence Res* 2004;**16**: 51–59.

4 Rosen RC, Diamond LE, Earle DC, *et al.* Evaluation of the safety, pharmacokinetics and pharmacodynamic effects of subcutaneously administered PT-141, a melanocortin receptor agonist, in healthy male subjects and in patients with inadequate response to Viagra®. *Int J Impotence Res* 2004;**16**:135–142.

5 Wessels H, Padma-Nathan H, Rajfer J, *et al.* At-home efficacy of an intranasal administered melanocortin receptor agonist, PT-141, in men with erectile dysfunction (ED). *J Urol* 2004;**171**:Suppl, 316 Abstr 1197.

6 Diamond LE, Earle DC, Spana C. Co-administration of low doses of intranasal PT 141, a melanocortin receptor agonist, and sildenafil to men with erectile dysfunction results in an enhanced erectile response. *J Urol* 2005;Suppl, 287, Abstr 1057.

7 Melis MR, Argiolas A, Gessa GL. Oxytocin-induced penile erection and yawning: sites of action in the brain. *Brain Research* 1986;**415**:98–104.

8 Argiolas A, Melis MR, Stancampiano R. Role of central oxytocinergic pathways in the expression of penile erection. *Regulatory Peptides* 1993;**45**:139–142.

9 Lidberg L. The effect of syntocinon on patients suffering from impotence. *Pharmacopsychiatry* 1972;**5**:187–190.

10 Lidberg L, Sternthal V. A new approach to the hormonal treatment of impotentia erectionis. *Pharmacopsychiatry* 1977;**10**:21–25.

11 Jevremovic M, Micic S, Terzic M. The influence of oxytocin on reproductive functions and sexual behavior in males. *Int J Impotence Res* 1994;**6** Suppl.1:P 97.

12 Rehman J, *et al.* Modification of sexual behaviour of Long-Evans male rats by drugs acting on the 5 HT_{1A} receptor. *Brain Res* 1999;**821**:414–425.

13 Rössler A-S, Bernabé J, Alexandre L, *et al.* Facilitation of proprioceptivity/sexual motivation in female rats by a serotonin 2A/2C (5-HT 2A12C)receptors agonist. *J Urol* 2005;**173**:292,Abstr 1077.

14 Hayes ES, Doherty PS, Hanson LA, *et al.* Pro-erectile effects of novel serotonin agonists. *Int J Impotence Res* 2000;**12** Suppl 3: S62.

15 Song Y, Rajasekaran M. Characterization of hippocampal glutamate receptor subtypes in the central regulation of penile erection. *J Urol* 2004;**171** Suppl, 380:Abstr 1442.

16 Argiolas A, Melis MR, Deghenghi R. EP 91073 prevents EP 80661 induced penile erection: evidence for a specific receptor mediating penile erection for EP peptides in the rat paraventricular nucleus. *Int J Impotence Res* 2001;**13** Suppl 4:S15.

17 Giuliano F, Argiolas A, Bernabé J, *et al.* Comparison of the pro-erectile effect of two hexarelin analogues EP80661 and EP 91072 with apomorphine after intravenous or intraparaventricular nucleus delivery in anaesthetized rats. *Int J Impotence Res* 2001;**13** Suppl 4:S15.

18 Paick JS, and the DA study group. Efficacy and tolerability of DA-8159 in patients with erectile dysfunction. *J Sex Med* 2004;**1**:Suppl 1, 46 O56.

19 Lewis RW, Hellstrom WJG, Gittelman M, *et al.* Rigiscan evaluation of TA 1790, a novel PDE-5 inhibitor for the treatment of men with erectile dysfunction. *J Urol* 2004;Suppl, 316,Abstr 1196.

20 Padma-Nathan H, Kim ED, McMurray JG, *et al.* A novel topical alprostadil cream for the treatment of erectile dysfunction (ED): Combined analysis of two phase 3 pivotal studies. *J Urol* 2004;**171** Suppl, 316 Abstr:1198.

21 Saenz de Tejada I,Cuevas P, Cuevas B, *et al.* S-nitrosylated alpha-blockers as potential drugs for the treatment of impotence:Biological activity of NMI-187 and NMI-221.*Int J Impotence Res* 8,1996, No 3,103.

22 Cellek S, Kalsi JS, Kell PD, *et al.* NCX-911,a novel nitric-oxide–releasing PDE-5 inhibitor relaxes rabbit corpus cavernosum in the absence of endogenous nitric oxide. *Int J Impotence Res* 2003;**15** Suppl. 6:S25.

23 Christ GJ. Editorial: Membrane bound guanylyl cyclase as a potential molecular target for the treatment of erectile dysfunction. *J Urol* 2003;**169**:1923.

24 Küthe A, Reinecke M, Ückert S, *et al.* Expression of guanylyl cyclase B in the human corpus cavernosum penis and the possible involvement of its ligand C-type natriuretic polypeptide in the induction of penile erection. *J Urol* 2003;**169**:1911–1917.

25 Bischoff E, Schramm M, Straub A, *et al.* BAY 41-2272 a stimulator of soluble guanylyl cyclase induces NO-dependent penile erection in vivo. *Int J Impotence Res* 2002;**14** Suppl 3,S43:BSP 10.

26 Brioni JD, Nakane M, Hsieh GC, *et al.* Activators of soluble guanylate cyclase for the treatment of male erectile dysfunction. *Int J Impotence Res* 2002; **14**:8–14.

27 Kalsi JS, Rees RW, Hobbs AJ, *et al.* Bay 41-2272, a novel nitric oxide independent soluble guanylate cyclase activator, relaxes human and rabbit corpus cavernosum in vitro. *J Urol* 2003;**169**:761–766.

28 Kalsi JS, Ralph DJ, Madge DJ, *et al.* A comparative study of sildenafil, NCX-911 and BAY 41-2272 on the anococcygeus muscle of diabetic rats. *Int J Impotence Res* 2004;**16**:479–485.

29 Chitaley K, Webb RC, Mills TM. The ups and downs of Rho-kinase and penile erection: upstream regulators and downstream substrates of Rho-kinase and their potential role in the erectile response. *Int J Impotence Res* 2003;**15**:105–109.

30 Sjunnesson J, Hedlund P, Mizusawa H, Andersson K-E. Inhibition of Rho-associated kinases by Y-27632 produces erectile responses in the mouse. *J Urol* 2002;**167** No 4 Suppl, 238:933.

31 Chang S, Hypolite JA, Changolkar A, *et al.* Diabetes associated erectile dysfunction: role of endothelin and Rho kinase. *J Urol* 2002;**167** No 4 Suppl 237:932.

32 Wilkes N, White S, Rajasekaran M. PDE-V inhibitors synergizes Rho-kinase antagonism and enhances erectile response in male hypertensive rats. *J Urol* 2003; **169**:No 4 Suppl, 360:1346.

33 Zheng Y, Chang S, Wein AJ, *et al.* Upregulation of Rho kinase in a human corpus cavernosum smooth muscle cell line in response to hypoxia. *J Urol* 2004;**171** Suppl, 376: Abstr 1429.

34 Mills TM, Chitaley K, Lewis RW. Vasoconstriction in erectile physiology. *Int J Impotence Res* 2001;**13** Suppl. 5:S29–S34.

35 Wilkes N, White S, Cosgrove DJ, Rajasekaran M. Y-27632, an inhibitor of Rho-kinase, improves erectile response in male hypertensive rats. *J Urol* 2002;**167** No 4 Suppl, 238:935.

36 Dai Y, Chitaley K, Webb RC, *et al.* Topical application of a Rho-kinase inhibitor in rats causes penile erection. *Int J Impotence Res* 2004;**16**:294–298.

CHAPTER 10

Future Treatment Aspects of Erectile Dysfunction: Gene Therapy and Tissue Engineering

Wayne J.G. Hellstrom

Introduction

Gene therapy in urology initially focused on urinary tract malignancies such as bladder and prostate cancer. However, in the last half decade new research endeavors in tissue engineering, and gene and cell-based therapies, have become more widespread for the treatment of erectile dysfunction (ED). Tissue engineering aims to replace complete tissues or organs, while gene and cell-based therapies act at the cellular level to improve specific cellular and enzymatic functions [1].

Tissue Engineering and ED

Various surgical techniques have been developed to restore genital abnormalities, e.g. epispadias, micropenis, penile carcinoma, genital trauma, corporal fibrosis, and Peyronie's disease. In many of these cases there is a limited amount of cavernosal tissue and surgeons have relied on prosthetic devices to recover the patient's erectile function [2].

Reconstruction of normal erectile tissue using autologous cells, derived from the patient's own body, is an intriguing concept for the treatment of this severe form of ED. Atala and colleagues have proposed a tissue regeneration approach that involves patching isolated cells to support structures that possess suitable surface chemistry for guiding cell reorganization and growth [3].

Initial experiments were performed in order to determine the feasibility of creating corporal smooth muscle and endothelial cells *in vivo*, using cultured human corporal smooth muscle cells seeded onto biodegradable polymers [4]. Their results were confirmed with human corporal smooth muscle and endothelial cells seeded on acellular matrices processed from donor rabbit corpora cavernosa [5].

Three and six months after implanting these tissue-engineered constructs into the corpora cavernosa of the animals from which the respective cells had been harvested, animals with tissue-engineered corporal segments exhibited much better functional and morphologic results compared to unseeded control animals, as assessed by cavernosography, cavernosometry, mating behavior, cell-specific immunochemistry, and Western blot analyses. Currently, this group has been working on engineering corporal tissue for the purposes of phallic reconstruction, and tunical tissue for reconstruction of severe cases of Peyronie's disease.

Gene Therapy and ED

Basic science research on erectile physiology has focused on the pathogenesis of ED and has provided convincing evidence that ED is predominantly a disease of vascular etiology. The oral phosphodiesterase-5 (PDE-5) inhibitors are uniformly recommended as first-line therapy because of their convenience and high rate of efficacy in a diverse population of ED patients. Unfortunately, not all ED patients benefit from PDE-5 inhibitor therapy, and the development of new approaches, including gene and cell-based therapies, is required.

Initially, gene therapy had been reserved for the treatment of life-threatening disorders, including cancer, hereditary and acquired diseases. Although there have been some concerns and regulatory changes due to the loss of a young volunteer who was treated with the intrahepatic administration of a recombinant adenoviral vector containing ornithine transcarbamylase in 1999, there are still hundreds of gene therapy trials being conducted worldwide [6,7]. Gene therapy is an attractive therapeutic possibility for the treatment of ED. A simple concept about ED is that in most men only a very small alteration in the balance between contracting and relaxing stimuli can cause significant effects on cavernosal and penile vascular smooth muscle tone [8,9] (Fig. 10.1). The penis is also a convenient tissue target for gene therapy because of its external location, the ubiquity of endothelial-lined spaces, and low level of blood flow.

The objective of gene therapy is to introduce new or repair damaged genetic materials (DNA or RNA) into the cells of a target (i.e. the penis) in order to recover the organ's function.

The ideal vector for gene transfer is one that allows for efficient transduction and long-term stable transgene expression while having few or no adverse effects, such as risk of infection, immunogenicity, or host-cell mutagenesis. Various vectors, such as viral vectors (adenovirus, adeno-associated virus, adeno-myoblast, and retrovirus) and nonviral vectors (naked DNA, plasmid DNA, liposomes, and myoblast-mediated), have been used to date for the transfer of genetic material to the target cell or tissue

[10]. Each has advantages and disadvantages with regards to their safety, efficiency, and immunogenicity (Fig. 10.2).

The essential component of the mechanism for penile erection is cavernosal smooth muscle relaxation. Therefore all molecules and enzyme systems that are involved in signal transduction for either relaxing or inhibiting contraction of corporal smooth muscle are potential targets for gene therapy to the penis. Many research centers have conducted or are conducting studies to exploit this recognized mechanism (Table 10.1).

Gene therapy can be divided into two simplistic strategies:

1 Increase the supply of stimulus, by increasing the expression of endogenous vasomodulators.

2 Alter the demand, such that the end organ or receptor becomes more sensitive to relaxatory stimuli. Therefore, gene therapy restores the normal

Table 10.1 Potential applications of gene therapy for ED.

Plasmid or naked DNA
- *hSlo* (maxi-K channel)*
- pnNOS

Viral mediated gene transfer
- iNOS
- eNOS
- pnNOS
- Anti-PIN
- BDNF
- VEGF
- Anti-Arginase
- EC-SOD
- CGRP
- T19NRhoA

Proteins
- VEGF
- bFGF
- BDNF
- IGF & growth hormone

Cell-based
- Endothelial Cell
- Adeno-Myoblast iNOS

* Initiated FDA-approved Phase I clinical trial.

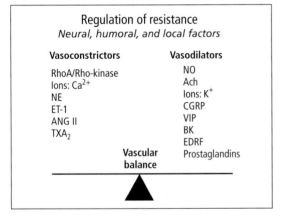

Fig. 10.1 Balance between vasoconstrictors and vasodilators determine penile vascular smooth muscle tone.

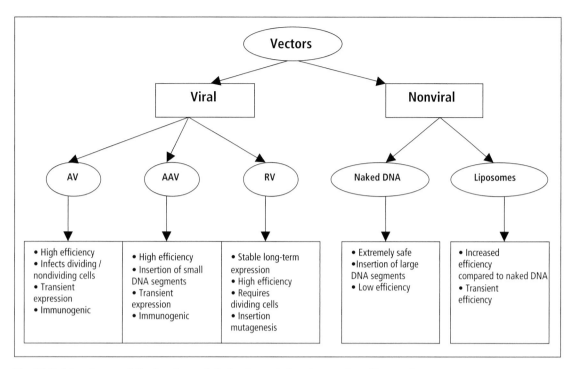

Fig. 10.2 Advantages and disadvantages of viral and nonviral vectors employed in gene therapy.

balance between contracting and relaxing stimuli to the cavernosal smooth muscle.

Since the first preclinical study in an *in vivo* rat model using iNOS [11], a variety of gene therapy trials have been conducted for the treatment of ED. Because of its significant role in the physiology of normal erectile function, many gene therapy studies have focused on the NO/GC/cGMP pathway. The rationale for this target is that overexpression of important endogenous cavernosal smooth muscle relaxants and vasodilators could assist with the diminished erectile response, as witnessed in men suffering from ED. Follow-up approaches suggest other means of genetic manipulation: nerve and vascular growth factors, (e.g. brain-derivated nerve growth factor [BDNF], vascular endothelial growth factor [VEGF]), the cyclic adenosine monophosphate (cAMP) cascade (i.e. calcitonin gene-related peptide [CGRP] receptor), the calcium sensitization pathway, and K+ channel gene expression (a cellular convergence point for mediating the effects of all of the above).

Cell-Based Approaches and ED

One of the most important recent discoveries in biomedical research is that stem cells are found in many tissues of adults that can provide new cells for normal tissue turnover and can regenerate damaged and diseased tissue [12]. Marrow stromal cells (mesenchymal stem cells) are adult stem cells from bone marrow that have multilineage differentiation potential and contribute to the regeneration of mesenchymal tissues, including bone, cartilage, muscle, and fat [13]. As marrow stromal cells are relatively easy to isolate, expand *ex vivo*, and gene engineer, genetically modified marrow stromal cells with desired genes have recently been used for gene delivery and tissue regeneration in the treatment of various diseases, including ED, with little or no host immune response [14].

Another potential application for ED is the (re)-implantation of genetically modified cells into the corpus cavernosum. The aim is to seed the corpora cavernosa with cells having desired, genetically modified physiologic characteristics. Endothelial cells have the ability to adhere and self-aggregate once they are transplanted into another organ, such as the penis [15]. Wessels *et al.* first demonstrated that autologous endothelial cells could be transplanted into the corpus cavernosum, and undergo cell adherence and persistence in the cavernosal sinusoids for up to two weeks and eventually become part of the sinusoidal lining of the penis [16]. This is the basis for the rationale of cell-based gene therapy for the treatment of ED. Studies have documented that muscle cell-mediated gene therapy was even more efficacious in delivering iNOS into the corpus cavernosum [17]. Transplanted cells are of considerable interest, and future studies using marker genes and functional transgenes will further our knowledge about the survival, replication, and function of endothelial cells within the corpus cavernosum.

Current Status of Human Erectile Dysfunction Therapy Trials

Because of limitations of current ED therapies, there is a clinical demand and a scientific interest in gene transfer therapy for ED. The safety and efficacy of many of the vectors used to allow for delivery of the gene of interest is of paramount importance to the regulatory bodies. These concerns, for the most part, have limited the widespread application and progress in the field of gene therapy for ED. (Table 10.2).

At the time of writing, there is only one ongoing human clinical trial of gene transfer for the treatment of ED [18]. The group from Albert Einstein in New York City has exploited the mechanism of action of ion channels over the last decade.

Unlike gene transfer therapy for cancer, where 100% of the cells must be affected, only a small percentage of cells in the corpora need to be transfected with the gene of interest in order to obtain the desired erectile response. Because of gap junctions, a small stimulus can be rapidly propagated from cell to cell in a collective syncytial response. This has relevance in a number of clinical situations (e.g. radical prostatectomy and diabetes mellitus) where the neural signaling may be impaired, but the local cavernous response may be intact.

Table 10.2 Gene therapy approaches for the treatment of erectile dysfunction.

Supply side	Increase NO
	eNOS
	nNOS
	Superoxide dismutase
	Increase nerve supply
	BDNF
	Increase vascular supply
	VEGF
	Increase CGRP
Demand side	Decrease amount of stimulus required for relaxation
	Alter potassium/calcium channels (via *hSlo*)
	Alter calcium sensitization (via RhoA)

The vector that meets both efficacy and FDA safety requirements is the maxi-K methodology. Though naked DNA has poor transduction efficiency, only a small amount is needed for obtaining the required response. Additionally, naked DNA does not cause an allergic or immune response as witnessed with viral vectors, and it is not integrated into host chromosomes.

The preclinical evidence employing the maxi-K vector injected intracavernosally as naked DNA has demonstrated efficacy and long duration of action in both diabetic and aging rat model experiments [19,20,21].

The USFDA approved a human trial studying *hSlo* maxi-K under an investigational application in August 2003. A phase I sequential dosing trial was initiated in early 2004 and enrollment has proceeded slowly, mainly because of the unknown issues of gene therapy.

A total of 15 men were screened for this trial and the preliminary results after transfer in six men at two dose levels was recently published [18]. At this time, three dose levels (500, 1000, and 5000 mg) were administered into three groups of men each [22]. Preliminary data has revealed no gene transfer-related serious adverse events in any of the trial participants. There has been no evidence of transfer of any *hSlo* maxi-K into the semen as measured by polymerase chain reaction analysis (an impor-

Table 10.3 Gene therapy approaches for the treatment of erectile dysfunction.

- NO/cGMP System
- Ion Channels and Gap Junctions
- Control of Oxidative Stress
- Growth Factors
- RhoA/Rho kinase System
- Stem Cells

---

tant requirement by the FDA). In the first two groups of 500 and 1000 mg (suboptimal dosing as per comparative rat model studies where 10–20-times higher doses were safely used for efficacy), there was no evidence of efficacy as determined by the international index of erectile function (IIEF) and Rigiscan data. However, in the third group (5,000 mg), one participant reported significant improvement as per Q3 and Q4 of the IIEF at three months after transfer. This benefit has been corroborated by his partner. These investigators plan sequential instillations at two higher doses in the near future. The efficacy and safety of this first gene transfer study will undoubtedly direct future research efforts in the field of gene therapy for ED in the years to come.

Conclusion

The past decade has seen an explosion of information regarding the physiology, pathophysiology, and pharmacology of the erectile mechanism. Creative research in the coming decades will stimulate new applications in tissue engineering that will complement our surgical reconstructive endeavors. The introduction of gene- and cell-based therapies for the treatment of ED will attract more scientific and media attention. Though one may simplistically codify a number of current gene-based approaches (Table 10.3), only time and data generated from human controlled trials will provide the answers.

References

1 Schultheiss D. Regenerative medicine in andrology: Tissue engineering and gene therapy as potential treatment options for penile deformation and erectile dysfunction. *Eur Urol* 2004;**46**:162.

2 Kwon GK, Yoo JJ, Atala A. Autologous penile corpora cavernosa replacement using tissue engineering techniques. *J Urol* 2002;**168**:1754.

3 Atala A. Tissue engineering applications for erectile dysfunction. *Int J Impot Res* 1999;**11** (Suppl 1):S41.

4 Falke G, Yoo JJ, Machado MG, Moreland R, Atala, A. Formation of corporal tissue architecture in vivo using human cavernosal muscle and endothelial cells seeded on collagen matrices. *Tissue Eng* 2003;**9**:871–879.

5 Kershen R, Yoo JJ, Moreland RB, Krane RJ, Atala A. Novel system for the formation of reconstitution of human corpus cavernosum smooth muscle tissue in vivo. *Tissue Eng* 2002;**8**:515.

6 Scollay R. Gene therapy: a brief overview of the past, present, and future. *Ann N Y Acad Sci* 2001;**953**:26.

7 Ferber D. Gene therapy. Safer and virus-free? *Science* 2001;**294**:1638.

8 Azadzoi KM, Kim N, Brown ML, Goldstein I, Cohen RA, Saenz de Tejada I. Endothelium-derived nitric oxide and cyclooxygenase products modulate corpus cavernosum smooth muscle tone. *J Urol* 1992;**147**:220.

9 Lerner SE, Melman A, Christ GJ. A review of erectile dysfunction: new insights and more questions. *J Urol* 1993;**149**:1246.

10 Bivalacqua TJ, Hellstrom WJ. Potential application of gene therapy for the treatment of erectile dysfunction. *J Androl* 2001;**22**:183.

11 Garban H, Marquez D, Magee T, Moody J, Rajavashisht T, Rodriguez JA, Hung A, Vernet D, Rajfer J, Gonzalez-Cadavid NF. Cloning of rat and human inducible penile nitric oxide synthase. Application for gene therapy of erectile dysfunction. *Biol Reprod* 1997;**56**:954.

12 Gerlach JC, Zeilinger K. Adult stem cell technology–prospects for cell based therapy in regenerative medicine. *Int J Artif Organs* 2002;**25**:83.

13 Pittenger MF, Mackay AM, Beck SC, Jaiswal RK, Douglas R, Mosca JD, Moorman MA, Simonetti DW, Craig S, Marshak DR. Multilineage potential of adult human mesenchymal stem cells. *Science* 1999;**284**:143.

14 Van Damme A, Vanden Driessche T, Collen D, Chuah MK. Bone marrow stromal cells as targets for gene therapy. *Curr Gene Ther* 2002;**2**:195.

15 Stopeck AT, Vahedian M, Williams SK: Transfer and expression of the interferon gamma gene in human endothelial cells inhibits vascular smooth muscle cell growth in vitro. *Cell Transplant* 1997;**6**:1.

16 Wessells H, Williams SK. Endothelial cell transplantation into the corpus cavernosum: moving towards cell-based gene therapy. *J Urol* 1999;**162**:2162.

17 Tirney S, Mattes CE, Yoshimura N, *et al.* Nitric oxide synthase gene therapy for erectile dysfunction: comparison of plasmid, adenovirus, and adenovirus-transduced myoblast vectors. *Mol Urol* 2001;**5**:37.

18 Melman A, Bar-Chama N, McCullough A, Davies K, Christ G. The first human trial for gene transfer therapy for the treatment of erectile dysfunction: Preliminary Results. *Eur Urol* 2005;**48**:314–318.

19 Christ GH, Rehman J, Day N, *et al.* Intracorporal injection of hSlo cDNA in rats produced physiologically relevant alterations in penile function. *Am J Physiol* 1998;**275** (2 pt 2): H600–8.

20 Melman A, Zhao W, Dzvies KP, Bakal PR, Christ GH. The successful long-term treatment of age related erectile dysfunction with hSlo cDNA in rata in vivo. *J Urol* 2003;**170**(1):285–290.

21 Christ GJ: Gene therapy treatments for erectile and bladder dysfunction. *Curr Urol Rep* 2004;**5**(1):52–60.

22 Melman A. Personal communication, August 2005.

CHAPTER 11

Vacuum Constriction Devices

Sidney Glina and Hartmut Porst

History

The concept of vacuum device therapy in the treatment of erectile dysfunction (ED) goes back as early as 1874 when the American physician John King described a method of improving erections by a small vacuum pump. The first patent for a vacuum device was granted in 1914 in Germany and 1917 in US to Otto Lederer. In 1960 the American entrepreneur Geddings Osbon started to produce a vacuum device and founded his own company for manufacturing the device he had invented. Finally in 1982 he was granted permission from the Food and Drug Administration to produce this device, which was named Erec-Aid® [1]. Nadig *et al.* published the first report on efficacy and safety of vacuum constriction devices (VCD) in 1986 [2].

Indications for Treatment of Erectile Dysfunction with VCD

Compared to other therapeutic options for ED the major advantage of VCD is that it can be applied successfully for nearly all etiologies of ED [2]; but its success clearly depends on adequate instruction [3].

After the launch of the phosphodiesterase type 5 inhibitors, the first effective oral treatment for broad spectrum ED populations, VCD became a second-line therapy along with intracavernosal self-injection and intraurethral therapy with vasoactive substances [4]. VCD may be offered mainly to elderly patients with occasional intercourse attempts, as younger patients show limited acceptance because of its mechanism resulting in a more unnaturally perceived erection [5]. On the other hand there may be couples preferring VCD, as was reported by Chen *et al.*, with one-third of men, who had been successfully treated with VCD and who had tried sildenafil with satisfactory erections, finally opting for VCD [6].

Vacuum therapy may also be used in conjunction with other therapies to enhance results. So, for example, the addition of 100 mg sildenafil with VCD improved sexual satisfaction and penile rigidity in patients unsatisfied with VCD alone, after radical prostatectomy [7]. Combination treatment of psychotherapy and VCD showed greater beneficial response in men with ED than either therapy alone [8].

Technique of VCD (Fig. 11.1a, 11.1b)

Nearly all commercially available vacuum devices share a common mechanism of action: a plastic cylinder, whose lower edge is made airtight with the application of a lubricant gel, is applied over the penis in a standing position and then firmly pressed against the body (see Fig. 11.1a). Then a vacuum is created manually via a pump that is either separately connected to the cylinder with a tube or is directly integrated in the distal end (top) of the cylinder and is then battery operated (see Figs 11.1a, 11.1b). The erection obtained with VCD is not a natural-like erection. The vacuum pressure passively draws blood into the sinusoidal spaces of the cavernous bodies of the penis, whose diameters double after negative pressure distension, but with maintenance of the

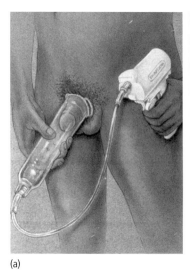
(a)

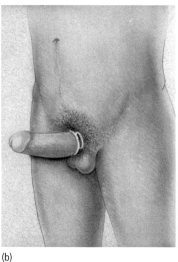
(b)

Fig. 11.1 Technique of vacuum device therapy (the conventional "two-piece" Osbon Erec-Aid® system).

cavernous artery flow [9]. Once an adequately rigid erection has been achieved a rubber constriction ring, previously rolled onto the cylinder prior to the vacuum maneuver, is now rolled off the base of the penis preventing the escape of the artificially entrapped blood. The application of the constriction ring should be limited for up to 30 minutes to avoid ischemic damages of the cavernosal tissue. Sometimes two constriction rings must be applied to maintain a rigid erection. Vacuum pressures between 100 mm Hg and 225 mm Hg is necessary to achieve erection [10]. Compared to naturally occurring erections, VCD-derived erections are perceived differently by both the men and their partners. Because the constriction ring can be applied only to the base of the penis, the proximal third of the cavernous bodies, i.e. the crura, are not involved in VCD erections. This non-involvement of the crura penis in VCD-induced erection causes some degree of instability at the penis' base, quite often requiring manual assistance while inserting the penis into the vagina. Due to the passively entrapped venous blood, the VCD-erected penis looks more cyanotic, is perceived to be much cooler, and not always enjoyed by the partners, in addition to the increased glans volume [11].

Results of VCD therapy (Table 11.1)

Among the available literature on VCD publications,

most series are reporting on the outcome of the Osbon VCD devices (Osbon Erec-Aid®) and its successor (Osbon Esteem®), and only few smaller series are published with the devices of other manufacturers such as Innovital System, Post-T, VED, and the Synergist System.

When analyzing the data of VCD therapy a striking feature of many published series is the discrepancy between the numbers of VCD users or men to whom VCD was prescribed, respectively, and those finally being eligible for assessment. So, for example, in the large series as published by Witherington [13] and Lewis [11], only 10–17% of all VCD owners were considered or eligible, respectively, for evaluation of the outcome, which is in marked contrast to all other ED therapies such as oral therapy, self-injection therapy, or even penile implants. In these series, in which a majority of primarily recruited patients were eligible, 40–60% failed to continue with VCD therapy [18,19,21]. The generally low acceptance of VCD therapy was shown in the series of Graham *et al*; among 1236 new ED patients who were subject to all diagnostic work-up and to whom all therapeutic modalities available at that time were offered to only 323 (27%), requested a two-week trial period and only 74 (6% of the total population) finally went for a VCD prescription [20]. In a German VCD series it was obvious that the acceptance rate of VCD was markedly higher in non-responders to pharma-

Table 11.1 Overview of the literature on VCD therapy outcome.

Author	Device	N	Evaluable	Mean age (years)	Follow-up (months)	Satisfaction
Nadig[12] 1987	Osbon ErecAid	302	81% (244)	?	up to 72	83%
Witherington[17] 1989	Osbon ErecAid	15,000	10% (1517)	64	8.6	92% good erections
Blackard[14] 1993	Osbon ErecAid	47	96% (45)	?	?	42%
Derouet[15] 1993	Osbon ErecAid	90	100%	32–75	?	37%
Baltaci[16] 1995	Osbon ErecAid	61	80% (49)	?	12.8	67%
Lewis[11] 1997	Osbon ErecAid	34,777	17% (5847)	?	1974–1992	65–83%
Meinhardt[17] 1993	Post-T VED	74	100%	55	3 weeks	30%
Fedel[18] 1995	Innovital	100	40%	52.4	6	90%
Cookson[19] 1993	?	216	53% (115)	65	29	84%
Graham[20] 1998	?	323	100%	61	2 weeks	23%
Droupy[21] 1998	?	53 (RRP)	55% (29)	66.5	27	52%
Opsomer[22] 1998	?	170	?	66	48	55%

cotherapy compared to responders (45% vs. 22%) [15].

Contraindications

Contraindications in the use of vacuum therapy are few and primarily include patients with a tendency for spontaneous priapisms/prolonged erections [11]. Originally, bleeding disorders were considered a contraindication [11], but a prospective trial showed that the adverse effects of vacuum therapy, especially hematoma and petechiae, in patients on warfarin, did not exceed those observed in the general urologic population [23]. In addition VCD therapy is contraindicated in severe penile anomalies, especially in marked penile deviations—either congenital or acquired—as a consequence of Peyronie's disease.

Complications

Side effects such as occasional numbness, pain, penile bruising, or petechiae, are the most common complications of VCD. Painful ejaculation, due to the constriction ring, has been commonly reported [11,13]. As mentioned, although VCD are able to give sufficient penile rigidity in the majority of patients, vaginal penetration can be impaired because of the instability of the phallus at the penis base, and ejaculation is achieved in less than two-thirds of men due to the fact that passage through the urethra is blocked by the constriction ring [11]. In addition, satisfaction with sexual intercourse may be impaired because the whole situation may not be accompanied by a subjective state of physical or mental sexual arousal. Thus, the mere physical presence of an erection does not seem to evoke bodily or mental feelings of sexual arousal, especially in the partners [24].

Rarely, the use of VCD has been associated with Peyronie's disease [25]. In a prospective trial the use of VCD for spinal cord-injured men with erectile dysfunction did not increase the risk of adverse events [26]. Other anecdotal complications linked to

VCD were skin necrosis and urethral bleeding [27]. Sometimes, continuous use of VCD may result in hyperpigmentation of the penile skin due to repeated skin bruising, with subsequent hemosiderin deposition. It is important to advise patients to use only prescription devices. Others devices have no pressure control or safety valves to release the pressure, which can increase the rate and severity of complications [25].

Acceptance, Long-term Use and Drop-out Rates of VCD

Although VCD therapy is able to produce erections sufficient for sexual intercourse in more than 75% of users [29], the main reasons for discontinuation of VCD therapy were ineffectiveness, side effects, the time-consuming nature of the procedure, lack of acceptance by patient and partner, and the relatively high costs of the devices [28]. Once VCD turned out to be effective, significant increase in frequency of intercourse, sexual arousal, coital orgasm and sexual satisfaction was reported by patients' partners [30].

In a minority of patients (8–16%) the continuing use of VCD therapy may result in recovery of spontaneous erections [11,16,18,19,21].

Present Role of VCD in the Era of Oral Pharmacotherapy

Treatment of ED with the vacuum constriction devices should be utilized as an alternative to intracavernous drug-induced erection therapy when oral therapy fails or is contraindicated. Elderly males with a stable partner are the main indication for this therapy [31.32].

Its main advantage is that almost every case, regardless of the underlying ED etiology, may be managed successfully with VCD, regarding the establishment of an erection [29]. Efficacy depends on correct individual instruction and it needs at least two teaching sessions for patient learning [11,33].

Although VCD therapy is presently not considered a first-line treatment, it is used in many countries worldwide [3]. The successful use of VCD was repeatedly reported in patients after removal of penile prostheses, to prevent penile scarring and shortening [30,31]. Chronic intermittent stretching with a vacuum erection device was used in a small trial to lengthening shortened penises caused by severe Peyronie's disease, after venous grafting [36].

Moreover, as mentioned before, VCD may be used successfully in conjunction with self-injection therapy, and may add to its efficacy [37,38].

References

1 Lederer O. Vorrichtung zur künstlichen erektion des penis. Patentschrift Nr. 268874, Klasse 30d, Gruppe 15. Kaiserliches Patentamt 1914. Available from European patent office, Den Haag, The Netherlands, 1914.

2 Nadig PW, Ware JC, Blummof R. Noninvasive device to produce and maintain an erection-like state. *Urology* 1986;**27**:126–131.

3 Tan HL. Economic cost of male erectile dysfunction using a decision analytic model: for a hypothetical managed-care plan of 100,000 members. *Pharmacoeconomics* 2000;**17**(1):77–107.

4 Montague DK, Jarow JP, Broderick RR, *et al.* Chapter 1: Management of erectile dysfunction: AUA Update. *J Urol* 2005;**174**:230–239.

5 Hakim LS, Kim C, Krongrad A, *et al.* Intracavernosal injection of prostaglandin E1 versus the vacuum erection device: A comparative analysis of the early effects on corporeal blood chemistry and blood flow. *J Urol* 1999;**161**(No.4 Suppl):270.

6 Chen J, Mabjeesh NJ, Greenstein A. Sildenafil versus the vacuum erection device: patient preference. *J Urol* 2001;**166**(5):1779–1781.

7 Raina R, Agarwal A, Allamaneni SS, Lakin MM, Zippe CD. Sildenafil citrate and vacuum constriction device combination enhances sexual satisfaction in erectile dysfunction after radical prostatectomy. *Urology* 2005;**65**:360–364.

8 Wylie KR, Jones RH, Walters S. The potential benefit of vacuum devices augmenting psychosexual therapy for erectile dysfunction: a randomized controlled trial. *J Sex Marital Ther* 2003;**29**(3):227–236.

9 Broderick GA, McGahan JP, Stone AR, White RD. The hemodynamics of vacuum constriction erections: assessment by color Doppler ultrasound. *J Urol* 1992; **147**:57–61.

10 Marmar JL, DeBenedictis TJ, Praiss DE. Penile plethysmography on impotent men using vacuum constriction devices. *Urology* 1988;**32**:198–203.

11 Lewis RW, Witherington R. External vacuum therapy for erectile dysfunction: use and results. *World J Urol* 1997;**15**(1):78–82.

12 Nadig PW. Osbon ErecAid. Letters to the Editor. *J Urol* 1987;**138**:630.

13 Witherington R. Vacuum constriction device for management of erectile impotence. *J Urol* 1989;**141**: 320–322.

14 Blackard E, Borkon WD, Lima JS, *et al.* Use of vacuum tumescence device for impotence secondary to venous leakage. *Urology* 1993;**41**:225–230.

15 Derouet H, Zehl U. Die behandlung der erektilen dysfunktion mittels vakuum-saugpumpen (EHS). *Urologe A* 1993;**32**:312–315.

16 Baltaci S, Aydos K, Kosar A, *et al.* Treating erectile dysfunction with a vacuum tumescence device: a retrospective analysis of acceptance and satisfaction. *Br J Urol* 1995;**76**:757–760.

17 Meinhardt W, Lycklama á Nijeholt AAB, Kropman RF, *et al.* The negative pressure device for erectile disorders: when does it fail? *J Urol* 1993;**149**:1285–1287.

18 Fedel M, Sudhoff F, Andreeßen R, *et al.* Vakuumerektionshilfesysteme in der behandlung der erektilen dysfunktion. *Akt Urol* 1995;**26**:339–343.

19 Cookson MS, Nadig PW. Long-term results with vacuum constriction device. *J Urol* 1993;**149**:290–294.

20 Graham P, Collins JP, Thijssen AM. Popularity of the vacuum erection device in male sexual dysfunction. *Int J Impotence Res* 1998;**10**(Suppl.3):S6.

21 Droupy S, Amar E, Thiounn N, *et al.* Acceptance and efficacy of vacuum constriction device for the treatment of erectile dysfunction after radical prostatectomy. *Int J Impotence Res* 1998;**10**(Suppl.3):S24.

22 Opsomer RJ, Wese FX, van Langh PJ. Long-term results with vacuum constriction device. *Int J Impotence Res* 1998;**10**(No.3):S49.

23 Limoge JP, Olins E, Henderson D, Donatucci CF. Minimally invasive therapies in the treatment of erectile dysfunction in anticoagulated cases: a study of satisfaction and safety. *J Urol* 1996;**155**(4):1276–1279.

24 Delizonna LL, Wincze JP, Litz BT, Brown TA, Barlow DH. A comparison of subjective and physiological measures of mechanically produced and erotically produced erections (or, is an erection an erection?). *J Sex Marital Ther* 2001;**27**(1):21–31.

25 Hakim LS, Munarriz RM, Kulaksizoglu H, Nehra A, Udelson D, Goldstein I. Vacuum erection associated impotence and Peyronie's disease. *J Urol* 1996; **155**(2):534–535.

26 Seckin B, Atmaca I, Ozgok Y, Gokalp A, Harmankaya C. External vacuum device therapy for spinal cord injured males with erectile dysfunction. *Int Urol Nephrol* 1996; **28**(2):235–240.

27 Ganem JP, Lucey DT, Janosko EO, Carson CC. Unusual complications of the vacuum erection device. *Urology* 1998;**51**:627–631.

28 Meuleman EJ. Experiences with a vacuum apparatus in the treatment of erection disorders. *Ned Tijdschr Geneeskd* 1993 20;**137**(8):412–416.

29 Montague DK, Barada JH, Belker AM, Levine LA, Nadig PW, Roehrborn CG, Sharlip ID, Bennett AH. Clinical guidelines panel on erectile dysfunction: summary report on the treatment of organic erectile dysfunction. The American Urological Association. *J Urol* 1996; **156**(6):2007–2011.

30 Althof SE, Turner LA, Levine SB, Bodner D, Kursh ED, Resnick MI. Through the eyes of women: the sexual and psychological responses of women to their partner's treatment with self-injection or external vacuum therapy. *J Urol* 1992;**147**:1024–1027.

31 Hatzimouratidis K, Hatzichristou DG. A comparative review of the options for treatment of erectile dysfunction: which treatment for which patient? *Drugs* 2005; **65**:1621–1650.

32 Nunez Mora C, Rios Gonzalez E, Martinez-Pineiro Lorenzo L, Julve Villalta E, Pastor Arquero T, Cortes Guiseris R, Cuervo Blanco E, de la Pena Barthel J. Treatment of erectile dysfunction with vacuum devices. *Arch Esp Urol* 2000;**53**:819–825.

33 Willard BA. An assessment of a vacuum constriction device in treating erectile dysfunction. *Urol Nurs* 1998;**18**(1):33–37.

34 Hakim LS, Green JT, Nehra A. Use of the vacuum erection device to minimize corporal fibrosis and shortening following removal of penile prosthesis for infection. *Int J Impotence Res* 1998;**10**(Suppl.3):S43.

35 Moul JW, McLeod DG. Negative pressure devices in the explanted penile prosthesis population. *J Urol* 1985;**142**:729–731.

36 Lue TF, El-Sakka AI. Lengthening shortened penis caused by Peyronie's disease using circular venous grafting and daily stretching with a vacuum erection device. *J Urol* 1999;**161**(4):1141–1144.

37 Chen J, Godschalk MF, Katz PG, *et al.* Combining intracavernous injection and external vacuum as treatment for erectile dysfunction. *J Urol* 1995;**153**: 1476–1477.

38 Marmar JL, DeBenedictis TJ, Praiss DE. The use of vacuum constrictor device to augment a partial erection following an intracavernous injection. *J Urol* 1988;**140**:975–979.

CHAPTER 12

Surgical Treatment of Erectile Dysfunction

Vascular Surgery of the Penis

Michael Sohn

Introduction and History

It was probably Leonardo Da Vinci who first recognized the importance of blood supply for penile erection [1]. In 1923 the French surgeon Leriche first described arterial vascular impotence in the syndrome of thrombotic obliteration of the aortic bifurcation [2,3]. During the following years several operative strategies were developed to save or reconstruct the internal iliac artery during abdominal vascular surgery for the purpose of maintaining or restoring erectile function [4].

It was in 1973 that the Czech surgeon Vaclav Michal performed direct anastomosis of the inferior epigastric artery to the cavernous body. This original penile revascularization technique has been named the Michal I procedure [5]. During the following years, many modifications of penile revascularization, all using the inferior epigastric artery (IEA) as the donor vessel were developed. Direct anastomoses to corpus cavernosum were soon abandoned and refined microsurgical techniques made it technically possible to anastomose the IEA to the dorsal penile vessels (arteria dorsalis penis, vena dorsalis penis). These techniques were developed in the 1970s and 1980s. Despite the passage of many years, no further important technical change has occurred in the field of penile revascularization and still no

consensus exists concerning the value of penile revascularization.

The same problem exists for venous surgery in the treatment of erectile dysfunction (ED). The idea that pathologic venous outflow from the corpora during sexual excitement may cause ED was initiated some 140 years ago when the Italian dermatologist Parona published the first report on percutaneous scarification of the dorsal penile vein in ED believed to be of venogenic origin [6].

At the turn of the 20th century, surgical venous ligation or resection was practiced by several surgeons [7]. Crural plication techniques for so-called proximal penile venous leakage were developed by Lowsley. In 1953 he published a series of more than 1000 patients in whom he performed this procedure [8]. With the new possibilities for investigation of vasculogenic ED after the introduction of drug-induced erection, these venous ligation and resection procedures were reintroduced into the therapy of ED in the 1980s. The surgical procedure over time has been expanded from simple deep dorsal vein ligation to extensive surgical exposure and excision, ligation or crural plication, and spongiolysis between the glans and corpora alone, or in combination [9]. At the same time, antegrade or retrograde embolization with microcoils, sclerosing agents, or cyanocrylate, was reported as a less invasive radiologic procedure, which could be used alone, or in combination with open operative procedures [4]. Even arterialization of the deep dorsal penile vein was used for the therapy of venogenic impotence [10].

All these procedures for venous ligation or resection were developed more than 15 years ago. Sufficient time for long-term follow up assessment has passed and we are still confronted with contradictory results. Indications, surgical technique, and prognostic criteria are not clearly defined, and are still debated in the literature [4].

Penile Revascularization Procedures

Rationale and technical considerations

The simplest approach to penile revascularization is a direct anastomosis of an arterial donor vessel to the corpus cavernosum. But, with this approach most patients develop high-flow priapism in the early postoperative phase, followed by fibrosis of cavernous tissue due to the supraphysiologic intracavernous pressure. Even a venous interposition graft between the femoral artery and cavernous body does not solve this dilemma [2].

Several authors have reported on an end-to-side anastomosis between the IEA and the deep cavernous artery. Theoretically this approach is the most direct way to improve intracorporal blood supply, but long-term results of this operation are not satisfactory, because the cavernous artery is so small that the microsurgical anastomosis between it and the IEA is prone to thrombosis. In addition, intensive intracorporal scarring often resulted from the operative procedure [1,2]. In the face of these difficulties, it became obvious that anastomoses of the IEA had to be performed to recipient vessels outside the corpora cavernosa.

Currently, three principal surgical approaches for penile revascularization are in clinical use (Fig. 12.1). These are:

1 Anastomosis of the IEA to the dorsal penile arteries (end-to-end or end-to-side)

2 Anastomosis of the IEA to the deep dorsal vein and deep dorsal artery (arterio-venous shunt)

3 Anastomosis of the IEA to the deep dorsal vein with additional proximal and/or distal vein ligation.

1. After the Michal I procedure was abandoned, direct anastomoses of the IEA to the dorsal penile artery (DPA) was proposed. This has been called the Michal II operation. This was a logical step because the cavernosal artery is a branch of the DPA. Most stenoses of the common penile artery due to trauma

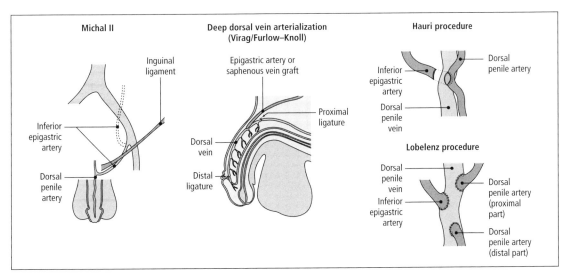

Fig. 12.1 Three principal surgical approaches for penile revascularization in clinical use.

or arteriosclerosis occur proximal to its bifurcation into cavernosal and dorsal artery. Only a small cohort of six patients have been re-evaluated by angiography after a Michal II procedure. This small study showed improved perfusion of cavernosal and helicine arteries [53].

The Michal II procedure probably works best in young patients with post-traumatic arteriogenic erectile dysfunction. In patients with systemic arteriosclerotic disease, arterial run-off is limited by multiple peripheral stenoses, and low flow rates will lead to early anastomotic thrombosis. As most candidates for revascularization procedures have systemic arteriosclerosis, an alternative to pure arterio–arterial bypasses was needed [15].

2. In 1986, Hauri published the results of an arterio–arterial anastomosis of the IEA to the dorsal artery including the deep dorsal vein into the anastomosis. The "triple anastomosis" permits an additional arterio–venous shunt with good arterial run-off and high flow rates [12]. This type of anastomosis was later modified by Löbelenz and published in 1992 [13]. Lobelenz preferred a simple end-to-side anastomosis between donor vessel and deep dorsal vein, and added two end-to-side anastomoses of the interrupted dorsal artery to the arterialized deep dorsal vein (see Fig. 12.1). The inclusion of the deep dorsal vein as a shunt vessel theoretically improves neo-arterial run-off, enabling the surgeon to apply penile revascularization to patients with systemic arteriosclerotic lesions or to patients with uncertain peripheral arterial conditions. Follow-up examinations have revealed patency rates with this operation of more than 75% [4,21]. However, the only experimental study on postoperative flow characteristics in the animal model did not detect neo-arterial flow in the dorsal arteries included in the anastomoses. All of the neoarterial run-off went into the venous system [14].

3. The idea of pure venous arterialization of the deep dorsal vein was first published by Virag in 1980 [16]. Virag developed various modifications of his original technique (Virag I–VI). The modifications involve distal and proximal ligation of the arterialized vein or creation of a window between vein and corpus cavernosum (Virag V–VI). The Virag procedures have been further modified by other authors [17,18,19] (see Fig. 12.1). These further modifications involve ligation of circumflex and emissary collaterals or destruction of valves in the dorsal vein. The rationale of all these procedures is to create retrograde filling of the corpora with arterial blood through emissary veins. At the same time, venous outflow is reduced, making these techniques theoretically applicable to patients with arteriogenic, venogenic and mixed arteriogenic and venogenic erectile dysfunction [17]. However, there is no study in peer-reviewed journals, which objectively demonstrates enhanced arterial inflow into the corpora with these procedures [4,20,21,22,23]. In the animal model, an intracorporal pressure rise could only be shown only after creation of an artificial window between the arterialized dorsal vein and the corpus cavernosum [14].

Results of penile revascularization

The literature on results of penile revascularization has been summarized for several consensus meetings on ED. The first relevant consensus statement was extracted from the consensus conference on ED at the National Institutes of Health (NIH) in 1993 [35]. This review evaluated 34 studies with more than 1700 patients, which were detailed in two further publications [20,21]. Reported success rates were found to range between 33 and 100%, with a median of 72%. Only seven studies included objective follow-up parameters. It was concluded that only highly selected patients may benefit from these operations, which should only be performed in an investigational setting in specialized centers. In 1996 the ED Guideline Committee of the AUA stated: "For venous and arterial surgery, the measures of success are nonstandardized and unpredictable" [36]. The 2005 AUA ED guideline recommends that: "Arterial reconstruction is a treatment option only in healthy individuals with recently-acquired erectile dysfunction secondary to a focal arterial occlusion and in the absence of any evidence of generalized vascular disease" (http://auanet.org/timssnet/products/guidelines/main_reports/edmgmt/chapter1.pdf). During the Second International Consultation on Erectile and Sexual Dysfunction in 2003 a Medline® based literature research on penile revascularization of

Table 12.1 Outcome data table for penile revascularization from 1996–2005 [4].

Study	No Pts	Procedure	Age	Follow-up month (Range)	% Success (Unassisted)	% Success (Assisted)	Over all Intercourse	Notes
Jarow 1996	11	Dorsal Artery DDVA 9	n/a	50 (12–84)	64%	28%	92%	10/11 patent
DePalma 1997	12	Dorsal Artery	n/a	33 (12–48)	27%	n/a	n/a	—
DePalma 1997	12	DDVA (F-F)	n/a	35 (12–84)	33%	47%	90%	—
Lukkarinen 1997	24	V5 6 Hauri 4 F-F 14	n/a	n/a	46%	33%	77%	No difference in outcomes by age at operation
Manning 1998	62	Virag 7 Hauri 55	48 (19–70)	41 (18–72)	34%	20%	54%	Patency: 92%
Manning 1998	42	DDVA (Mannheim)	n/a	n/a	31%	26%	57 5	<50 years. 83% success
Kawanishi 2000	18	Dorsal art. 1 Hauri 5 F-F 13	33 (18 > 50 yo)	32 (4–80)	94%	0%	04%	17/19 patent
Sarramon 1997	114	Dorsal art. 44 DDVA 70	47.5 (20–74)	17 (1–20)	48%	15%	63%	No diff. in outcome by procedure (p = 0.064)
Sarramon 2001	38	DDVA (F-F)	52	61	25% (IIEF EF > 26)	n/a	n/a	28% IIEF: 22–25
Vardi 2002	61	n/a	20–50	60 (24–120)	48%	n/a	n/a	CVOD success: 64% Art. Dx. success: 44%
Kawanishi 2004	51	Hauri proc. 26 Furlow (Virag5) 23	21–49	36–60	n/a	n/a	85.9% (3 years) 65.5% (5 years)	No difference between techniques

the literature from 1993 to 2003 was evaluated [4]. Eight studies were selected for evaluation (see Table 12.1). In Table 12.1 one further study, which appeared in 2004, is included [38].

The goal of an invasive vascular procedure for ED is to provide a durable and satisfying spontaneous erection with sexual stimulation without relying on pharmacologic augmentation. Using these strict criteria, success in these studies ranged from 27 to 94% for all procedures with no identified difference in success among the different techniques [4].

The best instrument for evaluating subjective success is the international index for erectile function (IIEF). This instrument has only been used in one study [34] and only for the *postoperative* evaluation. The IIEF was not administered to patients before surgery in this study.

In view of these data, it is impossible to draw definite conclusions concerning selection criteria for penile revascularization. If the arterial blood supply to the penis is impaired by systemic arteriosclerotic disease, no vascular reconstruction is appropriate because there are significant abnormalities in intracavernous structures [31]. Many authors have drawn conclusions concerning their own selection criteria, which are based on their personal experience. Advanced age (>50 years), smoking and the presence of severe corporal veno-occlusive dysfunction (CVOD) have been identified to have a signifi-cant negative impact on postoperative results [15,16,31,40,41,42]. The ideal candidate for penile revascularization is a young man with localized interruption of penile arterial supply after pelvic or straddle trauma, and without concomitant neural damage. Apart from the fact that these patients are very rare, the only published multicenter study in such a highly selected subgroup of patients showed a disappointing success rate of only 22% [21,43].

Complications of penile revascularization

Complications occur in up to 25% of patients after penile revascularization [4,37,39]. Glans hyperemia is the most common complication after these procedures. Inguinal hernia formation and postoperative hematoma have occurred in up to 25% of patients as well [4].

Venous ligation procedures: rationale and technical considerations

The previous terms venous leakage, venous vasculogenic dysfunction or venogenic ED have been replaced by the more precise term CVOD [11]. CVOD may be due to structural alterations in the corporal smooth muscle, trabecular framework or tunica albuginea. The location and degree of venous leakage is variable and can occur anywhere along the tunica albuginea of the corpus cavernosum. Hypercholesterolemia and arterosclerotic-induced ischemia can be associated with alterations in the fibroelastic components of the trabeculae [24]. A strong correlation has been demonstrated between measures of cavernosal venous leakage and trabecular smooth muscle content [25].

In addition, congenital anomalies and post-traumatic changes in the tunica albuginea can produce localized venous leakage [26,50]. Localization and severity of veno-occlusive dysfunction may be determined by invasive dynamic intracavernosal cavernosometry and cavernosography (DICC) [27]. A less invasive screening test for patients with suspected CVOD is color-coded duplex sonography of the penile vessels with artificial erection stimulated by intracavernous injection of vaso-active drugs such as alprostadil or papaverine. Duplex sonography should be considered prior to DICC [28].

Ligating or resecting penile veins is symptomatic treatment but does not cure the underlying disease. Most methods of penile venous surgery were invented before basic research defined the pathophysiologic mechanisms of CVOD. The extensive collateral venous drainage of the penis is probably a major reason that these surgical procedures fail [29]. With respect to the disappointing long-term results of venous ligation and resection procedures discussed later in this chapter, these operations are no longer recommended by several panels [4,30] and authors [31,32]. Nevertheless, better preoperative selection of young patients with rare congenital or post-traumatic isolated crural leakage, and the use of more sophisticated operative techniques for crural ligation or banding, may offer better long-term results in the future [50].

On the other hand, the concept of deep dorsal vein arterialization is still appealing for the treatment of

CVOD [10,33,34], because in this operation venous ligation is combined with improved arterial inflow into the corpora, producing hypothetical beneficial effects on damaged intracavernosal tissue [34].

Recently, a new extraperitoneal laparoscopic approach to venous ligation has been suggested. With this approach, it is easy to gain access to the deep dorsal vein complex overlying the anterior prostatic surface. Suture ligation can be performed quite easily without damaging the dorsal penile structures. However, no long-term success data are available for this new approach to penile venous ligation [54].

Results

As in penile revascularization, the literature on the results of venous surgery has been repeatedly reviewed for several consensus meetings. During the NIH consensus meeting in 1993, it was recommended that penile venous surgery should be used only in investigational settings in experienced centers with prospective outcome evaluation [35]. In 1994, a Medline®-based literature research revealed 30 studies with short-term follow up (<12 months) and a range of subjective success rates between 10 and 95% (median 62.3%) [21]. Twenty-two studies were found with long-term follow up data of more than 12 months. The success rates ranged from 13 to 74% with a median 41.4%. Only 12 studies compared short and long-term results. In these studies, the median short-term success rate dropped from 70 to 37.3% [21]. The AUA guideline panel recommendations from 1996 were not significantly different from the NIH recommendations in 1993 [36]. The updated 2005 AUA ED guideline recommends: "Surgeries performed with the intent to limit the venous outflow of the penis are not recommended" (http://auanet.org/timssnet/products/guidelines/main_reports/edmgmt/chapter1.pdf). During the Second International Consultation on Erectile Dysfunction in Paris 2003, it was concluded that meaningful data comparison between surgical series is not possible due to the varying diagnostic criteria, selection criteria, surgical techniques and length of follow-up and outcome assessment [4]. Six studies with a follow up of more than one year between 1997 and 1999 again showed success rates between 11.2 and 74% [4]. In Table 12.2, three recent studies are added to the original six studies from reference [4].

Several authors have tried to identify selection criteria, which might produce better results after penile venous surgery. In one study, only young, non-smoking patients with mild to moderate CVOD were selected, excluding those with significant smooth muscle degeneration and arterial pathology. But even in these patients success rates dropped to less than 50% after more than one year of follow up [4,45,46]. Even extensive ligation and resection procedures show the same steep decline in success after longer follow-up [32]. Perhaps there is a specific subgroup of young, otherwise healthy patients with trauma-induced or congenital circumscribed veno-occlusive dysfunction who might profit from venous resection or plication procedures [26,48,50]. However at the present time, the weight of evidence is that no clear indication for venous surgery can be identified [4,30]. The weight of evidence against the value of penile venous surgery is so strong that single center reports showing excellent long-term results must be interpreted with caution [47,50].

Venous embolization has the advantage of being minimally invasive. It also allows immediate proof of venous ablation and obstruction [4,49]. Overall short-term results after venous embolization or ablation show the same range of success between 26 and 73% as open procedures. There is no agreement on indications and techniques for this approach to the treatment of CVOD.

Long-term results on laparoscopic suture ligation of the deep dorsal vein complex are not yet available. Early follow-up data using IIEF for evaluation of success reveal promising results in a small patient group [54].

Venous arterialization of the dorsal penile artery has been investigated as a treatment for CVOD [10,34]. In these two studies, the IIEF score was used for success evaluation but the results must be interpreted with caution. In Sarramon's study, postoperative, but not preoperative, IIEF evaluation was done in 55% of patients. In Kayigil's study, only 18% were evaluable for postoperative controls. Sarramon and Kayigil reported subjective success rates of 55% and 75%, respectively, but success declined with length of follow-up.

Table 12.2 Outcome data of penile venous ligations surgery for CVOD. From [4,32,46,50].

Study	Date	No. of pts.	Age	Technique	Follow-up	Success Evaluation	Outcome
Sasso	1999	23	20–50 (mean 41)	Superficial deep dorsal, Circumflex and emissary vein ligation	12 months, long-term	Not specified	74% spontaneous erections at 12 months 55% long-term
Popken	1999	122	19–78 (mean 49)	Superficial, deep and circum-flex vein ligation	70 months	Questionnaire	14% spontaneous erections 19% ICI response
Al Assal	1998	325	18–162 (mean 45)	Ligation of DDV, abnormal veins, cavernosal veins, cavernosal-spongiosum shunts	1–13 years	Not specified	Age < 40 years:76% "cured" Age > 40 years: 58% "cured"
Lukkarinen	1998	21	NA	Ligation DDV, +/– cavernosal veins	>1 yr	Patient report	29% "good" 52% ICI-response
Basar	1998	26	NA	Venous ligation	25 months	Not specified	6 months 15% complete erection 23% partial erection
Schultheiss	1997	147	NA	DDV ligation	NA	Patient report, questionnaire	11.2% spontaneous erection
Rahman	2005	11	22–39 (mean 28)	Crural ligation	34 months	IIEF score	80% subjective success score from 8.9 to 17.5 (median)
Cakan	2004	134	21–72 (mean 39)	Extended ligations (no crural vein ligation)	54 months	Patient report	25.7% spontaneous or PDE5-supported erections
Da Ros	2000	32	23–66 (mean 55)	Extended ligations (occasionally crural plication)	>36 months	Patient report	22% spontaneous erections

Complications

Complications of penile venous surgeries are significant and numerous. Wound infections, penile curvature or shortening, skin necrosis, and painful erection, as well as loss of glans, and shaft sensitivity, have been reported [4]. A recent report showed a complication rate of 23.9% in 134 patients [46]. When venous arterialization has been applied to patients with CVOD, up to 32% of patients have experienced complications. This includes 8% who had glans hyperemia [10].

Conclusions

The application of penile revascularization procedures even in highly selected patients performed by well-trained experienced surgeons results in a variable and unpredictable outcome. The precise mechanism by which these procedures yield their potential benefit has not been fully elucidated. In the 2005 update of the AUA ED guideline, narrow criteria were chosen for outcome evaluation. These criteria were well-circumscribed arterial occlusive disease without obvious cavernous myopathy. Only four studies with a total of 50 subjects who fit these criteria could be found in the literature. *The panel concluded, that a patient population of 50 is too small to determine whether arterial reconstructive surgery is efficacious or not* [30]. This conclusion coincides with the final recommendation of the Second International Consultation on Erectile Dysfunction from 2004 [4].

Several tasks for future research in the field of penile revascularization can be identified. The potential mechanisms of improvement in penile blood supply after venous arterialization are not yet sufficiently understood. Contradictory and confusing results from human clinical studies, animal experience and post-mortem studies must be resolved [14]. A recently developed model for erectile mechanisms could be of help [44]. New modalities like CT–angiography should be examined for potential use in detecting hemodynamic changes after penile revascularization [38]. For subjective success evaluation, examiner-independent validated instruments such as the IIEF should be used preoperatively and postoperatively to achieve evidence-based data [4].

The vast majority of patients with CVOD have intracavernosal myopathy as the underlying cause of venous leakage [31]. The well-known capacity of venous collateralization after venous resection may also explain the rapid decline of postoperative success. Only carefully selected young patients with isolated congenital or post-traumatic CVOD, and without other concomitant pathologies, may benefit from individualized ligation procedures. The same restrictions are valid for percutaneous embolization techniques and for the application of venous arterialization procedures in CVOD patients.

After a careful analysis of literature on this subject, the most recent recommendation of the erectile dysfunction guideline panel of the AUA concluded that *surgeries performed with the intent to limit the venous outflow of the penis are not recommended* [30].

Further research should focus on diagnostic possibilities to differentiate isolated venous leakage from systemic intracavernosal disease. Results of evidence-based medicine meta-analyses in surgery of the venous system should be integrated in our future approaches [29]. Basic research on intracorporal hemodynamics should be pursued [44,51, 52,53].

For future clinical studies, validated survey instruments such as the IIEF should be administered both pre- and post-operatively to determine long-term success [4].

References

1 Hauri D. Development of surgical procedures in the treatment of erectile dysfunction. A historical overview. *Urol Int* 2003;**70**:124–131.

2 Hauri D. Penile revascularization surgery in erectile dysfunction. *Andrologia* 1999;**31**:65–76.

3 Leriche R. Désoblitération artérielles hautes (désoblitération de la terminaison de l'aorte) comme cause des insuffisances circulatoires des membres inférieurs. *Bull Soc Chir* Paris 1923;**49**:1404.

4 Mulcahy JJ. Implants, mechanical devices and vascular surgery for erectile dysfunction. In: Lue TF, Basson R, Rosen R, Giuliano F, Khoury S, Montorsi F, eds. *Sexual Medicine: Sexual Dysfunctions in Men and Women.* Paris: 2nd International Consultation on Sexual Dysfunctions, 2004, Chapter 14, pp. 469–498.

5   Michal V, Krama R, Pospichal J, Hejhal L. Direct arterial anastomosis on corpora cavernosa penis in the therapy of erective impotence. *Rozhl Chir* 1973;**52**:587–590.

6   Parona F. Imperfect penile erection due to varicosity of the dorsal vein: Observation. *Giornale Italiano delle Malattie Veneree e della Pelle* 1873;**14**:71–76.

7   Das S. Early history on venogenic impotence. *Int J Impot Res* 1994;**6**:183–189.

8   Lowsley OS, Rudea EA. Further Experience of an Operation for the cure of certain types of impotence. *J Int Coll Surg* 1953;**19**:69–77.

9   Lue TF. Surgery for crural venous leakage. *Urology* 1999;**54**:739–741.

10 Kayigil Ö, Ahmed, Ahmet SJ, Metin A. Deep dorsal vein arterialization in pure cavernooclusive dysfunction. *Eur Urol* 2000;**37**:345–349.

11 Goldstein I. Overview of types and results of vascular surgical procedures for impotence. *Cardiovas Intervent Radiol* 1988;**11**:240–244.

12 Hauri D. A new operative technique in vasculogenic impotence. *World J Urol* 1986;**4**:237.

13 Lobelenz M, Jünemann KP, Kohrmann KU, Seemann O, Rassweiler J, Tschada R, Alken P. Revascularization in nonresponders to intracavernous injections using a modified surgical technique. *Eur Urol* 1992;**21**:120–125.

14 Floth A, Paick JS, Suh JK, Lue TF. Hemodynamics of revascularization of the corpora cavernosa in an animal model. *Urol Res* 1991;**19**:281–284.

15 Grein U, Schubert GE. Arteriosclerosis of penile arteries: histological findings and their significance in the treatment of erectile dysfunction. *Urol Int* 2002;**68**:261–264.

16 Virag R, Zwang G, Dermange H, Legman M, Penven JP. Exploration et traitement chirurgical de l'impuissance vasculaire. *J Mal Vasc* 1980;**5**:205–209.

17 Mulcahy JJ, Lewis RW, Lue TF, Melman A, Padma-Nathan H. In pursuit of the best candidates and procedures for penile revascularization. *Contemporary Urology* **1993**;27–43.

18 Sarramon JP, Malavaud B, Braud F, Bertrand N, Vaessen C, Rischmann P. Evaluation of male sexual function by the International Index of Erectile Function after deep dorsal vein arterialization of the penis. *J Urol* 2001;**166**:576–580.

19 Furlow WL, Fischer J. Deep dorsal vein arterialization. Clinical experience with a new technique. *J Urol* 1998;**139**:289A.

20 Sohn M. Current status of penile revascularization for the treatment of male erectile dysfunction. *J Androl* 1994;Vol**15**(No.3):183–186.

21 Sohn M, Barada JH. Ergebnisse der penilen gefäßchirurgie bei erektiler impotenz. *Akt Urol* 1994;**25**:133–142.

22 Sohn M, Sikora R, Bohndorf K, Bohndorf K, Gunther R. Objective follow-up after penile ravascularization. *Int J Impot Res* 1992;**4**:73–84.

23 Wespes E, Corbusier A, Delcour C, Vandenbosch G, Struyven J, Schulman CC. Deep dorsal vein arterialization in vascular impotence. *Brit J Urol* 1989;**64**:535–540.

24 Fourner G, Jünemann KP, Lue TF. Mechanism of venous occlusion during canine penile erection: an anatomic demonstration. *J Urol* 1987;**137**:163–167.

25 Nehra A, Goldstein I, Pabby A, *et al.* Mechanisms of venous leakage: a prospective clinicopathological correlation of corporeal function and structure. *J Urol* 1996;**156**:1320–1323.

26 Tsao CW, Lee SS, Meng E, Wu ST, Chuang FP, Yu DS, Chang SY, Sun GH. Penile blunt trauma induced veno-occlusive erectile dysfunction. *Archives of Andrology* 2004;**50**:151–154.

27 Yu GW, Schwab FJ, JMelograna FS, DePalma RG, Miller HC, Rickholt AL. Preoperative and postoperative dynamic cavernosometry and cavernosography: Objective assessment of venous ligation for impotence. *J Urol* 1997;**147**:618–622.

28 Altinkilic B, Hauck EW, Weidner W. Evaluation of penile perfusion by color-coded duplex sonography in the management of erectile dysfunction. *World J Urol* 2004;**22**:361–364.

29 Hardy SC, Riding G, Abidia A. Surgery for deep venous incompetence. Cochrane Database Syt. *Rev* 2005;**2**.

30 Montague DG, Jarow JP, Broderick GA, Dmocowski RR, Heaton PW, Lue TF, Milbank AJ, Nehra A, Sharlip ID. The management of erectile dysfunction: An AUA update. *J Urol* 2005;**174**:230–239.

31 Wespes E, Wildschutz T, Roumeguere T, Schulman CC. The place of surgery for vascular impotence in the third Millennium. *J Urol* 2003;**170**:1284–1286.

32 Da Ros CT, Telöken C, Antonini CC, Sogari PR, Souto CAV. Long-term results of penile vein ligation for erectile dysfunction due to cavernovenous disease. *Techniques in Urology* 2000;Vol**6**(3):172–174.

33 Sha RS, Kulkarni VR. Penile Revascularization: An Overview. *Annals Academy of Medicine* 1995;Vol**24** (No.5):749–754.

34 Sarramon JP, Malavaud B, Braud F, Bertrand N, Vaessen C, Rischmann P. Evaluation of male sexual function by the International Index of Erectile Function after deep dorsal vein arterialization of the penis. *J Urol* 2001;**66**:576–580.

35 Consensus development conference statement National Institutes of Health on impotence. *Int J Impot Res* 1993;**5**:181–189.

36 Montague DK, Barada JH, Belker AM, Levine LA, Nadig PW, Roehrborn CG, Sharlip ID, Bennett AH. Clinical guidelines panel on erectile dysfunction: Summary report on the treatment of organic erectile dysfunction. *J Urol* 1996;**156**:2007–2011.

37 Bleustein CB, Melman A. Hypervascularity of the glans penis diagnosed with cutaneous temperature measurements. *Int J Imp Rse* 2002;**14**:543–544.

38 Kawanishi Y, Kimura K, Nakanishi R, Kojima K, Numata A. Penile revascularization surgery for arteriogenic erectile dysfunction. The long-term efficacy rate calculated by survival analysis. *BJU Int* 2004;**94**:361–368.

39 Lukkarinen O, Tonttila P, Hellström P, Leinonen S. Non-prosthetic surgery in the treatment of erectile dysfunction. *Scand J Urol Nephrol* 1998;**32**:42–46.

40 Vardi Y, Gruenwald I, Gedalia U, Nassar S, Engel A, Har-Shai Y. Evaluation of penile revascularization for erectile dysfunction: a 10-year follow-up. *Int J Impot Res* 2004;**16**:181–186.

41 Manning M, Jünemann KP, Scheepe JR, Braun P, Krautschick A, Alken P. Long-term follow-up and selection criteria for penile revascularization in erectile failure. *J Urol* 1998;**160**:1680–1684.

42 Zumbé J, Grozinger K, von Pokrzywnitzki W. Selektionskriterien zur penilen revaskularisation bei arteriell bedingter erektiler dysfunktion. *Akt Urol* 1995;**26**:114–118.

43 Barada JH. The changing role of impotence surgery. *J Urol* 1993;**149**(Suppl.1):99A.

44 Gillon G, Barnea O. Erection mechanism of the penis: A model-based analysis. *J Urol* 2002;**168**:2711–2715.

45 Rao DS, Donatucci CF. Vasculogenic impotence: Arterial and venous surgery. *J Urol Clin NA* 2001;**22**:309–319.

46 Cakan M, Yalcinkaya F, Demirel F, Özgünay T, Altug U. Is dorsale penile vein ligation (dpvl) still a treatment option in veno-occlusive dysfunction? *Int Urol Nephrol* 2004;**36**:381–387.

47 Chen SC, Hsieh CH, Hsu GL, Wang CJ, Wen HS, Lilng PY, Huang HM, Tseng GF. The progression of the penile vein: Could it be recurrent? *J Androl* 2005;**26**:53–60.

48 Mulhall JP, Martin D, Ergin E, Kim F. Crural ligation surgery for the young male with venogenic erectile dysfunction: *Techniques in Urology* 2001;**7**(No.4): 290–293.

49 Basche St, Egre C, Elsebach K, Ulshöfer B. Venookklusive dysfunktion als ursache der erektilen impotenz: therapie des venösen lecks durch retrograde embolisation der V. pudenda interna. *VASA* 2003;**32**:47–50.

50 Rahman NU, Dean RC, Carrion R, *et al.* Crural ligation for primary erectile dysfunction. A case series. *J Urol* 2005;**173**:2064.

51 Hsieh CH, Wang CJ, Hsu GL, Chen SC, Ling PY, Wang T, Fong TH, Tseng GF. Penile veins play a pivotal role in erection: the hemodynamic evidence. *Int J Androl* 2005;**28**:88–92.

52 Davila HH, Rajfer J, Gonzalez-Cadavid NF. Corporal veno-occlusive dysfunction in aging rats. Evaluation by cavernosometry and cavernosography. *Urology* 2004;**64**:1261–1266.

53 Mulhall JP, D'Agostino R, Pagan-Marin H, Krane RJ, Goldstein I. Post-operative follow-up arteriography in microvascular arterial bypass surgery for impotence. *Int J Imp Res* 1996;**8**(Suppl.1):152.

54 Scheplev P, Kadirov Z. Aliev A, *et al.* Extraperitoneal laparoscopic ligation of veins of periprostatic venous plexus for veno-occlusive erectile dysfunction. *J Sex Med* 2006;**P-07-347**(Suppl.1):112.

Penile Prosthetic Surgery

Michael Sohn and Antonio Martín-Morales

Introduction and History

Impotence, or in modern terms erectile dysfunction (ED), has afflicted human males since ancient times, if not since the very beginning of human existence. External supports intended to aid the inadequate erection, a precursor of the modern prosthesis, were known in the Ancient World. In the Roman theatre, actors wore oversized cases made of leather or wood, which were fastened to the actors' hips to produce the appearance of a large penis. These external devices originated in China and Japan. Ambroise Parée, the famous surgeon of the Renaissance, designed one of the first exterior penile prostheses. It was intended for disabled war veterans. Its advantage was to enable the user to micturate in an upright position. It was also popular with obese men whose penis was partially covered or totally hidden by pre-pubic and infra-pubic fat. Another device, dating to the turn of the 20th century, was a box for support, which provided the patient with something like an erection, the ejaculate being drained off by a separate tube.

The internal prosthesis is a copy from nature: some animals are equipped with a penile bone or baculum. Men whose ED followed trauma or partial penile amputation were the original target group for this treatment method. In a pioneering report of 1936, Bogoras [1] described his technique in a patient after traumatic penile amputation. Reconstruction was achieved with the help of a pedicled skin flap, which was supported by a piece of costal cartilage. If we believe him, the patient thereafter was able to reproduce. Somewhat later in time, Bergmann [2] implanted costal cartilage between the existing remnants of the proximal cavernous bodies, hiding the cartilage in a tubed flap. He reported normal micturition and satisfactory sexual intercourse by four months postoperatively. Other reports by various authors followed; however, long-term results of these techniques were not good. There was a slow resorption of the cartilage and insufficient rigidity of the phallus to permit coitus [3]. Therefore, there was a need for better material. In 1952 Goodwin [4] was among the first to implant two acrylic rods in the reconstructed penis after amputation. He published four case reports, two of which had to be explanted during a two-year follow-up period because of patients' intolerance to the rods. Later on, the acrylic rods were implanted outside the cavernous bodies [5] in patients with an intact penis but with ED due to priapism. Meanwhile, in the 1960s, more and more patients began to complain of ED and the demand for a durable penile device grew. In 1966, Beheri [6], an Egyptian surgeon, made a major advance in the field by using the intracavernosal spaces for implantation of a penile prosthesis. His pioneering idea was to implant polyethylene rods, which are more flexible and can be fashioned to the anatomy of the corpora cavernosa, in order to lower the risk of perforation that occurred with acrylic material. Beheri performed 700 implantations; subsequently, other investigators substituted silicone for polyethylene to reduce the risk of perforation [7,8]. Penile prostheses underwent continual improvement over a period of many years [9–12], with eventual improvement in the appearance of tumescence and detumescence.

The development of the hydraulic penile prosthesis–a far better copy of nature–in 1973 by Scott [13] represented a landmark in penile prosthetics. These new prostheses subsequently underwent several modifications, but the underlying principle however remained the same.

Types of Penile Prosthesis

Penile implants are currently available in a variety of forms, which can be categorized into two major types: semi-rigid, or inflatable, with a silicon or polyurethane jacket. Details of the available length and diameters can be found on the websites of the two manufacturing companies: American Medical Systems at www.visitams.com; and the Mentor Corporation at www.mentorcorp.com. When implanted into the corpora cavernosa, they can be manipulated by the patient to fit his needs. The Jonas implant, produced in Germany, has a silver core and a silicone covering [12]. A soft silicone implant was introduced by Subrini. Currently these devices are manufactured in France and sold under the names "SSDA" and "Virilis" in many countries [15]. These implants may be indicated in the presence of residual spongy erectile tissue, which permits tumescence and complimentary girth expansion around the central silicone support.

The only "mechanical" prosthesis on the market is the Dura II, which has articulating segments of polyethylene held together by a central spring. These articulating segments are covered by a polytetrafluoroethylene sleeve surrounded by a silicone jacket. The Dura II prosthesis is a product of the American Medical Systems (AMS). A similar device, called "Genesis", with a hydrophilic coating is planned by the Mentor Corporation. This design provides positional memory, allowing the prosthesis to remain concealed when not in use, yet rigid during intercourse [25]. These semi-rigid implants are cheaper than inflatable prostheses and easier to implant because there is no pump or reservoir to place. Semirigid prostheses may be implanted through a subcoronal, infrapubic or scrotal incision. Local anesthesia may be used if the corpora cavernosa are not too fibrotic and their dilatation is expected to be easy.

Inflatable implants are available in two-piece or three-piece models. Two-piece implants are made by AMS and by the Mentor Corporation. The AMS Ambicor prosthesis consists of a pair of inflatable cylinders, which are implanted into the corpora cavernosa, and a pump, which is implanted into the scrotum. The cylinders and pump are preconnected during the manufacturing process and the system is prefilled with sterile saline. To achieve an erection, the scrotal pump is squeezed and released several times. This inflates the cylinders by transferring saline solution from a small reservoir located at the

end of each cylinder into each cylinder shaft. The newly developed Mentor two-piece penile prosthesis is called the Excel Resist® device. It consists of a pair of inflatable cylinders, which are implanted into the corpora cavernosa, and a resi-pump that is implanted into the scrotum. The cylinders and resi-pump are preconnected and filled with sterile saline during the manufacturing process. The volume of fluid in the reservoirs of both two-piece inflatable penile prostheses is less than in the reservoir of the three-piece prostheses. The lesser volume of the two-piece reservoirs diminishes the difference between rigidity and flaccidity of these systems, compared to the three-piece systems.

Three-piece inflatable implants are composed of two cylinders, a scrotal pump and a reservoir, which is typically positioned either in the retrovesical space or within the peritoneal cavity. Three-piece implants manufactured by AMS are the 700 CX, 700 CXR and Ultrex devices. The CXR cylinders have a narrow base and come in shorter lengths than the CX cylinders. CX and CXR cylinders have a three-layer design consisting of an inner layer of elastic silicone, a middle layer of woven Dacron–Lycra and an outer layer of silicone. The inner layer fills with fluid to provide rigidity, the outer layer allows for capsule formation around, but not into, the prosthesis, and the middle layer permits controlled expansion of the cylinders. The recently introduced parylene coating of the cylinders diminishes the risk of aneurysmal dilatation of cylinders. In the CX and CXR cylinders, the middle layer is woven unidirectionally, permitting girth expansion but not length expansion. It is commonly agreed that although very satisfactory results may be obtained in all subsets of patients, the CX implant is particularly useful for patients with Peyronie's disease or any form of severe organic ED. Patients who have significant scarring of the corpora cavernosa, e.g. after priapism or with extensive Peyronie's disease, or having a re-implant after previous removal of an infected prosthesis, may benefit from an inflatable implant with narrow cylinders such as the CXR, which requires dilation of the corpora cavernosa to only 10 mm. The only penile prosthesis that can lengthen with inflation is the AMS Ultrex prosthesis. This prosthesis also has three layers, but the middle layer of Dacron–Lycra has a bi-directional weave that permits both length and girth expansion of the cylinders. However, the Ultrex prosthesis is not appropriate for patients with Peyronie's disease because these patients need greater stiffness than is provided by the Ultrex prosthesis.

Three-piece inflatable implants manufactured by the Mentor Corporation share a similar design to the previously described models. The main difference is that the Mentor implants are made based of an inert aromatic polyurethane polymer called Bioflex™. Compared to silicone, Bioflex™ has increased abrasion resistance and higher tensile strength. An additional feature of the current Mentor "Titan" or three-piece inflatable prostheses, is a lockout valve that reduces the common phenomenon of auto-inflation of the prosthesis [16]. The lockout valve is also used in the two-piece Excel Resist® device. The Titan prostheses are also available in a narrow-base version, which is best used in patients with severe fibrosis of the corpora cavernosa, as described above for the AMS CXR prosthesis.

As infection is the most feared complication of penile prosthetic surgery, two- and three-piece implants specifically modified to reduce this risk have been recently introduced into clinical practice. The InhibiZone™ prostheses by AMS are coated with a combination of rifampicin and minocycline to inhibit bacterial growth. In these prostheses, the surfaces of the prostheses, which come into contact with the adjacent tissue, are impregnated with quantifiable doses of these antibiotics that elute into the area surrounding the prosthesis after surgery. Both drugs elute initially at high rates, with a significant decrease in rifampicin after one and minocycline after seven days. The inhibitory effect of the Inhibi-Zone™ treatment is greatest for *Staphylococcus epidermidis* and *Staphylococcus aureus* [17,8].

Mentor has also developed a method to reduce penile prosthetic infection. This method uses an intensely hydrophilic coating called Resist™ that is applied to the Titan and Excel prostheses. Its increased lubrication has been shown to decrease bacterial adherence in vitro. Furthermore this coating absorbs antibiotics that can elute into surrounding tissues over 24 to 72 hours to further decrease infection. An antibiotic-soaking solution, which has been tested both in laboratory experi-

Table 12.3 Implant rates of all manufacturers. (Personal data with permission of AMS, Germany [22].)

Year	Overall	USA	Europe
1994	23.280	19.400	3.880
1995	23.760	19.800	3.960
1996	24.360	20.300	4.060
1997	20.760	17.300	3.460
1998	17.640	14.700	2.940
1999	24.960	20.800	4.160
2000	26.600	22.000	4.400
2001	28.800	23.800	5.000
2002	31.100	25.700	5.400

ments and in clinical use, is composed of 2 g of gentamycin and 100 000 units of bacitracin in 1000 ml of saline [17,21].

Reduced infection rates have been reported recently for the AMS InhibiZone™ and the Mentor Resist™ products [18,19,20]. The three-piece implants of AMS and Mentor can be seen with their coatings in Figure 12.2. The two-piece device of Mentor is also available with hydrophilic coating, while the AMS two-piece Ambicor device is not.

Notably, to avoid elution of the coating prior to implantation, the various components should not be soaked in saline or other solutions for a prolonged period. However, conventional parenteral prophylactic antibiotic protocols should be maintained.

Penile prosthesis implantation is a frequent operation performed worldwide. The implant statistics over the last years are summarized in Table 12.3.

The introduction of PDE5 inhibitors into the market in 1998 initially caused a significant drop in implant rates worldwide, but in more recent years a constant increase of implants has been noted. Seventy-five percent of penile implant sales are in the United States, where 90% of implants are three-piece and two-piece devices. Outside the United States 40% of all implants are non-hydraulic devices [55].

Patient and Implant Selection

It is of critical importance to offer this treatment only to properly selected patients, and furthermore to

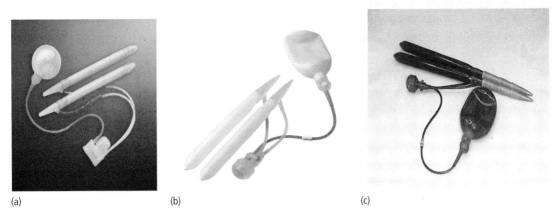

Fig. 12.2 (a) AMS 700CX InhibiZone™. (b) Mentor-Alpha 1. (c) Mentor Titan with Resist™-Coating (here, colour-enhanced with methylene-blue).

select the model that best fits the patient's needs and anatomy. Patients who are eligible for a penile implant should be assessed with a detailed systemic medical and sexologic history [14]. Candidates for penile prosthesis implantation should fulfill the following criteria:

- Good general health
- Failure of medical therapy for ED or,
- Contra-indication to medical therapy of ED
- Psychologic stability
- Patient and partner fully informed
- Informed consent for surgery
- Unsuccessful trial of vacuum devices or at least consideration of these devices [14,55]

The complete medical assessment may include the following elements if they are available:

- The international index of erectile function (IIEF) or other validated questionnaires to objectively assess severity of ED and subsequent postoperative outcome
- Penile colour Doppler sonography with intracorporal pharmacologic injection
- Nocturnal penile tumescence test, especially when the initial medical evaluation suggests the possibility that the patient's ED is predominantly psychogenic
- In cases with medico–legal questions, a comprehensive diagnostic work up should be done [14]

A thorough physical examination is very important. This should include an assessment or actual measurement of the length of the penis. The length after prosthetic implantation is usually similar to the length of a completely stretched flaccid penis. It is worthwhile to spend time with the patient illustrating this concept because, commonly, patients have unrealistic expectations of penile length that cannot be met by any form of therapy. The physical examination may also allow the detection of areas of significant scarring within the corpora cavernosa. Patients with Peyronie's disease may not report a penile bend even though they may have extensive corporal fibrosis, which can ultimately limit the intraoperative dilatation of the penis. In such cases, the final penile length and girth may be unsatisfactory to the patient [55]. Preoperative identification of corporal fibrosis and other factors that impact on postoperative results, plays a very important role in reducing or eliminating patients' disappointment with postoperative length and girth. During the physical examination, the manual dexterity of the patient should be assessed, as it must be sufficient when an inflatable prosthesis is used. Obesity may be a factor making the use of any prosthesis more difficult; this is a physical feature that must be addressed [14].

In patients with poorly-controlled or treated diabetes mellitus, it is wise to obtain a preliminary diabetologic consultation to normalize their glucose metabolism. There is controversy as to whether abnormally high serum glycosylated hemoglobin is a marker for higher risk of postoperative infection.

Several investigators suggest that patients with uncompensated diabetes mellitus may have an implant placed safely [23,55,57].

A critical point in the evaluation of the candidate for an implant is to identify active infections at the time of surgery. A urine culture is mandatory in all patients. Patients who have infectious lesions in the genital area or other local infections, and patients who have active systemic infections, should defer surgery until the infection has resolved. It has been suggested that patients should scrub their genitalia with an antiseptic solution during the five days prior to hospital admission, and should take an oral quinolone during the same period [14].

When an AMS three-piece implant is planned for a patient with long penile length, the CX device should be used because CX devices provide better rigidity than Ultrex devices at longer penile length [56]. Patients with limited dexterity should be offered malleable devices. If the limited dexterity is due to a neurologic condition in which there is reduced penile sensation, there is an increased risk of urethral or cutaneous erosion of the implant. In such cases, the surgeon should consider implanting somewhat shorter cylinders, to reduce the risk of erosion. In patients with severely scarred corpora, CXR or Mentor narrow-based devices should be used. If patients are disappointed postoperatively with their penile length, they can be advised that daily inflation of the prosthesis may produce corporal dilatation, and that surgical replacement with longer cylinders may be possible at a later time [24]. In patients undergoing secondary or repeat prosthesis implantation, the Ultrex device may be considered if preoperative physical examination reveals a 2 cm or more difference between the non-stretched and stretched penile length. However, Ultrex cylinders should not be used in patients with Peyronie's disease.

In patients who have had retropubic prostatectomy, cystectomy or other causes of perivesical scarring, two-piece implants offer the advantage of not requiring retropubic placement of an implant reservoir. However, the difference in rigidity and girth between the inflated and deflated states of two-piece penile prostheses is limited compared to three-piece implants. Alternatively, intra-abdominal, rather than retropubic, placement of the reservoir of a three-piece device can be chosen for the patient with retropubic fibrosis [25].

Technical Considerations in Penile Prosthetic Surgery

Preoperative considerations

Patients are admitted to the hospital either the evening before or the morning of the operation. The shorter the hospital stay, the smaller the risk of contracting infections from hospital contamination. The urine culture should be negative at the time of surgery [14,55].

Antibiotic prophylaxis is used routinely. Intravenous administration of the first dose of the antibiotic should be completed at least one hour before the skin incision to ensure having adequate serum concentrations of the antibiotics at the time of surgery. There is no general agreement on the antibiotic regimen to be used. It is advisable to use the antibiotic recommendations of the hospital in which the surgery is performed. The most common germs involved are *Staphylococcus* species, particularly *Staphylococcus epidermidis*, and gram negative enteric bacteria. One commonly used antibiotic regimen is a cephalosporine during the hospital stay followed by oral ciprofloxacine for one week after discharge [55]. Some clinicians prefer to use vancomycin and rifampicin [14]. Other clinicians use other combinations.

Genital shaving should be performed in the operating room immediately prior to surgery to avoid contamination of the incision. Shaving should be followed by a fifteen minute surgical scrub with iodopovidone [55]. Traffic within the operating room should be minimized to reduce the risk of infection. Proper sterile technique, minimizing tissue trauma, short operating time and effective wound closure, are also well known to reduce the risk of perioperative infections [26].

Operative considerations

The surgical approach may differ according to the type of implant used, the surgeon's preference and the previous surgical history of the patient. Semirigid prostheses may be implanted either subcoronally, infrapubically or scrotally. Inflatable implants may be implanted either infrapubically or scrotally. There is no evidence that any one surgical approach is best [27]. The transverse scrotal approach allows excellent exposure of most of the length of the corpora cavernosa. With this approach, the crura of the corpora cavernosa may be easily exposed as far back as the ischial tuberosities. This posterior exposure may be important when there is severe scarring of this segment of the corpora. At the same time, the distal part of the corpora may be easily exposed by degloving the penis from the surgical incision [14]. A ring retractor with hooks placed at the skin edges significantly facilitates the exposure of the surgical field. This retractor should be available during these procedures. Placement of a urethral catheter may be of help in identifying the urethra. In addition, if the reservoir is placed in Retzius' space, the bladder should be emptied first to minimize the risk of inadvertent bladder injury. During the procedure the surgical field should frequently be irrigated with an antibiotic solution such as gentamycin. Dilating the corpora cavernosa is a key step of the procedure. Different dilators are available; each surgeon should use the one with which he or she feels most comfortable. Hegar and Brooks dilators are useful in most cases, while Rossello dilators are of particular value when managing fibrotic corpora cavernosa [28]. The narrow base three-piece implants mentioned above are helpful in these cases, as they only require dilation up to 10 mm. A major advantage of using narrow-base implants is that they avoid the need for a synthetic patch to close the corporotomy. This may occur, when a conventional three-piece implant has been placed in severely fibrotic corpora cavernosa.

Measuring the length of the corpora cavernosa is important to avoid developing penile deformities after surgery. The use of the Furlow inserter to measure the length of the distal and proximal part of the corpora cavernosa is very helpful. The sum of the proximal and distal measurements minus 1 cm is the length of cylinder that should be implanted. Generally the shorter length should be chosen when there is doubt between measured lengths (e.g. choose an 18 cm cylinder if the length of the corpus cavernosum is 18.5 cm). Montague *et al.* [29,56] have proposed that the length of cylinders should be 2 cm less than the measured corporal length in order to avoid pain and deformities from over-sizing of the cylinders. Ultrex cylinders, which can lengthen with inflation should be sized 1 cm less than measured corporal length. Semi-rigid rods should be sized about half a centimeter less than the measured corporal length [25]. Proper prosthesis width is also critical for optimal support for erection. If the 12 mm dilator is snug, it is more appropriate to use a narrow cylinder, as the fully expanded standard inflatable cylinders reach at least 18 mm in girth [25].

Rear tip extenders may be used to achieve the desired length of the cylinders. In cases of severe fibrosis of the crura, it is better to choose a shorter cylinder and add several centimeters of rear tip extenders to achieve the desired length. The smaller size of the rear tip extenders will facilitate their insertion into the narrow crura. Once the cylinders are in place, they should be inflated to check for adequate positioning and sizing. Filling of the devices can be done with 0.9% NaCl solution or with iso-osmolar dilute contrast agents. In Europe, contrast material is preferred, while in the United States surgeons prefer NaCl solution. The corporotomy incisions should be closed with 2-0 polydioxanone running suture. The input tubing of inflatable cylinders may be positioned intracorporally and exit from the corpora at a convenient location or the tubing may exit directly where the tubing comes off the cylinder. If there is extensive scar tissue in the corpora, inflation and deflation of the cylinder may cause erosion of the cylinders where the tubing presses against the thickened tunica [25,56].

Placing the reservoir blindly into the retrovesical area from a scrotal incision requires special care. The superficial inguinal ring should be palpated and then elevated with a Deaver retractor. The index finger should be passed medial to the spermatic cord and should gently perforate the fascia transversalis, thus reaching the Retzius space. The use of an extra-long nasal speculum to open the space facilitates reservoir placement using a long clamp with no teeth. The reservoir should be filled adequately and the tubing connected using a specifically dedicated "quick" connector system. Blind placement of the reservoir should not be attempted when there is perivesical scarring, as may occur after cystectomy or prostatectomy. In such cases, the reservoir should be placed by a second pararectal skin incision.

Adequate filling of the reservoir can be achieved with less than the maximum reservoir capacity of 50, 65 or 100 ml, but the filling volume should be at least 10 cm more than the maximum filling volume of both cylinders. The implant should then be activated and the wound closed, leaving the cylinders fully inflated. This improves hemostasis and reduces the risk of hematoma formation. The use of a drain is controversial. Some surgeons prefer to use a drain to reduce the risk of hematoma while other surgeons believe that an indwelling drain increases the risk of infection. The infrapubic approach has the advantage of implanting the reservoir under direct view. However, the infrapubic approach has the disadvantages of possible damage to the dorsal nerves of the penis with sensory loss, limited corporal exposure and lack of ability to fix the pump in the scrotum. If a urethral catheter is used, it should be removed on the first morning after surgery. The cylinders should be deflated to half their maximum volume on the first morning after surgery, when the patient usually is discharged from the hospital [14].

Anesthesia

Penile implants may be placed under general or regional anesthesia. For the implantation of semi-rigid rod or soft silicone cylinders, a penile block with a local anesthetic may be sufficient. After tourniquet placement, about 25 cm^2 of 1% lidocaine are additionally instilled into each corpus cavernosum. Alternatively, surgery can be done with a pudendal block without the need of corpus cavernosum instillation [55]. For placement of hydraulic devices, penile blocks combined with pudendal blocks are preferred by some surgeons; most surgeons recommend general or spinal anesthesia [56].

Postoperative management

Most patients are discharged on the first day after surgery and intravenous antibiotics are stopped at that time. At home, patients are usually prescribed one week of oral quinolones.

Patients are instructed to start activating and deactivating the implant as soon as the local pain has subsided enough to allow this. In most cases this takes

place during the first follow-up visit appointment seven to ten days after surgery. Sexual activity is not allowed until six weeks after the procedure, when the second outpatient visit should take place. Ideally, validated instruments, including the IIEF, should be used at three, six and/or 12 months after surgery to produce objective outcome data once the patient has resumed sexual activity on a regular basis. Particular care should be taken in assessing penile length and sensitivity, which represent two possible patient complaints [14].

Complications of penile prosthetic surgery and their management
Intraoperative complications

The typical complication that may occur during dilation of the corpora cavernosa is perforation of the tunica albuginea. Typically the perforation occurs during the initial step of dilatation; if this is the case, interrupting the dilatation on that side and completing the same procedure contralaterally will show the real length of the crus. With a size nine Hegar dilator in place in the corpus cavernosum contralateral to the perforation, the surgeon should go back to the crus affected by the perforation and use only large dilators to complete the dilation. After completing the dilatation and placing the cylinders, a polydioxane suture may be passed through the rear tip of the cylinder and then through the tunica albuginea at the most proximal end of the corporotomy to anchor the cylinder in proper place. Alternatively a Dacron sock can be sutured to the rear tip of the prosthesis and fixed to the wall of the tunica with one or two sutures.

Proximal corporal perforations do not mean that surgery must be terminated. If there is a distal perforation, most experienced surgeons agree that surgery should be interrupted to prevent prosthesis infection. Although termination of surgery is the most prudent course in most distal perforations, in special cases such as extremely fibrotic corpora, primary suture of the albuginea with or without grafting may render good results. In such cases, after suturing the urethral perforation and inserting the cylinders, use of a suprapubic cystostomy tube or Foley catheter for one month has produced a successful outcome in a few reports [14].

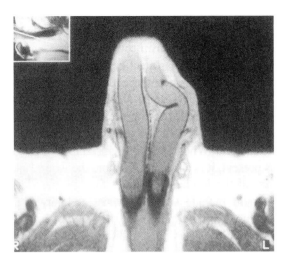

Fig. 12.3 Penile buckling due to overized left cylinder in MRI imaging.

Postoperative complications

The most significant postoperative complication associated with implant surgery is prosthetic infection, which occurs in 1 to 3% of cases [25]. Other important complications include distal and proximal perforation of the tunica albuginea, SST deformity, "S-shaped" deformity of the penis, erosion of a component, and mechanical malfunction of the device [30]. The best way to manage complications is to prevent them from happening by adequate sterile handling and correct sizing of the cylinders.

Diagnosis of complications is based on clinical history and physical examination, but imaging techniques may be useful to plan a surgical approach. MRI is the most valuable imaging technique for diagnosis of penile prosthesis complications [31]. MRI is radiation-free, demonstrates penile anatomy in three orthogonal planes, and is superior to any other imaging method in demonstrating soft tissue contrast [30,31,56] (see Figure 12.3). All penile implants except the now-discontinued Omniphase and Duraphase models, are compatible and safe with MRI field strength Tesla 1.5 and 3.0. The Omniphase or Duraphase prostheses are unsafe during MRI scanning due to their metallic components [60,61].

Prosthetic infection should be suspected when there is increasing postoperative pain, fever, erythema of the incision or genitalia, and/or cutaneous fixation of prosthesis components, such as the pump to the scrotal skin [25]. This is the most feared complication after penile implant surgery. The use of antibiotics alone has not been successful in eradicating postoperative infections. It is difficult, if not impossible, for antibiotics to penetrate the area of a postoperative infection because the pseudo-capsule, which forms around the device, the relatively poor blood supply in the area, and the biofilm or slime produced by *Staphylococci* and other bacteria that provide a protected cavity in which bacteria can proliferate. When an infection develops around a portion of the implant, it may easily migrate to all other parts along the connecting tubes, as well as any foreign body, such as polytetrafluoro-ethylene or permanent sutures in the immediate area.

In the face of infection the surgeon has two options. The first is to remove the prosthesis and reinsert it at least three months or more later. If this option is chosen, the penis will be noticeably shorter and the reinsertion procedure more difficult because of the scar tissue that forms during that interval. The second option is to use a salvage procedure, which entails removing the prosthesis and all foreign materials, cleaning the wound with a series of antiseptic solutions and reinserting a new prosthesis at the same operation. Mulcahy [32] reported a success rate of 85% with the salvage procedure. There are several circumstances in which salvage should not be considered. These include prosthesis infections in patients with diabetic ketoacidosis, life-threatening sepsis, and frank tissue necrosis or urethral erosion of the cylinders in the fossa navicularis. If one excludes these conditions, a salvage approach is a reasonable procedure. According to a technique first described by Mulcahy [32,33], all prosthetic parts and foreign materials are removed; the wound is irrigated with a series of seven antibiotic solutions; the drapes, instruments, gloves and gowns are then changed, and a new prosthesis system placed in the wound.

Also a delayed form of salvage therapy using primary removal of the prosthesis, continuous antibiotic irrigation for several days, and secondary prosthesis reimplantation, ideally after 72 hours, has been published [25]. If salvage procedures are planned, it seems wise to treat the patient with systemic antibiotics for up to 48 hours prior to the salvage surgery, especially if fluid is available for culture and antibiotic testing [30].

If mechanical problems in an inflatable device develop after surgery, a trend to remove and replace the entire device has emerged recently. Common mechanical failures are tubing fracture, cylinder or reservoir leak, cylinder aneurysm, or connector disruption. Most urologists consider that replacing the entire device will give the patient added longevity in all parts [14,30]. Certainly after two or three years, it is prudent to replace all the prosthesis components because there can be significant wear of the device within that period. In addition, repeated penile incisions to change cylinders may shorten the penile length [34]. Furthermore, bacteria-positive cultures of clinically uninfected penile prostheses have been found in 70% of tested implants. In some patients, more than one organism grew, and in some patients the pump culture was negative but the biofilm was positive [35]. This may explain the higher infection rate that occurs with revision surgery [36,37,38]. Combining complete implant removal with a modified salvage protocol leads to a markedly decreased incidence of infection in patients with a penile prosthesis who are undergoing revision for non-infectious reasons [39].

A correct procedure in a properly selected patient does not necessarily result in a satisfactory outcome for the patient. A common reason for patient dissatisfaction is the lack of adequate engorgement of the glans during sexual activity. Typically, the patient reports that the corpora cavernosa are perfectly rigid after activating the implant but the glans remains soft, interfering with the patient's sexual satisfaction. Mulhall *et al.* [40] recently reported a beneficial effect of oral sildenafil on glans engorgement in patients with penile implants complaining of lack of glans engorgement. By using the IIEF, the authors also showed that sildenafil caused a statistically significant improvement in implant assisted intercourse. Similar results with the use of 500µg of intra-urethral alprostadil were reported by Chew and Stuckey [41] in a patient who had been treated with a Dynaflex prosthesis.

In case of impending distal protrusion of cylinders,

a new pocket for the tip of the cylinder within the distal corpus cavernosum should be created after hemicircumcision. Also windsock techniques with synthetic materials have been described for this condition. In some patients, an SST deformity develops, also termed "floppy glans". This condition is best treated by a circumcising incision, dissection of the glans from underlying tissue, and non-absorbable suture fixation of the glans to the tips of the corpora [56].

Re-operations

The reimplantation of an inflatable three-piece prosthesis in a patient with severe corporeal fibrosis is a surgical challenge. The worst fibrosis develops as a result of previous removal of an infected implant. Penile shortening results and dilatation of the scarred corporal bodies may be tedious and time-consuming. Wilson published an excellent review on special tools and techniques for these patients [28]. Correct cylinder sizing is of special importance in these cases. Sometimes it is prudent to implant a smaller device and exchange it for a larger device, after several months of active tissue expansion by regular and frequent use of the device. While the implantation of synthetic graft material is sometimes unavoidable, it is important to remember that the risk of infection during any penile prosthesis surgery correlates with duration of the procedure and amount of synthetic material that is implanted [56].

Results of penile prosthetic surgery

Generally penile implant surgery is associated with a high success rate [42]. In a recent study, the satisfaction rates of erectile function in patients treated with sildenafil, intracavernosal alprostadil injections, or three-piece inflatable penile prosthesis, were compared [43]. Patients enrolled in this study had failed initial sildenafil therapy. They were reinstructed on proper dosing and timing of sildenafil or directed to an alternative treatment. Satisfaction from treatment was assessed by a validated instrument, the Erectile Dysfunction Inventory for Treatment Satisfaction (EDITS), and erectile function was checked by the erectile function domain score of the IIEF. Total satisfaction and erectile function scores were significantly better in patients who had received the penile implant than in those treated with sildenafil or intracavernosal injection therapy. Mulhall *et al.* [44] assessed the effect of two- or three-piece inflatable implants in a series of men who used the IIEF and EDITS questionnaires at baseline and postoperatively. At one year follow-up, all assessments of erection, ejaculation, orgasm, and sexual satisfaction were significantly better than baseline values.

Several authors have reported their long-term results in studies published prior to 2000. In 1997, Daitch *et al.* [45] reported a five-year actuarial mechanical failure rate of 9.1% for AMS CX three-piece devices and 17.1% for Ultrex devices. This study suggested that mechanical failure is correlated with patient dissatisfaction, but this suggestion should be interpreted cautiously because some patients with surviving implants may also have little satisfaction. In 1999 Wilson *et al.* [46] reported the results of a prospective study of 1383 Mentor Alpha-1 penile implants and determined the mechanical survival of 410 original and 971 enhanced models. The five-year device survival rate increased from 75.3% for the original to 92.6% for the enhanced model overall, and from 75.3 to 93.6% for first-time implants only. The estimated failure rate was 5.6% for the original model and 1.3% for the enhanced model. Carson [47] reported a long-term multi-center study of the 700CX three-piece inflatable prosthesis, focusing on patients' satisfaction with a median follow-up of almost 48 months. At follow-up, 79% of the patients were using the implant at least twice monthly and 88% stated that they would recommend an implant to a friend with ED.

In a recently conducted multi-center study assessing the long-term reliability of three-piece AMS prostheses including the CX, CXR and Ultrex cylinders [48], at a mean follow up of 59 months, 92.5% of patients were still engaging in sexual intercourse with a mean frequency of 1.7 times weekly. Patients and partners reports of erection were excellent, satisfactory or poor in 48, 50, and 2%, and 17, 66, and 17%, respectively. Levine *et al.* [49] studied 112 patients who had an Ambicor two-piece prosthesis and 91 of their partners at a mean of four years after surgery. This study included a modified EDITS instrument, which showed that the procedure met the expectations of 87% of the patients, and that

they were very confident with the device. A recent report of a head-to-head comparison of three-piece inflatable prostheses by Mentor and AMS did not reveal significant differences between the devices [50]. Data was collected by a computer-assisted telephone interview consisting of 37 questions. The overall satisfaction rate was 69% and 72%, and respondents reported that they would have the surgery performed again.

In another study, a psychosexual questionnaire was used to assess psychosexual benefits after implant surgery. Patients perceived an improvement in erectile ability and libido [51], and concerns about achieving and maintaining an erection during intercourse were significantly alleviated.

Montorsi *et al.* [14] reported an increase in the frequency of sexual activity, and improved satisfaction with sexual life in men with penile implants.

Only a few authors have reported long-term results of semi-rigid prostheses. Salama [52] reported that 70% of patients and 57% of partners were satisfied with their semi-rigid AMS 650 or Mentor Accu-Form prostheses. There was an increase in the frequency of intercourse, sexual desire and ability to achieve orgasm. Of note, dislike for the device was the most common cause for dissatisfaction among patients, while a sense of unnaturalness was the most common cause for dissatisfaction for partners.

In another recent study, Ferguson and Cespedes [53] reported five to seven year follow-up results with Dura-II penile prostheses. No mechanical defects were found in the 9% of men who had the device later explanted. Satisfactory rigidity was reported by 76% of the patients and ease of use was reported by 87%. A limitation of malleable implants is the potential for insufficient penile girth. Most of the patients having a semi-rigid penile implant have some form of penile vascular failure. Over time, spontaneous filling of the corporal tissue surrounding the cylinders tends to reduce. This may create the condition called "pencil-like erection", which is unsatisfactory to most patients [14].

Regardless of the type of prosthesis used, meticulous surgical technique and the surgeon's experience are the most important factors in determining the final outcome of the procedure. In addition, it is clear that the greatest chance for achieving satisfactory long-term results is at the time of the first implant. This underlines the importance of adhering to proven principles of patient selection, pre- and post-operative management and surgical technique, including meticulous observation of antiseptic procedures [54]. A recent paper has reported that the revision rate for penile prostheses may be much higher for inexperienced surgeons compared to experienced surgeons, and that inexperienced surgeons tend to select simple prosthetic devices, which may not fit the patients' expectations [59].

Conclusions and Recommendations

An important step forward has been achieved with the antibiotic coating of penile prostheses. Nevertheless, implant infection remains a threatening complication, especially in re-operations and for patients having simultaneous penile reconstruction and penile prosthesis implantation. It would be useful to define standard operating procedures for systemic antibiotic therapy and local antiseptic measures for penile implant operations. At the present time, there exists consensus on the general need for preoperative prophylactic antibiotic coverage against Gram–negative and Gram–positive bacteria, and the prohibition of prosthetic surgery when systemic, cutaneous or urinary tract infections are present [60].

Manufacturers of penile prostheses are continually trying to decrease mechanical failure rates. New devices with modified pump systems and cylinder coating will have to prove their value in future studies after at least five year follow-up. From the literature [46], suggestions have been made regarding the correlation between mechanical reliability and patient satisfaction, as well as patient confidence in the device [49]. Patients and possibly their partners should be informed preoperatively about the various types of prostheses, the possible complications and the differences in both the flaccid and erect states between the normal penis and the penis that has an implant. They should also know about the potential compromise of the effectiveness of other therapies should the device be removed subsequently [60]. Most patients who have had multiple penile implant surgeries suffer from corporal fibrosis and reduced

penile length and girth. If advances in penile enlargement surgery become possible in the future, they should be translated to penile implant surgery [24]. A similar problem has to be solved for patients with severe Peyronie's disease, who require incision or resection of their plaques during the implant surgery. The ideal graft material to cover defects in the tunica has yet to be found. It should have tensile strength and stretching characteristics similar to those of healthy tunica albuginea. Future advances should also include tissue welding techniques to replace time-consuming suturing [24].

Penile prosthesis implantation is a highly successful treatment for ED. In order to get evidence-based data, which can guide us to even better outcomes, standard survey tools should be used for all studies. A survey tool based on the IIEF and/or EDITS, but developed specifically for follow-up in prosthesis implantation, would be an important addition to future studies. In all these outcome studies partner evaluation should be included.

References

1 Bogoras N. Über die volle plastische wiederherstellung eines zum koitus fähigen penis (penisplastica totalis). *Zentralbl Chir* 1936;**63**:1271.

2 Bergmann RT, Howard A, Barnes RW. Plastic reconstruction of the penis. *J Urol* 1948;**59**:1174.

3 Hauri D. Development of surgical procedures in the treatment of erectile dysfunction. A historical overview. *Urol Int* 2003;**70**:124–131.

4 Goodwin WE, Scott WW. Phalloplasty. *J Urol* 1952; 68–903.

5 Löffler RA, Sayegh ES. Perforated acrylic implants in management of organic impotence. *J Urol* 1960;**84**: 559.

6 Beheri GE. Surgical treatment of impotence. *Plast Reconstr Surg* 1966;**38**:92.

7 Pearman RO. Treatment of organic impotence by implantation of a penile prosthesis. *J Urol* 1967;**97**:716.

8 Apfelberg DB, Maser MR, Lash H. Surgical management of impotence. *Am J Surg* 1976;**132**:336.

9 Morales PA, Suares JB, Delgado J, Whitehead ED. Penile implantation for erectile impotence. *J Urol* 1973;**109**:641.

10 Small MP, Carrion HM, Gordon JA. Small-carrion penile prosthesis: New implant for management for impotence. *Urology* 1975;**5**:479.

11 Finney RP. New hinged silicone penile implant. *J Urol* 1977;**118**:585.

12 Jonas U, Jakobi GH. Silicone-silver penile prosthesis: Description, operative approach and results. *J Urol* 1980;**123**:865.

13 Scott FB, Bradley WE, Timm GW. Management of erectile impotence: Use of implantable inflatable prosthesis. *Urology* 1973;**2**:80.

14 Montorsi F, Dehó F, Salonia A, Briganti AA, Bua L, Fantini GV, Gallina A, Saccá A, Mirone V, Rigatti P. Penile implants in the era of oral drug treatment for erectile dysfunction. *BJU International* 2004;**94**:745–751.

15 Subrini L. Subrini penile implants: Surgical, sexual and psychological results. *Eur Urol* 1982;**8**:222.

16 Wilson SK, Henry GD, Delk JR, Cleves MA. The Mentor Alpha 1 penile prosthesis with reservoir lock-out valve. Effective prevention of auto-inflation with improved capability for ectopic reservoir placement. *J Urol* 2002; **168**:1475–1478.

17 Carson CC. Diagnosis, treatment and prevention of penile prosthesis infection. *Int J Impotence Res* 2003; **15**(Suppl.5):S139–S146.

18 Carson CC. Efficacy of antibiotic impregnation of inflatable penile prostheses in decreasing infection in original implants. *J Uol* 2004;**171**:1611–1614.

19 Droggin D, Shabsigh R, Anastasiadis AG. Antibiotic coating reduces penile prosthesis infection. *J Sex Med* 2005;**2**:565–568.

20 Hellstrom WJG, Walter C, Rajpurkar A, *et al.* Hydrophilic-coated inflatable penile prosthesis: One year experience. *J Sed Med* 2005;**2**(Suppl.1): 16–17.

21 Hellstrom WJG, Hyun JS, Human L, Sanabria JA, Bivalacqua TJ, Leungwattanakij S. Antimicrobial activity of antibiotic-soaked, resist(-coated Bioflex). *Int J Impotence Res* 2003;**15**:18–21.

22 Martinez Portillo FJ, Jünemann KP, Sohn M. Operative therapie der erektilen dysfunktion. *Urol A* 2003;**42**: 1337–1344.

23 Carson CC. Penile prosthesis implantation and infection for Sexual Medicine Society of North America. *Int J Impotence Res* 2001;**13**(Suppl.5):S35–S38.

24 Montague DK, Angermeier KW. Future considerations: advances in the surgical management of erectile dysfunction. *Int J Impot Res* 2002;**12**(Suppl.4):140–143.

25 Mulcahy JJ, Austoni E, Barada JH, Choi HK, Hellstrom JG, Krishnamurti S, Moncada I, Schultheiss D, Sohn M, Wessells H. The penile implant for erectile dysfunction. *J Sex Med* 2004;**1**:98–109.

26 Carson CC. Diagnosis, treatment and prevention of

penile prosthesis infection. *Int J Impotence Res* 2003; **15**(Suppl.5):139–146.

27 Montague DK, Angermeier KW. Surgical approaches for penile prosthesis implantation: penoscrotal vs. infrapubic. *Int J Impotence Res* 2003;**15**(Suppl.5): 134–135.

28 Wilson SK. Reimplantation of inflatable penile prosthesis into scarred corporeal bodies. *Int J Impotence Res* 2003;**15**(Suppl.5):125–128.

29 Montague DK, Angermeier KW. Cylinder sizing: less is more. *Int J Impotence Res* 2003;**15**(Suppl.5):132–133.

30 Moncada I, Martinez-Salamanca JI, Allona A, Hernandez C. Current role of penile implants for erectile dysfunction. *Current Opinion in Urology* 2004;**14**:375–380.

31 Moncada I, Jara J, Cabello R, Monzo JI, Hernandez C. Radiological assessment of penile prosthesis: the role of magnetic resonance imaging. *World J Urol* 2004;**22**: 371–377.

32 Mulcahy JJ. Long-term experience with salvage of infected penile implants. *J Urol* 2000;**163**:481–482.

33 Mulcahy JJ. Treatment alternatives for the infected penile implant. *Int J Impotence Res* 2003;**15**(Suppl.5): 147–149.

34 Mulcahy JJ. Surgical management of penile prosthesis complications. *Int J Impotence Res* 2000;**12**(Suppl.4): 108–111.

35 Penile prosthesis cultures during revision surgery: A multicenter study. *J Urol* 2004;**172**:153–156.

36 Licht MR, Montague DK, Angermeier KW, Lakin MM. Cultures from genitourinary prostheses at re-operation: questioning the role of *Staphylococcus epidermidis* in periprosthetic infection. *J Urol* 1995; **154**:387.

37 Wilson SK, Delk JR. Inflatable penile implant infection: predisposing factors and treatment suggestions. *J Urol* 1995;**153**:659.

38 Jarow JP. Risk factors for penile prosthetic infection. *J Urol* 1996;**156**:402.

39 Gerard D, Henry, StK, Wilson JR, Delk II, Culley C, Carson J, Wiygul C, Tornheil M, Cleves MA, Silverstein CA, Donatucci CF. Revision washout decreases penile prosthetic infection in revision surgery. A multicenter study. *J Urol* 2005;**173**:89–92.

40 Mulhall JP, Jahoda A, Aviv N, Valenzuela R, Parker M. The impact of sildenafil citrate on sexual satisfaction profiles in men with a penile prosthesis in situ. *BJU Int* 2004;**93**:97–99.

41 Chew KK, Stuckey BGA. Use of transurethral alprostadil (MUSE) (prostaglandin E1) for glans tumescence in a patient with penile prosthesis. *Int J Impotence Res* 2000;**12**:195–196.

42 Jarow JP, Nana-Sinkam P, Sabbagh M, Eskew A. Outcome analysis of goal directed therapy for impotence. *J Urol* 1996;**155**:1609–1612.

43 Rajpurkar A, Dhabuwala CB. Comparison of satisfaction rates and erectile function in patients treated with sildenafil, intracavernous prostaglandin E1 and penile implant surgery for erectile dysfunction in urology Practice. *J Urol* 2003;**170**:159–163.

44 Mulhall JP, Ahmed A, Branch J, Parker M. Serial assessment of efficacy and satisfaction profiles following penile prosthesis surgery. *J Urol* 2003;**171**:1429–1433.

45 Daitch JA, Angermeier KW, Lakin MM, Ingleright BJ, Montague DK. Long-term mechanical reliability of AMS 700 series inflatable penile prostheses: comparison of CX/CXM and Ultrex cylinders. *J Urol* 1997; **158**:1400–1402.

46 Wilson SK, Cleves MA, Delk JR. Comparison of mechanical reliability of original and enhanced Mentor Alpha 1 penile prostheses. *J Urol* 1999;**162**:715–718.

47 Carson CC. Penile prosthesis implantation in the treatment of Peyronie's disease. *Int J Impotence Res* 1998; **10**:125–128.

48 Montorsi F, Rigatti P, Carmignani G, *et al.* AMS three-piece inflatable implants for erectile dysfunction: a long-term multi-institutional study in 200 consecutive patients. *Eur Urol* 2000;**37**:50–55.

49 Levine LA, Estrada CR, Morgentaler A. Mechanical reliability and safety of and patient satisfaction with the Ambicor inflatable penile prosthesis: results of a 2-center-study. *J Urol* 2001;**166**:932–934.

50 Brinkman MJ, Henry GD, Wilson SK, Delk WJ, Denny GA, Young M, Cleves MA. A survey of patients with inflatable penile prostheses for satisfaction. *J Urol* 2005;**174**:253–257.

51 Tefilli MV, Dubocq F, Rajpurkar A, Gheiler EL, Tiguert R, Barton C. Assessment of psychosexual adjustment after insertion of inflatable penile prosthesis. *Urology* 1998;**52**:1106–1109.

52 Salama N. Satisfaction with the malleable penile prosthesis among couples from the Middle East: is it different from that reported elsewhere? *Int J Impotence Res* 2004;**16**:175–180.

53 Ferguson KH, Cespedes RD. Prospective long-term results and quality of life assessment after Dura-II penile prosthesis placement. *Urology* 2003;**61**: 437–441.

54 Lota Y, Roehrborn CG, McConnell JD, Hendin BN. Factors influencing the outcomes of penile prosthesis surgery at a teaching institution. *Urology* 2003;**62**:918–921.

55 Dos Reis JM, Glina S, Da Silva MF, Furlan V. Penile prosthesis surgery with the patient under local regional anesthesia. *J Urol* 1993;**150**:1179–1181.

56 Mulcahy JJ. Implants, mechanical devices and vascular surgery for erectile dysfunction. In: Lue TF, Basson R, Rosen R, Giuliano F, Khoury S, Montorsi F, eds. *Sexual Medicine: Sexual Dysfunctions in Men and Women.* Paris: 2nd International Consultation on Sexual Dysfunctions, 2004, Chapter 14, pp. 469–498.

57 Montague DK, Angermeier KW. Penile Prosthesis Implantation. *Urol Cl N Am* 2001;**28**:355–361.

58 Wilson SK, Carson CC, Cleves MA, Delk II Jr. Quantifying risk of penile prosthesis infection with elevated glycosylated haemoglobin. *J Urol* 1998;**159**: 1537–1540.

59 Summerton D. The urological prosthetic surgeon? Should the implantation of both penile prostheses and artificial urinary sphincters only be performed by a small number of surgeons, based in designated centers? *J Sex Med* 2006;**P-06–279**(Suppl.1):91–92.

60 Montague DK, Jarow JP, Broderick GA, *et al.* Chapter1: The management of erectile dysfunction: an AUA update. *J Urol* 2005;**174**:230–239.

61 Shellock FG. *Reference Manual of Magnetic Resonance Safety, Implants, and Devices.* Los Angeles: Biomedical Research Publishing Group, 2006, pp. 476–478.

CHAPTER 13
Hypoactive Sexual Desire in Men

Eusebio Rubio-Aurioles

Hypoactive sexual desire (HSD) is a condition that is characterized by the absence or notable decrease in the frequency in which the man experiences desire for sexual activity.

In contrast with other conditions related to the sexual life, the key clinical determinants of this diagnosis are not as concrete and readily identified as erection or ejaculation for instance, in the case of HSD these clinical features refer to a variety of expressions of sexual desire, since the occurrence of sexual desire is an internal and subjective experience. Because of this, HSD has been historically either not identified [1], or erroneously diagnosed and presented (and treated) as other sexual dysfunctions like erectile dysfunction [2].

Hypoactive sexual desire was first defined as a clinical entity in 1977 [3], and recognized as a valid clinical diagnosis with the publication of the Diagnostic and Statistical Manual of Mental Disorders, third edition (DSM III) in 1980 [4]. In recent publications, the importance of this condition has been highlighted [2,5].

The DSM IV, in its current edition, defines HSD disorder as persistently or recurrently deficient (or absent) sexual fantasy and desire for sexual activity, leading to marked distress or interpersonal difficulty [6]. However, since the DSM IV is a psychiatric classification, its definition excludes HSD when it is caused by another medical disorder, or even another sexual dysfunction. There is some discussion in the literature as to this requirement, as the clinical practice illustrates, that the co-existence of HSD disorder with other sexual dysfunctions such as erectile dysfunction is rather common [5], and the management of the combined conditions often requires specific clinical decisions and actions.

Epidemiology and Risk Factors

There are two reports in the literature that merit commentary when attempting to answer the question: how prevalent is HSD?

Data from a probability sample study of sexual behavior in a demographically representative, 1992 cohort of US adults, known as the National Health and Social Life Survey, and that included 1749 women and 1410 men aged 18 to 59 years at the time of the survey, was analyzed by Laumann and colleagues [7]. A latent class analysis (LCA) was used to evaluate the syndromal clustering of individual sexual symptoms. Latent class analysis is a statistical method well suited for grouping categoric data into latent classes [8]. Latent class analysis tests, whether a latent variable, or specified as a set of mutually exclusive classes, accounts for observed covariation among manifest, categoric variables [9]. This study reports a 5% prevalence of low sexual desire, which should be compared to the 5% prevalence reported for erectile dysfunction. Table 13.1 presents the risk factors reported for this population.

In a more recent report, named the Global Study of Sexual Attitudes and Behaviors (GSSAB)—an international survey of various aspects of sex and relationships among adults aged 40 to 80 years—an estimate of the prevalence and correlates of sexual problems in 13 882 women and 13 618 men from 29 countries is reported by Laumann and co-workers [10]. Although the figures for low sexual desire are derived exclusively from the participant's response to a single question, the report has the value of including a rather large variation in countries and cultures. Depending on the geographic area, prevalence of "lack of sexual interest", a category where

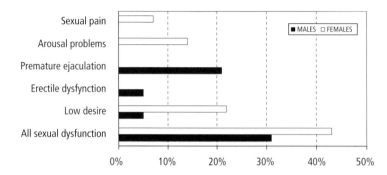

Fig. 13.1 Prevalence of hypoactive sexual desire disorder compared to other sexual dysfunctions prevalence as reported by Laumann *et al.* [7].

Table 13.1 Risk factors for low desire among males as reported by Laumann *et al.* [7]. All predictors included in the table are significant above $p \le 0.10$.

Predictor	Adjusted Odds Ratio	(95% CI)
Health and lifestyle		
Daily alcohol consumption	2.24	(0.89–5.64)
Poor to fair health	3.07	(1.38–6.81)
Emotional problems or stress	3.20	(1.81–5.67)
Sexual experience		
Thinks about sex less than once a week	3.63	(1.57–8.40)
Any same sex activity ever	2.51	(1.10–5.74)
Partner had an abortion ever	1.98	(0.92–4.23)
Sexually touched before puberty	2.23	(1.10–4.56)

Table 13.2 Risk factors for low sexual desire in men as reported in the Global Study of Sexual Attitudes and Behaviors [10].

Risk factor	Odds Ratio variation across regions of the world (minimum–maximum)
Older age	0.5 to 10.6
Depression	1.5–2.9
Poor health	0.8–2.6

respondents answering "occasionally, periodically or frequently" were included, varied from 12.5% to 28.0%. The risk factors that in this study reached statistical significance in a more or less consistent way across the different regions of the world, are reported as summarized in Table 13.2.

The Components of Sexual Desire

Sexual desire is not a single phenomenon. Anyone can say he is experiencing sexual desire for several reasons that do not correspond necessarily to the physiology of desire. In this respect Levine has suggested an interesting division; according to his view it

is clinically useful to think of desire as consisting of drive (biologic), motive (individual and relationship psychology), and wish (cultural) components [11]. The drive component of desire is what we could expect to be explained (some day) by the neurochemical mechanisms in the brain. The motivational component of desire might be a result of the interaction of the couple, for instance: "I want to have sex with her, otherwise she will leave". And the cultural component of desire can be best represented by what is considered a highly desirable partner in a culture, with whom the man needs to have desire in order to conform to the cultural demand of a "true man". Both in clinical practice and in the general surveys that explore the level of sexual desire the three components are always interwoven.

Molecules promoting sexual drive

Table 13.3 presents, in a short format, the various molecules that are thought to participate in the regulation of the biologic component of sexual desire, after a review by Meston [12].

Table 13.3 Molecules that have been reported to influence sexual desire (modified after Meston and Frohlich) [12].

Class Molecule	Effect on sexual desire: ↑ = increase 0 = no change ↓ = decrease	Kind of population studied	Author/year	Reference number
Hormones				
Testosterone	↑	Hypogonadal or castrated men	Davidson, *et al.* 1982 Kwan M, *et al.* 1983 Skakkeoaek NE, *et al.* 1981.	13,14,15
Testosterone	↑	Adolescent boys	Halpern CT, *et al.* 1994 Udry JR, *et al.* 1985	16,17
Testosterone	0	Normal range testosterone levels	Schiavi RC & White D, 1976	18
Estrogen	↓	Sex offenders	Bancroft J, *et al.* 1974	19
Progesterone	↓	Normal males and hyperactive sexual desire males	Heller CG, *et al.* 1958 Money J, 1970	20,21
Prolactin	↓	Hyperprolactinemia	Bancroft J, 1984 Bancroft J, *et al.* 1984 Buckman MT & Kellner R, 1984 Dornan WA & Malsbury CW, 1989 Muller P, *et al.* 1979	22,23,24,25,26
Cortisol	↓	Cushing syndrome	Starkman MN, *et al.* 1981	27
Pheromones	↑	Normal men	Cutler WB, *et al.* 1998	28
Neurotransmitters				
Serotonin	0, reported as ↓ probably because of interference with arousal and orgasm	Use of Monoamine oxidase inhibitors, Selective serotonin reuptake inhibitors and antipsychotic medication users	Montejo-Gonzalez AL, *et al.* 1997	29
Dopamine	↑	Apomorphine/levodopa Parkinson disease patients	Uitti RJ, *et al.* 1989	30
Histamine	↓	Cimetidine and ranitidine users	White JM & Rumbold GR, 1988	31

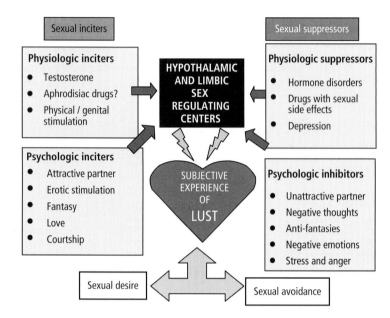

Fig. 13.2 A conceptual model of the integration of biologic and psychologic factors in sexual desire (after Kaplan, 1995) [35].

The role of testosterone, and perhaps several other androgens, appears to be necessary for the experience of sexual desire in its drive component [32]. It appears that a minimum level of androgen is required for the man to be able to experience sexual desire; however the relationship is not completely linear, as the higher level of androgen in blood does not correlate with higher level of sexual desire [18]. In addition to the molecules mentioned in Table 13.3, there has been some speculation on the role of oxytocin [33] and, in a recent report [34], the role of thyroid hormone has been suggested.

Integrating the components of desire

One conceptual model that is helpful to integrate both physiologic and psychologic factors of sexual desire has been proposed by Helen Kaplan [35]. Although this model still requires empirical validation, it represents an interesting tool for the understanding of the dynamics of a man with HSD. The model is summarized in Figure 13.2.

Etiology of Hypoactive Sexual Desire

Hypoactive sexual desire is a condition that many times is part of another disease or disorder. Other times, the decrease or absence of sexual desire occurs with no other sexual dysfunction or recognizable pathology. In any event, it is critical that the clinician identifies this condition; lack of success in treatment of other sexual dysfunctions, like erectile dysfunction, can sometimes be explained by the presence and lack of proper treatment of HSD. The list included in Table 13.4, taken from Meuleman & Van Lankvled (2005) [2], is a summary of the causes of HSD seen frequently in clinical practice.

Hypoactive sexual desire is frequent in men with erectile dysfunction. In a series of 428 men with erectile dysfunction, Corona and co-workers (2004) [5] reported that 43.3% of their participants had the condition. This group found no correlation for patient or partner's age. Men with HSD in this study were not diagnosed as hypogonadic more frequently than men without HSD; however ANOVA showed a significant ($P < 0.005$) difference of total, free testosterone and prolactin levels among patients with different severities of HSD. No significant correlation was found for: follicle-stimulating hormone (FSH) ($r = 0.04$), luteinizing hormone (LH) ($r = 0.04$), thyroid-stimulating hormone (TSH) ($r = 0.06$), or testis volume ($r = -0.08$). No correlation was found for: prostate specific antigen (PSA), blood pressure, lipid profile, glycemia, and parameters derived from

Table 13.4 List of medical and psychologic factors that can cause HSD [2].

- Androgen deficiency
- Hyperprolactinemia
- Anger and anxiety
- Depression
- Relationship conflict
- Stroke
- Antidepressant therapy
- Epilepsy
- Post-traumatic stress syndrome
- Renal failure
- Coronary disease and heart failure
- Ageing
- HIV
- Body-building and eating disorders

Table 13.5 Clinical indicators of sexual desire.

- Sexual frequency
  However, sometimes frequency ≠ desire: activity can occur with no desire
- Sexual fantasies
- Sexual thoughts
- Initiation of sexual activity

echo color Doppler. The psychologic correlates found were: free-floating anxiety, somatic symptoms, obsessive–compulsive traits, and depressive symptoms.

Diagnosis of Hypoactive Sexual Desire

The diagnosis of HSD is not difficult if the clinician asks directly about desire or interest for sexual activity. Most patients identify with ease a change in their usual pattern, and this is the way in which the condition is identified most of the time in clinical practice. Sometimes, it is necessary to investigate the indicators of sexual desire, which, although not as direct as the expression of desire, are often good clinical indicators. Table 13.5 shows a list of clinical indicators of sexual desire.

The question of how much is too little has not been answered with enough precision. However, some re-

ports in the literature give some light to this. In a group of non-dysfunctional couples, LoPiccolo and Friedman reported that the majority of the participants both desired and had sexual activity between once and four times a week [36]. In a research setting, Schiavi [37] suggested a criteria of sexual activity occurring less than once every two weeks, for persons 55 years or younger, suggests HSD.

Some patients present themselves as having low sexual desire, which in fact is a result of another sexual dysfunction. Erectile dysfunction is sometimes confused by the patient as a sign of diminished desire. Likewise, the avoidance pattern that follows the frustration generated by a persistent dysfunction, like severe premature ejaculation or erectile dysfunction, can also be reported as absence of desire. These clinical situations demand a careful evaluation from the clinician before arriving at a clinical diagnosis.

Laboratory Testing

In addition to identifying the condition, it is recommended that the main causes of HSD be screened during the initial consultation. The evaluation should include the measurement of serum total testosterone and prolactin as a minimum and, depending on the additional clinical signs, further endocrinologic testing might be appropriate.

Depression and Relationship Conflict Detection

Identification of depression and the presence of relationship conflict should also be part of the initial evaluation. Both can be identified through the clinical interview; however, in many instances the use of screening tools can be useful and helpful.

There are several scales that have been developed for depression detection. A short and useful tool, developed for the geriatric population, might be of help for the clinician unfamiliar with depression or with restricted time during consultation, and is included in Table 13.6 [38,39]. The briefness of the scale (only five items) and good psychometric properties make this a useful instrument for the detection of depression among older men.

Positive answers for depression screening are

Table 13.6 Five-item version of the Geriatric Depression Scale [38,39].

---

1. Are you basically satisfied with your life?
2. Do you often get bored?
3. Do you often feel helpless?
4. Do you prefer to stay home rather than going out and doing new things?
5. Do you feel pretty worthless the way you are now?

Table 13.7 Quebec 2000 Abbreviated Dyadic Adjustment Scale [40].

---

1. Do you and your partner agree or disagree on displays of affection?
2. Do you often think about getting a divorce or separation, or ending your current relationship?
3. In general, would you say that everything is fine between you and your partner?
4. Do you confide in your partner?
5. Do you ever regret getting married (or living together)?
6. How many times do you and your partner calmly discuss something?
7. How many times do you and your partner work together on something?
8. Circle the number that best corresponds to your level of happiness as a couple (rate between 1 and 7, 7 being perfectly happy).

"yes" to questions 2, 3, 4 and 5, and a "no" to question 1. A score of 0 to 1 positive answers suggest the patient is not depressed; a score 2 or higher indicates possible depression.

Conflict in relationships is easy to identify if the right questions are asked. Sometimes asking directly about the quality of the relationship will give enough information. The questions included in Table 13.7 can provide good clinical information about the quality of the relationship. Although they were developed in a research setting, the scale provides a good guideline on what to investigate when a couple is being evaluated.

As in many other areas of medical diagnosis, identifying a condition does not necessarily mean treating the condition. Many of the depressed patients or the distressed couples will have to be referred for proper treatment. However, when these conditions are not identified by the treating physician, the clinical managing of the case cannot be successful.

Treatment of Hypoactive Sexual Desire

Treatment of HSD is directed to the putative cause of the condition. There are no effective symptomatic treatments for HSD, as there are for erectile dysfunction (i.e. phosphodiesterase-5 (PDE-5) inhibitors). Bupropion, an antidepressant medication that has an effect in the re-uptake of dopamine and norepinephrine [41], has been studied, and it has shown a modest effect on women with HSD when compared to placebo (using the slow-release form starting 150 mg/day for one week and then 300 mg/day) [42,43]. An early report by Crenshaw and co-workers [44] included men and women who were not depressed, but who had some form of psychosexual dysfunction (inhibited sexual desire, inhibited sexual excitement or inhibited orgasm), and indicated some positive effect on patient's rated libido and global improvement, which was statistically significant compared to placebo; unfortunately, it is not clear from the report how many men responded. The response rates, though statistically significant when compared with placebo in all these studies, is low compared with the efficacy of PDE-5 treatment for erectile dysfunction; therefore the clinical use of this alternative is limited.

Testosterone replacement can be of benefit if the patient has hypogonadism [45]. In any event, testosterone replacement therapy should be established with the criteria outlined in the chapter "Hormones, Metabolism, Aging and Men's Health" of this book. Likewise, cases of hyperprolactinemia should be further studied and treated; the same chapter in this book offers guidelines for this treatment.

If depression is identified, then appropriate treatment for it should be established. A number of antidepressant medications exist, with demonstrated efficacy and safety. Likewise, if a conflict in the relationship is encountered, proper treatment should be established. As mentioned earlier, antidepressant therapy can in its turn decrease sexual desire [29]. This is sometimes a clinical situation that requires careful evaluation. If the antidepressant medication is considered as having a causative role in the low desire condition, changing the dose or considering a different medication might be helpful.

Sometimes, troubled relationships could benefit from relatively simple interventions. Simple suggestions can improve partner interaction for some couples and this can be done in the primary care setting. They include: use of open communication on sexual issues with an open and honest approach; increase of time dedicated to physical intimacy; increase of time dedicated to talk about intimacy issues; and sharing of feelings [46]. Severe conflict should be referred to specialized professionals.

Psychotherapy has a role in the treatment of depression and in conflicted relationships. Specific psychotherapeutic interventions for HSD have been described as having the following components (1): *affectual awareness*, that basically strives for identification of positive and negative emotions related to sexual interaction and desire; *insight and understanding*, where a framework to understand the problem is offered to the patient; *cognitive and systemic therapy*, when individual psychologic causes are addressed and interaction factors are addressed and corrected; and finally, *behavioral intervention*, where a number of strategies are utilized to gradually overcome obstacles to sexual interaction.

A very important part of proper management in the primary care scenario is to refer to another professional when the indicated treatment cannot be provided. A referral should be done if either the etiology of HSD cannot be identified, and/or if proper treatment cannot be provided.

References

1 Pridal CG, Lopiccolo J. Multi element treatment of desire disorders: integration of cognitive, behavioral, and sytemic therapy In: Leiblum SR, Rosen RC, eds. *Principles and Practice of Sex Therapy*, 3rd edn. New York: The Guilford Press, 2000.

2 Meuleman EJ, Van Lankvled J. Hypoactive sexual desire disorder: an underestimated condition in men. *BJU Int* 2005;**95**:201–296.

3 Lief HI. Hypoactive sexual desire. *Medical Aspects of Human Sexuality* 1977;**7**:94–95.

4 American Psychiatric Association. *Diagnostic and Statistical Manual of Mental Disorders,* 3rd edn. Washington DC: American Psychiatric Association, 1980.

5 Corona G, Mannucci E, Petrone L, Giommi R, Mansani R, Fei L, Forti G, Maggi M. Psycho-biological correlates of hypoactive sexual desire in patients with erectile dysfunction. *Int J Impot Res* 2004;**16**:275–281.

6 American Psychiatric Association. *Diagnostic and Statistical Manual of Mental Disorders,* 4th edn. Washington, DC: American Psychiatric Association, 2000.

7 Laumann EO, Paik A, Rosen RC. Sexual dysfunction in the United States: Prevalence and predictors. *JAMA* 1999;**281**(6):537–544.

8 Clogg CC. Latent class models. In: Arminger G, Clogg CC, Sobel ME, eds. *Handbook of Statistical Modeling for the Social and Behavioral Sciences.* New York, NY: Plenum Press, 1995 pp. 311–359.

9 McCutcheon AL. *Latent Class Analysis*. Newbury Park, Calif: Sage Publications, 1987.

10 Laumann EO, Nicolosi A, Glasser DB, Paik A, Ginge C, Moreira E, Wang T. Sexual problems among women and men aged 40–80 yrs: prevalence and correlates identified in the Global Study of Sexual Attitudes and Behaviors. *Int J Imp Res* 2005;**17**:39–57.

11 Levine SB. The nature of sexual desire: a clinician's perspective. *Arch Sex Behav* 2003 Jun;**32**(3):279–285.

12 Meston CM, Frohlich PF. The neurobiology of sexual function. *Arch Gen Psychiatry* 2000;**57**:1012–1030.

13 Davidson JM, Kwan M, Greenleaf WJ. Hormonal replacement and sexuality. *Clin Endocrinol Metab* 1982;**11**:599–623.

14 Kwan M, Greenleaf WJ, Mann J, Crapo L, Davidson JM. The nature of androgen action on male sexuality: a combined laboratory/self-report study on hypogonadal men. *Clin Endocrinol Metab* 1983;**57**:557–562.

15 Skakkeoaek NE, Bancroft J, Davidson DW, Warner P. Androgen replacement with oral testosterone undecanoate in hypogonodal men: a double-blind controlled study. *Clin Endocrinol* 1981;**14**:49–61.

16 Halpern CT, Udry JR, Campbell B, Suchindran C, Mason GA. Testosterone and religiosity as predictors of sexual attitudes and activity among adolescent males: a biosocial model. *J Biosoc Sci* 1994;**26**:217–234.

17 Udry JR, Billy JO, Morris NM, Groff TR, Raj MH. Serum androgenic hormones motivate sexual behavior in adolescent boys. *Fertil Steril* 1985;**43**:90–94.

18 Schiavi RC, White D. Androgen and male sexual function: A review of human studies. *J Sex Marital Ther* 1976;**2**:214–228.

19 Bancroft J, Tennent G, Loucas K, Cass J. The control of deviant sexual behavior by drugs. I: Behavioral changes following oestrogens and anti-androgens. *Br J Psychiatry* 1974;**125**:310–315.

20 Heller CG, Laidlaw WM, Harvey HT, Nelson WO. Effects of progestational compounds on the reproductive processes of the human male. *Ann N Y Acad Sci* 1958;**71**:649–665.

21 Money J. Use of an androgen-depleting hormone in the treatment of male sex offenders. *J Sex Res* 1970;**6**: 165–172.

22 Bancroft J. Hormones and human sexual behavior. *J Sex Martial Ther* 1984;**10**:3–21.

23 Bancroft J, O'Carroll R, McNeilly A, Shaw R. The effects of bromocriptine on the sexual behavior of a hyperprolactinaemic man: a controlled case study. *Br J Psychiatry* 1984;**21**:131–137.

24 Buckman MT, Kellner R. Reduction of distress in hyperprolactinemia with bromocriptine. *Am J Psychiatry* 1984;**6**:351–358.

25 Dornan WA, Malsbury CW. Neuropeptides and male sexual behavior. *Neurosci Biobehav Rev* 1989;**13**:1–15.

26 Muller P, Musch K, Wolf AS. Prolactin: variables of personality and sexual behavior. In: Zichella L, Pancheri P, eds. *Psychoneuroendocrinology in Reproduction*. Amsterdam, the Netherlands: Elsevier/North Holland Biomedical Press, 1979, pp. 357–372.

27 Starkman MN, Schteingart DE, Schork MA. Depressed mood and other psychiatric manifestations of Cushing's syndrome: relationship to hormone levels. *Psychosom Med* 1981;**43**:3–18.

28 Cutler WB, Friedmann E, McCoy NL. Pheromonal influences on sociosexual behavior in men. *Arch Sex Behav* 1998;**27**:1–13.

29 Montejo-Gonzalez AL, Llorca G, Izquierdo JA, Ledesma A, Buosono M, Calcedo A, Carrasco JL, Ciudad J, Daniel E, De La Gandara J, Derecho J, Franco M, Gomez MJ, Macias JA, Martin T, Perez V, Sanchez JM, Sanchez S, Vicens E. SSRI-Induced sexual dysfunction: fluoxetine, paroxetine, sertraline, and fluvoxamine in a prospective, multicenter, and descriptive clinical study of 344 patients. *J Sex Marital Ther* 1997;**23**:176–193.

30 Uitti RJ, Tanner CM, Rajput AH, Goetz CG, Klawans HL, Thiessen B. Hypersexuality with antiparkinsonian therapy. *Clin Neuropharmacol* 1989;**12**:375–383.

31 White JM, Rumbold GR. Behavioral effects of histamine and its antagonists: a review. *Psychopharmacology* 1988;**95**:1–14.

32 Morales A, Buvat J, Gooren LJ, Guay AT, Kaufman JM, Kim YC, Tan HM, Torrres LO. Endocrine Aspects of Men Sexual Dysfunction. In: Lue TF, Basson R, Rosen R, Guiliano F, Khoury S, Montorsi F, eds. *Sexual Medicine: Sexual Dysfunction in Men and Wome: 2nd International Consultation on Sexual Dysfunctions. Paris*: Health Publications,2004.

33 Dei M, Verni A, Bigozzi L, Bruni V. Sex steroids and libido. *European Journal of Contraception & Reproductive Health Care* 1997 Dec;**2**(4):253–258.

34 Carani C, Isidori AM, Granata A, Carosa E, Maggi M, Lenzi A, Jannini EA. Multicenter study on the prevalence of sexual symptoms in male hypo- and hyperthyroid patients. *J Clin Endocrinol Metab* 2005;**90**: 6472–6479.

35 Kaplan HS. The sexual desire disorders: dysfunctional regulation of sexual motivation. New York: Brunner/Mazel, 1995.

36 LoPiccolo J, Friedman J. Broad spectrum treatment of low sexual desire: integration of cognitive, behavioral and systemic therapy. In: Lieblum S, Rosen R, eds. *Sexual Desire Disorders*. New York: The Guilford Press, 1988.

37 Schiavi RC. Interview, psychometric and psycho physiologic strategies to assess sexual disorders. *J Clin Psychiatr Monogr* 1992;**10**, No. 19.

38 Hoyl MT, Alessi CA, Harker JO, *et al.* Development and testing of a five-items version of the Geriatric Depression Scale. *J Am Geriatr Soc* 1999;**47**:873–878.

39 Rinaldi P, Mecocci P, Benedetti C, Ercolani S, Bregnocchi M, Menculini G, Catani M, Senin U, Cherubini A. Validation of the five-item geriatric depression scale in elderly subjects in three different settings *J Am Geriatr Soc* 2003 May;**51**(5):694–698.

40 Begin C, Sabourin M, Bovin E. Frénetté. Paradis. The Couple -Part 1- Couple distress factors associated with evaluating the spousal relationship. In: *Quebec Longitudinal Study of Child Development (QLSCD 1998–2002) From Birth to 29 Months*. Québec: Institut de la statistique du Québec, Vol 2 No. 11.

41 Ferris RM, Cooper BR, Maxwell RA. Studies of bupropion's mechanism of antidepressant activity. *J Clin Psychiact* 1983;**44**:74–78.

42 Segraves RT, Croft H, Kavoussi R, Ascher JA, Batey SR, Foster VJ, Bolden-Watson C, Metz A. Bupropion sustained release (SR) for the treatment of hypoactive sexual desire disorder (HSDD) in nondepressed women. *J Sex Marital Ther* 2001 May–Jun;**27**(3): 303–316.

43 Segraves RT, Clayton A, Croft H, Wolf A, Warnock J. Bupropion sustained release for the treatment of hypoactive sexual desire disorder in premenopausal women. *J Clin Psychopharmacol* 2004 Jun;**24**(3): 339–342.

44 Crenshaw TL, Goldberg JP, Stern WC. Pharmacologic modification of psychosexual dysfunction. *J Sex Marital Ther* 1987;**13**(4):239–252.

45 Wang C, Swerdloff RS, Iranmanesh A, Dobs A, Snyder PJ, Cunningham G, Matsumoto AM, Weber T, Berman N, and the testosterone gel study group. Transdermal testosterone gel improves sexual function, mood, muscle strength, and body composition parameters in hypogonadal men. *J Clin Endocrinol Metab* 2000;**85**: 839–853.

46 Rosen RC. Psychogenic erectile dysfunction. Classification and management. *Urol Clin North Am* 2001 May;**28**(2):269–278.

CHAPTER 14

Peyronie's Disease

Pathophysiology and Medical Management

Ajay Nehra

Introduction

Peyronie's disease (indurato penis plastica) is an inflammatory condition that is characterized by the formation of fibrous, noncompliant nodules within the tunica albuginea [1–8]. These plaques impede tunical expansion during erection, resulting in penile bending. In some extreme cases, these plaques can induce a collar-like or an hourglass-like appearance in the erect penis. Unlike normal wound healing following trauma, plaques in patients with Peyronie's disease do not resolve. Subsequent to inflammation and cessation of pain, in the chronic stages of the disease, the plaques may ossify [1–7].

One can sub-classify Peyronie's patients into three categories: (1) patients with asymptomatic plaques or some penile bending, which does not affect intercourse; (2) patients whose plaques exacerbate penile bending to the point that intercourse is either painful and/or no longer physically possible; and (3) patients whose Peyronie's disease is also associated with erectile dysfunction [8]. In patients with erectile dysfunction, penile arterial inflow is usually unimpeded, with the major abnormality observed being venous leakage, usually at the site of the plaque [9,10].

Genetics and Occurrence

The search for a genetic link for Peyronie's disease has yet to identify a genetically-predisposed population. However, there are reports associating this condition and Paget's disease of the bone [11], Dupuytren's contracture [12], and specific human leukocyte antigen (HLA) subtypes [12–14]. In all of these studies, patients reporting one of the traits (Paget's disease of the bone, Dupuytren's contracture, or specific HLA subtypes), did not always report symptoms of Peyronie's disease. Studies of Peyronie's patients have implicated an autoimmune component. It was shown that Peyronie's disease patients had at least one abnormal immunologic test (75.8%), alterations in cell-mediated immunity (48.5%), and in markers of autoimmune disease (37.9%) [15]. Another study found higher than normal levels of anti-elastin antibodies in the serum of patients with Peyronie's disease, suggesting an autoimmune etiology [16]. It is likely that a certain proportion of men in this age group respond to mechanical tunical stress and microvascular trauma [4–6] with an aberrant or hyperactive wound healing response [17]. Thus, there may be a subpopulation whose genetic background is such that response to wound healing predisposes development of Peyronie's plaques.

There are few reports examining the incidence and prevalence of Peyronie's disease. The incidence is estimated to be 0.4 to 3.2% [53–59]. Unfortunately multi-national, multi-institutional data is lacking. However, there are some insights relating to a higher incidence. A thirty-five year retrospective study in Rochester, Minnesota, is notable [18]. In this study, comprised primarily of Caucasian men, the average age of onset was 53 years old, with a prevalence of 388.6/100 000 (0.4%), and an age-adjusted annual incidence rate of 25.7/100 000 men (0.3%) [18]. At the time of the study nine years ago, this translated into 32 000 new cases in the United States annually, with approximately 423 000 men with Peyronie's disease at any given time [18]. Contrary to the genetic studies described above, there was no significant association between Dupuytren's contracture and Peyronie's disease. Further, over the thirty-five year period, both total Peyronie's disease, and Peyronie's disease associated with pain and impotence, increased. This may be an actual increase in disease occurrence or due to heightened patient awareness and seeking of medical attention. Interestingly, rheumatoid arthritis ($p < 0.0001$) and hypertension ($p < 0.01$) were the most commonly associated conditions reported in this group of Peyronie's disease patients [18]. It should be noted that the study described above probably underestimates the true prevalence of Peyronie's disease, as indicated by autopsy studies [19]. In a study of 100 men who had no known Peyronie's disease, 22/100 had asymptomatic, fibrotic lesions of the tunica albuginea [19]. This suggests that in the natural course of aging and sexual activity, these asymptomatic lesions may develop. The prevalence of Peyronie's disease is probably much higher than 0.4% if one includes subclinical, asymptomatic cases [17,18]. Regardless, the number of patients presenting with Peyronie's disease in the United States is expected to increase as the "baby boom" generation progresses through ages 50 to 70.

Therapeutics and the Molecular Pathology of Peyronie's Disease

How do these mechanisms correlate with current therapeutic treatment of this disease? There are two basic categories of pharmacotherapeutics that have been used in Peyronie's disease: anti-oxidants and collagen synthesis inhibitors. As described briefly above, it has been hypothesized that oxidative damage may be causal in the initiation and progression of tissue fibrosis [20].

Presently, non-surgical options for the treatment of Peyronie's disease are based on anecdotal experiences with studies limited by a small number of patients, limited follow-up, the absence of placebo-control groups, and no objective measures to represent improvement. The historical reporting of spontaneous remission rates ranges from seven to 29%.

Oral Therapies

A number of oral therapies have been investigated for the treatment of Peyronie's disease.

Vitamin E

Mechanism of action: Antioxidant properties. First investigated by Scott and Scardino [21] in 1948, vitamin E was theorized to be of clinical efficacy secondary to its anti-oxidant activities. The use of vitamin E today continues and remains a choice for many practicing urologists, predominantly due to the minimal adverse event profile and the low cost. However, most studies do not address the natural history of the disease, nor have they included a control arm. Gelbard *et al.* [22] investigated vitamin E therapy in comparison to the natural history of Peyronie's disease in 86 patients, and revealed no significant difference between the treatment and control groups for curvature, pain, and the ability to have intercourse.

Colchicine

Mechanism of action: Inhibition of collagen synthesis and anti-fibrotic effects. Colchicine was first proposed by Akkus and colleagues [23] in 1994 where, in 19 patients, a progressively increasing dose was given over a three to five month period. Alterations in curvature were noted in 36% of the patients (n = 7) and palpable plaque improvement in 63% (n = 12). Erectile quality was improved in 78% (n = 7); however, no placebo or control arm was used in the studies. In a subsequent control study by Kadioglu [24], 60 patients were evaluated with Colchicine 1 mg twice a day, with mean follow up of 11 months. Pain improvement in 95% (n = 57), with reduction in curvature in 30% (n = 19) and progressive worsening of curvature in 22% (n = 13), were noted. *Adverse events*: Severe diarrhea.

Potassium amino benzoid (Potaba, Glenwood)

Potaba is historically used in dermatologic patients—particularly scleroderma, dermatomyositis, and pemphigus.

Mechanism of action: Increasing activity of monoamine oxidase in tissues, a subsequent decrease in serotonin levels, and thus a reduction in fibrogenesis, with subsequent decreased scar tissue formation.

The use of potassium amino benzoid was described initially by Zarafonatis in 1959 [25]. A large, pooled European study in 1978 involving 2653 patients, reported a 57% success rate with complete resolution in 9% [26]. However, this study had no study arm or placebo group, nor were any objective parameters assessed. Weidner *et al.* [27] reported a randomized prospective double-blind trial of potassium amino benzoid at a dose of 3 mg four times per day for one year, versus oral placebo. Statistically, an improvement between the two groups was noted in plaque size that did not correlate with a reduction in the curvature. *Adverse events*: Severe gastrointestinal side effects.

Tamoxifen citrate (Nolvadex, Astrozenica)

Mechanism of action: The potential benefit is based on its effect on the release of transforming growth factor beta (TGF-β) from fibroblasts, and blocking the TGF-β receptor sites, resulting in decreased fibrogenic activity.

This was first introduced by Ralph *et al.* in 1992 [28], at a dose of 20 mg given twice a day for three months in 36 patients. The results demonstrated a reduction in pain in 80% of patients (n = 29), reduction in curvature in 35% of patients (n = 13), and a decrease in plaque size in 34% (n = 12). However, a control trial by Teloken *et al.* [29] in 1999 at a similar dose revealed no significant improvement between

the treatment groups compared with the placebo arm.

Carnitine (Carnitor, Sigma-Tau)

Mechanism of action: Inhibition of acidyl coenzyme-A. Published initially by Biagiotti *et al.* [30] in 2001, 48 patients were randomized to receive either carnitine or tamoxifen. The first group received tamoxifen 20 mg twice daily for three months, while the second group received acetyl-L-carnitine at a dose of 1 mg twice daily for three months. While the authors reported a greater benefit with respect to curvature in the carnitine arm, no objective parameters were measured.

Topical Therapies

Mechanism of action: Increased extracellular matrix collagenic secretion, and decreased collagen and fibronectin synthesis and secretion. Martin and co-workers in 2002 [31] investigated tissue concentrations in men who applied verapamil topically. While this drug was found to be present in urine samples, no verapamil was detected in the tunica albuginea specimens obtained at the time of penile prostheses implantations. The authors subsequently concluded that topical application of verapamil had no scientific basis, and given the fact that no control trial has been performed, the current use of topical verapamil is not recommended.

Intra-lesional Therapies

Steroids

Mechanisms of action: Anti-inflammatory and reduction in collagen synthesis. Proposed in 1954 by Teasley [32] in 29 patients, with results that were at best equivocal. Subsequently in 1954, Boedner *et al.* [33] reported successful outcomes in 17 patients who were treated with intra-lesional hydrocortisone and cortisone injections. A study by Winter and Khanna [34] in 1975 demonstrated no statistical difference between patients treated with intra-lesional dexamethasone injections, when compared with the natural history of the disease in their general patient population. A prospective study by Williams and Green [35] in 1980 using intra-lesional triamcinolone revealed only 3% had spontaneous resolution of symptoms at one year with observation, and, following the administration of triamcinolone every six weeks for 36 weeks, 33% of patients reported improvement in particular pain and plaque size. At present, the use of intra-lesional steroid injections is not encouraged.

Collagenase

Mechanism of action: Collagen degradation. The use of collagenase was initially demonstrated in vitro by Gelbard *et al.* in 1982 [36]. An objective improvement in 64% of patients (n = 20) was demonstrated within four weeks with collagenase injections. However, a decade later in 1993 [37], they reported their findings from a double-blind trial of collagenase injections in 49 men. Following stratifying patients based on a severity of curvature, a statistically significant improvement was noted in curvature in the collagenase-treated groups, with maximum improvement ranging from 15 to 20%. The data subsequently showed a limited result, a limited improvement, and may potentially be suited for a long-term trial.

Verapamil

Mechanism of action: Increases extracellular matrix collagenase secretion and decreases collagen and fibronectin synthesis and secretion. Verapamil was initially used as an intra-lesional injection by Levine *et al.* in 1994 [38]. Fourteen patients received biweekly injections of verapamil into the plaque for six months. Subjectively, there was an improvement in plaque-associated waist deformity in all patients, and curvature in 42% (n = 6). An objective decrease in plaque volume of greater than 50% was noted in 30% (n = 4), and plaque softening was noted in all patients. Subsequently Rehman and colleagues [39] published the first randomized single blind trial of intra-lesional injection of verapamil where 14 patients were evaluated. Significant differences were noted in the subjective improvement in the quality of erections, as well as in objective measurements of plaque volume in the verapamil-treated arm. A non-significant improvement trend was noted in the degree of curvature in the verapamil group. Recently Levine *et al.* [40] published in a non-placebo control trial involving 156 men with intralesional vera-

pamil. These patients (77%) had failed prior oral therapies with vitamin E, Potaba, and/or colchicine. One hundred and twenty eight men completed the initial study, with an 84% resolution of pain. Curvature improvement was noted in 62% (n = 79); eight percent (n = 10) had worsening of their initial curvature. Improvements in girth, rigidity, and sexual performances were noted in 83%, 80%, and 71%, respectively. In patients being evaluated based on duration and severity of disease (greater than or less than one year), no differences in the two groups were noted with respect to curvature, rigidity, sexual function, and girth.

Interferons

Mechanism of action: In vitro decrease in the rate of proliferation of fibroblasts, and decreased production of extra-cellular collagen, with increased production of collagenases. Interferons were first demonstrated as a potential viable therapeutic arm by Duncan *et al.* in 1991 [47]. The initial clinical trials by Wegner *et al.* in 1995 [42] and 1997 [43] demonstrated low rates of improvement with high side effects, in particular fever and myalgia. Most promising results with interferons were demonstrated by Ahuja *et al.* [44] in a non-randomized sample of 20 men who received 1×10^6 units biweekly for six months. Patients demonstrated penile plaque softening in 100% of men, 90% had subjective improvement, and 55% had subjective reduction in plaque size. Recently Dang *et al.* [45] objectively demonstrated improvements in curvature using pharmacologic simulation and a protractor of greater than 20% in 67% (n = 14) of the study participants. Hellstrom and colleagues in 2003 [46] demonstrated a single blind multi-center placebo-controlled study with encouraging results. Curvature improvement of greater than 20% was demonstrated in 69% of the treatment group versus 37% of the control group. Pain was not statistically significant between the two groups. Further investigation of trials may be warranted with the use of intra-lesional therapy.

External Energy Therapy

Shock wave therapy

Mechanism of action: Local penile electro shockwave

therapy (ESWT) has been potentially recommended to induce inflammatory response leading to plaque lyses and improved vascularity.

Most studies on the efficacy of ESWT are limited to subjective reports of improvements of deformity, plaque size, or pain. Hauck *et al.* [47] in a controlled trial, randomized 43 men to ESWT or an oral placebo for six months. No significant effect of treatment was noted on curvature, plaque size, or subjective improvements in sexual function or rigidity.

Iontophoresis

Several studies have recently investigated the efficacy of topically-applied verapamil, with or without dexamethasone, with enhanced penetration using iontophoresis (electromotive drug administration).

Di Stasi and associates [48,49] randomized 96 patients to treatment with verapamil 5 mg plus dexamethasone 8 mg, using electromotive drug administration. Of the 73 patients who completed the study, 43% in the verapamil oblique dexamethasone noted improvement objectively in plaque size, as measured by ultrasonography, and curvature as noted by photography. No change in parameters in the Lido cream group was noted. Preliminary results of iontophoresis with verapamil versus saline were reported at the 2003 meeting of the American Urologic Association, with similar results in both groups. Further investigation in this modality may be warranted.

Combination Therapies

Various combinations of therapies have been evaluated and investigated as potential treatments for Peyronie's disease. A controlled study by Pieto Castro *et al.* [50] randomized 45 patients to receive vitamin E plus colchicine and/or ibuprofen (placebo). Patients in the treatment group reported a higher percentage of pain relief, although the difference was not significant. Mirone *et al.* [51] examined two populations of patients with Peyronie's disease: electromotive drug administration plus perilesional verapamil, versus electromotive drug administration alone. A 52% improvement in plaque size was noted for the ESWT group only, compared to 19% in the combination arm. Authors have randomized patients to receive intralesional verapamil plus oral car-

nitine, or intralesional verapamil plus oral tamoxifen as well. Cavalini *et al.* [52] demonstrated no significant difference in pain between the two groups.

Summary

Peyronie's disease is a fibrotic disorder of the tunica albuginea involving potential trauma to the penis and an inflammatory response. The fibrotic plaques that form are produced most likely by tunical fibroblasts in response to cytokine stimulation. Of the candidate cytokines, TGF-β1 and possibly platelet-derived growth factor (PDGF) play a role. To date, pharmacotherapy has not been effective or widely accepted, and surgery to either remove the plaque or insert penile prostheses remains the mainstay of treatment. A better understanding of the molecular pathology of this disease is expected to improve pharmacotherapeutic strategies to treat this condition.

The investigation for medical options in the management of Peyronie's disease currently lacks controlled clinical trials with standardized assessments and objective measurements of improvement in curvature, circumferential deformities, and/or sexual function. Research into the pathophysiology of this disorder is likely to yield new insights into potential treatment options. At the present time, no ideal non-surgical cure is noted.

References

1 Gelbard M. Peyronie's disease. In: Hashmat AI, Das S, eds. *The Penis.* Philadelphia: Lea and Febiger, 1993, pp. 244–365.

2 Carrier S, Lue TF. For Peyronie's disease, act conservatively. *Contemporary Urol* 1994;**9**:54–65.

3 Pryor JP. The management of Peyronie's disease. In Porst H, ed. *Penile Disorders. Proceedings of the International Symposium on Penile Disorders, Hamburg, Germany, January 26–27, 1996.* Berlin: Springer Verlag, 1997, pp. 75–86.

4 Devine CJ, Horton CE. Peyronie's disease. *Clin Plast Surg* 1988;**15**:405–409.

5 Jarow JP, Lowe FC. Penile trauma: An etiologic factor in Peyronie's disease and erectile dysfunction. *J Urol* 1997;**158**:1388–1390.

6 Devine CJ, Somers KD, Jordan GH, Schlossberg SM. Proposal: Trauma as a cause of Peyronie's lesion. *J Urol* 1997;**157**:285–290.

7 Vande Berg JS, Devine CJ, Horton CE, Somers KD, Wright GL, Leffel MS, Dawson DM, Gleischman SH, Rowe MJ. Mechanisms of calcification in Peyronie's disease. *J Urol* 1982;**127**:52–54.

8 Krane RJ. The treatment of loss of penile rigidity associated with Peyronie's disease. *Scand J Urol Nephrol Suppl* 1997;**179**:147–150.

9 Gasior BL, Levine FJ, Howannesian A, Krane RJ, Goldstein I. Plaque-associated corporal veno-occlusive dysfunction in idiopathic Peyronie's disease: a pharmacocavernosometric and pharmacocavernosographic study. *World J Urol* 1990;**8**:90–97.

10 Lopez JA, Jarow JP. Penile vascular evaluation of men with Peyronie's disease. *J Urol* 1993;**149**:53–55.

11 Lyles KW, Gold DT, Newton RA, Parekh S, Shipp KM, Pieper CF, Krishan R, Carson CC. Peyronie's disease is associated with Paget's disease of the bone. *J Bone Miner Res* 1997;**12**:929–934.

12 Nyberg LM, Bias WB, Hochberg MC, Walsh PC. Identification of an inherited form of Peyronie's disease with an autosomal dominant inheritance and association with Dupuytren's contracture and histocompatability B7 cross-reactive antigens. *J Urol* 1982;**128**:48–52.

13 Ralph DJ, Schwartz G, Moore W, Pryor JP, Ebringer A, Bottazzo GF. The genetic and bacteriological aspects of Peyronie's disease. *J Urol* 1997;**157**:291–294.

14 Leffell MS. Is there an immunogenetic basis for Peyronie's disease? *J Urol* 1997;**157**:295–297.

15 Schiavino D, Sasso F, Nucera E, Alcini E, Gulino G, Milani A, Patriarca G. Immunologic findings in Peyronie's disease: a controlled study. *Urology* 1997;**50**:764–768.

16 Stewart S, Malto M, Sandberg L, Colburn KK. Increased serum levels of anti-elastin antibodies in patients with Peyronie's disease. *J Urol* 1994;**152**:105–106.

17 Diegelmann RF. Cellular and biochemical aspects of normal and abnormal wound healing: an overview. *J Urol* 1997;**157**:298–302.

18 Lindsay MB, Schain DM, Grambsch P, Benson RC, Beard CM, Kurland LT. The incidence of Peyronie's disease in Rochester, Minnesota, 1950 through 1984. *J Urol* 1991;**146**:1007–1009.

19 Smith BH. Subclinical Peyronie's disease. *Am J Clin Pathol* 1969;**52**:385–390.

20 Zarafonetis CJD, Horran TM. Treatment of Peyronie's disease with potassium para-aminobenzoate (POTABA). *J Urol* 1959;**81**:770–772.

21 Scott WW, Scardino PL. A new concept in the treatment of Peyronie's disease. *South Med J* 1948;**41**:173–177.

22 Gelbard MK, Dorey F, James K. The natural history of Peyronie's disease. *J of Urol* 1990;**144**(6):1376–1379.

23 Akkus E, Carrier S, Rehman J, *et al.* Is colchicine effective in Peyronie's disease? A pilot study *Urology* 1994;**44**(2):291–295.

24 Kadioglu A, Tefekli A, Koksal T, *et al.* Treatment of Peyronie's disease with potassium oral colchicine: Long-term results and predictive parameters of successful outcome. *Int J Impot Res* 2000;**12**(3):169–175.

25 Zarafonetis CJ, Jorrax TM. Treatment of Peyronie's disease with potassium para-aminobenzoate (Potaba). *J of Urol* 1959;**81**(6):770–772.

26 Hasche-Klunder R. Treatment of Peyronie's disease with para-aminobenzoacidic potassium (Potaba) (author's transl). *Urologe A* 1978;**17**(4):224–227.

27 Weidner W, Schroeder-Printzen I, Rudnick J, *et al.* Randomized prospective placebo-controlled therapy of Peyronie's disease (IPP) with Potaba (aminobenzoate potassium). *J Urol* 1999;**6**(4 suppl):205. Abstract 785.

28 Ralph DJ, Rooks MD, Bottazzo GF, *et al.* The treatment of Peyronie's disease with tamoxifen. *Br J Urol* 1992;**70**(6):648–651.

29 Teloken C, Rhoden EL, Grazziotin TM, *et al.* Tamoxifen versus placebo in the treatment of Peyronie's disease. *J Urol* 1999;**162**(6):2003–2005.

30 Biagiotti G, Cavallini G. Acetyl-L-camitine versus tamoxifen in the oral therapy of Peyronie's disease: A preliminary report. *BJU Int* 2001;**88**(1):63–67.

31 Martin DJ, Badwan K, Parker M, *et al.* Transdermal application of verapamil gel to the penile shaft fails to infiltrate the tunica albuginea. *J Urol* 2002;**168**(6):2483–2485.

32 Teasley GH. Peyronie's Disease: A new approach. *J Urol* 1954;**71**(5):611–614.

33 Bodner H, Howard AH, Kaplan JH. Peyronie's disease: cortisone-hyaluronidase-hydrocortisone therapy. *J Urol* 1954;**72**:400–431.

34 Winter CC, Khanna R. Peyronie's Disease: Results with demo-jet injection of dexamethasone *J Urol* 1975;**14**:898–900.

35 Williams G, Green NA. The non-surgical treatment of Peyronie's disease. *Br J Urol* 1980;**52**:392–395.

36 Gelbard MK, Walsh R, Kaufman JJ. Collagenase for Peyronie's disease: Experimental studies *Urol Res* 1982;**10**:135–140.

37 Gelbard MK, James K, Riach P, *et al.* Collagenase versus placebo in the treatment of Peyronie's disease: A double-blind study. *J Urol* 1993;**149**(1):56–58.

38 Levine LA, Merrick PF, Lee RC. Intralesional verapamil injection for the treatment of Peyronie's disease. *J Urol* 1994;**151**(6):1522–1524.

39 Rehman J, Benet A, Melman A. Use of intralesional

verapamil to dissolve Peyronie's disease plaque: A long-term single-blind study. *Urology* 1998;**51**(4):620–626.

40 Levine LA, Goldman KE, Greenfield JM. Experience with intraplaque injection of verapamil for Peyronie's disease. *J Urol* 2002;**168**(2):621–625.

41 Duncan MR, Berman B, Nseyo UO. Regulation of the proliferation and biosynthetic activities of cultured human Peyronie's disease fibroblasts by interferons-alpha, -beta, and -gamma. *Scand J Urol Nephrol* 1991;**25**(2):89–94.

42 Wegner HE, Andresen R, Knispel HH, *et al.* Treatment of Peyronie's disease with local interferon-alpha 2b. *Eur Urol* 1995;**28**(3):236–240.

43 Wegner HE, Andresen R, Knispel HJ, *et al.* Local interferon-alpha 2b is not an effective treatment in early-stage Peyronie's disease. *Eur Urol* 1997;**32**(2):190–193.

44 Ahuja S, Bivalacqua TJ, Case J, *et al.* A pilot study demonstrating clinical benefit from intralesional interferon alpha 2b in the treatment of Peyronie's disease. *J Androl* 1999;**20**(4):444–448.

45 Dang G, Matern R, Bivalacqua TJ, *et al.* Intralesional interferon-alpha 2b injections for the treatment of Peyronie's disease. *South Med J* 2004;**97**(1):42–46.

46 Hellstrom W, Eichenberg C, Pryor JL, *et al.* A single-blind, multi-center, placebo-controlled study to assess the safety and efficacy of intralesional interferon alpha-2b in the non-surgical treatment of Peyronie's disease. *J Urol* 2003;**169**(4 suppl):274 Abstract 1065.

47 Hauck EW, Altinkilic BM, Ludwig M, *et al.* Extracorporeal shock wave therapy in the treatment of Peyronie's disease: First results of a case-controlled approach. *Eur Urol* 2000;**38**(6):663–669.

48 Di Stasi SM, Giannantoni A, Cappeli G, *et al.* Transdermal electromotive administration of verapamil and dexamethasone for Peyronie's disease. *BJU Int* 2003;**91**(9):825–829.

49 Di Stasi SM, Giannantoni A, Stephen RL, *et al.* A prospective, randomized study using transdermal electromotive administration of verapamil and dexametha-sone for Peyronie's disease. *J Urol* 2004;**171**(4):1605–1608.

50 Prieto Castro RM, Leva Vallejo ME, Regueiro Lopez JC, *et al.* Combined treatment with vitamin E and colchicine in the early stages of Peyronie's disease. *BJU Int* 2003;**91**(6):522–524.

51 Mirone V, Palmieri A, Granata AM, *et al.* Ultrasound-guided ESWT in Peyronie's disease plaques. *Arch Ital Urol Androl* 2000;**72**(4):384–387.

52 Cavallini G, Biagiotti G, Koverech A, *et al.* Oral propi-onyl-l-carnitine and intraplaque verapamil in the ther-apy of advanced and resistant Peyronie's disease. *BJU Int* 2002;**89**(9):895–900.

53 Ciancio SJ, Kim ED. Penile fibrotic changes after radical retropubic prostatectomy. *BJU Int* 2000;**85**:101–106.

54 Schwarzer U, Sommer F, Klotz T, Braun M, Reifenrath B, Engelmann U. The prevalence of Peyronie's disease: Results of a large survey. *BJU Int* 2001;**88**:727–730.

55 Rhoden E, Teloken C, Ting H, Lucas M, Teodosio D, Ros C, Ary Vargas Souto C. Prevalence of Peyronie's disease in men over 50 years old from southern Brazil. *Int J Impot Res* 2001;**13**:291–293.

56 La Pera G, Pescatori E, Calabrese M, Boffini A, Colombo F, Andriani E, Natali A, Vaggi L, Catuogno C, Giustini M, Taggi F, SIMONA study group. Peyronie's disease: prevalence and association with cigarette smoking. A multicenter population-based study in men aged 50–69 Years. *Eur Urol* 2001;**40**:525–530.

57 Sommer F, Schwarzer U, Wassmer G, Bloch W, Braun M, Klotz T, Engelmann U. Epidemiology of Peyronie's disease. *Int J Impot Res* 2002;**14**:379–383.

58 Perinchery G, El-Sakka A, Angan A, Nakajima K, Dharia A, Tanaka Y, Lue T, Dahiya R. Microsatellite alterations and loss of heterozygosity in Peyronie's disease. *J Urol* 2000;**164**:842–846.

59 Mulhall J, Thom J, Lubrano T, Shankey T. Basic fibro-glast growth factor expression in Peyronie's disease. *J Urol* 2001;**165**:419–423.

Surgical Treatment of Peyronie's Disease

John Mulhall

Guidelines for Surgical Management of Peyronie's Disease

Clinical guidelines

Defining candidacy for Peyronie's disease surgery

Correction of penile deformity due to Peyronie's disease is surgically challenging and is required in the minority of patients with this condition [1]. Surgery is considered only after stabilization of the fibrotic process. The committee recommends that men be considered candidates for surgical correction if they have had Peyronie's disease for at least 12 months and have had stable deformity (that is, no change in deformity) for a duration of at least three months. Surgical reconstruction is typically reserved for men with deformity that precludes satisfactory sexual intercourse, causes pain for themselves or their partners during sexual relations, or because of distress due to the presence of penile deformity [2]. While many men with Peyronie's disease can physically accomplish sexual intercourse, many are dissatisfied with relations because their deformity precludes spontaneity, or requires certain positions/dynamics that detract from satisfaction.

- *It is recommended that surgical reconstruction be reserved for patients who have had Peyronie's disease for more than 12 months and have had stable deformity for more than 3 months.*

Preoperative assessment

Prior to any surgery it is advisable to define:
1 Nature of deformity
2 Magnitude of deformity
3 Penile length
4 Erectile hemodynamics

An accurate assessment of the nature of the patient's deformity is a key factor in planning the surgical approach. Is this a simple curvature? Is the curvature uniplanar or multiplanar? Is this pure hourglass de-

formity? Is there any associated instability (hinge effect)? Is there waisting at the point of maximum curvature? The presence of multiplanar curvature or pure hourglass deformity is generally not correctable by plication procedures. Having a clear idea what magnitude of deformity exists is also important, as larger degrees of curvature may preclude plication type surgeries. The nature and magnitude of penile deformity can be assessed in a variety of ways, including self-photography, vacuum device, and administration of an intracavernosal injection agent. While poorly documented in the literature, the use of photography is not without problems; specifically, assessing penile rigidity with a photograph may be difficult and given the correlation between penile rigidity and degree of deformity, and a photograph taken with less than a fully rigid erection may lead to underestimation of deformity. Vacuum devices have been purported to be associated with sufficient subcutaneous venous congestion that it may partially obscure the deformity. Intracavernosal injection therapy has as a problem the requirement for a penile injection; but as a technique it permits excellent deformity assessment, although some patients may require more than one injection to generate maximum rigidity.

One of the primary concerns of patients preoperatively is penile length loss. At presentation many men complain of loss of penile length, and by the time many patients have reached comfort level with surgical intervention most have already experienced this problem. Thus, any further loss of length is a major concern. In patients with penile curvature, an assessment at full rigidity of penile length on the concave and convex sides may give a crude estimate of the potential for length loss if plication-type procedures are employed. Furthermore, having penile length documented preoperatively permits comparison to postoperative length in men who complain of postoperative length loss. Most authorities agree that an assessment of erectile hemodynamics preoperatively is an essential part of preoperative evaluation and this can be accomplished with either duplex Doppler penile ultrasound or dynamic infusion cavernosometry.

- *It is recommended that an adequate assessment of penile deformity and erectile hemodynamics be performed prior to surgical reconstruction.*

Surgical options

Surgical intervention may be sub-divided into three groups (or families) of operations, namely:
1 Plication-type procedures.
2 Plaque manipulation and grafting procedures.
3 Penile prosthetic surgery.

Plication procedures

This group of procedures addresses the side of the penile shaft opposite the location of the plaque and is best utilized for patients not concerned about length loss and with:
1 Uniplanar curvature
2 Mild-moderate magnitude of curvature
3 Combined penile dysfunction/erectile dysfunction responsive to oral or intracavernous erectogenic pharmacotherapy
4 Congenital penile deviation

- *Plication-type procedures are considered treatment of choice for congenital penile deviation.*

This group of procedures may be further subdivided into tunical incising and imbrication (nonincising) procedures. Advantages of these approaches include short surgical time, no significant negative effect on erectile hemodynamics, good cosmetic outcomes, simple, safe and effective, regarding straightening. The major disadvantages are shortening of the penis, and this group of procedures does not address the issue of hourglass deformity; lateral indentations, when present, and the presence of multiplanar curvature, may be difficult to correct adequately with this form of procedure.

Tunical incising procedures involve making incisions in the tunica and excising a wedge/ellipse (Nesbit procedure), or leaving an intervening segment of tunica intact and covering it over with a suture line connecting the two tunical incisions (modified corporplasty), or fashioning a longitudinal incision and closing it in a Heineke–Miculicz fashion transversely (Yacchia procedure). The advantages of these procedures are that the repair heals by primary intention. However, the repair does require an incision in the tunica, thus theoretically putting erectile tissue at risk. The Nesbit procedure was originally developed for congenital curvature. It is worth noting at this juncture, that many series reporting outcomes of this procedure have included patients with both Peyronie's disease and congenital curvature. These are non-identical conditions and caution in interpreting these series is warranted. First, the tunica albuginea of young men with congenital curvature is not diseased, as is the case in Peyronie's disease, and generally they have excellent penile stretch and do not have penile length loss at presentation. Second, congenital penile curvature results from corporal disproportion and most men have a gentle bowing of the penis without any specific point of angulation.

Imbrication procedures do not involve making a tunical incision but rather fold the tunica, thus the integrity of the curvature correction is dependent upon the strength of the suture used to imbricate the tunica (Essed–Schroeder, 16-dot procedures). A review of outcomes for tunical incising (Nesbit type) procedures for Peyronie's disease is presented in Table 14.1.

A review of outcomes for imbrication procedures for Peyronie's disease and congenital penile deviation are presented in Tables 14.2 and 14.3.

- *Tunica-incising plication procedures may give better long-term results than imbrication procedures in the correction of penile deformity in Peyronie's disease.*

Plaque manipulation and grafting

These procedures address the plaque directly and are best utilized for patients with:
1 Complex deformities
2 Hourglass deformity
3 Short penile length
4 All degrees of curvature
5 Normal erectile function
The advantages of this group of procedures are that they generally preserve penile length (approxi-

Table 14.1 Outcomes with Nesbit surgery in Peyronie's disease (1994 to 2005).

Author	Year	No. of Patients	Mean Follow-up	Satisfied	Shortening	Post-Op ED	Recurrence
Bokarica [9]	2005	40	81 m		100%	5%	—
Rolle [10]	2005	50 (32C, 18P)	—	94% P	—	—	—
Navalon [11]	2005	21 (12C, 9P)	—	95%	—	—	—
Savoca [12]	2004	218	89 m	83.5%	17%	13%	—
Portillo-Martin [13]	2003	59 (44C, 15P) 39N, 12RC, 8ES	12 m	86%	—	—	—
Rodriguez [14]	2003	45	—	87%	—	—	—
Syed [15]	2003	42	84 m	76%	50%	—	10%#
Savoca [16]	2000	157	72 m	88%	14%	—	—
Pryor [17]	1998	—	21 m	—	—	—	11%
Rehman [18]	1997	32 (26P, 6C)	—	100% C, 78% P	—	—	22%
Ralph [19]	1995	185	—	90%	—	—	3%
Sulaiman [20]	1994	78	50 m	79%	—	18%	4%

C, congenital; ES, Essed–Schroeder; P, Peyronie's disease; RC, Ruiz–Castane.

mately a 10% risk of penile shortening) and are useful in men with complex deformities. It is worth noting that some case series of plaque incision and grafting have included men who had counterplication maneuvers to achieve complete straightening, and these adjuvant maneuvers may be the reason for penile shortening. The disadvantages include worsening erectile function, dorsal nerve neuropraxia (if the neurovascular bundles require elevation) leading to prolonged sensory disturbances (anesthesia, dysthesiae). It is believed that the erectile function alterations may be related to the inflammatory reaction/fibrosis that occurs beneath the graft, leading to corporal smooth muscle damage. Historically, plaque excision was performed but this has been supplanted more recently by plaque incision, although some authorities also trim some of the plaque tissue prior to grafting.

Grafts are subdivided into three groups:

1 Synthetic
2 Autologous
3 Pre-packaged biological

• *Autologous and pre-packaged biological grafts are considered graft materials of choice for plaque incision/excision and grafting.*

Synthetic grafts are almost historical because of the literature supporting autologous grafts, such as vein, dermis, crural tunica albuginea, or flaps, such as penile dermal, shaft tunica albuginea and tunica vaginalis. Autologous materials provide a readily-available, reliable, well-tolerated and easily obtained graft, and also provide a resilient yet compliant graft that is easy to tailor and suture in place. Host reaction is minimal and the infection risk low. However, dermal, venous, buccal mucosa, crural albuginea, and tunica vaginalis grafts require additional operative

Table 14.2 Outcomes with plication procedures in Peyronie's disease (1994 to 2005).

Author	Year	No. of patients	Follow-up	Satisfied	Shortening	Post-op ED	Recurrence
Rolle [10]	2005	50	—	94%	—	—	—
Van der Horst [21]	2004	50 (28P, 22C)	30 m	78%	74%	—	—
Gholami [22]	2002	124	2.6 y	—	41%	—	15%
Van der Drift [23]	2002	59 (31P, 28C)	—	75% C 58% P	64% 90%	0% 29%	—
Chahal [24]	2001	44	49 m	52%	90%	—	—
Thiounn [25]	1998	60 (29P, 25C)	—	87%	—	—	—
Levine [26]	1997	22	—	—	—	9%	91%
Kummerling [27]	1995	54	36 m	90%	—	—	10%
Nooter [28]	1994	33	42 m	64%	—	—	5%
Klevmark [29]	1994	57	20 m	82%	—	—	5%

C, congenital; ED, erectile dysfunction; P, Peyronie's disease.

Table 14.3 Outcomes with plication procedures for congenital curvature (1987 to 2004).

Author	Year	No. of patients	Follow-up	Satisfied	Shortening	Post-op ED	Recurrence
Chertin [30]	2004	83	—	—	—	0%	0%
Chien [31]	2003	22	18 m	95%	18%	—	—
Hauck [32]	2002	23	34 m	—	65%	—	26%
Ebbehoj [33]	1987	140	—	—	—	—	4%

ED, erectile dysfunction

time to harvest. There is minimal outcome data on buccal mucosa or crural tunica grafts. One of the concerns about these two grafts is the inability to get enough graft material for complex curvatures where large defects are present. Vein graft has been purported to be associated with the least amount of intracavernosal fibrosis and has been proposed as the best material available for tunical patching, although no comparative analysis in humans exists for the different graft types [3]. The veins most often utilized are the greater saphenous or deep dorsal veins. The disadvantage of these grafts is that they result in extra operating time due to vein harvest and graft construction, and a second incision is required for saphenous vein harvesting. Most recently, pre-packaged grafts have been utilized with increasing frequency, primarily because of their ease-of-use and reduction in operating room time. While no comparative analysis has been conducted between autologous and biological grafts, the outcomes data appear comparable. The two biological materials most commonly utilized are human cadaveric pericardium (some areas utilize bovine pericardium because of non-availability of the human counterpart)

Table 14.4 Outcomes with plaque incision and grafting in Peyronie's disease (1995 to 2005).

Author	Year	No. of patients	Graft material	Complete correction	Post-op EF change	Sensory loss	Length loss
Kalsi [34]	2005	113	Vein	80%	23%	—	35%
Shioshvili [35]	2005	26	BM	92%	8%	—	15%
Levine [36]	2003	40	HP	98%	30%	—	—
Hatzichristou [37]	2002	17	TA	100%	0%	—	47%
Schwarzer [38]	2003	16	TA	75%	—	—	—
Hsu [39]	2003	24	Vein	96%	—	12%	—
Egydio [40]	2002	33	BP	88%	0%	—	—
Sampaio [41]	2002	40	DA	95%	15%	2.5%	—
Adeniyi [42]	2002	51	Vein	82%	8%	—	35%
Hauck [43]	2002	13	Vein	—	31%	—	54%
Knoll [44]	2001	12	IS	92%	0%	0%	0%
Akkus [45]	2001	58	Vein	86%	7%	—	22%
Teloken [46]	2000	7	TA	86%	—	0%	—
Montorsi [47]	2000	50	Vein	80%	6%	—	40%
Kadioglu [48]	1999	20	Vein	75%	5%	—	—
El-Sakka [49]	1998	113	Vein	96%	12%	—	17%
Krishnamurti [4]	1995	14	Dermal flap	100%	0%	—	0%

TA, tunica albuginea; HP, human cadaveric pericardium; BP, bovine pericardium; DA, dura mater; BM, buccal mucosa; IS, intestinal submucosa; EF, erectile function.

and animal intestinal submucosa. Outcomes data for plaque manipulation and grafting procedures are presented in Table 14.4.

Penile Prosthesis Surgery

Penile prosthesis placement for Peyronie's disease is best reserved for men with combined Peyronie's disease and erectile dysfunction, in particular those men with erectile dysfunction that are non-responsive to oral or local pharmacotherapy. Some authorities have suggested that men with hourglass deformity be considered for penile implant surgery because of anecdotally-based reports of poorer outcomes for patients undergoing lateral plaque incision

and grafting procedures. The advantages of penile prosthesis surgery in the Peyronie's disease patient include excellent rigidity and, in patients with mild to moderate curvature, excellent deformity correction without the need for intraoperative adjuvant maneuvers (vide infra). The disadvantages of this approach are the complications of penile prosthesis surgery (see section on penile prosthetic surgery).

The committee recommends that for all penile reconstructive surgical procedures, success be defined as end–of–operation residual curvature ≤15°. For patients with residual curvature greater than this, consideration should be given to performance of intra-operative maneuvers aimed at straightening the residual curvature. Such maneuvers include

Table 14.5 Outcomes with penile prosthesis surgery in Peyronie's disease (1996 to 2005).

Author	Year	No. of patients	Device	Manual modeling	Tunica incision/excision +/– graft	Complete correction	Patient satisfied
Akin-Olugbade [50]	2005	18	Alpha-1	20%	30%	100%	60%
Usta [51]	2003	42	—	74%	26%	88%	84%
Levine [52]*	2001	16	Ambicor	—	—	96%	96%
Wilson [8]	2001	104	700CX, Alpha-1	100%	—	—	—
Levine [53]	2000	46	2/3PI	54%	46%	100%	—
Carson [54]*	2000	63	700CX	—	—	—	88%
Ghanem [55]	1998	20	M	—	—	65%	87%
Morganstern [56]	1997	309	700CX	—	—	98%	—
Marzi [57]	1997	21	M, S	—	38%	—	—
Montague [7]	1996	72	34 700CX 38 Ultrex	—	—	100% 74%	—
Montorsi [58]	1996	23	700CX	—	40%	70%	79%

2PI, 2-piece inflatable; 3PI, 3-piece inflatable; M, malleable; S, Soft;
* Peyronie's disease patients as part of a larger prosthesis study

manual modeling (molding) and plaque incision, with or without grafting. Mulhall *et al.* demonstrated that, in 36 men undergoing (inflatable) penile prosthesis surgery for Peyronie's disease, all men with preoperative curvatures ≤30° had complete correction of curvature [5]. Eighty-six per cent of patients with preoperative curvatures ≥45° required adjuvant maneuver for complete curvature correction. Wilson *et al.* has popularized the technique of "molding" with excellent results [6]. This technique forcibly bends the semi-inflated implant over the plaque, in essence cracking the plaque. In his original series, Wilson demonstrated an 86% success rate using penile modeling. Montague *et al.* showed that all of the patients in their series (34 patients undergoing AMS 700CX device implantation) had correction of penile curvature with modeling [7]. In a long-term follow-up of his patients, Wilson demonstrated that at five years (using Kaplan–

Meier analysis) modeling resulted in long-term curvature correction and there was no higher incidence of device revision in this population compared to those men who had implant surgery without modeling [8] (Table 14.5).

Guidelines for Research in the Surgical Management of Peyronie's Disease

Defining surgical outcomes has been hampered by a number of factors including studies containing small patient numbers, lack of standardization of patient populations being studied, lack of a uniform definition of successful outcome, and absence of comparative outcomes between procedures. The committee suggests that every effort be made to define the patient population being studied in detail; in particular, defining the magnitude of baseline deformity, presence of associated deformities, and preoperative erectile hemodynamics status. Furthermore, patients with Peyronie's disease should be separated from patients with congenital penile curvature when assessing outcomes with plication-type procedures. The committee encourages all authors to declare the degree of residual deformity after penile reconstructive surgery. It was felt that residual deformities greater than 15 degrees were unacceptably high and warranted secondary procedures intraoperatively. Investigators are encouraged to define erectile function postoperatively using validated instruments. It is hoped that the future will see the development of a validated instrument specifically for Peyronie's disease, and especially for the assessment of postoperative patient satisfaction levels.

References

1 Ralph DJ, Minhas S. The management of Peyronie's disease. *BJU Int* 2004;**93**:208.

2 Hellstrom WJ, Usta MF. Surgical approaches for advanced Peyronie's disease patients. *Int J Impot Res* 2003;**15 S5**:S121.

3 Chang JA, Gholami SS, Lue TF. Surgical management: saphenous vein grafts. *Int J Impot Res* 2002;**14**:375.

4 Krishnamurti S. Penile dermal flap for defect reconstruction in Peyronie's disease: Operative technique and four years' experience in 17 patients. *Int J Impot Res* 1995;**7**:195.

5 Mulhall JP, Ahmed A, Anderson M. Penile prosthetic surgery for peyronie's disease: defining the need for intra-operative adjuvant maneuvers. *J Sex Med* 2004;**1**:318.

6 Wilson SK, Delk JR, 2nd. A new treatment for Peyronie's disease: modeling the penis over an inflatable penile prosthesis. *J Urol* 1994;**152**:1121.

7 Montague DK, Angermeier KW, Lakin MM, *et al.* AMS 3-piece inflatable penile prosthesis implantation in men with Peyronie's disease: comparison of CX and Ultrex cylinders. *J Urol* 1996;**156**:1633.

8 Wilson SK, Cleves MA, Delk JR, 2nd. Long-term followup of treatment for Peyronie's disease: modeling the penis over an inflatable penile prosthesis. *J Urol* 2001;**165**:825.

9 Bokarica P, Parazajder J, Mazuran B, *et al.* Surgical treatment of Peyronie's disease based on penile length and degree of curvature. *Int J Impot Res* 2005;**17**:170.

10 Rolle L, Tamagnone A, Timpano M, *et al.* The Nesbit operation for penile curvature: an easy and effective technical modification. *J Urol* 2005;**173**:171.

11 Navalon Verdejo P, Zaragoza Fernandez C, Sanchez Ballester F, *et al.* Correction of the penile curvature in ambulatory surgery. *Actas Urol Esp* 2005;**29**:217.

12 Savoca G, Scieri F, Pietropaolo F, *et al.* Straightening corporoplasty for Peyronie's disease: a review of 218 patients with median follow-up of 89 months. *Eur Urol* 2004;**46**:610.

13 Portillo Martin JA, Correas Gomez MA, Rado Velasquez MA, *et al.* Corrective surgery of penile inward curvature. *Actas Urol Esp* 2003;**27**:97.

14 Rodriguez Tolra J, Franco Miranda E, Prats Puig JM, *et al.* Treatment with the Newbit technique in patients with Peyronie's disease. *Actas Urol Esp* 2003;**27**:803.

15 Syed AH, Abbasi Z, Hargreave TB. Nesbit procedure for disabling Peyronie's curvature: a median follow-up of 84 months. *Urology* 2003;**61**:999.

16 Savoca G, Trombetta C, Ciampalini S, *et al.* Long-term results with Nesbit's procedure as treatment of Peyronie's disease. *Int J Impot Res* 2000;**12**:289.

17 Pryor JP. Correction of penile curvature and Peyronie's disease: why I prefer the Nesbit technique. *Int J Impot Res* 1998;**10**:129.

18 Rehman J, Benet A, Minsky LS, *et al.* Results of surgical treatment for abnormal penile curvature: Peyronie's disease and congenital deviation by modified Nesbit plication (tunical shaving and plication). *J Urol* 1997;**157**:1288.

19 Ralph DJ, al-Akraa M, Pryor JP. The Nesbit operation for Peyronie's disease: 16-year experience. *J Urol* 1995;**154**:1362.

20 Sulaiman MN, Gingell JC. Nesbit's procedure for penile curvature. *J Androl* 1994;**15 S**:54S.

21 Van Der Horst C, Martinez Portillo FJ, Seif C, *et al.* Treatment of penile curvature with Essed–Schroder tunical plication: aspects of quality of life from the patients' perspective. *BJU Int* 2004;**93**:105.

22 Gholami SS, Lue TF. Correction of penile curvature using the 16-dot plication technique: a review of 132 patients. *J Urol* 2002;**167**:2066.

23 van der Drift DG, Vroege JA, Groenendijk PM, *et al.* The plication procedure for penile curvature: surgical outcome and postoperative sexual functioning. *Urol Int* 2002;**69**:120.

24 Chahal R, Gogoi NK, Sundaram SK, *et al.* Corporal plication for penile curvature caused by Peyronie's disease: the patients' perspective. *BJU Int* 2001;**87**:352.

25 Thiounn N, Missirliu A, Zerbib M, *et al.* Corporeal plication for surgical correction of penile curvature. Experience with 60 patients. *Eur Urol* 1998;**33**:401.

26 Levine LA. Treatment of Peyronie's disease with intralesional verapamil injection. *J Urol* 1997;**158**: 1395.

27 Kummerling S, Schubert J. Peyronie's disease. Investigation of staging, erectile failure and operative management. *Int Urol Nephrol* 1995;**27**:629.

28 Nooter RI, Bosch JL, Schroder FH. Peyronie's disease and congenital penile curvature: long-term results of operative treatment with the plication procedure. *Br J Urol* 1994;**74**:497.

29 Klevmark B, Andersen M, Schultz A, *et al.* Congenital and acquired curvature of the penis treated surgically by plication of the tunica albuginea. *Br J Urol* 1994;**74**:501.

30 Chertin B, Koulikov D, Fridmans A, *et al.* Dorsal tunica albuginea plication to correct congenital and acquired penile curvature: a long-term follow-up. *BJU Int* 2004;**93**:379.

31 Chien GW, Aboseif SR. Corporeal plication for the treatment of congenital penile curvature. *J Urol* 2003;**169**: 599.

32 Hauck EW, Bschleipfer T, Diemer T, *et al.* Long-term results of Essed–Schroeder plication by the use of non-absorbable Goretex sutures for correcting congenital penile curvature. *Int J Impot Res* 2002;**14**:146.

33 Ebbehoj J, Metz P. Congenital penile angulation. *Br J Urol* 1987;**60**:264.

34 Kalsi J, Minhas S, Christopher N, *et al.* The results of plaque incision and venous grafting (Lue procedure) to correct the penile deformity of Peyronie's disease. *BJU Int* 2005;**95**:1029.

35 Shioshvili TJ, Kakonashvili AP. The surgical treatment of Peyronie's disease: replacement of plaque by free autograft of buccal mucosa. *Eur Urol* 2005;**48**:129.

36 Levine LA, Estrada CR. Human cadaveric pericardial graft for the surgical correction of Peyronie's disease. *J Urol* 2003;**170**:2359.

37 Hatzichristou DG, Hatzimouratidis K, Apostolidis A, *et al.* Corporoplasty using tunica albuginea free grafts for penile curvature: surgical technique and long-term results. *J Urol* 2002;**167**:1367.

38 Schwarzer JU, Muhlen B, Schukai O. Penile corporoplasty using tunica albuginea free graft from proximal corpus cavernosum: a new technique for treatment of penile curvature in Peyronie's disease. *Eur Urol* 2003;**44**:720.

39 Hsu YS, Huang WJ, Kuo JY, *et al.* Experience of surgical treatment of peyronie's disease with deep dorsal venous

patch graft in Taiwanese men. *J Chin Med Assoc* 2003;**66**:487.

40 Egydio PH, Lucon AM, Arap S. Treatment of Peyronie's disease by incomplete circumferential incision of the tunica albuginea and plaque with bovine pericardium graft. *Urology* 2002;**59**:570.

41 Sampaio JS, Fonseca J, Passarinho A, *et al.* Peyronie's disease: surgical correction of 40 patients with relaxing incision and duramater graft. *Eur Urol* 2002;**41**: 551.

42 Adeniyi AA, Goorney SR, Pryor JP, *et al.* The Lue procedure: an analysis of the outcome in Peyronie's disease. *BJU Int* 2002;**89**:404.

43 Hauck EW, Bschleipfer T, Diemer T, *et al.* Long-term results of plaque thinning with carbide burs, small incisions and venous grafting for correcting complex penile curvature in Peyronie's disease: poor results of an "ideal" approach. *J Urol* 2002;**167**:2070.

44 Knoll LD. Use of porcine small intestinal submucosal graft in the surgical management of Peyronie's disease. *Urology* 2001;**57**:753.

45 Akkus E, Ozkara H, Alici B, *et al.* Incision and venous patch graft in the surgical treatment of penile curvature in Peyronie's disease. *Eur Urol* 2001;**40**:531.

46 Teloken C, Grazziotin T, Rhoden E, *et al.* Penile straightening with crural graft of the corpus cavernosum. *J Urol* 2000;**164**:107.

47 Montorsi F, Salonia A, Maga T, *et al.* Evidence based assessment of long-term results of plaque incision and vein grafting for Peyronie's disease. *J Urol* 2000;**163**: 1704.

48 Kadioglu A, Tefekli A, Usta M, *et al.* Surgical treatment of Peyronie's disease with incision and venous patch technique. *Int J Impot Res* 1999;**11**:75.

49 El-Sakka AI, Rashwan HM, Lue TF. Venous patch graft for Peyronie's disease. Part II: outcome analysis. *J Urol* 1998;**160**:2050.

50 Akin-Olugbade Y, Ahmed A, Parker M, Patricia Guhring, Mulhall JP. Determinants of patient satisfaction following penile prosthesis surgery. *J Sex Med* 2005.

51 Usta MF, Adams DM, Zhang JW, *et al.* Penile epithelioid sarcoma and the case for a histopathological diagnosis in Peyronie's disease. *BJU Int* 2003;**91**:519.

52 Levine LA, Estrada CR, Morgentaler A. Mechanical reliability and safety of, and patient satisfaction with the Ambicor inflatable penile prosthesis: results of a 2 center study. *J Urol* 2001;**166**:932.

53 Levine LA, Dimitriou RJ. A surgical algorithm for penile prosthesis placement in men with erectile failure and Peyronie's disease. *Int J Impot Res* 2000;**12**:147.

54 Carson CC. Penile prosthesis implantation in the treatment of Peyronie's disease and erectile dysfunction. *Int J Impot Res* 2000;**12 S4**:S122.

55 Ghanem HM, Fahmy I, el-Meliegy A. Malleable penile implants without plaque surgery in the treatment of Peyronie's disease. *Int J Impot Res* 1998;**10**:171.

56 Morganstern SL. Long-term experience with the AMS 700CX inflatable penile prosthesis in the treatment of Peyronie's disease. *Tech Urol* 1997;**3**:86.

57 Marzi M, Zucchi A, Lombi R, *et al.* Implant surgery in Peyronie's disease. *Urol Int* 1997;**58**:113.

58 Montorsi F, Guazzoni G, Barbieri L, *et al.* AMS 700 CX inflatable penile implants for Peyronie's disease: functional results, morbidity and patient-partner satisfaction. *Int J Impot Res* 1996;**8**:81.

CHAPTER 15
Priapism

Pathophysiology and Non-Surgical Management
Ajay Nehra

Introduction

Priapism describes a persistent erection arising from dysfunction of the mechanisms regulating penile tumescence and flaccidity. The erection of priapism is typically *not* the result of sexual excitement and, if associated with erotic stimulation, lasts well beyond the original stimulus and is not relieved by orgasm or ejaculation.

A diagnosis of priapism is a matter of urgency requiring identification of the underlying etiology because prompt therapy may successfully alleviate the condition and minimize potential morbidities.

Ischemic Priapism (Table 15.1)

Ischemic or low-flow priapism accounts for more than 95% of all priapism episodes. Ischemic priapism is typically associated with a rigid and painful erection with stasis of blood, and which is not relieved by ejaculation or orgasm. (Stuttering or intermittent priapism is a recurrent form of low-flow priapism whereby the painful erections occur repeatedly with periods of intervening detumescence.)

Sickle cell disease and other hematologic abnormalities are most often associated with low-flow priapism. Various drugs may precipitate an episode of ischemic priapism, such as trazodone, antihypertensive agents, alcohol, marijuana, cocaine, as well as intracavernous vasoactive agents such as papaverine, prostaglandin E1, phentolamine and others.

Physical examination typically reveals painful or tender complete rigidity of the corpus cavernosa, sparing the glans and spongiosum. Abdominal and genital examination may reveal evidence of prior trauma or malignancy. Laboratory evaluation, including complete blood count (CBC) and white blood count (WBC), to rule out infection and hematologic abnormalities, reticulocyte counts, hemoglobin electrophoresis when indicated, drug screening (e.g. cocaine and its metabolites), corporal blood gas testing, and duplex ultrasound (if available), should be performed. Cavernous blood gas findings in ischemic priapism may include $pO_2 < 30$ mm Hg, $pCO_2 > 60$ mm Hg, and pH < 7.25. Cavernous blood gas findings similar to arterial blood are found in patients with non-ischemic priapism.

Ischemic Priapism: Treatment

In general, immediate surgical intervention should be avoided while less invasive and often successful

Table 15.1 Key clinical findings in priapism. Adapted from AUA Guidelines on Management of Priapism, 2003.

Findings	Ischemic priapism	Non-ischemic priapism
Corpora cavernosa fully rigid	Usually	Seldom
Penile pain	Usually	Seldom
Abnormal cavernosal blood gas	Usually	Seldom
Blood abnormalities and malignancy	Sometimes	Seldom
Recent intracorporal injection	Sometimes	Seldom
Chronic, well-tolerated tumescence	Seldom	Usually
Perineal trauma	Seldom	Sometimes

alternatives are first attempted, especially in cases of less than six hours duration. Previous recommendations for priapism episodes associated with sickle cell disease included prolonged treatments with oxygen, analgesics, and intravenous hydration, prior to intracorporal therapy or surgical intervention, due to the often repetitive and self-limiting nature of their priapism episodes. Unfortunately, this regimen is often unsuccessful and results in an increased rate of corporal fibrosis and erectile dysfunction, and is no longer recommended. In very select cases of priapism associated with sickle cell disease, the successful use of exchange transfusions to reduce the fraction of abnormal HbS hemoglobin, and hypertransfusion with packed red blood cells to double the hematocrit and diminish the fraction of HbS present, has been described to achieve detumescence. Early hemoglobin electrophoresis to determine the fractional percentage of HbS present serves as a useful guideline for monitoring subsequent transfusion therapy. As with any transfusion of blood or blood products, the associated risks, including disease transmission and HIV, should be discussed with the patients prior to transfusion, and the potential benefits weighed against the disadvantages.

The AUA guidelines committee recommends the use of phenylephrine, an alpha-selective adrenergic agonist with no indirect neurotransmitter-releasing action. This agent minimizes the risk of cardiovascular side effects that are more commonly seen with other sympathomimetic agents. For intracavernosal use in adult patients, phenylephrine is diluted with normal saline to a concentration of 100 to 500 µg/mL. One mL injections are made every five minutes as needed, up to one hour. During treatment, patients should be observed for symptoms, such as acute hypertension, headache, reflex bradycardia, tachycardia, palpitations, and cardiac arrhythmia.

For children or those with severe cardiovascular disease, lower doses are recommended. In patients with severe cardiovascular disease, it is prudent to monitor blood pressure and pulse rate in a controlled surveillance setting.

The use of oral terbutaline, a beta-agonist, both for the preventive and active treatment of ischemic priapism has been suggested. However, there are no studies to date demonstrating clear efficacy over placebo, and their use in the management of priapism is not recommended.

For patients with recurrent or "stuttering" priapism, a monthly regimen of gonadotropin-releasing hormone analogues can be effective in decreasing the occurrence of priapism. Likewise, the use of oral digoxin at therapeutic levels has been shown to be safe and efficacious for decreasing the frequency of recurrent priapism episodes while allowing for normal sexual function and libido.

Associated Issues of Ischemic Priapism

1 Persistence and recurrence despite active intervention.
2 Erectile dysfunction. It is estimated that more than 25% of patients with priapism will have some degree of ED.

Non-Ischemic (High Flow) Priapism

Non-ischemic or high-flow arterial priapism is a form of priapism typically caused by traumatic cavernosal artery laceration, or injury that enables unregulated flow of arterial blood directly into the lacunar spaces of the corpora, bypassing the protective, high-resistance helicine arterioles. This constant unregulated flow results in the pathognomonic arterial–lacunar fistula (ALF) of high-flow priapism.

The clinical characteristics of non-ischemic priapism typically include a pre-morbid history of trauma, delayed onset of priapism following the trauma, incomplete rigidity of the phallus compared to pre-morbid sexually-stimulated erectile rigidity, and a constant erection that is painless, non-tender, of persistent partial rigidity throughout the day and night, with the potential for increase to full rigidity with sexual stimulation. Although spontaneous resolution may occur, with non-ischemic priapism the painless, partial erection will often continue unless "active" intervention is performed.

Selective internal pudendal arteriography has been the mainstay of diagnostic and therapeutic maneuvers for arterial priapism. The pathognomonic arteriographic finding is of an arterial–lacunar fistula—a characteristic intracavernosal cone-shaped blush of contrast at the site of the cavernosal artery laceration.

Unfortunately, these therapies have had little success in reversing the high-flow priapism state and are currently not recommended by the AUA guidelines for priapism therapy.

The current standard of intervention remains selective internal pudendal arteriography with transcatheter autologous clot embolization. The goal of this therapy is to induce temporary occlusion of the cavernosal artery in order to allow the injured site to heal. The temporary nature of this occlusion allows for the subsequent reestablishment of physiologically-controlled normal cavernosal blood flow, with preservation of erectile tissue viability and normal long-term erectile function. This form of minimally-invasive intervention has a high probability for resolution of the priapism with restoration of erectile potency compared to more invasive techniques, including permanent coil embolization and surgical ligation of the cavernosal artery.

Studies comparing perineal duplex ultrasound and concomitantly preformed selective internal pudendal arteriography have revealed excellent sensitivity in detecting the arterial–lacunar fistula that is seen angiographically on ultrasound (12 of 12 cases). In both the selective internal pudendal arteriography and perineal duplex study, the arterial lacunar fistula was noted at the same location. In fact, in one reported case where physical examination suggested incomplete return to flaccidity and post-embolization due to recurrent fistula, the negative perineal duplex Doppler ultrasound study correctly predicted the final clinical outcome of complete priapism resolution and full erectile function. Therefore if the follow-up clinical examination is equivocal for recurrence of the arterial lacunar fistula, perineal duplex Doppler ultrasound may better predict the need for repeat arteriography and embolization.

The current algorithm for the management of non-ischemic priapism is seen in Fig. 15.2. The algorithm emphasizes patient history, physical examination, pre-morbid and current erectile function status, and the use of perineal duplex Doppler ultrasonography for initial identification of the pathognomonic arterial–lacunar fistula. If an "active" course of treatment is chosen, selective internal pudendal arteriography and embolization with autologous clot, with or without Gelfoam should be employed. While complete detumescence is ideally seen immediately following selective embolization, partial tumescence at this time may be related to long-standing edema, reinforcing the concept that physical examination alone cannot be used to determine the endpoint of treatment or as the sole means of follow-up evaluation. Serial perineal and penile duplex studies over the days and weeks post-embolization should be part of the overall regimen to assure adequate resolution of the arterial lacunar fistula. If further intervention is required, perineal duplex studies can reduce the reliance upon multiple subsequent angiographic procedures and their associated risks.

Conclusion

The medico–legal aspect of priapism and its associated diagnostic and therapeutic interventions remains important in our litigious society. The physician should explain to the patient the natural history of the disease and the extremely high risk of developing erectile dysfunction, early or late, despite active or no intervention. Discussion should include the advantages and potential disadvantages of the various treatment alternatives, as well as the risks associated with no treatment at all. Documentation of this, in addition to any prior erectile dysfunction, and all counseling sessions, should be meticulous.

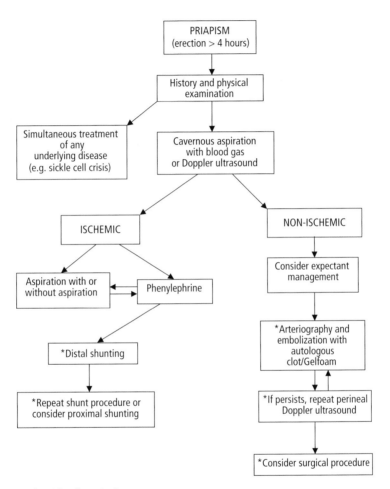

Fig. 15.1 Management algorithm for priapism.

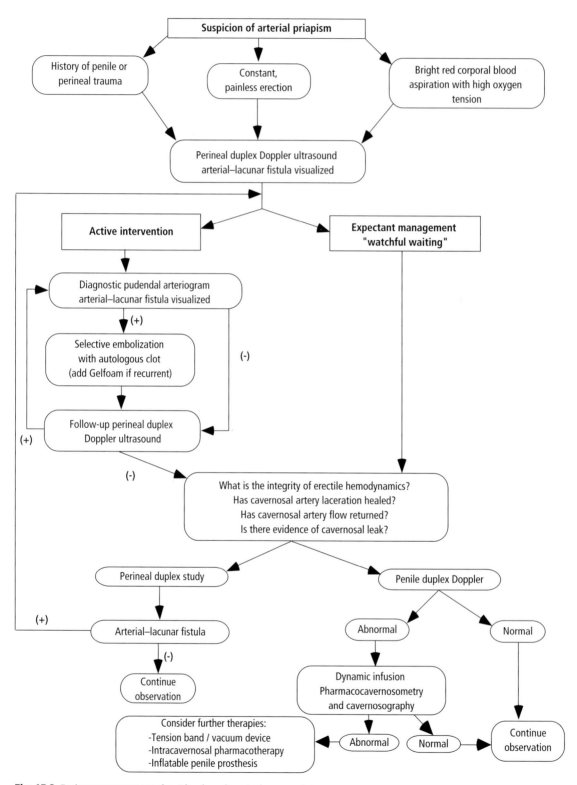

Fig. 15.2 Patient management algorithm based on study group data.

Suggested Reading

1 Witt MA, Goldstein I, Tejada IS, Greenfield A, Krane RK. Traumatic laceration of intracavernosal arteries: the pathophysiology of non-ischemic, high-flow, arterial priapism. *J Urol* 1990;**143**:129.

2 Bastuba MD, Saenz de Tejada I, Dinlenc CZ, Sarazen A, Krane RJ, Goldstein I. Arterial priapism: diagnosis, treatment and long-term follow-up. *J Urol* 1994;**151**:1231.

3 El-Bahnasawy M, Dawood A, Farouk A. Low-Flow priapism: risk factors for erectile dysfunction. *BJU Int* 2002;**89**:285.

4 Brock G, Breza J, Lue TF, Tanagho EA. High-flow priapism: a spectrum of disease. *J Urol* 1993;**150**: 968.

5 Hauri D, Spycher M, Bruhlmann W. Erection and priapism: a new physiopathological concept. *Urol Int* 1983;**38**:138.

6 Krane RJ, Goldstein I, Tejada IS. Impotence. *N Engl J Med* 1989;**321**:1648.

7 Lue TF, Hellstrom WJG, McAnich JW, Tanagho E. Priapism: a redefined approach to diagnosis and treatment. *J Urol* 1986;**136**:104.

8 Dahm P, Rao D, Donatucci C. Antiandrogens in the treatment of priapism. *Urology* 2002;**59**:138.

9 Levine L, Guss S. Gonadotropin-releasing hormone analogues in the treatment of sickle cell anemia-associated priapism. *J Urol* 1993;**150**:475.

10 Rourke K, Fischler A, Jordan G. Treatment of recurrent idiopathic priapism. *J Urol* 2002;**168**:2552.

11 Bookstein JJ. Penile angiography: The last angiographic frontier. *AJR* 1988;**150**:47.

12 Ji MX, He NS, Wang P, Chen G. Use of selective embolization of the bilateral cavernous arteries for post-traumatic arterial priapism. *J Urol* 1994;**151**:1641.

13 Wheeler GW. Angiography in post-traumatic priapism: A case report. *AJR* 1973;**119**:119.

14 Gudinchet F, Fournier D, Jichlinski P, Meyrat B. Traumatic priapism in a child: evaluation with color-flow Doppler sonography. *J Urol* 1992;**148**:380.

15 Feldstein VA. Post-traumatic high-flow priapism evaluation with color flow Doppler sonography. *J Ultrasound Med* 1993;**12**:589.

16 Walker TG, Grant PW, Goldstein I, Krane RJ, Greenfield A. High-flow priapism: treatment with super-selective transcatheter embolization. *Radiology* 1990;**174**:1053.

17 Steers WD, Selby JBJ. Use of methylene blue and selective embolization of the pudendal artery for high-flow priapism refractory to medical and surgical treatments. *J Urol* 1991;**146**:1361.

18 Puppo P, Belgrano E, Germinale F, Bottino P, Giuliani L. Angiographic treatment of high-flow priapism. *Eur Urol* 1985;**11**:397.

19 Levine FJ, Tejada IS, Payton TR, Goldstein I. Recurrent prolonged erections and priapism as a sequela of priapism: pathophysiology and management. *J Urol* 1991;**145**:764.

20 Crummy JB, Ishizuka J, Madsen PO. Post-traumatic priapism: successful treatment with autologous clot embolization. *AJR* 1979;**133**:329.

21 Berger R, Billups K, Brock G, Broderick GA, Dhabuwala CB, Goldstein I, Hakim LS, Hellstrom W, Honig S, Levine LA, Lue T, Munarriz R, Montague DK, Mulcahy JJ, Nehra A, Rogers ZR, Rosen R, Seftel AD, Shabsigh R, Steers W. AFUD Thought Leader Panel for evaluation and treatment of priapism. *Int J Impot Res* 2001;**13** (Suppl.5):S39–43.

22 Guideline on the Management of Priapism. American Urologic Association, 2003.

23 Hakim LS, Kulaksizoglu H, Mulligan R, Greenfield A, Goldstein I. Evolving concepts in the diagnosis and treatment of arterial high flow priapism. J Urol. 1996 Feb;**155**(2):541–8.

Surgical Management of Priapism

John Mulhall

Guidelines for the Surgical Management of Priapism

Clinical guidelines
Venocclusive (ischemic, low-flow) priapism

Venocclusive priapism is an emergency that requires urologic consultation. Time is of the essence in the preservation of erectile tissue integrity and erectile function. Failure to respond in a timely fashion may result in greater loss of erectile tissue and function.

Timing of surgical intervention

There is no data to answer at what time point after initiation of medical treatment (corporal aspiration and α-agonist administration) should a decision be made to perform a shunt, although many practitioners and the International Consultation Committee recommend attempting corporal aspiration and α-adrenergic agonist treatment for at least one hour prior to considering surgical intervention (see chapter on medical management of priapism). During this hour it is recommended that patients have their blood pressure and cardiac rate/rhythm monitored because of the risk for hypertension/reflex bradycardia in response to α-adrenergic agonist administration. In patients that have contraindications to α-agonist administration (malignant or poorly-controlled hypertension, use of monoamine oxidase inhibitor medications), an earlier decision regarding surgical intervention may be necessary. Failure of medical measures to result in permanent detumescence needs to be documented. Some authorities suggest that consideration be given to performing a repeat blood–gas analysis at the termination of corporal aspiration, or a Doppler penile ultrasound (to assess cavernosal artery inflow) prior to moving forward with surgical management. The conduct of the latter maneuvers is left to the discretion of the supervising clinician.

• *Corporal aspiration and α-agonist administration should be attempted prior to considering shunt surgery.*

Patient evaluation prior to surgical intervention

A comprehensive discussion should be held with the patient concerning the risks and benefits of the surgery, and clear documentation of this discussion and, in particular the risk of permanent erectile tissue damage and long-term erectile dysfunction, must be placed in the medical record, and an informed consent form signed by the patient or his guardian, preferably in the presence of a witness. It is recommended that all medical records should be both dated and timed because of the emphasis on chronology of events in medico–legal cases pertaining to priapism. Although it is universally accepted that the longer a priapism event the more likely a man is to experience long-term erectile dysfunction, at what time this becomes inevitable is unclear. There is evidence that 12 hours of priapism leads to overt histologic changes in corpus cavernosal smooth muscle, as seen by light microscopy.

• *The longer the venocclusive priapism event the greater the chance of permanent erectile dysfunction.*

Furthermore, at what time surgical intervention is no longer warranted is unclear. It is the committee's recommendation that shunting be considered for priapism events lasting ≤72 hours, that consideration be given to foregoing shunting in priapism events lasting >five days, in particular where no blood can be aspirated from the corporal bodies upon presentation. For priapism events lasting between three and five days, judgement regarding the value of shunt surgery is left to the discretion of the individual clinician. Some authorities suggest corporal smooth muscle biopsy be considered at the time of shunt surgery [1]. If biopsy is planned this should be delineated on the informed consent form.

• *Shunt surgery should be considered for all cases of venocclusive priapism lasting 72 hours or less.*

Surgical options

The primary purpose of shunt surgery is oxygenation of the corpus cavernosal smooth muscle (CCSM). Shunts do not always result in immediate detumescence, as the CCSM may remain paralyzed for some time and, depending upon the duration of the priapism event, significant tissue edema may be present, which will masquerade as penile tumescence/rigidity.

Shunt procedures are subdivided into four groups:

1 Percutaneous distal shunts (Winter, Ebbehoj)
2 Open distal shunt (Al-Ghorab)
3 Open proximal shunt (Quackles)
4 Saphenous vein (Grayhack)

It is recommended that a penile local anesthetic block be performed if percutaneous shunts are to be performed without general or spinal anesthesia. The Winter shunt is performed using a tru-cut (or analogous biopsy needle) [2]. Through a single stab incision (made with an 11 blade) in the glans, two passes are made on each side of the glans. The tip of the needle must be placed at a point beyond the termination of the corpus cavernosal tunica albuginea within the glans. Once the biopsy needle is fired, a piece of tunica albuginea is removed and a communication is made between glans (corpus spongiosum) and corpus cavernosum. The skin puncture usually does not require any suturing.

The Ebbehoj shunt differs in that, rather than using a tru-cut needle, an 11 blade is used. The blade is passed through the glans and the cavernosal tunica albuginea into the corporal body [3]. At this point, the blade is withdrawn and simultaneously rotated 90 degrees in an effort to maximize the size of the spongiosal-cavernosal communication. Little literature exists on the ability of these shunts to achieve permanent detumescence of the penis. Winter in his 1988 review of 105 cases cited a high likelihood of permanent detumescence. More recently, Nixon *et al.* reported on 28 patients with venocclusive priapism [2]. Patients were included in the analysis if

they had painful priapism more than four hours in duration that was refractory to conservative management, ultimately requiring a surgical shunt. Of the 28 patients included in the study, 13 (46%) required more than one operation for failed detumescence, of which 12 (92%) initially underwent a Winter shunt. Only 2/20 men (10%) with available follow-up reported preservation of pre-morbid erectile function. Three men (15%) achieved partial erection without the assistance of oral or injectable agents, while the remainder 15/20 (75%) had erectile dysfunction. In his original report on his procedure, Ebbehoj discussed 18 patients treated for priapism using his technique. Eleven obtained complete relief and follow-up examination of the 18 patients demonstrated normal erectile function in 11 cases [3].

Many authorities prefer to commence surgical management with an Al-Ghorab-type shunt [4]. This shunt is typically performed in an operating room setting. A curvilinear incision is made just distal to the coronal sulcus on the glans. The tunica albuginea is identified and a segment of tunica is excised leaving a generous communication between the corpora spongiosum and cavernosum on each side. One of the clear advantages of this approach is that dark blood and/or clot can be evaluated from corporal bodies through the fistulae and an assessment of blood color can be accomplished prior to wound closure. The glans incision is then sutured and the penis is gently wrapped with an absorbent dressing. There is no data comparing percutaneous and open distal shunt outcomes; however one of the factors involved in the success of shunts is shunt patency (the other is the degree of CCSM damage at presentation/pre-shunt surgery). Thus, it is likely if duration of priapism and CCSM status is controlled for, that open shunts are likely to result in higher shunt patency rates.

Prior to leaving the operating room, an assessment is required to define if the shunt is patent, thus promoting CCSM oxygenation—that is, that fresh blood is flowing into the corporal cavernosa. This can be accomplished in a number of ways:

1 Visualization of bright red blood emanating from the corpora cavernosa
2 Obtaining a corporal blood–gas analysis

3 Cavernosal artery Doppler ultrasound
4 Measurement of intracavernosal pressure
5 Penile compression maneuver

Documentation of one of these findings must be made in the operation report. The presence of bright red blood signifies that oxygenated blood is circulating through the corpora cavernosa, which is the main purpose of shunt surgery. This may be confirmed by sending a blood specimen for gas analysis. An intraoperative Doppler ultrasound can confirm arterial inflow through the cavernosal arteries. Some authorities have suggested that measurement of intracavernosal pressure may be predictive of permanent detumescence but data to support this concept is lacking. Finally, a simple maneuver can be used to document that the Al-Ghorab shunt is patent. Manual compression of the penile shaft from side to side proximal to the shunt that generates pressure greater than systolic blood pressure, thus occluding cavernosal arterial inflow, should result in immediate detumescence of the penis if the shunt is patent. It is important to avoid circumferential compression when doing this, as this will cause complete venocclusion, thus preventing efflux of blood from the penis.

• *Documentation of shunt patency at the completion of shunt surgery is recommended.*

In cases where a distal shunt fails, a proximal shunt is indicated. This decision may be made in the operating room after the completion of the distal shunt if patency cannot be established or if oxygenated blood is not present within the corporal bodies. Alternatively, a decision to proceed with a secondary procedure (proximal shunt) may be made within hours of performance of the distal shunt. The most commonly performed proximal shunt (Quackles) involves performing a transverse scrotal or perineal incision [5]. Prior to creation of the spongiosal–cavernosal communication, a urethral catheter is placed. The tunica albuginea of both corporal bodies is identified and communications are fashioned bilaterally between corpus spongiosum and corpus cavernosum. There is no data comparing bilateral and unilateral spongiosal–cavernosal shunts. It is, however, the recommendation of the committee that such shunts should be performed bilaterally. Typically, these communications are staggered; that is, right side and left side are separated by a distance of at least 1 cm in an effort to minimize the risk of urethral stricture at the point of fistulization. An ellipse of tunica is excised from the corpus cavernosum and a similarly-sized ellipse excised from the spongiosum. The edges of the ellipses are sutured in watertight fashion. This technique also allows "milking" of old blood and assessment of blood color prior to wound closure. After wound closure, the penis is gently wrapped with a dressing.

In cases where proximal shunt fails, some authorities advocate performing a saphenous vein bypass procedure (Grayhack procedure) [6], whereby the saphenous vein is interrupted below its junction with the femoral vein and tunneled subcutaneously for an anastomosis to one corporal body by excising an ellipse of tunica albuginea. The literature has a paucity of outcome analyses on the success of any of these procedures, but it is likely that their ability to achieve oxygenation of CCSM is related to the size of fistula between spongiosum and cavernosum, and their ability to lead to preservation of erectile function is related to duration of priapism event and the extent of CCSM structural changes at the time of the shunt procedure. Consideration may be given to urinary drainage by urethral or suprapubic catheter drainage in the immediate post-shunt period, in patients who have difficulty voiding or in those who have undergone Quackles shunting.

• *It is recommended to commence with a distal shunt and when this fails to perform a proximal shunt.*

Some authorities have suggested performing immediate penile prosthesis implantation for late-presentation priapism. The time point at which this becomes a reasonable option is unclear; however, the committee recommends that any discussion pertaining to early prosthesis insertion be documented and include a comprehensive review of the advantages (preservation of penile length) and disadvantages (infection, mechanical malfunction, urethral injury, device erosion). The Ralph group in London studied eight patients with priapism who underwent immediate penile prosthesis implantation [7]. Mean duration of priapism was 91 hours (range 32 to 192 hours). All patients had failed conservative management with the instillation of α-adrenergic agents, and four had already undergone shunt procedures elsewhere. Immediate management consisted of the insertion of a malleable prosthesis in six patients and an inflatable prosthesis in two. In this case series, there were no early complications, with all patients being satisfied with the end result, and seven being capable of having sexual intercourse.

The most obvious advantage of this approach is preservation of penile length, as priapism is associated with universal dramatic reduction in penile length due to collagenization and fibrosis of the corporal smooth muscle. This process leads to a difficult penile prosthesis insertion when performed in a delayed fashion. In the Ralph series, all patients maintained their penile length. Which implant type is optimal in this scenario depends primarily on availability and local financial considerations. The surgeon is forewarned that penile prosthesis insertion in the setting of a recent prior distal shunt (particularly, an Al-Ghorab shunt) may be associated with a higher incidence of distal corporal perforation because of the tunical defect at the distal end of the corpora cavernosa; likewise, penile prosthesis insertion in the setting of a proximal shunt may be associated with a higher incidence of urethral injury (at the point of the shunt). Thus, the surgeon is urged to exercise extreme caution during corporal dilation during these procedures and consideration may need to be given to buttressing or reconstruction of the tunica at the site of prior shunt surgery.

- *Early penile prosthesis insertion may be associated with an increased rate of tunical perforation at the site of a prior shunt.*

Postoperative management

Once the patient has exited the operating room, it is essential that repeated evaluation be conducted to ensure that the shunt remains patent. It is recommended that the patient be re-evaluated prior to leaving the recovery (post-anesthesia care) unit. Once the patient has been discharged to the surgical floor/ward, he needs to be re-evaluated in a serial fashion for the next 24 hours. At each assessment, shunt patency or corporal blood oxygenation needs to be defined. Relying on the degree of penile tumescence alone or patient-reported pain is unreliable. Oftentimes, despite good shunt patency, patients continue to have penile pain as a result of the penile trauma secondary to aspiration attempts and the shunt procedures themselves. Furthermore, residual penile tumescence due to CCSM edema is common in men whose venocclusive priapism event has lasted longer than 12 hours. Thus, patency evaluation should include either the penile compression maneuver (outlined above) for distal shunts, or corporal blood gas where distal shunt patency is in question, and for all proximal shunts. Adequate pain control should be prescribed. The patient should not be discharged from hospital until such time as a final determination has been made that either permanent detumescence has been achieved or that irreversible erectile tissue damage has occurred.

Following discharge from hospital, the patient should be followed-up within a few weeks for wound assessment. At further follow-up meetings, assessment of residual erectile function should be made. While postulated, the role of strategies for penile fibrosis minimization (oral colchicine) and penile length preservation (vacuum device) is unclear in the absence of outcomes data. Any conversation with the patient regarding the use of erectogenic medications (phosphodiesterase-5 (PDE-5) inhibitors, intra-urethral agents, intracavernosal injection agents) must include discussing the fact that men with a history of priapism using such agents must be carefully monitored. Patients using erectogenic medications must be monitored closely. While intriguing, the animal data supporting reduction in priapism events in sickle cell mice with chronic PDE-5 inhibitor administration is preliminary and no human studies have been conducted to date.

A number of case series evaluating outcomes of shunt surgery exist in the literature and these are presented in Table 15.2.

Many case reports exist and these are not reviewed. El-Bahnasawy *et al.* studied 35 patients (mean age 37.1 years, range 22 to 66) with a diagnosis of venocclusive priapism [8]. The median (range) duration of priapism was 48 (6 to 240) hours. Almost half the patients presented >48 h after the onset of

Table 15.2 Case series of shunt surgery for venocclusive priapism.

Author	Year	Patient number	Etiology of priapism	Duration of priapism	Shunt Type	Functional erections
Nixon [11]	2003	28	NM	NM	NM	25%
El-Bahnasawy [8]	2002	35	Idiopathic, ICI	48 h (6–240)	Various	43%
Lawani [12]	1999	17	NM	NM	NM	45%
Kulmala [9]	1996	124	Various	NM	Various	Overall, 69% 92% <24 h, 22% >7 days; 88% <30 years, 40% >50 years
Chakrabarty [10]	1996	5	SSD	NM	NM	Dependent on patient age and duration of priapism
Kaisary [13]	1986	14	NM	NM	Various	86% <12 h
Proca [14]	1979	6	NM	NM	NM	32%
Richard [15]	1979	8	NM	NM	Sapheno–cavernous	70%
Winter [2]	1978	105	NM	NM	NM	
Ebbehoj [3]	1977	18	NM	NM	NM	55%

ICI: intracavernosal injection therapy; NM: not mentioned; SSD: sickle cell disease

priapism. Sixteen patients (32%) reported a history of previous recurrent attacks, of whom seven had a history of previous treatments. The main cause of priapism was idiopathic or intracavernosal injection with papaverine. All patients were treated initially by corporal blood aspiration and injection with ephedrine; if this failed or if the priapism was prolonged (>48 h) various shunts were used. The hospital stay was significantly shorter among patients with papaverine-induced or brief priapism. In the long-term follow-up of 35 patients (mean 66.4 months, range 3 to 220) only 15 (43%) reported preserved erectile function, and this was more likely in patients with brief priapism (<48 h). Eight patients (23%) reported subsequent recurrent attacks of priapism; all were managed successfully as they presented shortly after their onset. Penile fibrosis was detected in 20 patients (57%), and was significantly more common in those with prolonged priapism (>48 h) or from causes other than papaverine. The 20 impotent men evaluated by Doppler ultrasonog-

raphy had severe echo-dense penile fibrosis and high end-diastolic velocities, suggesting veno-occlusive incompetence in all except two. In five men with shunts, cavernosography showed extensive venous leakage irrespective of site of the shunt. magnetic resonance imaging (MRI) in five patients with penile fibrosis showed heterogeneous areas of low signal intensity, corresponding with hemosiderin deposition and fibrosis. On univariate analysis the final result of management (complete detumescence or not), the duration of priapism and the presence of penile fibrosis, significantly influenced erectile function. On multivariate logistic regression only the first remained significant.

Kulmala *et al.* studied erectile function outcomes of 124 cases of priapism in previously potent patients [9]. Thirty-nine per cent of the patients became impotent. The duration of symptoms before treatment correlated markedly with the risk of impotence, in that 92% of those whose priapism had lasted less than 24 h remained potent, but only 22% of those for whom it had lasted longer than seven days did. The younger the patients the better the prognosis, so that 88% of those younger than 30 years preserved their potency but only 40% of those older than 50 years remained potent. The prognosis was poorest when heparin therapy or a combination of alcohol drinking and psychopharmaceuticals was the etiologic factor behind priapism. Only 31% of patients preserved their potency after conservative treatment for priapism, whereas 69% of those treated with small glanulo–corporal shunts did so.

Chakrabarty *et al.* retrospectively reviewed pediatric patients with sickle cell priapism and subsequently assessed erectile capabilities, subjectively by questionnaire, and objectively by RigiScan [10]. Of the 15 patients interviewed, five had undergone shunt procedures. The return of potency tended to vary inversely with patient age at onset and duration of priapism. Kaisary *et al.* analyzed 22 patients with priapism [13]. Fourteen various surgical shunts were carried out. Success of surgical treatment, as demonstrated by detumescence and maintenance of potency, was best achieved in those patients who were treated less than 12 hours following onset of priapism, irrespective of whichever venous shunting technique was used (6/7 patients, 86%). Richard *et al.* evaluated the records of 12 venocclusive priapism patients [15]. Treatment consisted of eight sapheno–cavernous shunts, achieving detumescence in seven cases, and preserving sexual potency in five. Moncada *et al.* reported on five patients with venocclusive priapism who underwent the Grayhack procedure. Two patients had no fibrosis of the CCSM yet had complete erectile dysfunction after the operation. Cavernosography revealed a patent shunt. Potency returned after ligation and division of the saphenous vein. In the other three cases cavernosography revealed thrombosis of the shunt. Fibrosis of the cavernous tissues was believed to be the cause of erectile dysfunction in these cases. The author suggested that in cases where erectile function does not return within three months of the Grayhack procedure, the shunt should be ligated.

Key recommendations

• *Document accurately, including timing and dating of all records.*

• *Obtain informed consent before surgical intervention.*
• *Ensure an adequate trial of corporal aspiration and α-agonist administration.*
• *Shunts must accomplish a wide fistula between spongiosum and cavernosum.*
• *Commence with a distal shunt.*
• *Define the patency of the shunt prior to sending patient to the surgical floor.*
• *Conduct serial postoperative examination to define maintenance of shunt patency.*
• *Perform repeat shunt (proximal) if patency cannot be established or is absent.*
• *Follow-up with patient on erectile function outcomes.*
• *Document discussion regarding erectile dysfunction drug use in men with priapism history.*
• *Closely monitor priapism patients using erectogenic drugs.*

Arterial (non-ischemic, high-flow) priapism

Arterial priapism is not a urologic emergency, as the corporal bodies remain oxygenated. The patient usually has little pain and the driving force behind a patient opting for intervention is embarrassment and the nuisance of living life with a permanent partial erection. Once a formal diagnosis has been made, any intervention must follow a comprehensive discussion with the patient regarding pros and cons and risks and benefits of any of the procedures advocated by the clinician. Expectant management is considered a reasonable option given the data that a minority of fistulae will close spontaneously. Surgical ligation of a fistula should occur only in patients who fail angioembolization, or in whom angioembolization is contraindicated (see chapter on medical management of priapism).

• *It is recommended that angioembolization be considered as first-line treatment in patients opting for intervention for arterial priapism.*

Surgical ligation procedures

In cases of long-standing arterial priapism, where the likelihood of a well-developed pseudocapsule around the fistula are greater (to aid localization), surgical ligation has been reported to be successful. No case series exist in the literature, although numerous case reports are cited. Currently, this intervention is reserved for patients who do not wish to pursue expectant management, and who are either poor candidates for angioembolization, do not want this procedure, or where it is not technically feasible or where angioembolization fails after at least one repeat attempt. Which clot material is optimal is a matter of debate without any robust data to answer this question.

Shapiro *et al.* reported on two cases requiring surgical ligation of the fistula. In each patient, angiographic embolization was attempted but abandoned because the distal artery feeding the fistula could not be safely catheterized. Both patients were definitively treated with surgical ligation of the arteriovenous fistula, guided by intraoperative ultrasound. Two surgical approaches were used, one extracorporal and the other transcorporal, with successful preservation of erectile function. Kim *et al.* reported on two patients with arterial priapism that occurred after blunt perineal trauma and lasted for a mean duration of 38 days. Cavernous arterial blushes were demonstrated on selective internal pudendal arteriograms and angioembolization was achieved by autologous clot. Both patients experienced return of pre-morbid erectile function and no local or systemic complications occurred.

Key recommendations

- *Document accurately, including timing and dating of all records.*
- *Obtain informed consent before surgical intervention.*
- *Arterial priapism is not emergent and may be managed conservatively.*
- *Diagnosis is best made by penile/perineal duplex Doppler ultrasound.*
- *Angioembolization represents first-line intervention.*
- *Where angioembolization fails or is contraindicated surgical ligation is reasonable.*

Guidelines for Research in Surgical Management of Priapism

As can be seen from the cited literature, outside of case reports and, generally, small case series, little data exist on outcomes following shunt surgery. While more data exists on outcomes from angioembolization, there is ample room for greater urologic involvement in this area.

There is a need for research in the surgical management of priapism in the following areas:
1 Outcomes analysis of shunt surgery as it pertains to erectile function
2 Defining the correlation between duration of priapism and erectile function
3 Outcomes analysis of immediate penile prosthesis surgery
4 Erectile function outcomes following ligation of arteriocavernous fistula

The committee recommends that erectile function outcomes following surgical intervention for venocclusive and arterial priapism be assessed using a validated instrument, with an attempt to have the patient document pre-priapism function and to follow this after the priapism event. It is believed that this is the only way in which we can accurately document the optimal approach to surgical management of these patients. There are a variety of questionnaires available, but at the time of writing the international index of erectile function (IIEF) is the most frequently utilized and is the questionnaire recommended for erectile function assessment. The committee hopes that erectile function analysis, as well as patient (as well as partner) satisfaction assessment, be conducted in patients who undergo post-priapism implant surgery, whether this be conducted in an early or a delayed fashion. Currently, there exists no satisfaction instrument specifically for penile prosthesis patients, thus no recommendation can be made as to which questionnaire should be used.

References

1 Pryor JP, Hehir M. The management of priapism. *Br J Urol* 1982;**54**:751.
2 Winter CC, McDowell G. Experience with 105 patients with priapism: update review of all aspects. *J Urol* 1988;**140**:980.
3 Ebbehoj J. A new operation for priapism. *Scand J Plast Reconstr Surg* 1974;**8**:241.
4 Borrelli M, Mitre AI, Alfer Junior W, Denes FT, Wroclawski ER, Castilho LN, de Goes GM. Surgical treatment of priapism using Al-Ghorab's technique. *Rev Paul Med* 1983;**101**:27.

5 Quackles R. Cure of a patient suffering from priapism by cavernos spongiosa anastomosis. *Acta Urol Belg* 1964;**32**:5.

6 Grayhack JT, McCullough W, O'Cnor VI, Trippel O. Venous bypass to control priapism. *Invest Urol* 1964;**1**:509.

7 Rees RW, Kalsi J, Minhas S, *et al.* The management of low-flow priapism with the immediate insertion of a penile prosthesis. *BJU Int* 2002;**90**:893.

8 El-Bahnasawy MS, Dawood A, Farouk A. Low-flow priapism: risk factors for erectile dysfunction. *BJU Int* 2002;**89**:285.

9 Kulmala RV, Lehtonen TA, Tammela TL. Preservation of potency after treatment for priapism. *Scand J Urol Nephrol* 1996;**30**:313.

10 Chakrabarty A, Upadhyay J, Dhabuwala CB, *et al.* Priapism associated with sickle cell hemoglobinopathy in children: long-term effects on potency. *J Urol* 1996;**155**: 1419.

11 Nixon RG, O'Connor JL, Milam DF. Efficacy of shunt surgery for refractory low flow priapism: a report on the incidence of failed detumescence and erectile dysfunction. *J Urol* 2003;**170**:883.

12 Lawani J, Aken' Ova YA, Shittu OB. Priapism: an appraisal of surgical treatment. *Afr J Med Med Sci* 1999;**28**:21.

13 Kaisary AV, Smith PJ. Aetiological factors and management of priapism in Bristol 1978–1983. *Ann R Coll Surg Engl* 1986;**68**:252.

14 Proca E. Venous shunts in the treatment of acute thromboses of the cavernous body]. *Rev Chir Oncol Radiol O R L Oftalmol Stomatol Chir* 1979;**27**:37.

15 Richard F, Fourcade R, Le Guillou M, *et al.* Etiological aspects and interest of early surgical management of priapism. *Eur Urol* 1979;**5**:179

CHAPTER 16

Ejaculatory Disorders

Chris G. McMahon, Marcel Waldinger, David Rowland, Pierre Assalian, Young Chan Kim,
Amado Bechara, and Alan Riley

Introduction

Ejaculatory dysfunction (EjD) is one of the most common male sexual disorders. The spectrum of EjD extends from premature or rapid ejaculation, through delayed ejaculation to a complete inability to ejaculate, anejaculation, and includes retrograde ejaculation and painful ejaculation. The sexual response cycle comprises four interactive, non-linear stages: desire, arousal, orgasm, and resolution. In males, the fourth stage of orgasm is usually coincident with ejaculation, but represents a distinct cognitive and emotional cortical event. Ejaculatory dysfunction is a disruption of the fourth stage of orgasm.

Physiology of Ejaculation

The physiology of ejaculation may be distinguished in the neurophysiology and neuropharmacology of ejaculation.

Neurophysiology of ejaculation

Both the central and peripheral neural system is involved in the ejaculatory process.

• *Central Nervous System*: The brain, brainstem and lumbospinal cord contain various areas that are involved in ejaculation. These areas have been identified in male rat studies. Specific information on areas in the human brain leading to ejaculation is mostly lacking. However, one positron electron tomography (PET) scan study in normal male volunteers has shown that during ejaculation a dopamine-rich area, the ventral tegmental area (VTA), becomes strongly stimulated [1].

• *Peripheral Nervous System*: The autonomic (peripheral) nervous system, and particularly the sympathetic nervous system, mediates ejaculation. The mechanism of ejaculation is divided into two phases: emission and expulsion.

• *Emission*: During emission, semen (e.g. sperm and seminal fluids) is deposited into the posterior urethra through contractions of the vasa deferentia, seminal vesicles, and prostate. At the same time, the internal sphincter of the urinary bladder is closed.

• *Expulsion (or true ejaculation)*: Emission is immediately followed by expulsion. During expulsion, semen is forcefully propelled along the urethra and out of the penis by clonic contractions of striated muscles of the pelvic floor.

It should be noted that compared to erection, human ejaculation has, until recently, been poorly investigated [2]. Although the neurophysiology of ejaculation is often described in absolute terms, a detailed, non-disputed physio–anatomic description of the mechanism of human ejaculation has still to be produced [2].

Neuropharmacology of ejaculation

Ejaculation is centrally mediated by both the serotonergic (5-hydroxytryptamine; 5-HT) and dopaminergic systems [3]. Animal studies have clearly demonstrated that activation of the 5-HT1A receptor facilitates ejaculation. Other animal studies suggest involvement of 5-HT2C and 5-HT1B receptors. It is assumed that in men these receptors have similar functions, but evidence-based data about their role in men is still lacking.

On the other hand the mechanism of action of serotonergic neurons is well known. Interference of these mechanisms by daily use of selective serotonin re-uptake inhibitor (SSRIs) drugs initially leads to only mild changes in the serotonergic content of their synapses. It is only after desensitization of 5-HT receptors, usually occurring within one to two weeks, that the 5-HT content of the synapse increases in a non-natural way, hereby stimulating various post-synaptic 5-HT receptors. The timing of interference may have consequences for the extent of clinical efficacy of on-demand and chronic use of SSRI drugs [4].

Premature Ejaculation

Although premature ejaculation (PE) is considered the most frequent self-reported male sexual dysfunction, there is a lack of a universally accepted definition [5]. This has led to a wide range of prevalence estimates and the development of proposed guidelines for the use of the varied psychologic and pharmacologic therapeutic interventions [6].

Premature ejaculation may affect the level of sexual satisfaction of both men and/or their partners. However, few studies have examined the impact of PE on the man, his partner, and/or their relationship [7,8]. Many patients are reluctant to seek help and to discuss this issue with their physician out of embarrassment and uncertainty whether effective treatment options are available. In many relationships, PE causes few if any problems. Couples may reach an accommodation of the problem through various strategies—young men with a short refractory period may often experience a second and more controlled ejaculation during a subsequent episode of lovemaking. Frequently however, PE eventually leads to significant relationship problems with partners regarding the man as selfish and developing a pattern of sexual avoidance. This only worsens the severity of the prematurity on the occasions when intercourse does occur.

Epidemiology

Premature ejaculation is claimed to be the most common male sexual disorder, affecting 5–40% of sexually-active men [9]. It is believed that there is a higher frequency of PE in adolescents or young adults. Premature ejaculation is more frequently reported by men in East Asia (China, Indonesia, Japan,

Korea and Malaysia), and less frequently by men in Middle Eastern and African countries (Algeria, Egypt, Morocco and Turkey). The European prevalence of PE is said to be between that of East Asia and Middle East and African countries [10].

The prevalence of self-reported PE is difficult to interpret, as non-quantified subjective complaints of PE may not have the same meaning in different cultures. In addition, it is unknown to what extent the role of, and the emancipation of, females determines the opinion of the men who self-report PE.

The current knowledge of the epidemiology of PE is limited by both the lack of a consensus definition of lifelong PE and a failure to consistently distinguish lifelong and acquired PE in most earlier studies. Medical literature contains several univariate and multivariate operational definitions of premature ejaculation. The lack of agreement as to what constitutes premature ejaculation has hampered basic and clinical research into the etiology and management of this condition.

Premature ejaculation has been defined in various ways. Masters and Johnson defined PE as ". . . the inability to delay ejaculation long enough for the woman to achieve orgasm fifty per cent of the time" [11]. On the other hand the American Psychiatric Association's DSM-IV-R classified PE as ". . . the persistent or recurrent ejaculation with minimal stimulation before, on, or shortly after penetration and before the person wishes it . . . the disturbance causing marked distress or interpersonal difficulty" [12]. The World Health Organisation's ICD-10 defines PE as ". . . an inability to delay ejaculation sufficiently to enjoy lovemaking" [13]. Recent quantification of the intravaginal ejaculation latency time (IELT) has introduced a more evidence-based approach to defining PE.

A cohort stopwatch study in a random sample of 491 men from five different countries (The Netherlands, the United Kingdom, Spain, Turkey, and the United States) demonstrated a positively-skewed distribution of the IELT, with a median IELT of 5.4 min (range 0.55–44.1 min) [14] (Figure 16.1). By applying the 0.5 and 2.5 percentiles as accepted standards of disease definition it appeared that the 0.5 percentile equated to an IELT of 0.9 min, and the 2.5 percentile to an IELT of 1.3 min. It was proposed that

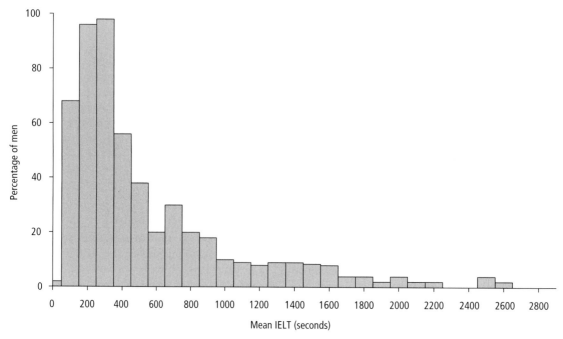

Fig. 16.1 Distribution of intravaginal ejaculatory latency times (IELT) values in a random cohort of 491 men [14].

men with IELT values <0.5 percentile have "definite" PE, and men between 0.5 and 2.5 percentile have "probable" PE. Large-scale international studies using the same methodology, which also include information about feelings of control, have been recommended by the authors to further clarify the epidemiologic distribution of the IELT and subjective complaints of PE [14,15].

Etiology and Risk Factors

Lifelong PE

For about a century it was thought that lifelong PE is mainly caused by psychologic factors. Several different psychologic mechanisms have been proposed.

• *Psychoanalytic theory*: Karl Abraham (1917) postulated that PE is due to unconscious hostile or anxious feelings towards women [16].

• *Psychosomatic theory*: In 1943 Bernard Schapiro suggested that PE be considered a psychosomatic disorder in which psychologic problems influence the activity of the genitals, which are thought to be weak in men with PE [17]. However both psychoanalytic

hypotheses and other hypotheses, suggesting a higher degree of neurotic symptoms or psychopathology in PE patients, have not been experimentally demonstrated.

• *Behavioral theory*: Masters and Johnson (1970) claimed that PE is due to learned behavior related to the occurrence of ejaculations at first intercourse [11]. However, they did not provide strong empirical evidence for their theory.

• *Sexual arousal theory*: Kaplan (1974) proposed that the central etiologic factor in PE was a lack of awareness of the level of sexual arousal and pre-orgasmic sensations [18]. This lack of sensory feedback, or "genital anaesthesia", prevents the man from achieving voluntary control of his ejaculatory reflex. However, this hypothesis has not been yet been adequately tested or strongly supported [7].

• *Hypersensitive sympathetic system*: Assalian (1988) postulated that premature ejaculation is related to a hypersensitivity of the sympathetic nervous system [19]. However, although this may have face validity, this hypothesis has not yet been adequately tested.

• *Ejaculation distribution theory*: Waldinger (1998) postulated that a dysregulation of the activation of some serotonergic receptor subtypes and/or genetic factors give rise to a biologic variation of the IELT in men. According to this theory, men with lifelong PE belong to the extreme left side of the IELT curve [20]. Recently such a biologic continuum of ejaculatory latency has been demonstrated in male rats and in a random population of men in different countries [14,21]. The use of the 0.5% and 2.5% as accepted medical standards of disease definition demonstrated that the 0.5% percentile equals a one minute IELT, and the 2.5% a 1.5 minute IELT. Although both animal and human studies have indeed clearly demonstrated the existence of an ejaculation time distribution and a key role of the serotonergic system in the motoric output of ejaculation, the core neurobiologic factors of PE, including genetic factors, remain to be discovered.

Acquired PE

In contrast to lifelong PE, much less attention has been paid to the research of acquired PE. However, in general, one can distinguish three main causes:
• *Urologic causes*: erectile dysfunction, prostatitis.
• *Psychologic causes*: feelings of insecurity towards the partner, or a sexual relationship with a new partner, may lead to PE. It is believed that PE in these cases tends to only exsist temporarily. Evidence-based studies however are lacking.
• *Endocrine causes*: Many patients with thyroid hormone disorders experience sexual dysfunction, which can be reversed by normalizing thyroid hormone levels. Jannini *et al.* reported acquired PE in 50% of men with hyperthyroidism and 7.1% in men with hypothyroidism, and acquired inhibited ejaculation (IE) in 2.9% of men with hyperthyroidism and 64.3% in men with hypothyroidism. After thyroid hormone normalization in hyperthyroid subjects, PE prevalence fell from 50% to 15%, while IE was improved in half of the treated hypothyroid men [22]. However, there appears to be no relationship between lifelong PE and thyroid hormone disorders [23].
• *Neurologic causes*: Cerebrovascular accidents and transient ischemic accidents in areas involved in the neural circuitry of ejaculation may give rise to PE.

Diagnosis

Diagnosis of PE in clinical practice is not difficult and is based on patient self-report, clinical history and examination findings alone. Men with PE should be evaluated with a detailed medical and sexual history, a physical examination, and appropriate investigations, to establish the true presenting complaint and any identifying obvious biologic causes, such as genital or lower urinary tract infection. Treating physicians must interpret patient self-report of PE with some caution as both PE and non-PE men tend to somewhat overestimate their intravaginal ejaculatory latency time (IELT) compared to stopwatch-recorded IELT. Pryor *et al.* reported that non-PE men, however, overestimate their IELT to a larger extent than PE men, and that IELT estimations for PE men correlate reasonably well with stopwatch-recorded IELT [24]. Although this observation has yet to be confirmed in other studies and differs from anecdotal observations of treating physicians, it does provide some evidence to suggest that PE patient estimation of IELT may be sufficient for the diagnosis of PE in clinical practice. It is clinically relevant to distinguish lifelong and acquired PE. Usually lifelong PE has a global manifestation, whereas acquired PE may occur situationally [25].

However, in a research setting, objective measurement of IELT by stopwatch and subjectively validated, reliable and consistent patient-reported outcome measures (PROs) of ejaculatory control, sexual satisfaction, and bother/distress, are essential in studies assessing treatment [26–28].

Although IELT self-estimations for PE men correlate reasonably well with stopwatch-recorded IELT and are sufficient for the clinical diagnosis of PE, there is no available data to suggest that men can reliably estimate the increases in IELT that occur with treatment. Each of the three criteria above has been operationalized, although not always with consistency [7]. Clinical trial outcome measures include the following:
• *Intravaginal Ejaculation Latency Time (IELT)*: The length of time between penetration and ejaculation; the IELT forms the basis of most current clinical studies on PE [29]. The IELT is measured with a stopwatch operated by the female partner, is expressed in

seconds or minutes and in case of ante-portal ejaculation, is equal to zero. Although it is not clear nowadays whether the use of a stopwatch is influenced by the cultural background of women, various studies, mainly conducted in Western countries, have shown that in general this assessment tool is accepted by study participants. There has been considerable variance of the latencies used to identify men with PE, with IELTs ranging from one to seven minutes, and none of the definitions were based on normative data or offer any supportive rationale for their proposed cut-off time [30–33]. However, a recent multinational, community-based, age-ranging study has provided previously lacking normative data [14]. This study demonstrates that the distribution of the IELT was positively skewed, with a median IELT of 5.4 min and a range of 0.55 to 44.1 minutes, and suggests that men with IELTs of less than 60 seconds and between 60 and 90 seconds have "definite" PE and "probable" PE, respectively.

• *Voluntary control*: Various authors have proposed the extent of voluntary control over ejaculation as an appropriate measure, suggesting minimal or absent control as defining PE [34–36]. However, the patient's feeling of ejaculatory control is a subjective measure and difficult to translate in quantifiable terms. Although feelings of ejaculatory control are part of the ejaculation process, diminished feelings of ejaculatory control are not exclusive for men suffering from PE. Consistent with this, attempts to operationalize the dimension of control has reported conflicting results, making comparison across subjects or across studies difficult [37–39]. Nevertheless the dimension of voluntary control over ejaculation has been found to differentiate men with PE from men without PE [39].

• *Distress*: Existing definitions of PE include distress as an important dimension of PE [12,40,41]. However, the word distress has negative social implications and its existence is denied by most men with PE. This dimension of PE is better captured by the word "bother". The extent of bother defines the severity of PE. One study reported that 64% of men with PE rated their extent of personal distress as "quite a bit" or "extremely", compared to 4% in a group of normal controls [39].

• *Sexual satisfaction*: Men with PE report lower levels of sexual satisfaction than do men with normal ejaculatory latency. A recent observational study reported sexual satisfaction ratings of "very poor" or "poor" in 31% of men with premature ejaculation, compared with 1% in a group of normal controls [39].

• *Questionnaires*: Subjective patient-reported outcomes (PROs) of ejaculatory control, sexual satisfaction and bother/distress may be important additional efficacy endpoints and can be evaluated using validated PRO instruments [26–28]. However, a meta-analysis of 35 drug treatment studies has confirmed that the variability of answers of spontaneous reports and questionnaire studies on the IELT are significantly higher than stopwatch assessments [29].

Clinical Trial Design

In the past decade the concept of evidence-based medicine (EBM) has strongly influenced the research of PE. The results of PE drug clinical trials are only reliable, interpretable and capable of being generalized to patients with the disorder studied when conducted in well-defined and consistent populations, using a double blind placebo-controlled study design with consistent objective physiologic measures or sensitive, validated outcome assessment instruments as study endpoints [41]. Optimal clinical trial design will facilitate subsequent meta-analysis of results, and is one of the goals of an evidence-based approach to medicine [29].

Clinical trial design differs between research into the methodology of diagnosis and research into treatment efficacy.

Methodology of Diagnostic Research

In PE studies, the study population should be well-characterized, representative of the overall patient population, and defined using a multivariate definition of PE. As the etiology, pathogenesis and treatment of lifelong and acquired PE is different, one should make a clear distinction in both types of PE. Accordingly this should be represented by a clear difference in inclusion and exclusion criteria. Men with lifelong and acquired PE should be treated as demographically and etiologically distinct disorders and analyzed as separate PE subgroups [42].

Subjects should be involved in a stable, monogamous heterosexual relationship, prepared to attempt intercourse on a regular basis, and provide written informed consent. The presence of comorbid erectile dysfunction (ED) should be evaluated using a validated instrument such as the international index of erectile function (IIEF), and patients with any degree of ED should be either excluded from the study or treated as a separate subgroup. Patients with hypoactive sexual desire or other sexual disorders, urogenital infection, major psychiatric disorders, a history of drug and alcohol abuse or contraindications to the study drug should be excluded from the study.

A very important issue is the definition of lifelong PE and acquired PE. In recent years most attention has focused on an adequate definition of lifelong PE and much less to acquired PE. For the diagnosis of lifelong PE both objective and subjective items have been proposed but none are universally accepted. As such, a consensus of a definition of lifelong PE has not been reached. There is general agreement that the DSM definition of PE is vague and multi-interpretable [12]. It contains mainly qualitative descriptions and not quantitative values, which makes the current DSM-IV definition inappropriate for scientific research. Research papers stating that PE is defined by the DSM-IV definition should therefore add more diagnostic information of the patients that are included in the study. Outcome measures such as the intravaginal ejaculation latency time (IELT), and patient subjective assessments of control, distress (bother), and sexual satisfaction, using validated patient reported instruments [26–28], form the basis of diagnostic research.

Methodology of Effectiveness of Treatment

Drug treatment trials should be performed according to standard rules of evidence-based medicine. That means the trials should be performed prospectively in a double-blind design in which patients are randomized into either drug or placebo groups. The trial should include a baseline period (usually of about four weeks duration) after which randomization occurs. The duration of the treatment phase is dependent on the aim of the study. A minimum six weeks treatment design is advised for daily SSRI studies as SSRIs need three to four weeks before receptor desensitization has occurred. On-demand studies may have a shorter duration, but should include days in which the drug is not taken, dependent of the half-life of the drug. It is advised that patients not only measure the IELT, but also the drug coitus interval time (DCIT) in order to assess after which period of time the drug is most effective in delaying ejaculation [43]. In studies that include restoration of ejaculatory control or relapse rate as outcome measures, study duration may need to be at least 6–12 months. For assessment of efficacy of drug treatment the items mentioned under methodology of diagnostic research should be applied.

Therapy

Pharmacologic treatment of premature ejaculation

Pharmacologic modulation of ejaculatory threshold represents a novel and refreshing approach to the treatment of PE and a radical departure from the psychosexual model of treatment, previously regarded as the cornerstone of treatment. The introduction of SSRIs has revolutionized the approach to, and treatment of, PE. Selective serotonin reuptake inhibitors encompass five compounds—citalopram, fluoxetine, fluvoxamine, paroxetine and sertraline—with a similar pharmacologic mechanism of action. Although the methodology of the initial drug treatment studies was rather poor, later double-blind and placebo-controlled studies replicated the genuine effect of clomipramine and SSRIs to delay ejaculation. In spite of a development towards more evidence-based drug treatment research, the majority of studies still lack adequate design and methodology [44]. A recent meta-analysis of all drug treatment studies demonstrated that only 14.4% had been performed according to the established criteria of evidence-based medicine, and that open design studies and studies using subjective reporting or questionnaires showed a higher variability in ejaculation delay than double-blind studies in which

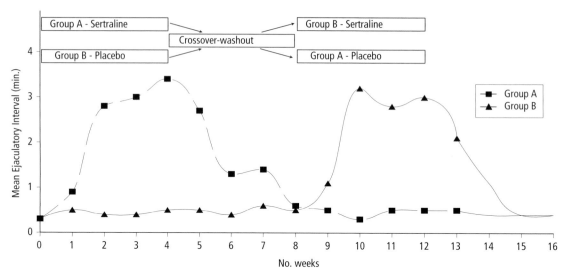

Fig. 16.2 Selective serotonin re-uptake inhibitors produce ejaculatory delay within 5 to10 days [46].

the ejaculation delay was prospectively assessed with a stopwatch [44].

Daily treatment with selective serotonin reuptake inhibitors

Daily treatment can be performed with paroxetine 20–40 mg, clomipramine 10–50 mg, sertraline 50–100 mg, and fluoxetine 20–40 mg [19,45,46] (Figure 16.2) Paroxetine appears to exert the strongest ejaculation delay, increasing IELT approximately 8.8-fold over baseline [44]. Ejaculation delay usually occurs within five to10 days, but may occur earlier. Adverse effects are usually minor, start in the first week of treatment, gradually disappear within two to three weeks and include fatigue, yawning, mild nausea, loose stools or perspiration. Diminished libido or mild erectile dysfunction is infrequently reported. Significant agitation is reported by a small number of patients, and treatment with SSRIs should be avoided in men with a history of bipolar depression.

On-demand treatment with selective serotonin reuptake inhibitors

Administration of clomipramine, paroxetine, sertraline, or fluoxetine, four to six hours before intercourse, is efficacious and well-tolerated, but is associated with less ejaculatory delay than daily treatment. Daily administration of an SSRI is associated with superior fold-increases in IELT compared to on-demand administration, due to greatly enhanced 5-HT neurotransmission resulting from several adaptive processes, which may include presynaptic 5-HT1A and 5-HT1B receptor desensitization [20]. On-demand treatment may be combined with either an initial trial of daily treatment or concomitant low-dose daily treatment [47–49].

A number of rapid acting short half-life SSRIs (Dapoxetine-Johnson & Johnson, UK-369,003-Pfizer) are under investigation as on-demand treatments for PE. Preliminary data suggest that dapoxetine (Johnson & Johnson) administered one to two hours prior to planned intercourse, is effective and well-tolerated, superior to placebo, and increases IELT two- to three-fold over baseline in a dose-dependent fashion [50]. In randomized, double-blind, placebo-controlled, multicenter, phase III, 12-week clinical trials involving 2614 men with a mean baseline IELT ≤ 2 minutes, dapoxetine 30 mg or 60 mg was more effective than placebo for all study endpoints [51]. Intravaginal ejaculatory latency time increased from 0.91 minutes at baseline to 2.78 and 3.32 minutes at study end with dapoxetine 30 and 60 mg, respectively. (Figure 16.3) Mean

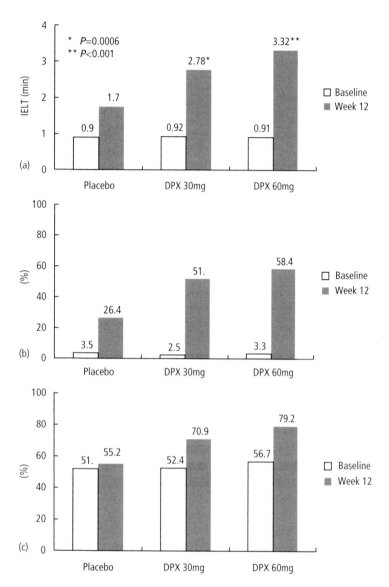

Fig. 16.3 (a) Dapoxetine increased intravaginal ejaculatory latency time (IELT) from 0.91 minutes at baseline to 2.78 and 3.32 minutes at study end with 30 and 60 mg, respectively. (b) Percentage of subjects rating control over ejaculation as fair, good, or very good, increased from 3.1% at baseline to 51.8% and 58.4% at study end with dapoxetine 30 and 60 mg, respectively. (c) Percentage of subjects rating sexual satisfaction as fair, good or very good increased from 53.6% at baseline to 70.9% and 79.2% with dapoxetine 30 mg and 60 mg, respectively (rating scale 0–5 scale, 0 = very poor & 5 = very good) [51].

patient rating of control over ejaculation as fair, good, or very good, increased from 3.1% at baseline to 51.8% and 58.4% at study end with dapoxetine 30 and 60 mg, respectively. Treatment-related side effects were uncommon, dose-dependent, included nausea, diarrhea, headache, and dizziness, and were responsible for study discontinuation in 4% (30 mg) and 10% (60 mg) of subjects.

Several in vitro and animal studies have demonstrated that the desensitization of 5-HT1A receptors, increased activation of postsynaptic 5-HT2C receptors, and the resultant higher increase in synaptic 5-HT neurotransmission seen in daily dosing of SSRI class drugs, can be acutely achieved by blockade of these receptors by administration of an on-demand SSRI and a 5-HT1A receptor antagonist [52–54]. Drug combinations such as this, or single agents that target multiple receptors, may form the foundation of more effective future on-demand medication.

Anesthetic topical ointments

The use of topical local anesthetics such as lidocaine and/or prilocaine as a cream, gel or spray is well established and is moderately effective in retarding ejaculation. They may be associated with significant penile hypo-anesthesia and possible transvaginal absorption, resulting in vaginal numbness and female anorgasmia unless a condom is used [55–57].

Type 5 Phosphodiesterase (PDE-5) inhibitors

Nitric oxide (NO) is becoming recognized as one of the important intracellular messengers in the brain [58]. Several studies suggest that elevation of extracellular NO in the medial pre-optic area (MPOA) accelerates dopamine release and facilitates male copulatory behavior of rats, whereas a decrease of NO reduces their copulatory behavior [59–61].

Several authors have reported their experience with PDE5 inhibitors alone or in combination with SSRIs as a treatment for PE [62–66]. The proposed mechanisms for the effect of sildenafil on ejaculatory latencies include a central effect involving increased NO and reduced sympathetic tone, smooth muscle dilatation of the vas deferens and seminal vesicles, which may oppose sympathetic vasoconstriction and delay ejaculation, reduced performance anxiety due to better erections, and down-regulation of the erectile threshold to a lower level of arousal so that increased levels of arousal are required to achieve the ejaculation threshold. Most of these studies are uncontrolled and the results are confusing and difficult to interpret. The only double-blind placebo-controlled multicenter study showed no significant difference in the IELT of sildenafil-treated subjects compared to placebo, but did demonstrate significant improvements in the ejaculatory control domain and the ejaculatory function global efficacy question. The latter is possibly consistent with the erectile response of sildenafil [67].

It is unlikely that PDE inhibitors significantly delay ejaculation in men with PE without erectile dysfunction. However, it may well be that PDE inhibitors may be beneficial in men with erectile dysfunction and secondary PE. Well-designed, placebo-controlled studies are a prerequisite to further study the efficacy of these compounds in delaying ejaculation.

Psychologic treatment of premature ejaculation

The outcome objective of treating PE is the prolongation of ejaculatory latency, leading to a better and preferably mutually-satisfying sexual relationship between the patient and his partner. As PE may result in sexual problems in the patient's partner or may lead to relationship problems, its treatment should be preceded by both a sexologic and relationship assessment.

Psychotherapy

A number of different psychotherapeutic approaches to PE have been described, but their efficacy have not been evaluated in properly controlled and adequately powered trials, and the different therapeutic modalities have not been compared in formal studies.

It is likely that only some men seeking treatment for PE require in-depth psychotherapy. In spite of hard evidence on the efficacy of psychotherapy, behavioral retraining is still often practiced by sexologists. Behavioral treatment is distinguished in the "stop-start" and the "squeeze" [11,68]. The basis of behavioral retraining is the hypothesis that PE occurs because the man fails to appreciate the sensations of heightened arousal and recognize the feelings of ejaculatory inevitability.

Stop-start method

In the first step of the "stop-start" process, the penis is manually stimulated until the man is fairly highly aroused at which point stimulation is stopped. When his arousal subsides, stimulation recommences and continues until a high level of arousal is again achieved when stimulation is stopped. This sequence is repeated at least four times before stimulation continues to ejaculation. The process is repeated three or more times a week. The aim is to increase the duration of stimulation the man can receive before needing to stop.

The second step is almost identical to the first. The only difference is that the patient's partner applies the manual penile stimulation and the patient tells her when he wants her to pause and then re-start. The next step is penile containment in the "quiet vagina". The woman sits astride the man and accepts the penis in her vagina without any thrusting. Artificial lubricant is used if necessary. The couple is encouraged to remain in this position, without any coital thrusting, for prolonged periods so the man can experience and learn to enjoy the feeling of being inside the vagina. The woman then starts gentle coital thrusting movement until the man tells her to stop because he is nearing ejaculation. She can vary the tempo and depth of thrusting to allow the man to discover what movements he finds over-stimulating and these can be avoided. Movements then stop until the feelings of imminent ejaculation subside, and the process is repeated at least four times before thrusting continues to ejaculation.

The squeeze technique

The squeeze technique is essentially the same as the stop-start process described above except that at the time stimulation is stopped, the penis is squeezed firmly between the thumb and the first two fingers applied to the ventral and dorsal aspects of the coronal sulcus with the thumb applied to the frenulum. During the final step of the programme when the penis is stimulated within the vagina, the woman lifts herself off the penis and applies the squeeze until the man's arousal subsides. The squeeze aims to facilitate loss of arousal but some men find it has the opposite effect, in which case the squeeze is abandoned.

Concurrent with practicing the stop-start process, the couple is encouraged to spend time in mutual pleasuring involving non-genital massage and caressing, following the programme known as "sensate focus". This is essential to reduce the genital-focused interaction of the ejaculatory control process. It is also essential for the man to be encouraged to satisfy the sexual needs of his partner during the training programme.

There are initiations on the use of these therapy processes. The man needs a cooperative partner and sufficient time to follow the programme properly. Manual penile stimulation must be culturally acceptable. The therapist should be experienced in treating PE and have sufficient time to assess the patient

and his partner, to teach the therapeutic processes, and to provide adequate follow-up.

Although success rates in the short term from 60% to almost 100% have been reported [11,69], the methodology and design of these studies have been weak and fail to meet the criteria of evidence-based research. In addition, long-term maintenance of ejaculatory control induced by these treatment has shown to be very low [70].

Surgery

Several authors have reported the use of surgically-induced penile hypo-anesthesia via selective dorsal nerve neurectomy, or hyaluronic acid gel glans penis augmentation, in the treatment of lifelong PE refractory to behavioral and/or pharmacologic treatment [71,72]. This is based on the hypothesis that some men with PE have penile hypersensitivity. In selective dorsal neurectomy, several branches of the dorsal nerve of the penis are severed. The exact role of selective dorsal nerve neurectomy in the management of PE remains unclear and is currently under investigation as one of the methods of reducing penile sensation in selected patients with penile hypersensitivity that do not like to use topical anesthetics.

Future aspects

The use of various SSRIs, clomipramine, and topical anesthetics, along with the development of new on-demand drugs for the treatment of PE, has drawn new attention to this age-old and benignly ignored problem. Drug combinations or single agents that target multiple 5-HT receptors may represent the next stage of PE drug development. The resulting spate of recent research is providing greater understanding of the problem, and equally important, the negative psychosocial effects of this dysfunction. However, until the neurobiologic, physiologic and psychologic mechanisms responsible for PE are better understood, treatment strategies for PE may fall short. Because ejaculation depends upon the complex interplay of central and peripheral somatic and autonomic nervous systems, and various neurochemical regulatory pathways, a complete understanding of PE undoubtedly lies some distance down the road.

The challenge will be to find ways to integrate drug treatment and behavioral psychotherapy into a multi-dimensional treatment plan. Both drug treatment and psychotherapy are limited in that they represent symptomatic treatments for controlling and delaying ejaculation. Furthermore, the irreversible nature of surgical procedures relegates them to last-resort strategies. The goal of treatment should be to improve the level of sexual satisfaction of both sufferer and partner by offering a variety of tools and treatment options that afford greater self-efficacy over their sexual response with their partner. To this end, further investigation into the ways in which biomedical and psychologic strategies can combine to achieve optimal outcomes is greatly needed.

Inhibited Ejaculation and Anejaculation

Epidemiology

Inhibited ejaculation (IE) is less common than PE. The prevalence of IE in the general male population was found to be 1.5 in 1000 [73]. The prevalence of acquired IE in men below the age of 65 years was 3 to 4% [73].

IE can be classified as either lifelong or acquired. It may be global, occurring with every sexual encounter and all sexual partners, or it may be intermittent and situational. Some men with acquired IE can masturbate to orgasm, whereas others will or cannot. Approximately 75% of a recent clinical sample could reach orgasm through masturbation [74]. As is the case with other types of sexual dysfunction, men with IE may report significantly higher levels of personal and relationship distress, sexual dissatisfaction, sexual performance anxiety and general health issues compared to sexually-functional controls [10,75]. A distinguishing characteristic of these men is that they typically have no difficulty attaining or keeping their erections, yet report lower levels of subjective sexual arousal compared with sexually-functional controls [76].

Etiology and risk

Any single or combination of psychologic or medical diseases, surgical procedure or drugs that interfere with either central control of ejaculation, the affer-

Table 16.1 Causes of delayed ejaculation, anejaculation and anorgasmia.

Psychogenic	Inhibited ejaculation
Congenital	Mullerian duct cyst
	Wolfian duct abnormality
	Prune belly syndrome
Anatomic Causes	Transurethral resection of prostate
	Bladder neck incision
Neurogenic Causes	Diabetic autonomic neuropathy
	Spinal cord injury
	Radical cystectomy or prostatectomy
	Proctocolectomy
	Bilateral sympathectomy
	Abdominal aortic aneurysmectomy
	Para-aortic lymphadenectomy
Infective	Urethritis
	Genito–urinary tuberculosis
	Schistosomiasis
Endocrine	Hypogonadism
	Hypothyroidism
Medication	Alpha-methyl dopa
	Thiazide diuretics
	Tricyclic and SSRI antidepressants
	Phenothiazine
	Alcohol abuse

ent or efferent nerve supply to the vas, bladder neck, pelvic floor or penis, can result in IE, anejaculation and anorgasmia (Table 16.1). However, the majority of men with IE have no clear somatic etiology. Rather than assuming a psychogenic etiology for these men, their classification should be verified through an appropriate psychosexual history. Similar to other sexual problems, most cases of IE result from a mix of organogenic and psychogenic factors.

Organogenic

In the discussion of organogenic causes of IE, it is essential to distinguish between "physiologic" and "pathophysiologic" factors. "Physiologic" refers to those that are biologically inherent to the system, perhaps "hardwired" through genetic and normal maturational processes. "Pathophysiologic" refers to

Table 16.2 Correlation of erection, ejaculation and intercourse with level and severity of spinal cord injury [81].

Cord lesion		Reflexogenic erections (%)	Psychogenic erections (%)	Successful coitus (%)	Ejaculation (%)
Upper motor	Complete	92	9	66	1
neuron	Incomplete	93	48	86	22
Lower motor	Complete	0	24	33	15
neuron	Incomplete	0	1	100	100

those that are medical and occur through disruption of the normal physiologic processes, through disease, trauma, surgery, medication and so on. Pathophysiologic causes of RE are far more readily identifiable and generally surface during a medical history and examination. They typically stem from predictable sources: anomalous anatomic, surgical, neuropathic, endocrine, and medication (iatrogenic). For example, surgical therapy for prostatic obstruction is likely to disrupt bladder neck competence during emission. All types of IE show an age-related increase in prevalence and increased severity, with lower urinary tract symptoms independent of age [77,78]. Commonly-used medications, particularly antidepressants, may centrally inhibit or delay ejaculation as well [79].

The ability to ejaculate is severely impaired by spinal cord injury (SCI) and is dependent upon the level and completeness of SCI [80]. Unlike erectile capacity, the ability to ejaculate increases with descending levels of spinal injury [81] (Table 16.2). Less than 5% of patients with complete upper motor neuron lesions retain the ability to ejaculate. Semen for use with artificial reproductive techniques may be obtained from men with SCI by vibratory stimulation, electro-ejaculation, or percutaneous aspiration of semen from the vas deferens [82–84]. Testicular biopsies in spinal cord injured men demonstrate a wide range of testicular dysfunction, and sperm density and motility are higher in men with incomplete lesions [85].

More difficult to identify are inherent physiologic factors that account for variation in ejaculatory latency and thus might play a role in IE (particularly primary anorgasmia). Low penile sensitivity, most often associated with aging, may exacerbate difficulty with reaching orgasm, but it is unlikely to be a primary cause [86,87]. Alternatively, variability in the sensitivity of the ejaculatory reflex may be a factor, as several studies have demonstrated shorter latencies and stronger bulbocavernous EMG and ERP responses in men with ejaculation. However, ejaculatory response and latency are more likely to result from an interaction between higher cortical (cognitive–affective–arousal), supraspinal, spinal, and peripheral neuron systems [88].

Psychogenic

Multiple psychosocial explanations have been offered for IE, with unconscious aggression, unexpressed anger, malingering, and fear of pregnancy, recurring as themes in the psychoanalytic literature. Religious orthodoxy may be a factor in some instances, the idea being that certain beliefs may limit the sexual experience necessary for developing the knowledge necessary to learn to ejaculate, or may result in an inhibition of normal function [11].

Although religious orthodoxy may play a role for some men (e.g. 35% of a recent clinical sample), the majority do not fall into this category [74]. A number of relevant behavioral, psychologic, and relationship factors appear to contribute to difficulty reaching orgasm for these men. For example, men with IE sometimes indicate greater arousal and enjoyment from masturbation than from intercourse [75]. This "autosexual" orientation may involve an idiosyncratic and vigorous masturbation style, carried out with high frequency, and is dissimilar to what the man experiences with a partner [74]. Apfelbaum labels this as a desire disorder specific to partnered sex [89]. Consistent with this idea, recent data indicate that, unlike sexually-functional men, or men with other sexual dysfunctions, men with IE report better erections during masturbation than during foreplay or intercourse [75]. Disparity between the reality of sex with the partner and the sexual fantasy (whether or not unconventional) used during masturbation, is another potential cause of IE [90]. This disparity takes many forms, such as partner attractiveness and body type, sexual orientation, and the specific sex activity performed. In summary, high-frequency, idiosyncratic masturbation, combined with fantasy/partner disparity, may well predispose men to experiencing problems with arousal and ejaculation [76].

The above patterns suggest that IE men, rather than withholding ejaculation as suggested by earlier psychoanalytic interpretations, may lack sufficient psychosexual arousal during coitus to achieve orgasm. That is, their arousal response to their partner cannot match their response to self-stimulation and self-generated fantasy. In this respect, IE is thought to be due to difficulties in psychosexual arousal. This is supported by psychophysiologic research demonstrating that although men with IE attain erections comparable to sexually-functional controls, or men with PE during visual and penile psychosexual stimulation, they report far lower levels of subjective sexual arousal [75,76]. Apfelbaum has suggested that the couple interprets the man's strong erectile response as erroneous evidence that he is ready for sex and capable of achieving orgasm [89].

Finally, the evaluative/performance aspect of sex with a partner often creates "sexual performance anxiety" for the man, a factor that may contribute to IE. Such anxiety typically stems from the man's lack of confidence to perform adequately, to appear and feel attractive (body image), to satisfy his partner sexually, and to experience an overall sense of self-efficacy [91,92]. The impact of this anxiety on men's sexual response varies depending on the individual and the situation, but in some men it may interfere with the ability to respond adequately. With respect to IE, anxiety surrounding the inability to ejaculate may draw the man's attention away from erotic cues that normally serve to enhance arousal. Apfelbaum,

for example, has emphasized the need to remove the "demand" (and thus anxiety-producing) characteristics of the situation, noting that men with IE may be over-conscientious about pleasing their partner [89]. This "ejaculatory performance" anxiety interferes with the erotic sensations of genital stimulation, resulting in levels of sexual excitement and arousal that are insufficient for climax (although more than adequate to maintain their erections).

Diagnosis and Evaluation

Although no clear operationalized criteria exist for IE, given that most sexually-functional men ejaculate within about three to eight minutes following intromission, a clinician might assume that men with latencies beyond 20 or 30 minutes (and who experience consequent distress), or men who simply cease sexual activity due to exhaustion or irritation, qualify for this diagnosis [39]. Such symptoms, together with the fact that a man and/or his partner decide to seek help for the problem, are usually sufficient for the IE diagnosis.

The diagnostic evaluation of ejaculatory dysfunction focuses on finding potential physical and specific psychologic/learned causes of the disorder. A medical (particularly genito–urinary) examination and history are critical, as these may uncover physical anomalies, various pathophysiologies, and iatrogenic procedures associated with the IE. In addition, concomitant or contributory neurologic, endocrinergic, or erectile disorders can be identified and addressed. Particular attention should be given to identifying reversible urethral, prostatic, epididymal, and testicular infections. Given the lack of understanding of basic physiologic mechanisms responsible for the timing of ejaculation, assessment procedures tapping into the basic physiology of the ejaculatory reflex (e.g. sensory thresholds or efferent reactivity) have to date not been particularly meaningful or useful for the management of this dysfunction.

A focused psychosexual evaluation, important even to a diagnosis that is primarily pathophysiologic, is critical for men with no obvious somatic etiology. Evaluation typically begins by differentiating this sexual dysfunction from other sexual problems (e.g.

terminating intercourse due to pain), and reviewing the conditions under which the man is able to ejaculate, (e.g. during sleep, with masturbation, with partner's hand or mouth stimulation, or infrequently, with varying coital positions). Domains related to the psychologic and relationship issues commonly associated with IE (identified in the previous section) require investigation. Thus, the developmental course of the problem, including predisposing issues of religiosity, and variables that improve or worsen performance, particularly those related to psychosexual arousal, should be noted. Coital and masturbatory patterns, perceived partner attractiveness, the use of fantasy during sex, and anxiety surrounding performance, require exploration. If orgasmic attainment had been possible previously, the clinician should review the life events/circumstances temporally related to orgasmic cessation events in question, which may be pharmaceuticals, illness, or a variety of life stressors and other psychologic factors previously highlighted in the section on etiology. Generally, a complete evaluation should identify all possible predisposing, precipitating, and maintaining factors for the dysfunction.

Since many men attempt their own remedies, the patient's previous approaches to improving ejaculatory response should be investigated, including the use of herbal or folk therapies, prior treatments, and home remedies (e.g. using particular cognitive or behavioral strategies). Information regarding the partners' perception of the problem and their satisfaction with the overall relationship is often helpful. Once this body of knowledge is complete, an appropriate treatment plan, developed in conjunction with the couple, can be implemented.

Therapy
Psychologic
The man who presents with inhibited ejaculation, in whom organic and pharmacologic causes have been eliminated by careful medical assessment and investigation, requires thorough psychosexual assessment. If he is in a relationship, his partner, and the quality of the relationship, also require evaluation. Numerous psychotherapeutic processes are described for the management of inhibited ejaculation, but none has been properly evaluated [11,18,89,93].

Therapists generally devise their own therapy approaches based on the following:

1 *Sex education.* Dispelling myths, sexual response and physiology, stimulation techniques, orgasm triggers (e.g. pelvic floor contraction, arching foot and pointing toes etc.).

2 *Reduction of goal-focused anxiety.* Prohibition of ejaculation during masturbation and/or partner-related sexual activity.

3 *Increased, more genitally-focused stimulation.* Some therapists advocate anal and rectal stimulation by finger or vibrator.

4 *Patient role-playing an exaggerated ejaculatory response on his own and in front of his partner.* This can be especially helpful where the man's inability to ejaculate arises from the embarrassment the patient thinks he will experience when he loses emotional control during ejaculation.

The man with situational inhibited ejaculation who is able to ejaculate on his own but not with a partner undergoes a desensitizing programme. First, he masturbates on his own imagining that his partner is present. He continues stimulation, by whatever means he usually uses, to high levels of sexual arousal. He is told to try not to ejaculate (to reduce goal-focused anxiety), but rather to prolong stimulation so that he can enjoy long periods of heightened arousal. After a few sessions he finds he is unable not to ejaculate. He repeats this exercise on three or four subsequent occasions. He then repeats the process in the following sequence of situations:

• He is in a room adjacent to the room occupied by his partner, with the door between the rooms shut
• He is in a room adjacent to the room occupied by his partner, with the door between the rooms open
• He is in the same room as his partner
• He is on the same bed as his partner; the partner is not involved in the stimulation process
• He begins to masturbate until nearing ejaculation when his partner takes over by providing manual or oral stimulation
• Partner takes over stimulation at progressively earlier times
• Patient masturbates with partner sitting astride him and she lowers herself on to his penis just before ejaculation so that ejaculation occurs between labia.
• As before but with deeper vaginal penetration

The success of treating inhibited ejaculation is difficult to assess from the literature, as most reports relate to single cases or small series of cases. Authors are more likely to publish cases with successful outcome than treatment failures.

Pharmacotherapy

A variety of drugs have been reported as treatments of drug-induced delayed ejaculation. [94–105] The drugs facilitate ejaculation by either a central dopaminergic or anti-serotonergic mechanism of action. However, there are no published placebo-controlled studies and most reports are anecdotal case reports/series of men with anti-depressant or anti-psychotic drug induced IE.

5-HT receptor antagonists

Cyproheptadine, a serotonin (5-HT) receptor antagonist has been shown to increase male sexual activity in the rat [106]. Several anecdotal case reports and small case series mention success of the use of cyproheptadine to reverse the anorgasmia induced by the SSRI antidepressants. However, controlled studies have not been published [94,97,98]. The case reports suggest an effective dose range of 2 to 16 mg, administration on a chronic or "on-demand" basis.

Dopaminergic drugs

Central dopamine activity can be increased by a variety of mechanisms ranging from the use of dopamine synthesis precursors, e.g. L-dopa or substitute neurotransmitters, to direct stimulation of central dopamine receptors.

Amantadine is an indirect stimulant of dopaminergic nerves both centrally and peripherally, and has been reported to stimulate sexual behavior, ejaculation and other sexual reflexes in rats [107,108]. Several authors have reported their experience with 100 to 200 mg amantadine in the reversal of SSRI antidepressant-induced anorgasmia [95–97, 99–101].

Apomorphine, a central and peripheral DA-2 receptor agonist, has been reported to induce early ejaculation in rats by several authors. Dopamine receptor antagonists block this effect [109,110].

Yohimbine is an α-2 antagonist, an α-1 agonist, a calcium channel blocker, and inhibits platelet aggregation. Price and Grunhaus reported reversal of clomipramine-induced anorgasmia with a dose of 10 mg administered 90 minutes prior to coitus [102]. In a placebo-controlled study of 15 patients with fluoxetine-induced anorgasmia, Jacobsen reported a 73% response rate to yohimbine [103]. The response to yohimbine is typically delayed, taking up to eight weeks, and is often associated with adverse effects including nausea, headache, dizziness, and anxiety. Careful dose titration is important as the extremes of dose have less pro-sexual effect.

5-HT1A receptor agonist

Buspirone is a 5-HT1A receptor agonist [111]. Othmer *et al.* reported normalization of sexual function in eight out of 10 men with a generalized anxiety disorder and associated sexual dysfunction, using a dose range of 15 to 60 mg daily [104].

Dopamine reuptake inhibitor

Bupropion is a dopamine reuptake inhibitor [112]. Ashton and Rosen described reversal of SSRI-induced anorgasmia in 66% of patients studied [105].

Future aspects

Inhibited ejaculation has been less well researched than PE, probably because fewer cases are seen. The etiology of inhibited ejaculation is multifactorial and includes organic and psychologic distur-bances; pharmacologic agents are also implicated. Improved techniques for clinical evaluation are required.

Except where a treatable organic cause has been identified or a drug known to impair ejaculatory function has been withdrawn, the mainstay of treatment is by psychotherapy, but this is not evidence-based, as the most successful psychotherapeutic intervention has not been established. Future research should address this shortcoming. A number of pharmacologic agents are reported to treat drug-induced delayed (inhibited) ejaculation, but these observations are not based on well-controlled and adequately powered studies, but rather on single cases or small series of cases. The pharmacotherapy of inhibited ejaculation requires proper evaluation.

Retrograde Ejaculation

Etiology and risk factors

Antegrade ejaculation requires a closed bladder neck and proximal urethra. Retrograde ejaculation (RE) may be caused by anatomic, neurologic, pharmacologic, or idiopathic factors [113–116].

• *Anatomic causes*: Anatomic causes include congenital (urethral valves, congenital defects of the hemitrigone, congenital dysfunction of the hemitrigone, or bladder exstrophy), or acquired (urethral stricture, bladder neck resection or fibrosis, and transurethral or open prostatectomy).

• *Neurologic causes*: These are usually secondary to disorders that interfere with the ability of the bladder neck to close during emission: spinal cord injury, multiple sclerosis, autonomic neuropathy (diabetes), retroperitoneal lymphadenectomy (usually performed for testicular cancer), sympathectomy, and colorectal and anal surgery.

• *Pharmacologic causes*: Multiple drug classes may be associated with retrograde ejaculation as an adverse effect. The mechanism usually involves paralysis of the bladder neck by certain types of medications including antihypertensive drugs (phenoxybenzamine, clonidine, guanethidine, thiazide diuretics), α1-blocking drugs (alfuzosin, phenoxybenzamine, prazosin, tamsulosin, terazosin), antipsychotics drugs (chlorpromazine fluphenazine, levomepromazine, thioridazine, trifluoperazine, thioxitene, zuclopenthixol), and all classes of antidepressant drugs.

• *Idiopathic causes*: Occasionally a clear etiology cannot be identified.

Diagnosis

The diagnosis of RE can be often made obviously with a history of previous surgical procedure. Retrograde ejaculation can be confirmed by demonstration of sperm in an analysis of a post-ejaculation urine sample [114]. Patients with absent and even low-volume ejaculate should be evaluated with a post-ejaculation urine specimen as retrograde ejaculation is frequently combined with antegrade ejaculation [117].

Examination of the post ejaculation urine is performed by centrifuging the specimen for 10 minutes at 300 g or more. In patients with absent ejaculation, the finding of greater than five to 10 sperm per high-power field in a post-ejaculation urine specimen confirms the presence of retrograde ejaculation. In patients with low-volume ejaculate, the finding of more sperm in the urine than in the antegrade ejaculate indicates a significant component of RE [117].

Treatment
Pharmacotherapy

The success of the treatment of the RE depends, to some extent, on the etiology. When RE is caused by a pharmacologic agent, withdrawal of the offending medication may reverse the RE. In other cases, medical treatment is based either on increasing the sympathetic tone of the bladder neck or decreasing the parasympathetic activity.

Pharmacotherapy has a particular place in the neurologic causes of RE; however its success is in direct relation with the magnitude (complete or partial) of the nerve damage (e.g. spinal cord injury, diabetes). In partial nerve damage medications may reverse RE. The most used drugs for the treatment of RE are adrenergic agents such as ephedrine (30 to 60 mg one hour before sexual activity), pseudoephedrine (60–120 mg two hours before sexual activity), or tricyclic antidepressant with anticholinergic effects such as desipramine (50 mg, one to two hours before sexual activity), or imipramine (25–75 mg three times a day) [113,114]. The success rate reported by different authors varied between 20 and 67% [115].

Surgery

When RE is due to surgical changes of the bladder neck, surgical techniques might be applied in attempt to treat this dysfunction. However, surgical treatment for RE are not commonly used, due to the success achieved with seminal fluid harvesting, sperm processing and assisted reproductive technology [118]. A few specific surgical techniques for treatment of RE have been reported [119–121].

Painful ejaculation

Painful ejaculation or odynorgasmia is a poorly-characterized syndrome and may be associated with benign prostatic hypertrophy (BPH), infection, or inflammation from acute prostatitis, chronic prostatitis/chronic pelvic pain syndrome, seminal vesiculitis, seminal vesicular calculi, or ejaculatory duct obstruction, a treatable cause of male infertility [122–125]. Nickel reported that 18.6% of men with lower urinary tract symptoms (LUTS) diagnosed with clinical benign prostatic hyperplasia reported painful ejaculation [123]. Men with BPH and painful ejaculation have more severe LUTS and reported greater bother, and had a higher prevalence of erectile dysfunction and reduced ejaculation, than men with LUTS only [78]. Treatment of men with LUTS with α-blocking drugs may be associated with painful ejaculation. A lower incidence of pain has been reported with the uroselective α-1 blocking drug, alfuzosin [126].

Painful ejaculation is a rarely reported side-effect of tricyclic and SSRI class antidepressants [127–129]. The severity of pain appears to be dose–dependent and may resolve with reduction of dose or use of a different drug. It has been suggested that partial blockade of peripheral sympathetic adrenergic receptors could interfere with coordinated contractions of smooth muscles involved in semen transport and thus induce painful spasms or retrograde ejaculation.

However no obvious etiologic factor can be found in a number of patients with painful ejaculation.

Future aspects

The development of new drugs for the treatment of BPH, hypertension, psychiatric disorders, among others, with selective action on central or peripheral receptors, should improve the therapeutic efficacy and minimize the adverse ejaculatory events. Careful anatomic studies should lead improvements in surgical techniques in order to decrease the incidence of RE as an unwanted side event. Examples of this are retroperitoneal lymph node dissection with nerve sparing, or trans-urethral resection of the prostate (TURP) with conservative of 1 cm of inframontanal urethra [116,130,131]. Last but not least, other important aspects to consider are the necessity to make good controlled clinical trials comparing different treatments, since the current data is

not clear enough in the criteria used to evaluate success.

Closing Comments

The diagnosis lifelong or acquired PE in daily clinical practice is not difficult and can be achieved with a careful medical and sexual history. Detailed evaluation with questionnaires or stopwatch is not required. Pivotal to the management of PE is the recognition that PE is a condition defined by the IELT and the dimensions of control, satisfaction and bother. Reliance on patient self-report is associated with a high level of false-positive diagnosis of PE, and consequential inappropriate treatment. However, the results of epidemiologic research, research for development of an evidence-based consensus of PE, and drug/psychotherapy treatment research, are only reliable, interpretable and capable of being generalized to patients with the disorder studied when conducted in well-defined and consistent populations, using a double-blind placebo-controlled study design, with consistent objective physiologic measures or sensitive, validated outcome assessment instruments as study endpoints.

The lack of agreement as to what constitutes PE has hampered basic and clinical research into the etiology and management of this condition. A consensus definition of PE should be evidence-based, trans-cultural and applicable in all parts of the world. The recent proposal for a definition of lifelong PE based on the 0.5 and 2.5 percentile of the IELT distribution in the general male population may contribute to a consensus, but more at-random IELT stopwatch studies should be conducted in the various parts of the world.

Although recent neuropharmacologic studies and animal research has deepened our understanding of neurobiology of PE and the mechanism of pharmacotherapy, a genuine understanding of the etiology of lifelong and acquired premature ejaculation is still lacking. Despite high levels of evidence from multiple well-controlled studies to support the efficacy of drug treatment strategies in lifelong PE, there is little or no evidence to support the role and longitudinal efficacy of behavioral therapy. As such, the place of behavioral therapy must be limited to a supportive role of pharmacotherapy in selected men and not as a first-line treatment. First-line treatment of lifelong PE is off-label daily use of some SSRIs—particularly paroxetine, sertraline and fluoxetine, and clomipramine, and the on-demand use of some SSRIs, clomipramine, and topical anesthetics, although the latter exert less ejaculation-delaying effects. Ejaculation-specific selective serotonin reuptake inhibitors (ESSRIs), such as dapoxetine, will clearly expand but not dominate or replace our current therapeutic armamentarium. Comparative studies are needed to investigate potential differences between both classes of SSRIs.

An effective treatment of lifelong inhibited ejaculation does not exist. It is therefore ethical to inform men at risk of developing IE secondary to surgery or drug treatment, and to discuss all treatment options for IE, emphasizing the lack of a universal response to psychotherapy.

References

1 Holstege G, Georgiadis JR, Paans AM, *et al.* Brain activation during human male ejaculation. *J Neurosci* 2003;**23**(27):9185–8193.

2 Levin RJ. The mechanisms of human ejaculation—a critical analysis. *Sex Rel Ther* 2005;**20**:123–131.

3 Giuliano F, Clement P. Physiology of ejaculation: emphasis on serotonergic control. *Eur Urol* 2005(in press).

4 Waldinger MD, Schweitzer DH, Olivier B. On-demand SSRI treatment of premature ejaculation: pharmacodynamic limitations for relevant ejaculation delay and consequent solutions. *J Sex Med* 2005;**2**:121–131.

5 Laumann EO, Paik A, Rosen RC. Sexual dysfunction in the United States: prevalence and predictors. *Jama* 1999;**281**(6):537–544.

6 Assalian P. Guidelines for the pharmacotherapy of premature ejaculation. *World J Urol* 2005;**12**:12.

7 Rowland DL, Cooper SE, Schneider M. Defining premature ejaculation for experimental and clinical investigations. *Arch Sex Behav* 2001;**30**(3):235–253.

8 Byers ES, Grenier G. Premature or rapid ejaculation: heterosexual couples' perceptions of men's ejaculatory behavior. *Arch Sex Behav* 2003;**32**(3):261–270.

9 St. Lawrence JS, Madakasira S. Evaluation and treatment of premature ejaculation: a critical review. *Int J Psychiatr Med* 1992;**22**:77.

10 Jannini EA, Lenzi A. Ejaculatory disorders: epidemiology and current approaches to definition, classification and subtyping. *World J Urol* 2005;**18**:18.

11 Masters WH, Johnson VE. *Human Sexual Inadequacy.* Boston: Little Brown, 1970, pp. 92–115.

12 American Psychiatric Association. *Diagnostic And Statistical Manual of Mental Disorders, DSM-IV,* 4th edn. Washington D.C., 1994, pp. 509–511.

13 World Health Organization. *International Classification of Diseases and Related Health Problems,* 10th edn. Geneva: World Health Organization, 1994.

14 Waldinger MD, Quinn P, Dilleen M, *et al.* A multinational population survey of intravaginal ejaculation latency time. *J Sex Med* 2005;**2**:492–497.

15 Waldinger MD, Zwinderman AH, Olivier B, Schweitzer DH. Proposal for a definition of lifelong premature ejaculation based on epidemiological stopwatch data. *J Sex Med* 2005;**2**(4):498–507.

16 Abraham K. Ueber Ejaculatio Praecox. *Zeitschr Aerztl Psychoanal* 1917;**4**:171.

17 Schapiro B. Premature ejaculation, a review of 1130 cases. *J Urol* 1943;**50**:374–379.

18 Kaplan HS. *The New Sex Therapy.* New York: Brunner/Mazel, 1974.

19 Assalian P. Clomipramine in the treatment of premature ejaculation. *J Sex Res* 1988;**24**:213–215.

20 Waldinger MD, Berendsen HH, Blok BF, Olivier B, Holstege G. Premature ejaculation and serotonergic antidepressants-induced delayed ejaculation: the involvement of the serotonergic system. *Behav Brain Res* 1998;**92**(2):111–118.

21 Pattij T, de Jong TR, Uitterdijk A, *et al.* Individual differences in male rat ejaculatory behavior: searching for models to study ejaculation disorders. *Eur J Neurosci* 2005;e-pub.

22 Carani C, Isidori AM, Granata A, *et al.* Multicenter study on the prevalence of sexual symptoms in male hypo- and hyperthyroid patients. *J Clin Endocrinol Metab* 2005;**90**(12):6472–6479.

23 Waldinger MD, Zwinderman AH, Olivier B, Schweitzer DH. Thyroid-stimulating hormone assessments in a Dutch cohort of 620 men with lifelong premature ejaculation without erectile dysfunction. *J Sex Med* 2005;**2**(6):865–870.

24 Pryor JL, Broderick GA, Ho KF, Jamieson C, Gagnon D. Comparison of estimated versus measured intravaginal ejaculatory latency time (IELT) in men with and without premature ejaculation (PE). incomplete 2005;ABSTRACT #126.

25 Grenier G, Byers S. Evaluating models of premature ejaculation: A review. *CJHS* 1992;**3**:115–122.

26 Symonds T, Althof SE, Rosen RC, Roblin D, Layton M. Questionnaire assessment of ejaculatory control: development and validation of a new instrument. *Int J Imp Res* 2002;**14**(suppl 4):S33:abstract PS-7-1.

27 Yuan YM, Xin ZC, Jiang H, *et al.* Sexual function of premature ejaculation patients assayed with Chinese Index of Premature Ejaculation. *Asian J Androl* 2004; **6**(2):121–126.

28 Rust J, Golombok S. The GRISS: a psychometric instrument for the assessment of sexual dysfunction. *Arch Sex Behav* 1986;**15**(2):157–165.

29 Waldinger MD, Zwinderman AH, Schweitzer DH, Olivier B. Relevance of methodological design for the interpretation of efficacy of drug treatment of premature ejaculation: a systematic review and meta-analysis. *Int J Impot Res* 2004;**16**(4):369–381.

30 Spiess WF, Geer JH, O'Donohue WT. Premature ejaculation: investigation of factors in ejaculatory latency. *J Abnorm Psychol* 1984;**93**(2):242–245.

31 Strassberg DS, Kelly MP, Carroll C, Kircher JC. The psychophysiological nature of premature ejaculation. *Arch Sex Behav* 1987;**16**(4):327–336.

32 Kilmann PR, Auerbach R. Treatments of premature ejaculation and psychogenic impotence: a critical review of the literature. *Arch Sex Behav* 1979;**8**(1):81–100.

33 Schover L, Friedman J, Weiler S, Heiman J, LoPiccolo J. Multiaxial problem-oriented system for sexual dysfunctions. *Arch Gen Psychiat* 1982;**39**:614–619.

34 Kaplan HS, Kohl RN, Pomeroy WB, Offit AK, Hogan B. Group treatment of premature ejaculation. *Arch Sex Behav* 1974;**3**(5):443–452.

35 McCarthy B. Cognitive-behavioural strategies and techniques in the treatment of early ejaculation. In: Leiblum SR, Rosen R, eds. *Principles and Practices of Sex Therapy*: Update for the 1990s. Guilford Press: New York, 1988, pp. 141–167.

36 Vandereycken W. Towards a better delineation of ejaculatory disorders. *Acta Psychiatr Belg* 1986;**86**(1): 57–63.

37 Grenier G, Byers ES. The relationships among ejaculatory control, ejaculatory latency, and attempts to prolong heterosexual intercourse. *Arch Sex Behav* 1997;**26**(1):27–47.

38 Waldinger M, Hengeveld M, Zwinderman A, Olivier B. An empirical operationalization of DSM-IV diagnostic criteria for premature ejaculation. *Int J Psychiatry Clin Pract* 1998;**2**:287–293.

39 Patrick DL, Althof SE, Pryor JL, *et al.* Premature ejaculation: An observational study of men and their partners. *J Sex Med* 2005;**2**(3):58–367.

40 Montague DK, Jarow J, Broderick GA, *et al.* AUA guideline on the pharmacologic management of premature ejaculation. *J Urol* 2004;**172**(1):290–294.

41 Lue TF, Basson R, Rosen RC, *et al.* Sexual Medicine-Sexual Dysfunctions in Men and Women. 2004.

42 McMahon CG. Long term results of treatment of premature ejaculation with selective serotonin re-uptake inhibitors. *Int J Imp Res* 2002;**14**(Suppl.3):S19.

43 Waldinger MD, Zwinderman AH, Olivier B. On-demand treatment of premature ejaculation with clomipramine and paroxetine: a randomized, double-blind fixed-dose study with stopwatch assessment. *Eur Urol* 2004;**46**(4):510–515.

44 Waldinger M. Towards evidenced-based drug treatment research on premature ejaculation: a critical evaluation of methodology. *J Impot Res* 2003; **15**(5):309–313.

45 Waldinger MD, Hengeveld MW, Zwinderman AH, Olivier B. Effect of SSRI antidepressants on ejaculation: a double-blind, randomized, placebo-controlled study with fluoxetine, fluvoxamine, paroxetine, and sertraline. *J Clin Psychopharmacol* 1998;**18**(4):274–281.

46 McMahon CG. Treatment of premature ejaculation with sertraline hydrochloride: a single-blind placebo controlled crossover study. *J Urol* 1998;**159**(6):1935–1938.

47 Strassberg DS, de Gouveia Brazao CA, Rowland DL, Tan P, Slob AK. Clomipramine in the treatment of rapid (premature) ejaculation. *J Sex Marital Ther* 1999; **25**(2):89–101.

48 Kim SW, Paick JS. Short-term analysis of the effects of as needed use of sertraline at 5 PM for the treatment of premature ejaculation. *Urology* 1999;**54**(3):544–547.

49 McMahon CG, Touma K. Treatment of premature ejaculation with paroxetine hydrochloride as needed: 2 single-blind placebo controlled crossover studies. *J Urol* 1999;**161**(6):1826–1830.

50 Hellstrom WJ, Gittelman M, Althof S. Dapoxetine HCl for the treatment of premature ejaculation: A Phase II, randomised, double-blind, placebo controlled study. *J Sex Med* 2004;**1**(suppl.1):59, 97.

51 Pryor JL, Althof SE, Steidle C, Miloslavsky M, Kell S. Efficacy and tolerability of dapoxetine in the treatment of premature ejaculation. *J Urol* 2005;**173**(4): 201, 740.

52 Cremers TI, De Boer P, Liao Y, *et al.* Augmentation with a 5-HT1A, but not a 5-HT1B receptor antagonist criti-

cally depends on the dose of citalopram. *Eur J Pharmacol* 2000;**397**:63–74.

53 Williamson IJ, Turner L, Woods K, Wayman CP, van der Graaf PH. The 5-HT1A receptor antagonist robalzotan enhances SSRI-induced ejaculation delay in the rat. *Brit J Pharmacol Biochem Behav* 2003;**138**(suppl1): PO32.

54 de Jong TR, Pattij T, Veening JG, *et al.* Citalopram combined with WAY 100,635 inhibits ejaculation and ejaculation-related Fos immunoreactivity. *Eur J Pharmacol* 2005;**509**(1):49–59. Epub 2005 Jan 21.

55 Berkovitch M, Keresteci AG, Koren G. Efficacy of prilocaine–lidocaine cream in the treatment of premature ejaculation. *J Urol* 1995;**154**(4):1360–1361.

56 Xin ZC, Choi YD, Lee SH, Choi HK. Efficacy of a topical agent SS-cream in the treatment of premature ejaculation: preliminary clinical studies. *Yonsei Med J* 1997; **38**(2):91–95.

57 Busato W, Galindo CC. Topical anaesthetic use for treating premature ejaculation: a double-blind, randomized, placebo-controlled study. *BJU Int* 2004; **93**(7):1018–1021.

58 Dawson TM, Snyder SH. Gases as biological messengers: nitric oxide carbon monoxide in the brain4. *J Neurosci* 1994;**14**:5147–5159.

59 Sato Y, Horita H, Kurohata T, Adachi H, Tsukamoto T. Effect of the nitric oxide level in the medial preoptic area on male copulatory behavior in rats. *Am J Physiol* 1998;**274**(1 Pt 2):R243–247.

60 Lorrain DS, Hull EM. Nitric oxide increases dopamine and serotonin release in the medial preoptic area. *Neuroreport* 1993;**5**(1):87–89.

61 Lorrain DS, Matuszewich L, Howard RV, Du J, Hull EM. Nitric oxide promotes medial preoptic dopamine release during male rat copulation. *Neuroreport* 1996; **8**(1):31–34.

62 Abdel-Hamid IA, El Naggar EA, El Gilany AH. Assessment of as needed use of pharmacotherapy and the pause-squeeze technique in premature ejaculation. *Int J Impot Res* 2001;**13**(1):41–45.

63 Salonia A, Maga T, Colombo R, *et al.* A prospective study comparing paroxetine alone versus paroxetine plus sildenafil in patients with premature ejaculation. *J Urol* 2002;**168**(6):2486–2489.

64 Chen J, Mabjeesh NJ, Matzkin H, Greenstein A. Efficacy of sildenafil as adjuvant therapy to selective serotonin reuptake inhibitor in alleviating premature ejaculation. *Urology* 2003;**61**(1):197–200.

65 Sommer F, Klotz T, Mathers MM. Treatment of premature ejaculation: a comparative Vardenafil and SSRI crossover study. *J Urol* 2005;**173**(4):202, abst.741.

66 Mattos RM, Lucon AM. Tadalafil and slow-release fluoxetine in premature ejaculation—a prospective study. *J Urol* 2005;**173**(4):239, abst.880.

67 McMahon CG, Stuckey B, Andersen ML. Efficacy of Viagra: Sildenafil citrate in men with premature ejaculation. *J Sex Med* 2005;**2**(3):368.

68 Semans JH. Premature ejaculation: a new approach. *South Med J* 1956;**49**(4):353–358.

69 Clarke M, Parry L. Premature ejaculation treated by the dual sex team method of Masters and Johnson. *Aust N Z J Psychiatry* 1973;**7**(3):200–205.

70 De Amicis LA, Goldberg DC, LoPiccolo J, Friedman J, Davies L. Clinical follow-up of couples treated for sexual dysfunction. *Arch Sex Behav* 1985;**14**(6): 467–489.

71 Kim JJ, Kwak TI, Jeon BG, Cheon J, Moon DG. Effects of glans penis augmentation using hyaluronic acid gel for premature ejaculation. *Int J Impot Res* 2004; **16**(6):547–551.

72 Choi HK, Rha KH. Premature ejaculation evaluation and treatment. In: Kim YC, Tan HM, eds. *APSIR Book on Erectile Dysfunction*. The Asia-Pacific Society for Impotence Research (APSIR), 1999, pp. 263–274.

73 Nathan SG. The epidemiology of the DSM-III psychosexual dysfunctions. *J Sex Marital Ther* 1986;**12**(4): 267–281.

74 Perelman M. Retarded ejaculation. *Curr Sex Hlth Rep* 2004;**1**(3):95–101.

75 Rowland DL, Van Diest S, Incrocci L, Slob AK. Psychosexual factors that differentiate men with inhibited ejaculation from men with no dysfunction or with another dysfunction. *J Sex Med* 2005;**2**:383–289.

76 Rowland DL, Keeney C, Slob AK. Sexual response in men with inhibited or retarded ejaculation. *Int J Impot Res* 2004;**16**(3):270–274.

77 Blanker MH, Bosch JL, Groeneveld FP, *et al.* Erectile and ejaculatory dysfunction in a community-based sample of men 50 to 78 years old: prevalence, concern, and relation to sexual activity. *Urology* 2001;**57**(4): 763–768.

78 Rosen R, Altwein J, Boyle P, *et al.* Lower urinary tract symptoms and male sexual dysfunction: the multinational survey of the aging male (MSAM-7). *Eur Urol* 2003;**44**(6):637–649.

79 Perelman MA, McMahon CG, Barada J. Evaluation and treatment of ejaculatory disorders. In: Lue TF, ed. *Atlas of Male Sexual Dysfunction*, Philadelphia: Current Medicine LLC, 2004, pp. 127–157.

80 Bors E, Comarr AE. Neurological disturbances of sexual function with special reference to 529 patients with spional cord injury. *Urol Surv* 1960;**10**:191.

81 Comarr AE. Sexual function among patients with spinal cord injury. *Urol Int* 1970;**25**(2):134–168.

82 Brindley GS. The fertility of men with spinal injuries. Paraplegia 1984;**22**(6):337–348.

83 Brindley GS. Sexual and reproductive problems of paraplegic men. *Oxf Rev Reprod Biol* 1986;**8**:214–222.

84 Hovatta O, von Smitten K. Sperm aspiration from vas deferens and in vitro fertilization in cases of non-treatable anejaculation. *Hum Reprod* 1993;**8**(10): 1689–1691.

85 Ohl DA, Bennett CJ, McCabe M, Menge AC, McGuire EJ. Predictors of success in electroejaculation of spinal cord injured men. *J Urol* 1989;**142**(6):1483–1486.

86 Rowland DL. Penile sensitivity in men: an overview of recent findings. *Urology* 1998;**52**(6):1101–1105.

87 Paick JS, Jeong H, Park MS. Penile sensitivity in men with premature ejaculation. *Int J Impot Res* 1998;**10**(4): 247–250.

88 Motofei IG, Rowland DL. The neurophysiology of ejaculation: developing perspectives. *BJU Int* 2005; in press.

89 Apfelbaum B. Retarded ejaculation: A much-misunderstood syndrome. In: Lieblum SR, Rosen RC, eds. *Principles and practice of sex therapy: Update for the 1990's* 2nd ed. New York: Guilford Press, 1989, pp. 168–206.

90 Perelman M. Sildenafil, sex therapy, and retarded ejaculation. *J Sex Educ Ther* 2001;**26**(1):13–21.

91 Zilbergeld B. *The New Male Sexuality*. New York: Bantam, 1992.

92 Althof SE, Lieblum SR, Chevert-Measson M, *et al.* Psychological and interpersonal dimensions of sexual function and dysfunction. In: Lue TF, Basson R, Rosen R, *et al.*, eds. *Sexual Medicine: Sexual Dysfunctions in Men and Women (2nd International Consultation on Sexual Dysfunctions)*. Paris: France, 2004, pp. 73–116.

93 McCarthy B. Strategies and techniques for the treatment of ejaculatory inhibition. *J Sex Ed Ther* 1981; **7**(2):20–23.

94 McCormick S, Olin J, Brotman AW. Reversal of fluoxetine-induced anorgasmia by cyproheptadine in two patients. *J Clin Psychiatry* 1990;**51**(9):383–384.

95 Balogh S, Hendricks S, Kang J. Treatment of fluoxetine-induced anorgasmia with amantadine. *J Clin Psychiatry* 1992;**53**(6):212–213.

96 Valevski A, Modai I, Zbarski E, Zemishlany Z, Weizman A. Effect of amantadine on sexual dysfunction in neuroleptic-treated male schizophrenic patients. *Clin Neuropharmacol* 1998;**21**(6):355–357.

97 Ashton K, Hamer R, Rosen R. Serotonin reuptake inhibitor-induced sexual dysfunction and its treatment: a large-scale retrospective study of 596 psychiatric outpatients. *J Sex Marital Ther* 1997;**23**(3):165–175.

98 Aizenberg D, Zemishlany Z, Weizman A. Cyproheptadine treatment of sexual dysfunction induced by serotonin reuptake inhibitors. *Clin Neuropharmacol.* 1995;**18**(4):320–324.

99 Balon R. Intermittent amantadine for fluoxetine-induced anorgasmia. *J Sex Marital Ther* 1996;**22**(4): 290–292.

100 Shrivastava R, Shrivastava S, Overweg N, Schmitt M. Amantadine in the treatment of sexual dysfunction associated with selective serotonin reuptake inhibitors. *J Clin Psychopharmacol* 1995;**15**(1):83–84.

101 Gitlin MJ. Treatment of sexual side effects with dopaminergic agents. *J Clin Psychiatry* 1995; **56**(3):124.

102 Price J, Grunhaus LJ. Treatment of clomipramine-induced anorgasmia with yohimbine: a case report. *J Clin Psychiatry* 1990;**51**(1):32–33.

103 Jacobsen FM. Fluoxetine-induced sexual dysfunction and an open trial of yohimbine. *J Clin Psychiatry* 1992; **53**(4):119–122.

104 Othmer E, Othmer SC. Effect of buspirone on sexual dysfunction in patients with generalized anxiety disorder. *J Clin Psychiatry* 1987;**48**(5):201–203.

105 Ashton AK, Rosen RC. Bupropion as an antidote for serotonin reuptake inhibitor-induced sexual dysfunction. *J Clin Psychiatry* 1998;**59**(3):112–115.

106 Menendez Abraham E, Moran Viesca P, Velasco Plaza A, Marin B. Modifications of the sexual activity in male rats following administration of antiserotoninergic drugs. *Behav Brain Res* 1988;**30**(3):251–258.

107 Ferraz MR, Santos R. Amantadine stimulates sexual behavior in male rats. *Pharmacol Biochem Behav* 1995; **51**(4):709–714.

108 Yells DP, Prendergast MA, Hendricks SE, Miller ME. Monoaminergic influences on temporal patterning of sexual behavior in male rats. *Physiol Behav* 1995; **58**(5):847–852.

109 Napoli-Farris L, Fratta W, Gessa GL. Stimulation of dopamine autoreceptors elicits "premature ejaculation" in rats. *Pharmacol Biochem Behav* 1984;**20**(1): 69–72.

110 Kaplan JM, Hao JX, Sodersten P. Apomorphine induces ejaculation in chronic decerebrate rats. *Neurosci Lett* 1991;**129**(2):205–208.

111 Witkin JM, Perez LA. Comparison of effects of buspirone and gepirone with benzodiazepines and antagonists of dopamine and serotonin receptors on punished behavior of rats. *Behav Pharmacol* 1989;**3**: 247–254.

112 Cooper BR, Hester TJ, Maxwell RA. Behavioral and biochemical effects of the antidepressant bupropion (Wellbutrin): evidence for selective blockade of dopamine uptake in vivo. *J Pharmacol Exp Ther* 1980; **215**(1):127–134.

113 Ralph DJ, Wylie KR. Ejaculatory disorders and sexual function. *BJU Int* 2005;**95**(9):1181–1186.

114 Colpi G, Weidner W, Jungwirth A, *et al.* EAU guidelines on ejaculatory dysfunction. *Eur Urol* 2004;**46**(5): 555–558.

115 Kamischke A, Nieschlag E. Treatment of retrograde ejaculation and anejaculation. *Hum Reprod Update* 1999;**5**(5):448–474.

116 Hendry WF, Althof SE, Benson GS, *et al.* Male orgasmic and ejaculatory disorders. In: Jardin A, Wagner G, Khoury S, *et al.*, eds. Erectile Dysfunction. Plymbridge, Plymouth UK; Paris, France: Health Publications Ltd., 2000, pp. 477–506.

117 Sigman M, Howards SS. Male infertility. In: Walsh PC, Retik AB, Darracott Vaughan Jr E, Wein AJ, eds. Campbell's Urology (7th ed). Philadelphia: WB Saunders Company, 1998.

118 Jimenez C, Grizard G, Pouly JL, Boucher D. Birth after combination of cryopreservation of sperm recovered from urine and intracytoplasmic sperm injection in a case of complete retrograde ejaculation. *Fertil Steril* 1997;**68**(3):542–544.

119 Abrahams JI, Solish GI, Boorjian P, Waterhouse RK. The surgical correction of retrograde ejaculation. *J Urol* 1975;**114**(6):888–890.

120 Ramadan AE, el-Demiry MI. Surgical correction of post-operative retrograde ejaculation. *Br J Urol* 1985; **57**(4):458–461.

121 Middleton RG, Urry RL. The Young-Dees operation for the correction of retrograde ejaculation. *J Urol* 1986; **136**(6):1208–1209.

122 Kochakarn W, Leenanupunth C, Muangman V, Ratana-Olarn K, Viseshsindh V. Ejaculatory duct obstruction in the infertile male: experience of 7 cases at Ramathibodi Hospital. *J Med Assoc Thai* 2001;**84**(8): 1148–1152.

123 Nickel JC, Elhilali M, Vallancien G. Benign prostatic hyperplasia (BPH) and prostatitis: prevalence of painful ejaculation in men with clinical BPH. *BJU Int* 2005;**95**(4):571–574.

124 Corriere JN, Jr. Painful ejaculation due to seminal vesicle calculi. *J Urol* 1997;**157**(2):626.

125 Weintraub MP, De Mouy E, Hellstrom WJ. Newer modalities in the diagnosis and treatment of ejaculatory duct obstruction. *J Urol* 1993;**150**(4):1150–1154.

126 van Moorselaar RJ, Hartung R, Emberton M, *et al.* Alfuzosin 10 mg once daily improves sexual function in men with lower urinary tract symptoms and concomitant sexual dysfunction. *BJU Int* 2005;**95**(4):603–608.

127 Aizenberg D, Zemishlany Z, Hermesh H, Karp L, Weizman A. Painful ejaculation associated with antidepressants in four patients. *J Clin Psychiatry* 1991; **52**(11):461–463.

128 Hsu JH, Shen WW. Male sexual side effects associated with antidepressants: a descriptive clinical study of 32 patients. *Int J Psychiatry Med* 1995;**25**(2):191–201.

129 Michael A. Venlafaxine-induced painful ejaculation. *Br J Psychiatry* 2000;**177**:282.

130 Hermabessiere J, Guy L, Boiteux JP. Human ejaculation: physiology, surgical conservation of ejaculation. *Prog Urol* 1999;**9**(2):305–309.

131 Hedlund H, Ek A. Ejaculation and sexual function after endoscopic bladder neck incision. *Br J Urol* 1985; **57**(2):164–167.

CHAPTER 17

Radical Pelvic Surgery-Associated Sexual Dysfunction

John Mulhall and Sidney Glina

While erectile dysfunction is the most well-appreciated radical pelvic surgery-associated sexual dysfunction, there are a number of others that deserve attention, namely penile length changes, Peyronie's disease and orgasm alterations.

Penile Length Alterations

There are a total of three analyses on this issue in the literature. Fraiman *et al.* studied 100 men less than six months after radical prostatectomy, and took preoperative and postoperative flaccid and erect measurements and demonstrated an overall mean reduction in erect penile length of 9% but a mean reduction in volume of 22 [1]. Munding *et al.* studied 31 men and measured penile length in the stretched flaccid state (accepted as equivalent to erect length) and showed that 71% had a decrease in penile length compared to preoperatively, with 48% of men demonstrating greater than a 1 cm loss and a range of loss of 0.5–4 cm [2]. Finally, Savoie *et al.* studied 63 patients with preoperative measurements followed by repeat measurement, at three months postoperatively, and demonstrated that 68% of patients had some degree of length loss. The authors also showed that in this population there was no difference between patients with erectile dysfunction (ED) and those without, postoperatively [3].

One of the commonest explanations given by urologists to patients is that the removal of the prostate results in shortening of the urethra, which leads to loss of penile length. However, the urethra is fixed at the urogenital diaphragm and cannot easily be retracted inwards and the bladder is in fact brought down to the urethra at this level for the fashioning of the vesico–urethral anastomosis. The reasons for penile volume changes may be related to three factors: (1) cavernous nerve injury associated structural alterations in the penis; (2) cavernosal hypoxia-induced structural changes in the penis; and (3) sympathetic hyper-innervation (competitive sprouting).

It is recognized that even in the hands of an experienced surgeon performing nerve sparing surgery, neuropraxia is likely to occur to the cavernous nerves. Some have suggested that the tunica albuginea may also undergo structural changes after radical prostatectomy; however, other than a small amount of data on post-radical prostatectomy (RP) Peyronie's disease, at this time there is no data to support tunical structural alterations [4]. It is recognized that neural injury leads to end-organ structural alterations. Carrier *et al.* in 1995 demonstrated that in a rat model of bilateral cavernous nerve transaction there was a significant reduction in nitric oxide synthase (NOS) staining of nerves as early as three weeks post-injury, and that these reductions were sustained at the six-month time point [5]. Shortly after, Klein *et al.* demonstrated that following cavernous nerve injury, the corporal smooth muscle demonstrated apoptotic changes [6]; these findings were confirmed by User *et al.* [7]. This latter group demonstrated that penile wet weight and DNA content were reduced in both unilateral and bilateral cavernous nerve injury models, the latter demonstrating greater changes. Of note, the apoptosis was mostly observed in the subtunical zone of the smooth muscle. Leungwattanaki *et al.* further demonstrated that cavernous neurotomy leads to upregulation of fibrogenic cytokines and collagenization of the corporal smooth muscle [8].

It has also been postulated that the chronic absence of erectile activity leads to a state of cavernosal hypoxia [9], although this concept is controversial and has not gained universal acceptance in the sexual medicine community. In the flaccid state, the corporal bodies have a venous pO_2, which has been shown in vitro to promote the secretion of fibrogenic cytokines such as transforming growth factor-β (TGF-β). During erection, the corporal smooth muscle is oxygenated and this results (in vitro at least) in the secretion of endogenous prostanoids (prostaglandin E_1, PGE_1), which in turn, switch off fibrogenic cytokine production [9]. Thus, the health of erectile tissue relies to some extent on the balance between erection and flaccidity. In the patient who has no erectile activity, such as frequently occurs in the earliest phases post-radical prostatectomy, the balance shifts in favor of hypoxia and collagen production. Sattar *et al.* have elegantly demonstrated that there may be a correlation between corporal smooth muscle content and intracavernosal pO_2 levels [10]. Moreland has published a large body of work demonstrating in cell culture models that corporal smooth muscle cells, when exposed to hypoxic conditions, preferentially secrete TGF-β, and this is altered to PGE_1 once the cells are exposed to normoxic conditions [11–12]. Sympathetic hyperinnervation (termed by some as competitive sprouting) refers to the concept that when autonomic nerves are injured, sympathetic fibers are biologically primed to recuperate from injury and regenerate more quickly, resulting in un-antagonized sympathetic tone in the end organ [13]. Following cavernous nerve injury, this phenomenon results in a state of hypertonia in the penis.

To synthesize these concepts into a working hypothesis, penile length changes can be divided into early and delayed changes. In response to the neural injury that occurs intraoperatively the cavernous nerves undergo Wallerian degeneration and, early on when sympathetic nerve function is in the ascendancy, as stated above, the penis is a hypertonic organ—an organ exhibiting sympathetic overdrive. Given the fact that the penile smooth muscle is highly contractile in response to adrenergic tone, this results in a penis that patients often refer to as "being drawn back in the body". A clinical scenario supporting this is the circumcised male whose penis early

after surgery appears incompletely circumcised or even uncircumcised. The clue that these changes are not the result of permanent structural sequelae is that upon gentle penile stretch the penis readily elongates from its buried position. It has been my experience that this hypertonic state is most pronounced within the first 3–6 months after surgery. More concerning are delayed structural changes. These result from true irreversible structural alterations in the corporal smooth muscle. These structural changes most probably result from a combination of factors (as described above)—neural injury-associated denervation, apoptosis, as well as cavernosal hypoxia-induced collagenization—in men who experience delayed return of erectile function. The difference between these changes and early hypertonicity is evidenced by the reduced or absent penile stretch in the group with permanent smooth muscle alterations. It is easy to appreciate how these alterations affect not only length but also girth. Finally, whether the institution of a pharmacologic penile rehabilitation program early after RP can abrogate these alterations, remains unanswered at this time.

Alterations in Orgasm

Most of the post-radical prostatectomy sexual dysfunction literature has focused specifically on erectile dysfunction, and changes in orgasm have been reported in post-prostatectomy patients [14–16]. Orgasm, which is often considered to be a goal and reinforcer of sexual behavior, remains the least understood phase of the sexual response cycle. Alterations in orgasm, and in particular its absence, are associated with significant reductions in emotional and physical satisfaction, which in turn may lead to sexual avoidance behavior and secondary relationship discord [17–18].

Barnas *et al.*, in a questionnaire–based analysis, demonstrated that orgasmic dysfunction is a relatively prevalent problem in the post-RP population [19]. The alterations identified in this study include complete absence of orgasm, alterations in intensity, and orgasmic pain. Decreased intensity of orgasm or the complete lack of orgasm was reported by 74% of the patients surveyed. Fourteen percent of the patient population experienced orgasmic pain (dysorgasmia) at some time after surgery. Goriunov *et al.* have reported on orgasm alterations in surgically-treated BPH patients [15]. This group reported that 188 of 818 (23%) such patients suffered from dysorgasmia after their surgery. Koeman reported pain during orgasm in 11% post-radical prostatectomy patients, and 82% complained of diminished orgasmic intensity after surgery [16]. Bergman's study of 43 men who had undergone cystoprostatectomy for bladder cancer found 25% of post-operatively sexually active men were unable to attain orgasm, and 17% of those able to achieve orgasm by masturbation found the sensation impaired [14]. Teg *et al.* reported that 36% post-prostatectomy patients who had benign prostatic hypertrophy (BPH) described their sensation of orgasm to be "different" after surgery [20].

The etiology of dysorgasmia is not well understood. It has been postulated that the physiologic bladder neck closure that occurs contemporaneous with orgasm in the men, translates into spasm of the vesico–urethral anastomosis, or pelvic floor musculature dystonia in the RP population. This phenomenon has been purported to be associated with penile and testicular pain in men with chronic pelvic pain disorder [21]. The latter group frequently reports orgasmic pain, and the similarity of the complaints between the two groups at this center are striking. The muscle spasm concept is supported by the experience that amelioration of dysorgasmia can be seen using the α-blocking agent tamsulosin (Boehinger-Ingelheim, Germany) [19]. In 98 patients, 77% patients reported improvement in pain and 8% noted complete resolution of their pain using tamsulosin, 0.4 mg po QD. Using a visual analog scale (0 to 10) for pain tamsulosin therapy resulted in a statistically significant decrease in pain, with a mean decrease of 2.7 points between pre- and post-treatment phases. Anorgasmia and decreased intensity of orgasm are most probably psychologic events, presumably related to the multiple issues that men with a diagnosis of prostate cancer and who have undergone major radical pelvic surgery experience.

Finally, recent attention has been focused on orgasm-associated urinary incontinence (OAI), what has become to be termed "climacturia". This troubling problem is a clear barrier to the resumption of satisfactory sexual relations for many couples. Lee *et al.* analyzed 42 sexually active men at least one year after RP [22]. All patients underwent IPSS score and uroflow analysis. Forty-five percent of men reported climacturia, 68% of these reported rare occurrence. Fifty-two percent of patients stated that this was not bothersome, but 21% said that this was bothersome to the partner. Age was not a predictor of climacturia. There was no association between Q max or IPSS and the incidence of climacturia ($P = 0.20$ and 0.15, respectively).

Aboussally *et al.* reported on the Cleveland Clinic experience of 200 patients evaluated, that 26 men experienced urine leak almost exclusively at the time of orgasm [23]. The average age of the patients was 62 years and there was no clear association with degree of nerve sparing or daytime continence level. Patients experienced anywhere from 3–120 ml of urine leak (by patient self-report) at the time of orgasm.

Most recently, Choi *et al.* at Memorial Sloan Kettering Cancer Center analyzed 392 patients for this problem [24]. Fourteen percent (47/392) reported orgasm-associated urine leak (OAI). No difference in OAI rates were noted based on nerve-sparing or type of radical pelvic surgery. Men reporting OAI were more likely to complain of penile length loss (44%) than men not reporting OAI (26%, $P < 0.01$). Likewise, they were more likely to report orgasm pain (18.5%) compared to men without OAI (2%, $p < 0.01$). On multivariate analysis, both factors remained predictive: reporting penile length loss, OR $= 2.25$, $P < 0.01$; orgasm pain, OR $= 10.42$, $P < 0.01$.

Peyronie's Disease

While not viewed as a classic risk factor of the development of Peyronie's disease, radical prostatectomy is being increasingly recognized as a potential correlate of acquired penile curvature. There is only a single report in the literature suggesting that men with ED following RP may also have Peyronie's disease [4]. Analyzing 100 men who presented with post-RP ED, 11% had what the authors termed fibrotic changes. Three-quarters of this latter group had palpable plaques. At 24 months after diagnosis, 50% were stable, 10% were improved from a deformity standpoint. Despite the dearth of literature on this issue it has been the experience at Memorial

Sloan Kettering Cancer Center that there is a distinct correlation between the performance of radical prostatectomy surgery and the development of Peyronie's disease. While some have suggested that spongiofibrosis may be the etiology secondary to catheter placement at the tie of surgery, the majority of patients have dorsal plaques—and think of the many thousands of men who have catheter placement intermittently or chronically (spinal cord injury) without Peyronie's disease development. Thus, it is possible that there is something unique about RP surgery and the development of Peyronie's disease. Might the neuropraxia that occurs at the time of RP in a genetically-susceptible patient result in tunical changes, just as can occur in corporal smooth muscle? Some have suggested that the sue of intra-cavernosal injections may be a precipitant of Peyronie's disease, yet most men at MSKCC who develop post-RP Peyronie's disease have plaques remote from the site of ICI. Furthermore, we see patients who present at eight weeks after surgery, having failed oral therapy, who have had no sexual activity since surgery, who wish to pursue ICI and upon their first injection have penile deformity without any plaque palpated preoperatively. Clearly, this is an area in which much new research will need to be conducted.

Erectile Dysfunction

It is estimated that 10% of all men presenting with erectile dysfunction suffer the condition as a result of surgical procedure—typically, radical pelvic surgery [25]. Major discrepancy exists in the literature regarding postoperative potency rates, with spontaneous erectile function cited as occurring in 30–80% of patients [26]. Thus, despite the advent of nerve-sparing techniques a significant percentage of men continue to suffer from erectile impairment following this operation. It is estimated that 50 000 men undergo radical prostatectomy in the USA alone each year. Given the long-term survival of post-radical prostatectomy, at any given time there may be more than one million men who live life following RP many of whom will experience long-term changes in sexual function after this operation.

Pathophysiology

Mechanistically, post-RP ED may be neurogenic, ar-

teriogenic, venogenic, mixed vascular (arterio–venogenic) or psychogenic in etiology and is generally multi-factorial in nature. Neurogenic impotence, while obviously occurring after cavernous nerve interruption, may also occur transiently following cavernous nerve traction and/or dissection. Even in the hands of expert nerve-sparing surgeons, temporary neural trauma may occur. It is believed that the primary mechanism of development of arteriogenic erectile dysfunction results from injury to accessory pudendal arteries [27]. Venogenic impotence (venocclusive dysfunction, venous leak) is based upon corporal smooth muscle collagenization and fibrosis, which is most probably the result of either apoptosis associated with neural injury, and/or disuse atrophy [7]. The venocclusive mechanism is a major determinant of success with vasoactive therapies. The venocclusive mechanism is dependent upon appropriate corporal smooth muscle expansion with resultant occlusion of the subtunical venules [28]. Failure to expand the corporal smooth muscle adequately because of structural alterations in the tissue results in failure to compress the subtunical venules present between the corporal smooth muscle and the tunica albuginea, resulting in venous leak.

In previous work, Mulhall *et al.* have examined the chronology of venous leak development post-radical prostatectomy, in patients with excellent preoperative erectile function who developed postoperative erectile dysfunction [29]. The incidence of venous leak, (suggestive of permanent, irreversible structural damage to the erectile tissue) was 8% <4 months postoperatively, 22% 4–8 months postoperatively, and 50% 8–12 months postoperatively. In this analysis no patient was treated with postoperative pharmacotherapy in any regimented fashion. More recent data, presented by Ohebshalom *et al.,* indicates that the post-RP penile vascular status is predictive of return of spontaneous erections, degree of erectile rigidity, and response to sildenafil [30]. These data also indicate that the prognosis is poor for the return of functional erections in the presence of abnormal end diastolic velocity values.

While psychogenic mechanisms receive very little attention [31,32], there is a group of men post-RP who suffer anxiety and/or erosion of self-confidence, over the 12–18 months postoperatively, and who experience poor sexual erections, but, with self-stimulation or nocturnally, have functional erections.

ED Minimizing Maneuvers

Nerve-sparing surgery

Nerve injury can occur at four time points during radical retropubic prostatectomy: at the time of urethral dissection, during lateral pedicle division, during dissection along the base of the prostate, and at the time of seminal vesicle dissection. Nerve trauma is classically thought of as occurring with cautery, ligation or avulsion; however, overly aggressive traction may lead to neuropraxia, and even this temporary trauma may result in structural sequelae in the corporal bodies that may limit the recovery of erectile function [7,8,33]. Donohue *et al.*, using a rat model of cavernous nerve injury, demonstrated that nerve exposure alone without any direct manipulation results in a significant reduction in erectile function as measured by intracavernous pressure generation in response to cavernous nerve stimulation [34]. There is a plethora of robust data supporting the concept that the greater the volume of nerve tissue preserved the better the spontaneous erectile function and the better the response to oral ED therapies [35–43].

Intraoperative neurostimulation

This technique was initially described by Lue [44] and was later formally developed as an intra-operative tool (CaverMap, Bluetorch Technologies, Ashland, MA) for nerve stimulation and tumescence monitoring. The tip of this device, which contains an array of electrodes, is placed over the (suspected) cavernous nerve and current is applied [45]. Tumescence is monitored by the presence of a penile strain gauge, which records changes in penile girth. The strain gauge system is sensitive enough that it can detect a 0.5% change (increase or decrease) in circumference. The initial study on Cavermap was reported by Klotz, in 21 men with functional erections prior to RP, who had application of the device intraoperatively. Postoperative erectile function assessment was performed using a questionnaire [45]. Of the 19 patients who had erectile function assessed postoperatively, the two men who had no intraoperative Cavermap response failed to have return of

functional erections after surgery. Ninety-four percent (16/17) who had a response had functional erections following surgery. This study demonstrated the feasibility of using intra-operative neurostimulation, and suggested that a Cavermap response may portend a better prognosis for postoperative erectile function.

Two years later, Klotz lead a Canadian-based multi-center study using nine different surgeons, which randomized men, in a single-blind fashion, to either use of Cavermap or no such use [46]. Erectile function was assessed using a questionnaire, and both penile tumescence and rigidity monitoring (Rigiscan™, Endocare); 53 patients were enrolled (26 patients in the control group, 27 in the Cavermap group) but only 35 were available for 12 month erectile function assessment. Of note, the margin positivity rate was 40%, although there was no difference in this rate between the two groups. Following prostate removal, 31/53 patients had a bilateral Cavermap response (+/+), 27/53 had a unilateral response (+/−), and 3/53 had no response (−/−) on either side. While there was no difference in the overall erectile rigidity between the groups, as assessed by Rigiscan (percentage of men with base rigidity ≥60%), the mean and median durations spent at ≥60% base rigidity was significantly higher in the positive response group: 15.9 and 3 minutes versus 2 and 1 minute, respectively. This work further supported the use of Cavermap.

In 2000, the Brendler group from University of Chicago, published their experience with Cavermap. 60 men with normal preoperative erectile function had Cavermap used during radical prostatectomy [47]. Postoperative erectile function was assessed using items extracted from the UCLA prostate cancer index (PCI). 80% of the entire group had a positive Cavermap response, 63% had a bilateral response, 26% unilateral, and 11% no response. At 12 months after surgery, 11/60 patients (18%) of patients had functional erections. In men with a +/+ response, 27% had functional erections, +/− 15%, and −/− no patient had return of functional erections.

The Vanderbilt group reported on their experience in 2001 [48]. Sixty-one patients underwent Cavermap stimulation during RP. BNS surgery was conducted in 76%, UNS in 8%, and NNS in 16%.

Following prostate removal 58% of the stimulations along the right NVB and 58% along the left NVB resulted in penile tumescence. However, 43% of stimulations along the bladder neck (non-specific stimulation) resulted in some change in penile girth. Based on these data the authors questioned the value of the device in the form (first generation) used at the time of this study. In follow-up to this work, Chang from the same center examined men who underwent prostatectomy with either BNS or NNS, coupled with intra-operative neurostimulation [49]. Twenty-two men underwent wide resection of the neurovascular bundles and all were impotent post-operatively. Intra-operatively, 16/22 had no response to neurostimulation; however, six patients demonstrated a response to the neurostimulator. Forty-one underwent bilateral nerve-sparing procedures and 27 were potent at one year of follow-up. Thirty of these 41 men had tumescence on intra-operative neurostimulation, with 24 of these 30 potent (80%) post-operatively. Thus, in this analysis, intra-operative Cavermap response predicted postoperative potency ($P = 0.017$).

In 2001, a multi-institutional study was published reviewing the experience of a group of acclaimed nerve-sparing prostatectomists [50]. Five surgeons enrolled a total of 50 patients for Cavermap stimulation during RP. All patients were <60 years of age and had clinically organ-confined prostate cancer. For inclusion, patients were required to score 4 or 5's on the erectile function domain of the IIEF questionnaire (4 refers to "most of the time", 5 to "always or nearly always", when questioned about the frequency of various parameters such as development of rigidity adequate for penetration, ability to maintain, satisfaction and confidence). Follow-up of the patients occurred at three, six and 12 months. Ninety percent of patients had BNS surgery, the remainder UNS surgery. This paper presents data in a similar fashion to the original Vanderbilt paper, in that it presents the number of stimulations attempted and the percentage that result in a positive Cavermap response: 336 for 100 NVB's (3.3 per nerve); 87.8% of all stimulations resulted in a positive response. Only 6.4% of all stimulations resulted in a tumescence response alone; 32.2% resulted in detumescence, and the remainder resulted in a combined tumescence/

detumescence response. Eighty-eight percent of all stimulations (295/336) elicited a positive response, while of 54 stimulations overlying nerve bundles that were resected (based on surgeon report), 29 (54%) resulted in no response. The authors concluded, based on these figures that Cavermap had a high sensitivity (88%) and a low specificity (54%). This work from a who's who of RP surgeons, based on specificity and sensitivity data, concluded that there was therefore little role for intra-operative neurostimulation.

The greatest limitation to the interpretation of Cavermap data is that the responses are compared to the surgeons' assessment of the integrity of the cavernous nerve that is being stimulated, and the latter is held as the gold standard. The Cavermap response tells us important information, that is, that there is some functional neural tissue present at the end of the case, but fails to quantify the degree of preservation and cannot account for postoperative factors that may be nerve threatening. Cavermap response may however indicate that this is a patient in whom oral phosphodiesterase-5 (PDE-5) inhibitor therapy may work. At this time, the use of intra-operative neurostimulation remains investigational until such time as a consensus can be arrived at regarding technical and interpretation issues.

Cavernous nerve interposition grafting

Resection of the neurovascular bundle (NVB) may be indicated in patients with high-grade disease, advanced unilateral or bilateral disease (multiple positive cores, length of positive core, high Gleason grade, suggestion of extracapsular extension on imaging), to decrease the risk of positive surgical margins. Positive surgical margins increase the chance of treatment failure. Extracapsular extension increases the risk of a positive margin and this occurs most frequently in the area of the NVB. Wide resection, which may include the NVB, decreases the risk of a positive surgical margin, but increases the chance of post-operative ED without intervention to restore continuity of the nerves. The initial experience using nerve grafts was in rodents over a decade ago [51]. Quinlan et al., at Johns Hopkins, used the genito–femoral nerve grafted between proximal and distal stumps of the rat cavernous nerve to demonstrate that this was technically feasible, and that it increased the chances of functional recovery of erections, although formal hemodynamic assessment of erectile response to cavernous nerve injury was not used then, as is currently standard. Following cavernous nerve resection, an assessment can be made of the ipsilateral or contralateral genito–femoral nerve (GNG) for caliber matching. If the caliber is acceptable then the GNG can be harvested and sutured with fine non-absorbable sutures between the two stumps of the cavernous nerve. If not, then the sural nerve can be harvested as described by Kim *et al.* [52].

The first report was by Kim *et al.* from Baylor discussing their experience with nine men, with excellent preoperative erectile function, who underwent non-nerve-sparing RP for locally extensive, high-grade prostate carcinoma [52]. All underwent bilateral sural nerve interposition grafting (SNG). Postoperative erectile function was assessed using patient interview, a questionnaire and Rigiscan™ analysis. Of the nine patients, one had spontaneously functioning erections at 14 months postoperatively. This experience demonstrated feasibility and encouraged these investigators to continue to accrue patients for SNG. The following year, they reported on their experience in 12 men in whom SNG and genito–femoral nerve interposition grafting (GNG) was performed [53]. The data from this analysis indicated that erections unassisted by medication and sufficient for sexual intercourse occurred in one third of patients; partial erections occurred in 42%, while the remainder had no return of erections. The mean IIEF erectile function domain scores for the three groups were 16 ± 10, 9 ± 10, and 7 ± 1, respectively. Erections with sildenafil use were achieved in 50% at 12 months after RP. Twelve potent men who had non-nerve-sparing surgery and had no grafting, acted as controls. In this latter group none had return of functional erections with or without sildenafil.

A follow-up study from the same group included 28 men who underwent bilateral cavernous nerve resection and SNG/GNG, 23 of whom had at least 12-month follow-up [54]. The data demonstrated that 26% of patients had spontaneous medically-unassisted erections sufficient for intercourse, 26% had partial erections, while 48% had no erectile activity whatsoever. In these three groups, the mean erectile function domain scores were 20 ± 6, 10 ± 5, and 6 ± 3, respectively. Of note, using sildenafil, the overall potency rate (ability to achieve vaginal penetration) was 43%. This contrasted to only 1/70 patients in their database who underwent bilateral nerve resection and who had return of functional erections.

The MD Anderson experience was published in 2003 [55]. Thirty men with functional erections preoperatively, underwent bilateral cavernous nerve resection and grafting. At a mean follow-up of 23 months, 18/30 (60%) had subjective and objective changes in penile tumescence with sexual stimulation. However, only 13 (43%) were capable of having sexual intercourse, seven without sildenafil (23%) and six (20%) with sildenafil.

One of the challenges to the propagation of interposition nerve grafting is the fact that bilateral deliberate nerve resection is uncommon, a point emphasized by Dr. Patrick Walsh in a recent journal editorial [56]. There is a dire need for the development and funding of randomized, controlled trials assessing the utility of nerve grafting. The question cannot be answered definitively in any other way, and the naysayers will continue to criticize until such data are available. In the world of prostate cancer however, this strategy ranks low on the list of priorities. The major criticisms of the data available thus far, besides the non-controlled nature of the studies, are the short duration of follow-up and the small patient numbers. Given the association between bilateral cavernous nerve resection and long-term failure to obtain spontaneous functional erections, or failure to gain a significant response to oral therapy, this technique appears to be a reasonable strategy to restore erectile function in men in whom bilateral nerve resection is either planned or is required intra-operatively. Thus, in the small group of men in whom bilateral cavernous nerve resection is required, it may be appropriate to offer cavernous nerve interposition grafting. However, at this time this procedure remains investigational.

Penile rehabilitation

The relationship between hypoxia and cavernosal fibrosis has been documented in at least two in vitro studies [9,57]. It is thought that hypoxia induces TGF-β1 expression that in turn accelerates collagenization of the corpus cavernosum smooth muscle, while at the same time decreasing the level of PGE_1, which may help protect from fibrosis. Since hypoxia of cavernous tissue is related to the blood supply, and the greatest blood supply occurs at time of erection, any neural damage that results in ED may expose the cavernous tissues to longer periods of hypoxia. Leungwattanakij et al. demonstrated in a cavernous neurotomy rat model that sharp neural injury resulted in an increase in hypoxia inducible factor-1 (HIF-1α) and TGF-$β_1$ as well as increase in cavernous tissue collagen synthesis [8]. In a landmark study, Montorsi et al. based a study on the assumption that the events of nocturnal erection supply the cavernous bodies with oxygenation that might protect them from developing fibrotic changes during the transient period of erectile dysfunction following nerve-sparing radical prostatectomy [58]. In their study they treated patients with three times per week intracavernosal injections of alprostadil. In this prospective study, 30 patients were enrolled, all potent, and all had nerve-sparing RP. Fifteen received three injections per week for 15 weeks; twelve completed the treatment. Despite the small sample size, the difference between treatment and control group was statistically significant. (Treatment group, 67% had erections good enough for intercourse; control group, 20%, $P < 0.01$.) However, this is to date the only evidence-based medicine for the role of penile rehabilitation with intracavernosal injections after radical prostatectomy; because of the small sample size used combined with the invasiveness of the treatment, there is a need for a larger confirmatory study.

A single human randomized, placebo-controlled study has been conducted examining the role of nightly sildenafil for six months following RP [59]. This analysis demonstrated the ability of this regimen to increase the rate of preservation of preoperative erectile function (based on validated inventory assessments) at 48 weeks in the sildenafil arm compared to the placebo arm (27% vs. 4%, respectively). In another non-controlled study, Schwartz et al. gave either 50 mg or 100 mg of sildenafil on alternate nights for six months after RP [60]. Patients had a percutaneous biopsy before RP and after six months of sildenafil treatment. Comparing the smooth muscle content of the post-treatment biopsy to the pre-

operative biopsy, no change was demonstrated in the 50 mg group, but an increase in smooth muscle content was noted in the 100 mg group. In an animal study, Donohue et al. used doses of 10 mg/kg and 20 mg/kg of sildenafil, given at induction of anesthesia and continued daily, which results in trough serum levels comparable to levels obtained with 50 mg and 100 mg tablets, respectively, in man [61]. Daily subcutaneous sildenafil administration at both doses showed an improvement in the mean ICP/MAP ratio compared to control. The control group demonstrated improvement in erectile function over time, with the ICP/MAP ratio rising from $18 \pm 6\%$ at three days to $31 \pm 9\%$ at 10 days, remaining relatively unchanged at 28 days ($32 \pm 5\%$). The 10 mg/kg group showed higher ICP/MAP ratios at all time points compared to control, but these changes were not statistically significant. Further improvement in a dose- and time-dependent manner was demonstrated by the 20 mg/kg group, with maximal improvement shown at 28 days with an ICP/MAP ratio of $45 \pm 6\%$ ($P = 0.01$) noted. Mean sham ICP/MAP ratios were 70%. Thus, there exists human and animal evidence that ICI and regular sildenafil (and possible PDE5 inhibitors in general) use may translate into greater preservation of erectile function. In the absence of a large, multi-center, randomized controlled trial assessing the utility of a formal penile rehab regimen, this approach to post-RP care remains investigational.

To date, there has been no formal analysis of what represents the optimal rehabilitation program and thus giving the reader formal guidelines is difficult. Figure 17.1 represents the approach at MSKCC, although this is not to say that this is the only approach. The algorithm is based on the animal and human data at this time that there is probably a value to erections, that there is probably an adjunctive value to regular PDE5 inhibitor use.

Neuromodulatory drugs

The term nerve sparing essentially means that the surgeon using his experience and expertise defines if the nerves are anatomically and macroscopically intact. This may have less than perfect correlation with the actual functional integrity of the cavernous nerves. In animal models there is a plethora of literature associating cavernous nerve injury with corpus cavernosal smooth muscle structural damage.

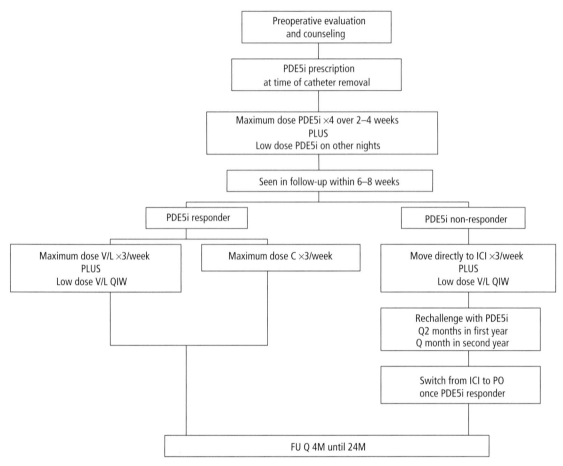

Fig. 17.1 Memorial Sloan Kettering Cancer Center approach to penile rehabilitation in the radical pelvic surgery patient. C, Cialis; ICI, intracavernosal injection therapy; L, Levitra; PDE5i, PDE5 inhibitor; QIW, four times per week; V, Viagra.

Carrier *et al.* demonstrated in 1995 that there is reduction in NOS-containing nerves after cavernous neurotomy in the rat model [33]. These authors demonstrated that animals that had bilateral neurotomy were far less likely to have return of NOS-staining nerves compared to animals that had undergone unilateral neurotomy. Numerous authorities have demonstrated that cavernous nerve injury results in apoptosis, but User *et al.* have demonstrated that both rat penile wet weight and DNA content were significantly reduced in animals who had bilateral cavernous neurotomy [7]. Furthermore, these authors demonstrated that apoptosis was most prominent in the subtunical area of the corpus cavernosum and they suggested that this was

the reason why patients develop venous leak post-prostatectomy. The Hellstrom group at Tulane have demonstrated very elegantly that cavernous neurotomy leads to up-regulation of cytokines in the penis which mediate fibrosis [8].

The concept of pharmacologic neuromodulation refers to the idea that patients could use pharmacologic agents that can either protect nerves from trauma or enhance nerve regeneration following injury. There is excellent animal data supporting this concept in facial, tibial, and sciatic nerve injury models. The most widely-studied group of compounds are immunophilin ligands. Immunophilins are found in immune tissue, but are in the range of 50–100-fold greater concentrations in neural tissue, both centrally and peripherally [62]. Cavernous nerves are combined sympathetic/parasympathetic, with the latter being erectogenic and the former being erectolytic. Immunophilins are proteins that act as receptors for immunosuppressive medications such as tacrolimus and cyclosporine. They mediate their effect through FK-binding proteins, the most important of which are FKBP12 and FKBP52 [62]. One of the great concerns about agents like tacrolimus is the immunosuppressant properties. Great interest has existed in the development of non-immunosuppressant, immunophilin ligands and Guildford Pharmaceuticals have developed a series of compounds. GPI-1046 has been shown in vitro to stimulate external growth from various neurons in cell cultures [63].

Burnett *et al.* are the first group to demonstrate that rats exposed to unilateral cavernous injury randomized to saline or FK506 have fared better when FK506 is used [64,65]. The use of this drug has resulted in greater intracavernosal pressure recovery and reduction in the structural changes within the cavernous nerve. This group has also shown that FK506 binding proteins are expressed in the major pelvic ganglion of the rat proximal to the cavernous nerve, and are upregulated close to normal after cavernous nerve injury. There is great interest in the development of this field, and not just FK506 and GPI compounds have been looked at; drugs such as rapamycin, minocycline and erythropoietin have also been explored. While there has been a suggestion that sildenafil (PDE-5 inhibitors) may have neuromodulatory effect, there is little evidence at this time to support this concept [61,66].

Treatment of Post-Radical Prostatectomy Erectile Dysfunction

Treatment of post-RP ED follows the same principles as for any other ED. The first therapeutic option is oral treatment with PDE-5 inhibitors (PDE-5i) or vacuum device, when there is a contraindication for the use of oral agents. Second-line treatment includes the intraurethral alprostadil suppository or intracavernosal injection therapy. When pharmacologic treatment does not restore the patient's erectile ability or there is a preference for a surgical treatment, penile implant may be the option. Although

the prevalence of post-RP ED is considerable, many patients remain untreated. Herkommer *et al.* reported that 59.3% of German patients with post-RP ED wished to be treated; however only 30.3% of the patients received long-term therapy: 19.8% of the patients using oral medication, 1.7% intraurethral alprostadil, 26.7% intracavernous injections, 50.9% a vacuum constriction device, and 0.9% a penile implant. Only 28.9% of the patients reported being satisfied with treatment [67].

Phosphosdiesterase Type 5 inhibitors

The efficacy of PDE-5i for the treatment of post-RP ED has only recently been studied. Sildenafil is the most studied PDE-5i in this subgroup of patients. However, despite this there does not exist data from a multi-center, randomized, placebo-controlled study evaluating sildenafil in patients with post-RP ED. Montorsi and McCullough found eleven studies in a systematic research on MEDLINE and CANCERLIT (1998–2004) with discrete data sets of post-prostatectomy patients with erectile dysfunction treated with sildenafil monotherapy [68]. From their analysis they concluded that with sildenafil, more than one-third of patients with post-RP ED achieved erections sufficient for intercourse. The odds of responding improved 12-fold with preservation of at least one neurovascular bundle. Early treatment failure does not necessarily imply lack of efficacy in the future, and patients should be encouraged to continue trying sildenafil, titrating up to 100 mg as needed.

Using multivariate analysis, Bennett *et al.* demonstrated predictors of failure to generate a penetration hardness erection with sildenafil post-RP [69]. In 187 patients with functional erections prior to RP ANOVA demonstrated statistical significance for IIEF erectile function domain improvement over time. Using sildenafil, at 18 months post-RP, 52% of men had functional erections, mean IIEF erectile function domain (EFD) score was 22 ± 9 and 21% had normalization of EFD score. Logistic regression analysis demonstrated statistically significant predictors of failure to respond to sildenafil post-RP included: patient age ≥ 60 years (RR = 2.8), ≥ 2 vascular comorbidities (RR = 1.9), duration ≤ 6 months post-RP (RR = 6.1).

Raina *et al.* reported a long-term effect of sildenafil

citrate on erectile dysfunction after radical prostatectomy with a follow-up of three years [70]. They enrolled 91 patients that had started on sildenafil at least three months after surgery. Initial dose was 50 mg, which was titrated up to 100 mg in case of an unsatisfactory response. At 12 months, 52.7% (48/91) reported having successful vaginal penetration. In patients who underwent a nerve-sparing radical prostatectomy, this rate increased to 71.7%. At three years, 31 (71%) of the 43 patients who had returned the second surveys were still responding to sildenafil.

Brock et al. reported on a double-blind study in which 440 men with ED after nerve sparing radical prostatectomy were randomized to take on-demand placebo, or 10 or 20 mg vardenafil for 12 months [71]. Improved erections were reported by 65.2% and 59.4% of patients on 20 and 10 mg vardenafil, respectively, and by only 12.5% of patients on placebo ($P < 0.0001$). Among men with bilateral neurovascular bundle sparing, improvement of erection rates were 71.1% and 59.7% of patients on 20 and 10 mg vardenafil, respectively, versus 11.5% of those on placebo ($P < 0.0001$). However the percentage of "yes" responses to the SEP Q3 was 9.5% for placebo, 37.2% for vardenafil 10 mg, and 34.2% for vardenafil 20 mg ($P < 0.001$).

Montorsi et al. reported on a double-blind, multi-center study in which 303 men who had undergone a BNS RP 12–48 months before study commencement were randomized to tadalafil 20 mg or placebo [72]. A subgroup of 201 patients reporting evidence of postoperative tumescence was analyzed. For all randomized patients who received tadalafil, the mean "yes" response to SEP Q2 was 54% vs. 32% for those who received placebo, and for SEP Q3 was 41% (19% for placebo). For the subgroup with evidence of postoperative tumescence these values were 69% vs. 42%, and 52% vs. 26%, respectively.

Vacuum constriction device (VCD)

VCD is probably the oldest described tool for treatment of ED. Cookson and Nadig (1993) reported long-term efficacy and high satisfaction rate for non-selected patients and couples treated with VCD [73]. However Dutta and Eid (1999) reported a dropout rate of 65% and most patients reported stopping the treatment within a mean of four months [74]. Raina

et al. published one the few papers on the subject VCD and post-RP erectile dysfunction [75]. To assess the efficacy of VCD following RP they conducted a prospective study; 74 patients were randomized to VCD use and 35 to observation without any erectogenic treatment. In the treatment arm 60/74 patients successfully used their VCD with a constriction ring for vaginal intercourse at a frequency of twice/week, with an overall spousal satisfaction rate of 55% (33/60). After a mean use of three months, 14/74 (18%) discontinued treatment. Also, VCD has been reported to be used in combination with sildenafil to improve erectile response in patients with post-RP ED [76].

Intraurethral alprostadil

Intraurethral delivery of alprostadil was first introduced by Padma-Nathan et al., in 1997, who claimed an overall efficacy rate of 44% for post-RP ED [77]. Raina et al. in a retrospective study, reported a 48% rate of significant improvement in all domains of the Sexual Health Inventory for Men (SHIM) after a mean of 2.2 years in 27 patients with post-RP ED treated with intraurethral alprostadil, although seldom reaching pre-operative scores, and 52% of patients had discontinued after a mean of eight months, mainly due to inadequate response or side effects [78]. Mulhall et al. reported a lack of consistency in the erectile response of patients treated with this therapy. They showed that only 51% of patients that had a rigid erection in an office-test could obtain the same response at home, although this was not confined to patients post-RP [79]. Intraurethral alprostadil is a safe alternative for the treatment of PRPED, but with a low efficacy, high dropout rate, and inconsistent results. Nehra et al. reported that combination therapy with intraurethral alprostadil and sildenafil was more efficacious in the salvage of patients who desire noninvasive therapy but in whom single-treatment modalities fail [80].

Intracavernosal injections

The use of intracavernosal injections to treat post-RP ED was first proposed by Dennis and McDougal in 1988 [81]. They reported a success rate of 85% (12/14 patients) with a mixture of papaverine and phentolamine. Intracorporeal injection therapy with alprostadil alone is effective in the majority of post-RP ED patients regardless of the status of their cavernosal nerves [82]. Gontero *et al.* evaluated the best regimen for starting intracavernosal injections in a series of patients who had undergone non-nerve sparing RP [83]. They demonstrated that when commenced within month three after the operation, a significantly higher proportion of patients had a successful response. Injections given in postoperative month one gave the best response rate but with poor patient compliance.

The main complaint of patients using intracavernosal alprostadil alone for the treatment of post-RP ED is penile pain, which can be minimized by the use of combination agents that permit reduction in alprostadil dose [84]. Claro *et al.* reported a efficacy rate of almost 95% in post-RP ED patients treated with self-injection therapy using papaverine/phentolamine/PGE$_1$ [85]. Raina *et al.* evaluated 102 patients treated with ICI [86]. They found that 68% of patients were satisfied with the treatment and 48% of patients continued for a mean of 3.5 years. The majority of the patients used alprostadil alone (61%) and the others the combination of alprostadil, papaverine and phentolamine.

Mulhall *et al.* mailed a questionnaire to 1424 nonselected patients who completed the office training and home use phases of a penile self-injection program to understand the major reasons for the high dropout rate that is common among ICI users [87]. The overall attrition rate was 31% of the 720 men who completed the questionnaire, with a mean follow-up of 38 months. The main reasons for dropout were cost of therapy, patient,\ and partner problems with the concept of penile injection, lack of partner availability, and spontaneous improvement in erections. Lack of efficacy of therapy was the primary reason for only 1/7 dropouts. Furthermore, adverse effects of penile injections (priapism, penile nodules, pain) appeared to be only minor contributors to dropout in the general population.

Penile prosthesis

Penile prosthetic surgery is an option for patients with post-RP ED who do not respond to more conservative treatments or prefer a surgical and definitive treatment. There is no randomized study on penile implant in this population, but overall satisfaction rates after penile implants in men with vari-ous causes of ED is usually high [78]. In a review of 504 implants, Minervinni *et al.* reported that 81% of the patients were satisfied with the outcome, and an even higher proportion were satisfied when an inflatable prostheses had been used. Dissatisfaction was mainly due to complications of the procedure [88].

Ramsawh *et al.* examined the satisfaction and quality of life (QOL) of patients who had simultaneous placement of a penile prosthesis at the time of RP [89]. Those patients reported greater overall QOL, erectile function and more frequent sexual contact than a comparison group of men who underwent RP alone. They proposed that placement of penile prosthesis at the time of radical prostatectomy may be an option for men with prostate cancer in whom a nerve sparing procedure may not be ideal.

Mulhall *et al.* studied 114 patients who underwent penile prosthesis surgery [90]. Sub-groups evaluated included patients with Peyronie's disease (24%), post-radical prostatectomy (38%), patients with body mass index (BMI) >30 (17%), partner age >70 years (10%), and patient age >70 years (28%). Patients with Peyronie's disease, a history of RP and BMI >30 had significantly lower scores on a global satisfaction question, IIEF satisfaction domain and EDITS questionnaire, compared to the general population.

References

1 Fraiman MC, Lepor H, McCullough AR. Changes in penile morphometrics in men with erectile dysfunction after nerve-sparing radical retropubic prostatectomy. *Mol Urol* 1999;**3**:109.

2 Munding MD, Wessells HB, Dalkin BL. Pilot study of changes in stretched penile length 3 months after radical retropubic prostatectomy. *Urology* 2001;**58**:567.

3 Savoie M, Kim SS, Soloway MS. A prospective study measuring penile length in men treated with radical prostatectomy for prostate cancer. *J Urol* 2003;**169**:1462.

4 Ciancio SJ, Kim ED. Penile fibrotic changes after radical retropubic prostatectomy. *BJU Int* 2000;**85**:101.

5 Carrier S, Zvara P, Nunes L, *et al.* Regeneration of nitric oxide synthase-containing nerves after cavernous nerve neurotomy in the rat. *J Urol* 1995;**153**:1722.

6 Klein LT, Miller MI, Buttyan R, *et al.* Apoptosis in the rat penis after penile denervation. *J Urol* 1997;**158**:626.

7 User HM, Hairston JH, Zelner DJ, *et al.* Penile weight and cell subtype specific changes in a post-radical prostatectomy model of erectile dysfunction. *J Urol* 2003;**169**: 1175.

8 Leungwattanakij S, Bivalacqua TJ, Usta MF, *et al.* Cavernous neurotomy causes hypoxia and fibrosis in rat corpus cavernosum. *J Androl* 2003;**24**:239.

9 Moreland RB. Is there a role of hypoxemia in penile fibrosis: a viewpoint presented to the Society for the Study of Impotence. *Int J Impot Res* 1998;**10**:113.

10 Sattar AA, Salpigides G, Vanderhaeghen JJ, *et al.* Cavernous oxygen tension and smooth muscle fibers: relation and function. *J Urol* 1995;**154**:1736.

11 Daley JT, Brown ML, Watkins T, *et al.* Prostanoid production in rabbit corpus cavernosum: I. regulation by oxygen tension. *J Urol* 1996;**155**:1482.

12 Moreland RB, Traish A, McMillin MA, *et al.* PGE1 suppresses the induction of collagen synthesis by transforming growth factor-beta 1 in human corpus cavernosum smooth muscle. *J Urol* 1995;**153**:826.

13 Zhou S, Chen LS, Miyauchi Y, *et al.* Mechanisms of cardiac nerve sprouting after myocardial infarction in dogs. *Circ Res* 2004;**95**:76.

14 Bergman B, Nilsson S, Petersen I. The effect on erection and orgasm of cystectomy, prostatectomy and vesiculectomy for cancer of the bladder: a clinical and electromyographic study. *Br J Urol* 1979;**51**:114.

15 Goriunov VG, Davidov MI. Sexual readaptation after the surgical treatment of benign prostatic hyperplasia. *Urol Nefrol* 1997;(Mosk):20.

16 Koeman M, van Driel MF, Schultz WC, *et al.* Orgasm after radical prostatectomy. *Br J Urol* 1996;**77**:861.

17 Perez MA, Skinner EC, Meyerowitz BE. Sexuality and intimacy following radical prostatectomy: patient and partner perspectives. *Health Psychol* 2002;**21**:288.

18 Snyder DK, Berg P. Determinants of sexual dissatisfaction in sexually distressed couples. *Arch Sex Behav* 1983;**12**:237.

19 Barnas JL, Parker M, Guhring P, Mulhall JP. The utility of alpha adrenergic blockade in the management of dysorgasmia, 2004.

20 Steg A, Zerbib M, Conquy S. Sexual disorders after an operation for benign prostatic hypertrophy. *Ann Urol* (Paris) 1988;**22**:129.

21 Hetrick DC, Ciol MA, Rothman I, *et al.* Musculoskeletal dysfunction in men with chronic pelvic pain syndrome type III: a case-control study. *J Urol* 2003;**170**:828.

22 Lee J, Fleshner N, Hersey K. Climacturia following radical prostatectomy: incidence and risk factors. *J Urol* 2005, **Abstract 1249**.

23 Abousassaly R, Gill I, Lakin M. Ejaculatory incontinence after radical prostatectomy: a review of 26 cases. *J Sex Med* 2005, SMSNA Annual Meeting Supplement.

24 Choi JM, Nelson C, Mulhall JP. Orgasm associated incontinence following radical pelvic surgery: prevalence and predictors. *J Urol* 2006.

25 Lue TF. Impotence after prostatectomy. *Urol Clin North Am* 1990;**17**:613.

26 Talcott JA, Rieker P, Propert KJ, *et al.* Patient-reported impotence and incontinence after nerve-sparing radical prostatectomy. *J Natl Cancer Inst* 1997;**89**:1117.

27 Aboseif S, Shinohara K, Breza J, *et al.* Role of penile vascular injury in erectile dysfunction after radical prostatectomy. *Br J Urol* 1994;**73**:75.

28 Lue TF. Erectile dysfunction. *N Engl J Med* 2000; **342**:1802.

29 Mulhall JP, Slovick R, Hotaling J, *et al.* Erectile dysfunction after radical prostatectomy: hemodynamic profiles and their correlation with the recovery of erectile function. *J Urol* 2002;**167**:1371.

30 Ohebshalom M, Parker M, Waters WB, Flanigan RC, Mulhall JP. Erectile hemodynamic status following radical prostatectomy correlates with erectile function outcomes. Presented at the Annual Meeting of the Sexual Medicine Society of North America, New York, 2005.

31 Canada AL, Neese LE, Sui D, *et al.* Pilot intervention to enhance sexual rehabilitation for couples after treatment for localized prostate carcinoma. *Cancer* 2005; **104**:2689.

32 Schover LR, Fouladi RT, Warneke CL, *et al.* Seeking help for erectile dysfunction after treatment for prostate cancer. *Arch Sex Behav* 2004;**33**:443.

33 Carrier S, Zvara P, Nunes L, *et al.* Regeneration of nitric oxide synthase-containing nerves after cavernous nerve neurotomy in the rat. *J Urol* 1995;**153**:1722.

34 Mullerad M, Donohue JF, Li PS, Scardino PT, Mulhall JP. Functional sequelae of cavernous nerve injury in the rat: Model dependency. *J Sex Med* 2005;**1**:39.

35 Bates TS, Wright MP, Gillatt DA. Prevalence and impact of incontinence and impotence following total prostatectomy assessed anonymously by the ICS-male questionnaire. *Eur Urol* 1998;**33**:165.

36 Begg CB RE, Bach PB, Kattan MW, Schrag D, Warren JL, Scardino PT. Variations in morbidity after radical prostatectomy. *N Engl J Med* 2002;**346**:1138.

37 Catalona WJ, Basler JW. Return of erections and urinary continence following nerve sparing radical retropubic prostatectomy. *J Urol* 1993;**150**:905.

38 Fowler FJ, Barry MJ, Lu-Yao G, *et al.* Patient-reported complications and follow-up treatment after radical prostatectomy. The national medicare experience: 1988–1990 (updated June 1993). *Urology* 1993; **42**:622.

39 Gralnek D, Wessells H, Cui H, *et al.* Differences in sexual function and quality of life after nerve sparing and non-nerve sparing radical retropubic prostatectomy. *J Urol* 2000;**163**:1166.

40 Litwin MS, Flanders SC, Pasta DJ, *et al.* Sexual function and bother after radical prostatectomy or radiation for prostate cancer: multivariate quality-of-life analysis from CaPSURE. Cancer of the Prostate Strategic Urologic Research Endeavor. *Urology* 1999;**54**:503.

41 Stanford JL, Feng Z, Hamilton AS, *et al.* Urinary and sexual function after radical prostatectomy for clinically localized prostate cancer. The prostate cancer outcomes study. *JAMA* 2000;**283**:354.

42 Talcott JA, Rieker P, Clark JA, *et al.* Patient-reported symptoms after primary therapy for early prostate cancer: results of a prospective cohort study. *J Clin Oncol* 1998;**16**:275.

43 Walsh PC, Marschke P, Ricker D, *et al.* Patient-reported urinary continence and sexual function after anatomic radical prostatectomy. *Urology* 2000;**55**:58.

44 Lue TF, Gleason CA, Brock GB, *et al.* Intraoperative electrostimulation of the cavernous nerve: technique, results and limitations. *J Urol* 1995;**154**:1426.

45 Klotz L, Herschorn S. Early experience with intraoperative cavernous nerve stimulation with penile tumescence monitoring to improve nerve sparing during radical prostatectomy. *Urology* 1998;**52**:537.

46 Klotz L, Heaton J, Jewett M, Chin J, Fleshner N, Goldenberg L, Gleave M. A randomized phase 3 study of intraoperative cavernous nerve stimulation with penile tumescence monitoring to improve nerve sparing during radical prostatectomy. *J Urol* 2000;**164**:1573.

47 Kim HL, Stoffel DS, Mhoon DA, Brendler CB. A positive Cavermap response poorly predicts recovery of potency after radical prostatectomy. *Urology* 2000;**56**:561.

48 Holzbeierlein J, Peterson M, Smith JJ. Variability of results of cavernous nerve stimulation during radical prostatectomy. *J Urol* 2001;**165**:108.

49 Chang SS, Peterson M, Smith JA. Intraoperative nerve stimulation predicts postoperative potency. *Urology* 2001;**58**:594.

50 Walsh PC, Marschke P, Catalona WJ, Lepor H, Martin S, Myers RP, Steiner MS. Efficacy of first-generation Cavermap to verify location and function of cavernous nerves during radical prostatectomy: a multi-institutional evaluation by experienced surgeons. *Urology* 2001;**57**:491.

51 Quinlan DM, Nelson RJ, Walsh PC. Cavernous nerve grafts restore erectile function in denervated rats. *J Urol* 1991;**145**:380.

52 Kim ED, Hampel O, Mill N, *et al.* Cavernous nerve grafting restores partial erections after non-nerve

sparing radical retropubic prostatectomy. *J Urol* 1999;**161**:188.

53 Kim ED, Kadmon K, Miles BJ, *et al.* Bilateral nerve grafts during radical retropubic prostatectomy: a one year follow-up. *J Urol* 2001;**165**:1950.

54 Kim ED, Scardino PT, Kadmon D, *et al.* Interposition sural nerve grafting during radical prostatectomy. *Urology* 2001;**57**:211.

55 Chang DW, Wood CG, Kroll SS, *et al.* Cavernous nerve reconstruction to preserve erectile function following non-nerve-sparing radical retropubic prostatectomy: a prospective study. *Plast Reconstr Surg* 2003;**111**:1174.

56 Walsh PC. Nerve grafts are rarely necessary and are unlikely to improve sexual function in men undergoing anatomic radical prostatectomy. *Urology* 2001;**57**:1020.

57 Moreland RB, Albadawi H, Bratton C, *et al.* O_2-dependent prostanoid synthesis activates functional PGE receptors on corpus cavernosum smooth muscle. *Am J Physiol Heart Circ Physiol* 2001;**281**:H552.

58 Montorsi F, Guazzoni G, Strambi LF, *et al.* Recovery of spontaneous erectile function after nerve-sparing radical retropubic prostatectomy with and without early intracavernous injections of alprostadil: results of a prospective, randomized trial. *J Urol* 1997;**158**:1408.

59 Padma-Nathan H, McCullough A, Giuliano F, *et al.* Nightly post-operative sildenafil dramatically improves the return of spontaneous erections following a bilateral nerve-sparing radical prostatectomy (abstract). *J Urol* 2003.

60 Schwartz EJ, Wong P, Graydon RJ. Sildenafil preserves intracorporeal smooth muscle after radical retropubic prostatectomy. *J Urol* 2004;**171**:771.

61 Donohue JF, Mullerad M, Paduch DA, Kobylarz K, Li PS, Scardino PT, Mulhall JP. The functional and structural consequences of cavernous nerve injury in the rat model are ameliorated by sildenafil citrate. *J Urology* 2005.

62 Snyder SH SD, Lai MM, Steiner JP, Hamilton GS, Suzdak PD. Neural actions of immunophilin ligands. *Trends Pharmacol Sci* 1998;**19**:21.

63 Burnett AL, Becker RE. Immunophilin ligands promote penile neurogenesis and erection recovery after cavernous nerve injury. *J Urol* 2004;**171**:595.

64 Sezen SF, Blackshaw S, Steiner JP, Burnett AL. FK506 binding protein 12 is expressed in rat penile innervation and upregulated after cavernous nerve injury. *Int J Impot Res* 2002;**14**:506.

65 Sezen SF, Hoke A, Burnett AL, Snyder SH. Immunophilin ligand FK506 is neuroprotective for penile innervation. *Nat Med* 2001;**7**:1073.

66 Zhang R, Wang Y, Zhang L, Zhang Z, Tsang W, Lu M, Zhang L, Chopp M. Sildenafil induces neurogenesis and

promotes fucntional recovery after stroke in rats. *Stroke*, 2002;**33**:2675.

67 Herkommer KNS, Zorn C, Gschwend JE, Volkmer BG. Management of erectile dysfunction after radical prostatectomy. Urologists' assessment vs patient survey responses. *Urologe A* 2005.

68 Montorsi FMA. Sildenafil citrate in men with erectile dysfunction following radical prostatectomy: a systematic review of clinical data. *J Sex Med* 2005;**2**:658.

69 Bennett NE, Donohue J, Parker M, Mulhall JP. Predictors of sildenafil citrate response following radical prostatectomy. *J Sex Med* Presented at The Annual Meeting of the Sexual Medicine Society of North America, 2005.

70 Raina RL MM, Agarwal A, Sharma R, Goyal KK, Montague DK, *et al.* Long-term effect of sildenafil citrate on erectile dysfunction after radical prostatectomy: 3-year follow-up. *Urology* 2003;**62**:110.

71 Brock G, Nehra A, Lipshultz LI, Karlin GS, Gleave M, Seger M, *et al.* Safety and efficacy of vardenafil for the treatment of men with erectile dysfunction after radical retropubic prostatectomy. *J Urol* 2003;**170**:1278.

72 Montorsi F, Nathan HP, McCullough A, Brock GB, Broderick G, Ahuja S, *et al.* Tadalafil in the treatment of erectile dysfunction following bilateral nerve sparing radical retropubic prostatectomy: a randomized, double-blind, placebo controlled trial. *J Urol* 2004;**172**:1036.

73 Cookson MD, Nadig PW. Long term results with vacuum constriction device. *J Urol* 1993;**149**:200.

74 Dutta TC, Eid JF. Vacuum constriction devices for erectile dysfunction: a long-term, prospective study of patients with mild, moderate, and severe dysfunction. *Urology* 1999;**54**:891.

75 Raina R, Agarwal A, Ausmundson S, Lakin M, Nandipati KC, Montague DK, *et al.* Early use of vacuum constriction device following radical prostatectomy facilitates early sexual activity and potentially earlier return of erectile function. *Int J impot Res* 2006;**18**:77.

76 Raina R, Agarwal A, Allamaneni SS, Lakin MM, Zippe CD. Sildenafil citrate and vacuum constriction device combination enhances sexual satisfaction in erectile dysfunction after radical prostatectomy. *Urology* 2005;**65**:360.

77 Padma-Nathan H, Hellstrom WJ, Kaiser FE, *et al.* Treatment of men with erectile dysfunction with transurethral alprostadil. *NEJM* 1997;**336**:1.

78 Raina R, Agarwal A, Zippe CD. Management of erectile dysfunction after radical prostatectomy. *Urology* 2005;**66**:923.

79 Mulhall JP, Jahoda AE, Ahmed A, *et al.* Analysis of the consistency of intraurethral prostaglandin E(1) (MUSE) during at-home use. *Urology* 2001;**58**:262.

80 Nehra A, Blute ML, Barrett DM, Moreland RB. Rationale for combination therapy of intraurethral prostaglandin E(1) and sildenafil in the salvage of erectile dysfunction patients desiring noninvasive therapy. *Int J Impot Res* 2002;**14**:S38.

81 Dennis RL, McDougal WS. Pharmacological treatment of erectile dysfunction after radical prostatectomy. *J Urol* 1988;**139**:775.

82 Briganti A, Salonia A, Zanni G, Fabbri F, Saccá A, Bertini R, *et al.* Erectile dysfunction and radical prostatectomy: an update. *EAU Update Series* 2004;**2**:84.

83 Gontero P, Fontana F, Bagnasacco A, Panella M, Kocjancic E, Pretti G, *et al.* Is there an optimal time for intracavernous prostaglandin E1 rehabilitation following non-nerve sparing radical prostatectomy? Results from a hemodynamic prospective study. *J Urol* 2003;**169**:2166.

84 Montorsi F, Guazzoni G, Bergamaschi F, Dodesini A, Rigati P, Pizzini G, *et al.* Effectiveness and safety of multidrug intracavernous therapy for vasculogenic impotence. *Urology* 1993;**42**:554.

85 Claro A, de Aboim JE, Maringolo M, Andrade E, Aguiar W, Nogueira M, *et al.* Intracavernous injection in the treatment of erectile dysfunction after radical prostatectomy: an observational study. *Sao Paulo Med* 2001;**5**:135.

86 Raina R, Lakin MM, Thukral M, Agarwal A, Ausmundson S, Montague DK, *et al.* Long-term efficacy and compliance of intracorporeal injection for erectile dysfunction following radical prostatectomy. *Int J Impot Res* 2003;**15**:318.

87 Mulhall JP, Jahoda AE, Cairney M, Goldstein B, Leitzes R, Woods J, *et al.* The causes of patient dropout from penile self-injection therapy for impotence. *J Urol* 1999;**162**:1291.

88 Minervini A, Ralph DJ, Pryor JP. Outcome of penile prosthesis implantation for treating erectile dysfunction: experience with 504 procedures. *BJU Int* 2006;**97**:129.

89 Ramsawh HJ, Morgentaler A, Covino N, Barlow DH, DeWolf WC. Quality of life following simultaneous placement of penile prosthesis with radical prostatectomy. *J Urol* 2005;**174**:1395.

90 Akin-Olugbade Y, Ahmed A, Parker M, Guhring P, Mulhall JP. Determinants of patient satisfaction following penile prosthesis surgery. *J Sex Med* (In Press), 2006.

CHAPTER 18

Hormones, Metabolism, Aging, and Men's Health

Jacques Buvat, Ridwan Shabsigh, André Guay, Louis Gooren,
Luiz Otavio Torres, and Eric Meuleman

Introduction

Hormone and metabolic disorders feature strongly in male sexual function and dysfunction. This chapter will discuss the direct implications of androgens in the areas of sexual desire and erectile function. Androgens are also implicated indirectly in sexual disorders through other metabolic derangements, such as obesity, insulin resistance, and the metabolic syndrome. We shall review the difficulties of defining androgen deficiency in aging men, when normal aging may produce similar symptoms, as may other aging changes, such as decreasing growth hormone levels. Diabetes mellitus is a hormonal disorder that embodies many hormonal and metabolic factors that may cause sexual dysfunction, such as hypertension, hyperlipidemia, obesity, and insulin resistance. It is little wonder, therefore, that the prevalence of sexual disorders is so high in this condition. Thyroid and adrenal disorders have a definite, though less pronounced and controversial role in the etiology of sexual dysfunction. The pituitary hormone—prolactin—when in excess, has a number of effects on sexual desire, erectile function, and androgen secretion. This review will attempt, in an evidence-based manner, to outline what is known, what is controversial, and what direction future research should take to understand these mechanisms better.

Hypogonadism

Many observations suggest that androgens play a critical role in human sexual behavior. Throughout life, the general pattern of their rise and decline cor-

responds to that of male sexual potency and activity. However the possibility of minimally-impaired sexual function in men with very low levels of testosterone (T), as well as the often disappointing results of T therapy used alone in men with sexual dysfunction and moderate hypogonadism, have cast doubt on the importance of androgens in sexual function. Actually the androgen deficiency that may be found during the work-up of a sexual dysfunction more often than not is only one element of a multifactorial causality.

On the other hand, it is now well established that the mean T level progressively decreases in healthy elderly men. The extent to which this contributes to clinical signs and symptoms of aging, and the potential merits of androgen replacement in aging men, constitute a very exciting but still much debated field.

The two main sections of this chapter are thus controversial areas. Evidence-based knowledge has considerably increased during the last few decades. Guidelines have been developed to help in practical management of the aspects which remain uncertain.

Levels of T are expressed either in pmol or nmol/L or in pg or ng/mL (1000 pg or pmol = respectively 1 ng or nmol. The conversion factors are nmol/L or pmol/L × 0.2884 = respectively ng/mL or pg/mL, and ng/ml or pg/ml × 3.467 = respectively nmol/L or pmol/L.

Definitions

Hypogonadism in men is deficient function of the testes. In this chapter its reproductive aspects will not be considered. This term will be used in the sense of deficiency of the testicular secretion of androgens mainly needed for virilization, anabolic effects, and expression of male sexual behavior. If the cause of hypogonadism lies in the testis itself, this is referred to as *primary* or *hypergonadotropic hypogonadism*. Hypothalamic or pituitary disorders of testicular dysfunction are grouped together under the term *secondary* or *hypogonadotropic hypogonadism* [1].

Late onset hypogonadism (LOH) is the term recommended by the International Society for the Study of the Aging Male (ISSAM), the International Society of Andrology (ISA), and the European Association of Urology (EAU), to replace the previous terminology of andropause, androgen deficiency of the aging male (ADAM), and partial androgen deficiency of the aging male (PADAM) [2]. It is a clinical and biochemical syndrome associated with advancing age and is characterized by typical symptoms and a deficiency in serum T levels. It may result in significant detriment in the quality of life and adversely affect the function of multiple organ systems.

Summary of androgen physiology
Mechanism of action and conversions

The testis has a dual function: spermatogenesis and the production of T. The latter takes places in the Leydig cells. The daily production of T in adulthood is about 5–7 mg. T diffuses passively into cells of the target organs of androgens. To exert its biologic action, it must bind to the androgen receptor, though there are also a number of biologic actions of T that do not require receptor activation. For some of its biologic actions T is a prohormone. After diffusion into the cell, T may be converted to 5 α-dihydrotestosterone (DHT) or estradiol. There are two types of 5 α-reductase enzymes that convert T to DHT. 5α reductase type 1 is predominantly located in skin, liver, and brain whereas 5α reductase type 2 is almost exclusively distributed in the classical androgen-dependent organs such as prostate, seminal vesicles, and testicles. DHT and T bind to the same androgen receptor, although DHT has an approximately tenfold greater affinity for the receptor and its dissociation is slower, resulting in a considerably higher biopotency than T. The conversion of T to DHT can be viewed as an androgen amplification mechanism in organs that require a strong androgen action, such as

the prostate. About 80% of DHT is produced in peripheral tissues and the remaining 20% is secreted directly by the testis. Furthermore, approximately 30–40 µg of estradiol is produced by the adult male, mainly in peripheral tissues, such as adipose tissue, bone, prostate, and brain. Insight into the biologic actions of estradiol in the male is rather recent. Estrogens have an important effect on the final phases of skeletal maturation and bone mineralization in puberty. In addition, from some studies in elderly men it appears that estrogen levels show a higher correlation with bone mineral density (BMD) than androgen levels [3]. Impaired estrogen action in men leads to dyslipidemia and to endothelial dysfunction. Observation in men with aromatase deficiency is linked to a complex dysmetabolic syndrome characterized by insulin resistance, diabetes mellitus type 2, acanthosis nigricans, steatosis hepatis, and signs of precocious atherogenesis, remedied by estrogen administration. Estrogen effects on the brain are also increasingly recognized [4]. Though the effects of estrogens in the male are undeniably biologically significant, estrogen deficiency as a clinical entity is sporadic in men. Since T is a precursor molecule for estradiol, it is usually associated with (severe) androgen deficiency.

Transport

Testosterone is a lipophilic molecule and its solubility in blood is limited. Only ± 2% of circulating T is free, non-bound to transport proteins, able to diffuse into cells, and immediately available for biologic action. Approximately 60% of circulating T is bound with high affinity to sex hormone binding globulin (SHBG), and ±38% is loosely bound and transported by albumin. The free fraction of T (FT, ±2%) and the albumin-bound fraction (±38%) have been termed bioavailable testosterone (BT), since these two fractions are readily available for biologic action. Testosterone has a high affinity with SHBG and changes in concentrations of circulating SHBG impact on the bioavailability of T. SHBG is produced by the liver and a number of conditions and hormones influence its production. Androgens and growth hormone decrease circulating SHBG, which increases BT, and amplifies the action of T along with the combined anabolic effects of growth hormone (GH) and T. Andro-

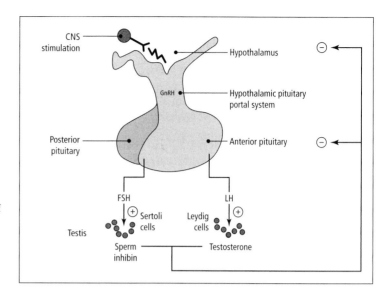

Fig. 18.1 Production and regulation of testosterone. CNS, central nervous system; FSH, follicle stimulating hormone; GnRH, gonadotropin-releasing hormone; LH, luteinizing hormone.

gen deficiency, estrogens, hyperthyroidism, and liver disease increase circulating SHBG, and consequently limit its biologic action. SHBG also binds estradiol but with lower affinity than T, such that certain conditions may be associated with signs of estrogen excess such as gynecomastia. Overweightness with its associated hyperinsulinism, corticosteroids, and hypothyroidism reduce circulating SHBG and result in low total plasma concentrations.

Secretion

T secretion follows a daily rhythm with highest T levels in the early morning hours, gradually declining to reach the lowest levels in the early evening. The biologic significance of this diurnal rhythm has not been established, and dissipates with aging. It is usually recommended to measure T in the early morning hours to avoid an erroneous diagnosis of hypogonadism, on the basis of the physiologically lower T levels in the afternoon. Two recent papers questioned this recommendation because they did not find any significant diurnal variation in men over 40 [6,7], contrary to younger healthy men in whom this variation was marked [7].

The secretion of T from the Leydig cell is stimulated by the pituitary hormone, luteinizing hormone (LH) (Fig. 18.1). Human chorionic gonadotropin (hCG) is

chemically largely identical with LH and is capable of stimulating T production. Follicle stimulating hormone (FSH) binds to the Sertoli cells and promotes spermatogenesis. The pituitary production of LH and FSH, in turn, is regulated by the hormone, luteinizing hormone releasing hormone (LHRH), also called gonadotropin-releasing hormone (GnRH), produced in the arcuate nucleus and the preoptic area of the hypothalamus under the stimulating and inhibitory influence of local neurotransmitters. LHRH is secreted in regular pulses, with peaks in adulthood every 90–120 minutes, due to the intrinsic capacity of LHRH neurons to secrete episodically. The pulsatility of LHRH is essential to its gonadotropin-releasing effect. Continuous stimulation of the pituitary by LHRH leads to desensitization and to a cessation of LH and FSH release. The hypothalamus is connected with the anterior pituitary through a portal system through which LHRH reaches the pituitary. Due to this anatomic situation the concentration of LHRH in peripheral blood is immeasurably low.

Feedback control

Testicular hormones exert a negative feedback control on the secretion of LH and FSH. Testosterone itself and also estradiol and DHT are involved in the negative feedback action, which is exerted both at the level of the hypothalamus (reducing LHRH pulse frequency and amplitude), and at the level of the pituitary by reducing production and release of LH and FSH. The negative feedback action of estrogens on the secretion of LH and FSH is evidenced by the resulting rise of LH and FSH following administration of agents that pharmacologically reduce estrogen action (anti-estrogens and aromatase inhibitors).

Aging

With aging the production of T declines and its bioavailibity is reduced. These are the results of age-related changes at all levels of the hypothalamic–pituitary–testicular axis. Testosterone production is less efficient in old age, with a lower response to stimulation with LH or hCG. The decline of circulating T is not always compensated by an increase in LH, which would be expected on the basis of a decreased negative feedback signal. So, it would seem that the pituitary has become more sensitive to the negative feedback action of T and its metabolites. A more important factor is probably the changes of the aging hypothalamic structures that produce LHRH. The pulsatile secretion of LHRH is attenuated and more disordered so that stimulation of the pituitary to produce LH is less efficient. Also the synchrony between an LH pulse and a T pulse is weakened in elderly men. Aging not only affects androgen production but also its bioavailability. The levels of the T-binding protein, SHBG, commonly rise with aging, but this is counterbalanced by obesity and hyperinsulinism, which reduce circulating SHBG. The rise in SHBG in the first instance is associated with lower FT levels. With a healthy hypothalamus–pituitary system this leads to a compensatory secretion of LH and subsequently of T. But the aging hypothalamus–pituitary system is not always capable of this response leading to lower levels of FT and BT [5].

The importance of receptivity

Many of the changes associated with aging, such as loss of bone and muscle mass, increased fat mass, and deterioration of physical, cognitive, and sexual capacities, are similar to the symptoms of classical hypogonadism in younger men. The decline in circulating T is not universal in elderly men and is of a lesser magnitude than in classical hypogonadism. To explain the androgen deficiency-like symptoms in aging in the presence of relatively mildly reduced T levels, it has been hypothesized that the efficacy of androgen action at the level of receptor and post-receptor mechanisms is diminished in old age compared to younger age. Arguing against this is that, with regard to the anabolic actions of T, elderly men are as responsive to T as young men [8]. While male sexual functioning in (young) adulthood can be maintained with lower-than-normal values [9,10], there are indications that the threshold required for behavioral effects of T increases with aging [11]. The fact that libido and erectile function require higher T levels in old age compared to younger age has been recently confirmed [12], and this is also apparent from clinical observation [13] and from meta-analysis [14].

It is of note that there are (subtle) genetic differences in androgen receptor properties in men. The androgen receptor gene contains a polymorphic trinucleotide in exon one—CAG repeats. The length of the (CAG) polymorphism of the gene is negatively associated with transcriptional activity of the androgen receptor. In other words, an androgen receptor with fewer CAG repeats mediates a stronger androgen effect than a receptor with more CAG repeats. Some studies have found that men with fewer CAG repeats, subject to enhanced androgen action, are more liable to develop prostate cancer. Other reports fail to confirm this (for review see [15]). Similar controversy surrounds the relevance of the number of CAG repeats for the severity of symptoms related to the age-associated decline of T [16]. For the time being, determination of the number of CAG repeats is not part of routine clinical assessment of the hypogonadal male, young or old.

Clinical picture of hypogonadism

The clinical picture of androgen deficiency is dependent on the age at which this deficiency appears, and on its extent [1]. Prenatally, depending on the phase of development, it may result in intersexuality, or in abnormal positioning of the testes and an abnormally small penis (micropenis). Congenital penile deviations may also be the result of a temporary T deficiency or androgen insensitivity during fetal development [17]. Between birth and puberty androgen production is minimal and hypogonadism will not manifest itself. Hypogonadism at the normal time of puberty will result in a typical syndrome of eunuchoidism. Epiphyseal cartilage does not stop growing, so the long bones continue to grow, resulting in a ratio of upper to lower body <1, and arms extending beyond the torso by over 5 cm. Voice does not deepen, and hair development remains of the feminine type: horizontal pubic hair line, no facial hair, no body hair. Fat distribution is also of the female type, with pronounced hips. The penis and testes remain child-like, the scrotum is only slightly wrinkled and not very pigmented, and the prostate is small. Libido and potency do not develop. Spermatogenesis is not initiated, resulting in aspermia and infertility.

After puberty, the clinical picture may vary considerably according to the time elapsed since puberty and the degree of the androgen deficiency. Body proportions, size of penis, and pitch of voice do not change. Body and facial hair may decrease. The main clinical signs are reduced sexual desire and potency, and infertility. Size and consistency of testes vary from normal to significantly reduced. Long-term androgen deficiency usually causes atrophy of muscle mass, osteoporosis, loss of strength and energy, normochromic and normocytic anemia, fatigue, and mood disturbances.

Role of hypogonadism in sexual dysfunctions

We look first at the prevalence of hypogonadism.

Prevalence of hypogonadism

Erectile dysfunction (ED)

Serum T is more often than not normal in ED. It was below 3 ng/mL in 12% of 7000 ED patients compiled from nine large series (including in 4% of 944 men < 50 years, and 14.7% of 4342 men > 50) [18–20]. The real prevalence of hypogonadism is probably lower because most of these patients had a single T determination. A repeat determination is recommended in cases of subnormal value, since it proves to be normal in as many as one-third of the patients [18–21]. In addition, some studies did not sample blood in the morning in every case even though the T level decreases after 11 am in normal men, at least up to the

age of 40 [6]. In one series of over 1000 ED patients in which the diagnosis of hypogonadism was based on two consecutive values <3 ng/mL before 11 am, the prevalence of hypogonadism was only 6.6%, including 4% before 50 years old, and 9% after 50 [18]. Determinations of the bioavailable fractions of T, FT, and BT, may find higher prevalences of low values (up to respectively, 37% and 24% of ED patients over 50 years old) [22–24]. In a narrow majority of the studies, the average values of total T (TT), FT, and BT are slightly but significantly lower in ED patients than in age-matched controls [22–26].

Other male sexual dysfunctions

Testosterone is also generally normal [23]. This is the case even in patients complaining of isolated hypoactive sexual desire [23,24,27], although in aging men one study has found that low sexual desire was associated with low T level [28].

Responsibility of hypogonadism

Sexual function of men with severe organic hypogonadism

Data accumulated in such men show that T is required for pubertal acquisition of gender characteristics as well as adult sexual behavior and functional capacity, including libido, ejaculation, and spontaneous erections. Administration of T during placebo-controlled studies demonstrated that sexual desire and arousal are T-dependent [13,29,30] and represent the main impact of T on sexual function of men. The frequency of sexual activity [13,30,31] and spontaneous erections (especially sleep related, i.e. morning and nocturnal) [13,29,32] are also clearly T-dependent. The psychic erections (i.e. in response to erotic stimuli) were initially thought to be androgen-independent [33], but are in fact partly T-dependent [34]. Ejaculations [31] and orgasm [35] are also partly androgen-dependent.

Threshold levels for testosterone effects on sexual function

The effects of T upon male sexual function are dose-dependent up to a serum level close to the lower limit of the normal adult range, at which they are maximum. Below this threshold sexual function is impaired. This threshold level is consistent within an individual [10,36], but markedly variable between individuals [10,31,36], and may be specific to each parameter of sexual function [37]. For example, in a study by Kelleher, the average T level from which hypogonadal males on testosterone pellet implants began to perceive androgen deficiency symptoms leading them to request a new implantation was 2.6 ng/mL (or 10 nmol/L), but the individual levels varied from less than 1 to 4.5 ng/mL. In another series of hypogonadal males on injectable T esters, the individual threshold level varied from 1.1 to 3.6 ng/mL [10,36]. Overall, levels below 2 ng/mL are in most cases associated with impairment of sexual function [10,31,36], and levels below 1.4–2 ng/mL with diminished nocturnal erections [38]. Conversely, from a ceiling level of 4.5–6 ng/mL, according to the studies [10,31,36,37], the effect of T is maximum and is not enhanced with additional T supplementation. In eugonadal males, a significant increase in sexual interest and arousal [27,39,40], along with rigidity and duration of the erections [41], was obtained in some studies by increasing the serum T level within or above the normal range. But others could not replicate these findings [42], and in the former the effect upon sexuality was too small to be clinically significant. Between these two thresholds levels of about 2 and 4.5–6 ng/mL, the impact of T on sexual activity may or may not be optimum according to the sensitivity to androgens of the individual.

Role of testosterone in control of erections
• *Data from experiments in animals:* Studies in rodents suggest that besides its well-known effects on the brain centers of sexual function, especially the hypothalamic preoptic area and arcuate nucleus, T plays a key role in the peripheral modulation of erectile function. It is well known that the nitric oxide (NO) pathway is critical for initiation and maintenance of erections. In animals, the expression of both the endothelial and neuronal NO synthases (NOS), and therefore the capacity for NO production, is regulated by androgens [43,44]. Androgen suppression via castration results in marked decrease in NOS activity and cyclic guanosine monophosphate (cGMP) formation, through both NOS-dependent and -independent mechanisms, as well as in profound structural changes in penile tissue (atrophy con-

comitant with alterations in dorsal nerve structure and endothelial morphology, reduction in trabecular smooth muscle content, increased deposition of extracellular matrix, and accumulation of adipocytes in the subtunical region of the corpus cavernosum) [45]. Thus androgens exert a direct effect on penile tissue to maintain erectile function, and androgen deficiency produces metabolic and structural imbalance in the corpus cavernosum, which results in venoocclusive dysfunction and ED, reversed by T administration [45,46].

• *Data from experiments in men:* In human males the main sites of the action of T upon sexual function are considered to be located in the brain. Positron emission tomography (PET) studies have begun to map them [47,48]. Until now a critical impact on the peripheral mechanisms of erection had not been demonstrated in men. However there are androgen receptors in the human corpus cavernosum [49], and some recent studies suggest T may modulate the vascular mechanisms of erection also in men. Peak systolic velocity was measured at the level of the cavernosal arteries with penile color Doppler ultrasound (CDU), following intracavernosal injection of alprostadil in ED patients with severe hypogonadism (serum T < 2 ng/mL) and no vascular co-morbidity [50]. It was significantly lower than in a control group of psychogenic ED patients, and increased up to the range of the later group following T-replacement for six months. In another study based on CDU of the cavernosal arteries, Aversa *et al.* found a highly significant correlation of the resistive index with the serum value of FT [51]. In a third study of arteriogenic ED patients with low–normal T—non-responders to sildenafil—T supplementation significantly enhanced the accelerating effect of sildenafil on peak systolic velocity measured in the cavernosal arteries [52]. However, more evidence is required before the hypothesis of a significant impact of T on the penile vascular mechanisms of men can be totally accepted.

• *Effects of T therapy in the hypogonadal ED patients:* Testosterone therapy consistently restores erectile function in young patients with organic hypogonadism [24]. A recent meta-analysis by Isidori *et al.* integrated 17 randomized controlled trials (RCTs) that had studied the effects of T on male sexual function in men of any age [53]. A significant improvement of all aspects of sexual function was found in men with low (<7 nmol/L, 2 ng/mL) and low–normal T (7–12 nmol/L, 2–3.46 ng/mL) receiving standard replacement doses of T, with respect to placebo. Concerning erectile function, the magnitude of the effect was inversely related to the baseline T concentration and was detectable only in studies with mean baseline T level < 12 nmol/L (3.46 ng/mL). No statistically significant effect on libido (though close to significance) or erections was found in studies with mean baseline T level above this. The type of T preparation used, the length of follow-up assessment, as well as the presence of ED and other co-morbidities (diabetes mellitus, hypertension, dyslipidemia), all influenced response to treatment. The effect of age was not studied in this meta-analysis. Although this data suggests a significant effect of T therapy on erectile function in cases of marked or moderate hypogonadism, the effects reported in the literature regarding this treatment have been mostly disappointing when it was used alone in middle-aged patients consulting for ED who are subsequently found to be hypogonadal. This situation may be quite different from that of men with organic hypogonadism, diagnosed earlier in life, who constitute the majority of the populations studied in RCTs. No controlled trial has been specifically devoted to such patients, but the compilation of eight observational studies totalling 259 cases (T < 3 ng/mL or 11.5 nmol/L) leads to the conclusion that only 36% were definitely improved regarding their erectile function [18,20,54–59]. Perhaps TT is a poor index of androgenicity, and only its bioavailable fractions should be taken into account. This speculation was not confirmed by the results of T therapy in ED patients with low levels of FT or BT, since the success rate was even poorer in this category, including cases that had low FT or BT and normal TT levels [23,60]. Probably the low T level of some ED patients is not the real, or at least the sole cause of their ED. The lability of serum T has to be considered, and every low result should be confirmed by a second determination. In addition, ED is often multifactorial, and the meta-analysis by Isidori et al. found that co-morbidities influence the effect of T therapy [53]. Significant vascular factors, such as obstruction of the penile arteries or venoocclusive dysfunction

were found in as many as 42% of ED patients with low T levels [18]. More subtle alterations such as endothelial dysfunction, probably exist due to many other medical co-factors, and this may also hamper the effects of T therapy. It is even probable that in certain cases low T is more a consequence than the cause of ED. In two studies the low serum T increased following successful non-hormonal ED therapies (such as intracavernosal or phosphodiesterase type 5 inhibitor (PDE5i) therapies) [25,26]. In such cases the reduction in T secretion was likely caused by reduced sexual activity (that has been shown to stimulate T secretion) [61], and by the stress and depression that often result from ED, through the well-known inhibitory impact of the two latter factors on the hypothalamic gonadotropic centers [62,63]. Carosa et al. observed a reduction in the bioavailability of LH in ED patients that could result from a spacing out of the LHRH pulses via a psychosomatic mechanism, since it was also reversible with successful non-hormonal ED therapies [64].

• *Possible requirement of a minimum serum T level for a complete effect of PDE5i in ED patients:* cGMP, the key intracavernosal signal for the relaxation of the cavernosal smooth muscle and thus erection, is inactivated by the enzyme PDE5, present in the cavernous bodies. This limits the effects of NO release on erection. By inhibiting PDE5, intracavernosal cGMP accumulation occurs, and that often improves the quality of erection. In rodents androgens modulate not only the expression of NOS but also that of PDE5 [65,66], as well as the response to electrostimulation of the corpora cavernosa [67]. In animal models, it was demonstrated that normal androgen levels are a prerequisite for proper functioning of PDE5i [67,68]. The critical importance of a normal T level for intra-penile mechanisms of erection has not been proved until now in humans, but the expression of PDE5 is T-dependent in humans too [66]. In addition in a group of ED patients without any other apparent cause of ED than severe hypogonadism, the PDE5i sildenafil failed to improve the blunted erectile response to visual sexual stimulation, as it did in eugonadal psychogenic ED patients. This response was subsequently restored following T substitution for six months [50]. Lastly in another study sildenafil improved sleep-related erections even in hypogonadal men, but the effect of sildenafil and T was greater than the sum of the two compounds alone [69].

Several uncontrolled studies recently reported an increased prevalence of low or low–normal T levels in ED patients who were non-responders to PDE5i, with a frequent improvement of their response following T substitution [70–72]. The speculation that hypogonadism was responsible for the PDE5i failure is supported by two controlled studies. Aversa *et al.* studied 20 patients (mean age 55) with arteriogenic ED and both TT and FT in the lower quartile of normal range [52]. These had been non-responders to six trials with 100 mg sildenafil and were randomized to T or placebo patches combined with sildenafil on demand. With respect to placebo, T-treatment significantly increased the arterial inflow to cavernous bodies (peak systolic velocity measured with CDU following sildenafil administration), as well as increased scores of the "erectile function," "intercourse satisfaction," and "overall satisfaction" domains of the international index of erectile function (IIEF). The Shabsigh *et al.* study (Fig. 18.2) involved more ED patients (75) with low or low–normal TT ($\leq$ 4 ng/mL)—non-responders to sildenafil 100 mg [73]. They were randomized to T or placebo gels combined with sildenafil on demand during this time, for 12 weeks. After four weeks the scores of the "erectile function," "orgasmic function," and "overall satisfaction" domains of the IIEF, as well as the number of patients reporting that their gel improved their response to sildenafil, were significantly higher in the T group. However the statistical differences between the T and placebo groups waned or disappeared at eight and 12 weeks, probably in part because of the small size of the patient sample and the rather high drop-out rate. However the speculation that a certain threshold level of T is required for a complete effect of PDE5i has still to be confirmed in larger studies.

Conclusions

What are the practical consequences of diagnosing hypogonadism in an ED patient? Hypogonadism is present in 5–15% of ED patients according to age. Although low T may not be the main cause of ED in many patients, due to the frequent multifactoriality of ED, and the preponderance of vascular factors, there are clearly benefits to screening for T deficiency:

• Achieving physiologic levels of T is one of the rare opportunities to restore spontaneous erections and save patients from having to plan sexual activity, as is the case with most other therapies of ED.

• Providing T therapy is the only possibility of restoring sexual desire [13,74], which is often low in such patients, especially since low sexual desire is a frequent cause of drop-out from PDE5i therapy.

• Replacing T may also improve other symptoms associated with hypogonadism, including lack of energy and mood disturbances [71,72].

• A threshold serum T level could be required to achieve full efficacy with PDE5i. Therefore if an ED patient does not satisfactorily respond to PDE5i, it is indicated to determine serum T if not already done. In case the level is low or low-normal ($\leq$4 ng/mL, 14 nmol/L), combining T therapy with PDE5i for at least two months is recommended.

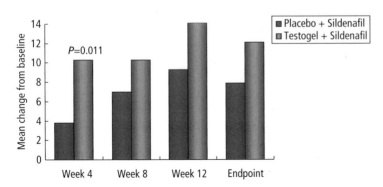

Fig. 18.2 Testosterone therapy (5 g testosterone gel/d/12 wk) converts sildenafil 100 mg non-responders to responders in men with hypogonadism (T <4 ng/mL) and erectile dysfunction. The figure represents the mean change in "erectile function" domain score. The difference was no longer significant from week eight. Source: Shabsigh R, *et al. J Urol* 2004; **172**:658–663 [73].

Role of late onset hypogonadism in male aging and effects of testosterone therapy
Nature and prevalence of late onset hypogonadism

In late onset hypogonadism (LOH) there is a variable decline predominantly involving non-SHBG-bound T. Several studies document that androgen levels decline with aging (for review see [75]). Longitudinal studies [76–78] have documented a statistical decline of serum T by approximately 30% in healthy men between the ages of 25 and 75 years. Since serum levels of SHBG increase with aging, plasma T not bound to SHBG decreases even more, by about 50%, over that period. Studies in twins have shown that genetic factors account for 63% of the variability of serum T levels, and for 30% of the variability in SHBG levels [79]. Also systemic diseases, increasing with age, are a cause of declining serum levels of T [78,80]. While it now has been shown beyond doubt, that serum T, and in particular BT and FT, decline with aging, it remains uncertain what percentage of men actually become T-deficient with aging, in the sense that they will suffer the clinical consequences of T deficiency, and will potentially benefit from T therapy. In a study of 300 healthy men between the ages of 20 and 100 years, Vermeulen, defining their reference range of total plasma T between 11 and 40 nmol/L, found one man with subnormal T in the age group 20–40 years, but more than 20% above the age of 60 years [81]. However, 15% of men above the age of 80 years still had T values above 20 nmol/L! It follows that only a certain proportion of men have lower-than-normal T values in old age.

What are the pitfalls of diagnosing LOH? There are several problems regarding LOH. For androgen deficiency it is difficult to rely on clinical symptoms, particularly in elderly men. In previously eugonadal adults, symptoms of T deficiency emerge only gradually and insidiously. Only the physical signs of long-standing T deficiency will be clinically recognized. Further, stringent criteria to diagnose T deficiency have not been formulated, neither in the young nor in the elderly male population. In the elderly population T deficiency is difficult to identify since symptoms of aging mimic symptoms of T deficiency and are also similar to growth hormone deficiency. It has not become clear whether other criteria for T deficiency in aging men should be different than those for younger men.

There are different threshold values for different biologic effects. Testosterone has a number of physiologic functions in the male. In adulthood it is responsible for maintenance of reproductive capacity and of secondary sex characteristics. T has positive effects on mood and libido, anabolic effects on bone and muscle, and affects fat distribution and the cardiovascular system. Threshold serum values of T for each of these functions are becoming established. The studies of Bhasin *et al.* and of Kelleher *et al.*, analyzing the dose-response relationships between serum T and biologic effects, show that low-to-mid-normal serum levels of T suffice for most biologic actions of T [8,36]. Another consideration is whether these threshold values change over the life cycle. Theoretically, it is possible that in old age normal androgen levels suffice for some but not for all androgen-related functions. With regard to anabolic actions, elderly men are as responsive to T as young men [8]. Conversely, as previously detailed in p. 228, the threshold required for libido and erectile function might increase with aging.

Correlations between androgen levels and symptoms of male aging and effects of testosterone therapy

Table 18.1 summarizes the clinical signs of androgen deficiency.

Body composition

Body composition is seriously affected by the aging process. Aging is almost universally accompanied by an increase in abdominal fat mass and a decrease of muscle mass. Androgens have a substantial impact on muscle mass and on fat distribution, and therefore the relationship between these signs of aging and T levels has been assessed.

Increase in fat mass

Several studies have convincingly documented an inverse correlation between abdominal fat mass and FT levels and this appears to be independent of age [82–84]. This finding has clinical relevance: the amount of visceral fat is highly significantly,

Table 18.1 Clinical signs of androgen deficiency.

Lean/muscle mass	↓ Muscle mass ↓ Muscle strength ↓ Global performance
Fat mass	↑ Abdominal and visceral fat ("beer belly")
Bone mass	↓ Bone mineral density Back pain ↑ Risk of fractures (femoral neck, body of a vertebra, radius) ↓ Height
Metabolism and cardiovascular system	↑ Total and LDL cholesterol, ↓ HDL ↑ Cardiovascular risk ?? (atherosclerosis) ↑ Insulin resistance
Blood	↓ Erythropoietin Anemia (fatigue, decreased performance)
Cognitive functions	↓ Spatial cognition and memory Depressive mood Irritability Sleep disturbances
Sexual functions	↓ Sexual desire ↓ Sexual arousal ↓ Erections, ED Retarded orgasm Diminished sperm production
Skin/hair	Atrophy (parchment skin) ↓ Secondary hair Sweating, flushes

ED, erectile dysfunction; HDL, high density lipoprotein; LDL, low density lipoprotein.

associated with an increased risk of cardiovascular disease, impaired glucose tolerance, and non-insulin-dependent diabetes mellitus (the so-called syndrome X) [85,86]. Whether the abdominal, and more specifically visceral, obesity is the consequence of the low T levels or vice versa, is not yet clear. It is clear, however, that visceral obesity leads to a decrease of T levels, mainly via a decrease in SHBG levels; hyperinsulinemia associated with visceral obesity suppresses SHBG levels, leading in the first instance to higher quantities of FT, which are subsequently rapidly metabolized since the half-life of FT in the circulation is short (15–20 minutes). In morbid obesity

(BMI > 35) there is also a decrease of FT. Fat mass decreased in 13 of 17 RCTs of T therapy in men over 50 [87]; although limited (1.5–2.5 kg), the decrease was statistically significant in 12 of the 14 RCTs of more than three months in duration. In one meta-analysis of 16 of these RCTs [88], an average of nine months of T therapy produced a mean reduction of 1.6 kg in total body fat (−6.2% of initial percentage body fat, $p < 0.001$). The effect was not different in men with baseline T < 10 nmol/L (1.46 kg) and then those with T > 10 nmol/L (1.5 kg).

Decline in muscle mass

There is an impressive age-associated decline in muscle mass (12 kg between age 20 and 70 years), which is most pronounced for the fast twitch type II fibres [89]. This loss of muscle mass is a major contributor to the age-associated decline in muscle strength and fatigue [90]. Maximal muscle strength shows a correlation with muscle mass, independently of age [91]. This is again related to the occurrence of falls and fractures and the consequent limitations of independent living. Lean mass, mainly muscle mass, increased in 13 of 15 RCTs in aging men, including 12 of the 13 exceeding 13 months [87]. The average increase was 1–3 kg, and no significant change occurred after six months. But higher plateau could be achieved with higher doses. In a meta-analysis of 17 RCTs in men over 50, T therapy produced an increase in fat-free mass of 1.6 kg (+ 2.7% over initial percentage of lean body mass ($p < 0.001$) [88].

Decline in muscle strength

The correlation between T levels and muscle mass appears stronger than the correlation with muscle strength. In a study of men aged 73–97 years, serum T levels were, independently of age, positively related to isometric grip strength and leg extension strength [92]. In institutionalized men, who have lower T concentrations than healthy elderly men, a correlation between T levels and severity of loss of muscle function could be established [93]. By contrast, two other studies failed to establish correlations between T and strength. In one in elderly men (65–97 years old), a significant correlation was found between FT and muscle mass, but not grip strength [94]. In the other, no correlation between T levels and muscle strength was found [95]. In most RCTs in men over 50, the increase in muscle mass was not associated with statistically significant improvements in muscle strength. Where improved, this effect was mainly seen in the upper limbs with a statistically significant increase in hand grip strength in four of eight studies [87]. Higher doses might give higher effects on muscle strength because the study in which the highest T doses were used (400 g T esters per month) resulted in statistically significant improvements in both upper and lower limbs. Improvement in overall physical function was also reported in a limited number of studies. These improvements were on timed stair climbing in two out of two studies: timed walking in one of two, and functional independence in one of two [87]. Finally, in one study T therapy was observed to prevent the perception of decreasing physical function that occurred over time with placebo in men >65 years old who wore scrotal patches containing either T or placebo for 36 months. In a meta-analysis of nine RCTs in men over 50, only the hand grip strength and knee extension in the dominant limbs showed a tendency towards improvement on T over placebo ($p = 0.06$ for both). No significant effect could be detected in the muscles of the non-dominant limbs nor in the knee flexion or leg extension in the dominant limbs [88].

It must be concluded that the correlation between T levels and muscle mass is readily demonstrable, whereas the relation with muscle strength is apparently less firm and could not be demonstrated in all studies. Factors other than androgens, such as growth hormone, probably play a significant role.

Bone mineral density

Decrease in bone mineral density

With aging there is an exponential increase in bone fracture rate [96,97], which carries a clear association with the age-related decrease of bone mineral density (BMD). In view of the significance of sex steroids in the maintenance of BMD at all ages, the question whether the partial androgen deficiency in aging males plays an important role in the decrease of BMD is pertinent. A pivotal role of androgens in the decrease of BMD has, however, been difficult to establish [98]. Not all scientific findings agree. Indeed, some studies find a significant, though weak, correlation between androgen levels and bone mineral density at some, but not all, bone sites [99–101]. Others are unable to establish a correlation [102–104]. There are some recent large-scale studies of several hundred elderly men [92,105,106] and they demonstrate that bone density in the radius, spine, and hip are correlated with levels of BT. Interestingly, the correlation with levels of bioavailable estradiol was much more prominent, probably pointing to the significance of estrogens in men, also in old age. The effects of T therapy on BMD of men over 50 have been studied in six RCTs of 12 ($n = 4$) to 36 months ($n = 2$) [87,88]. The T group behaved significantly better than the placebo group in five of these six trials. Pooled effects revealed that treatment effect was higher at the lumbar spine and femoral neck sites [88]. However, due to high baseline variability of the study population, the pooled effects failed to reach statistical significance. Only a trend towards significance was found at the lumbar spine site (estimated increase of 3.7%). In a study by Snyder *et al.*, increase in lumbar BMD was inversely correlated with pretreatment T concentrations suggesting that this effect mainly concerned the really hypogonadal subjects. A recent uncontrolled but large-scale study evaluating long-term effects of T treatment showed that BMD continues to increase at the lumbar spine after 18 and 30 months of treatment [107]. Meta-regression analysis performed at the lumbar spine and femoral neck revealed a significant effect of treatment preparation used, with the highest effect found with T esters [88]. Study of pooled effects of T therapy on bone markers used in eight RCTs found that T had a moderate effect in reducing bone resorption markers ($p < 0.01$) [88]. However the corresponding data showed significant heterogeneity. The only two individual markers that showed statistical reduction during T treatment were the N-telopeptides and the deoxypyridinoline/creatinine ratio (respectively, $P < 0.05$) [88]. No significant effect was found on bone formation markers. Until now no adequately powered trial has yet explored the impact of T administration on hip and vertebral fractures.

Role of aromatization

The suggestion presents itself that the effects of androgens, which decline in elderly males, are at least partially mediated via their aromatization to estrogens [108]. In line with the latter observation Barett-Connor *et al.* observed a significant negative and graded association between levels of total and bioavailable estradiol, but not of BT and fracture prevalence in males (median age 67 years, range 56–87 years) independently of age, body mass index, or exercise [109]. While the evidence for a significant role of estrogens in bone health is growing, the effects of T should not be dismissed. Levels of BT correlated with all regions of proximal femur BMD and total body BMD after adjustment for age [92]. It is to be remembered that estrogens are largely (>80%) products of peripheral aromatization of androgens.

In sum, the relevance of androgens (both in their own right and as precursors for the formation of estrogens) in age-associated osteopenia seems clear on the basis of these recent large-scale studies. However the extent of the effects of T therapy is limited with respect to what has been reported in young hypogonadal males.

Cardiovascular function
Steroids and vascular risk factors
Premenopausal women suffer significantly less from cardiovascular disease than men, and traditionally it has been thought that the relationship between sex steroids and cardiovascular disease is predominantly determined by the relatively beneficial effects of estrogens, and by the relatively detrimental effects of androgens on lipid profiles [101]. Nevertheless, the vast majority of cross-sectional studies in men are not in agreement with this assumption; they show a positive correlation between FT levels and HDL cholesterol [111–113], and a negative correlation, with fibrinogen, plasminogen activator inhibitor-1 [105], and insulin levels as well as with coronary heart disease [115,116], but not with cardiovascular mortality [117–119].

Recent research shows the effects of sex steroids on biologic systems other than lipids. Fat distribution, endocrine/paracrine factors produced by the vascular wall (such as endothelins, nitric oxide), blood platelets and coagulation, must also be considered in the analysis of the relationship between sex steroids and cardiovascular disease [120,121].

Low testosterone level in coronary artery disease
Premenopausal women, in comparison to men, are felt to be protected against cardiovascular disease by estrogens. It is then paradoxical that in cross-sectional studies of men, elevated levels of estrogens [115] and relatively low levels of T [116,122,123] appear to be associated with coronary disease and myocardial infarction. These studies suggest the intriguing possibility that, in spite of the prior assumption of overall negative effects of androgens on lipid profiles, a lower-than-normal androgen level in aging men is associated with an increase of atherosclerotic disease. In a study of geriatric male patients who had suffered a myocardial infarction, it was found that these patients had low T levels [116]. In addition four trials have found that pharmacologic doses of T relax coronary arteries when injected intraluminally, and modest but consistent improvement of exercise-induced angina and electrocardiographic ischemia have been observed following short-term T administration in at least five RCTs [123–127]. These results are encouraging but they await longer-term investigations. On the other hand no beneficial effect could be demonstrated on peripheral arterial disease, and possible effects on cerebrovascular disease have not been evaluated [124,126].

The apparently negative effect of androgens in old studies may have been due, in part, to the supraphysiologic levels of T achieved when injectable T esters were used. The explanation may also lie in the fact that T also exerts both beneficial and adverse effects on the vascular wall, and that a complex of risk factors for cardiovascular disease—termed syndrome X or the metabolic syndrome (comprising hypertension, insulin resistance, hypertriglyceridemia, and visceral obesity)—is associated with low T levels [83,84,115,128].

Testosterone effects on the arterial wall
Vascular cells contain T and estradiol (E2) receptors as well as converting enzymes needed for E2 production. Therefore T may regulate vascular physiology, directly or indirectly [126]. It may especially modulate vascular reactivity by both endothelium-dependent and -independent mechanisms. Physiologic doses reduce vasodilation through genomic actions. As already described, supraphysiologic

doses enhance vasodilation through non-genomic action. In addition, T exerts both pro-atherogenetic (rapid accumulation) and anti-atherogenetic effects (lipid secretion) on macrophage functions.

Role of metabolic syndrome and prospects of testosterone supplementation

Low T in men is a component of a plurimetabolic syndrome (syndrome X)-associated increase in abdominal fat, insulin resistance, type 2 diabetes, high blood pressure, hypertriglyceridemia, low HDL cholesterol, and a procoagulatory, antifibrinolytic state [124,126]. It could be the driving etiologic factor of this syndrome since following reassessment of the initial cohort of the MMAS study after 15 years, it appeared that low serum TT and SHBG at baseline were significant predictors of subsequent occurrence of metabolic syndrome in men with initially low BMI (<25), but not in those with BMI >25 (risk increase of 41%) [129]. The association of clinical symptoms of androgen deficiency doubled the risk of subsequent metabolic syndrome (OR 2.51), but only in lean men. The assumption that the effects of androgens on lipid profiles are only one factor in the relationship between androgens and cardiovascular disease is supported by Tchernof *et al.* who could demonstrate that, upon multivariate analysis, adjusting for visceral obesity, the correlation between androgen levels and lipid parameters loses its significance [84]. Given the fact that cardiovascular disease is associated with low plasma T levels, the question whether T supplementation in aging men can reverse these cardiovascular risks is very interesting (for review see [123]).

Effects of testosterone therapy

The first results of studies wherein T was actually administered to mildly hypogonadal aging men did not indicate negative effects on lipid profiles. In a double-blind, placebo-controlled, crossover study, Tenover found that administering T enanthate (100 mg per week) for three months to 13 healthy elderly men (with low serum total and non-SHBG-bound T levels) decreased total and LDL cholesterol without affecting levels of HDL cholesterol [130]. Results of a study by Morley *et al.* are in agreement with these findings [131]; administration of 200 mg of T enan-

thate every two weeks for three months decreased total cholesterol without affecting HDL cholesterol levels. The meta-analysis by Isidori *et al.* [88] pooled 16 RCTs performed in men over 50, including the two previous ones. Testosterone therapy significantly decreased serum total cholesterol whatever the baseline T level, but its effects were more pronounced in men with TT <10 nmol/L (average −0.42 mmol/L or 16 mg/dL) than in men with higher TT (average −0.14 mmol/L). T had no effects on LDL cholesterol. A small but significant reduction in HDL cholesterol was observed in the group of studies performed in men with baseline T >10 nmol/L (−0.09 mmol/L or −3.3 mg/dl, −4–6%, with respect to the baseline values), but not in men with lower T values; the effect over the whole of the studies (whatever the baseline T level) was not significant.

Overall T therapy has both beneficial and adverse metabolic effects: the decreases in visceral fat, Lp(a) lipoprotein, insulin resistance, fibrinogen, the fibrinolysis inhibitor PAI-1, and to a lesser degree triglycerides and, if any, LDL cholesterol, are probably beneficial. The decrease in HDL cholesterol may be adverse, though its final effect depends in fact on its mechanism, presently unknown. It would be beneficial if it reflected accelerated reverse cholesterol transport.

Conclusions

Conclusions about T therapy and cardiovascular function [87] are, first, that T exerts both apparently beneficial and deleterious actions on a multitude of factors implicated in pathogenesis of arteriosclerosis and cardiovascular disease. However, epidemiologic studies have found no consistent association of endogenous androgens with cardiovascular disease. In addition no cardiovascular overmortality has been reported during RCTs. But follow-up is too limited in these RCTs (36–48 months) to assess long-term risks. It has also to be remembered that overdosing T therapy exposes men to a risk of fluid retention that may result in heightened blood pressure or decompensation of cardiac insufficiency, and to polycythemia that may result in increased blood viscosity and thrombosis. But provided overdosing is avoided, current evidence suggests that therapeutic use of T in men need not be restricted by concerns over cardiovascular side effects. On the other hand, even if most T effects on vascular risk factors seem beneficial, and if a large amount of clinical data suggests the possibility of vascular benefits of T therapy, as concerns coronary artery disease, available data do not justify uncontrolled use of T for prevention of this disease [87,126,127].

Psychic functions

Cognitive functions

There is some evidence to suggest that T may influence performance on cognitive tasks [132,133], which is supported by the finding that T administration to older men enhances performance on measures of spatial cognition. The correlation between T levels and cognitive performance, such as spatial abilities or mathematical reasoning [134,135], has been confirmed in Western and non-Western cohorts of healthy males [135]. In a cross-sectional analysis of the MMAS data, while older age was associated with lower cognitive functioning (spatial ability, working memory, and speed/attention), no association of these cognitive measures with any hormone persisted after adjustment for age and covariates, and logged hormones did not mediate the age–cognition relationship [136]. However in the 10 years' longitudinal assessment of multiple cognitive domains and of T, SHBG, and free T index (FTI) of the Baltimore Longitudinal Study, higher FTI predicted better scores on visual and verbal memory, visuospatial functioning, and visuomotor scanning, and a reduced rate of longitudinal decline in visual memory [137].

While it is well known that T therapy significantly improves cognition, mood, energy, and well-being in young hypogonadal men, such effects are less clear in aging men. Among seven RCTs in men over 50 that assessed cognitive abilities, only three found statistically significant effects on spatial cognition (two of two), spatial and verbal memory (two of four) and working memory (one study) [87]. No significant effect over placebo was found for overall memory, recall, or verbal fluency. T therapy proved to increase energy more than placebo in three of four RCTs in aging men. Lastly, one or more of the measures of quality of life were improved in three of the five RCTs that assessed it, but the improvement concerned

only a minority of the assessed dimensions [87]. The cognitive benefits of T therapy thus seem limited, especially considering the mainly negative findings found in the two RCTs of longer duration. Nevertheless it has to be noted that the few positive results were obtained in men with impaired health or in a subset of men with manifestly low serum T [138].

Mood

Testosterone has also been associated with general mood-elevating effects. Some studies have found associations between lowered T levels and depressive symptoms [139,140]. Depression is not rare in aging men, and impairs their quality of life [139]; so the effects that declining levels of androgens may have on mood and on specific aspects of cognitive functioning in aging are well-worth researching. However, although low T was recently observed to predict incident depressive illness in older men in a longitudinal study [141], and a significant relation between depression and androgen receptor CAG repeat length has been reported in men aged 48–79 years [142], only two of the nine RCTs that have assessed the effects of T therapy on mood in aging men found a significant improvement in depression scores compared with placebo [87]. Combined therapy with T has also been observed to improve the efficacy of anti-depressant agents over placebo in small groups of younger men with refractory depression [143].

Role of aromatization

Earlier studies have questioned the relevance of estrogens in human male sexuality [144]. A recent study found that estrogen replacement in an aromatase-deficient man increased libidinous aspects of sexuality [145]. There is also a range of non-sexual effects of androgens on the brain and for (some of) these effects aromatization of androgen to estrogens might be relevant. Indeed, effects of estrogen on the brain are increasingly being recognized [146], though studies have mainly been carried out using animal models. Estrogens have been observed to influence many processes in many regions of the brain throughout the entire life span. These effects include those on cognitive function, co-ordination of movement, pain, and affective state, involving both the estrogen receptor (ER)-α and ER-β genes. Only some of the estrogen actions on the brain are intracellularly receptor-mediated, while others take place on the cell membrane, mediated via second messenger mechanisms, neuronal excitability, and ion channels [147].

Steroids and Alzheimer disease

With regard to Alzheimer disease, men are relatively protected in comparison to women. One intriguing possibility is the putative neuroprotective effect of estrogens in preventing or retarding this condition [147]. Estrogens increase choline acetyltransferase, the enzyme needed to synthesize acetylcholine [148]. The assumption that postmenopausal women enjoy protection from Alzheimer disease when they receive estrogen replacement therapy has been challenged by the recently discontinued Women's Health Initiative (WHI) study. The WHI Memory Study showed that the combination of conjugated equine estrogens and progestagens increased the risk of probable dementia in postmenopausal women aged 65 years or over [149]. This could be due to the antagonistic effects of medroxyprogesterone acetate on the positive effects of estrogens on cognitive functions [150], and not to estrogenic effects per se. There is evidence that androgens confer protection from Alzheimer disease in their own right [151]. So there may be an advantage in supplementing androgens in aging men whose T levels have fallen below a certain limit, thereby in fact substituting both androgens and estrogens. Not all studies in aging men are in agreement, however. A recent study [152] found only a link between cognition and estrogens in women but not in men, whereas Yaffe *et al.* found a correlation between cognitive functioning and BT, but not E2 [153].

Estrogens contribute to explicit (or declarative) memory function through their action on hippocampal neurons. The implication of this estrogen effect is improved (conscious) recall of facts, events, and autobiographic memories [153,154]. Explicit memory is considered the cognitive function that is most vulnerable to loss of estrogen. Women receiving estrogen replacement, and men whose estrogen levels are above those of postmenopausal women, score better on explicit memory tasks [155].

Summary

For the effects of androgens on sexual functioning, aromatization of T is probably not required; but for other effects on the brain the evidence is much stronger, and it seems recommendable that androgen-deficient men, including the androgen-deficient aging male, should receive an aromatizable androgen preparation.

It is of note that almost all the above studies are observational and in need of replication. Placebo-controlled studies proving the benefits of (aromatizable) androgens on cognitive functioning, and prevention or slowing of dementia, are lacking. Therefore, it is too early to recommend androgens to improve the age-related decline of cognition in men.

Sexual functioning

Aging is the most robust risk factor predicting erectile difficulties. It is obvious that aging per se is associated with a deterioration of the biologic functions mediating erectile function: hormonal, vascular, and neural processes. This is often aggravated by intercurrent disease in old age, such as diabetes mellitus, cardiovascular disease, and use of medical drugs. T is only one of the elements which may explain sexual dysfunction with aging.

It has been repeatedly shown in hypogonadal patients (with a wide age range) that sexual functions only require androgen levels below or at the lower end of reference values of T [8–10]. The relative androgen-independence of erections in response to erotic stimuli in the first studies [33], since then challenged in many others [156], and the relatively low androgen levels required, suggest that T was not a useful treatment for men with erectile difficulties whose T levels were usually only marginally low. This was reinforced with the advent of intracorporal smooth muscle relaxants (papaverine, prostaglandin E1), later superseded by the PDE5i, hailed as the ultimate successful treatment of ED.

As already detailed in p. 231, T therapy-replacement alone may not suffice to restore erectile potency in every case since ED is often multifactorial in aging patients. It is a matter of clinical judgment what type of treatment should be tried first, PDE5i or T, but it is important to remember that insufficient success of one type of treatment might require addition of the other, as well as treating the underlying medical risk factors.

Diagnosis: clinical symptoms and screening
Screening for hypogonadism in sexual dysfunctions

Several varieties of sexual dysfunction, mainly ED, may be the presenting symptom of hypogonadism, a condition that can reveal diseases with serious nonsexual consequences, such as pituitary tumors. In addition, missing a hypogonadism responsible for sexual dysfunction would deprive the patient of an etiologic therapy that would give him the best chance of success. This has led to the advocating of routine determination of T in several dysfunctions.

Erectile dysfunction

Several authors question the recommendation of routine T determination in ED because of the cost of hormone determinations, the low prevalence of hypogonadism in this population, and the limited success rate of T therapy in the hypogonadal ED patient [18,54]. They recommend screening only patients with low sexual desire or abnormal physical examination (small and soft testes, reduced body hair, and so on). However, in a study of routine determinations of TT in over 1000 ED patients, the specificity, sensitivity, and efficiency of low sexual desire in the detection of low T (<3 ng/mL, 10.4 nmol/L) were very low (66, 48, and 63%, respectively) [18]. By combining both clinical signs (low sexual desire, present in 29% of the ED patients, and/or physical signs of hypogonadism, present in 30%), sensitivity was only 59%. If T had been determined only in cases of low sexual desire or physical signs of hypogonadism, 40% of the men with low T would have been missed, including 37% of the hypogonadal patients who were subsequently markedly improved with androgen therapy alone. Today most published guidelines recommend routine determination of T in ED [2,24,157].

Other sexual dysfunctions

Routine determination of T is also recommended in case of isolated low sexual desire [24,168], although the prevalence of hypogonadism is low in the absence of associated ED [23]. Testosterone determination is not necessary in the other sexual dysfunctions, unless clinical signs of hypogonadism are associated. Some men using the 5α reductase inhibitor, finasteride, for benign prostate hyperplasia, experience an impact on sexual function, especially on ejaculation, although these effects are relatively rare [158].

Screening for late onset hypogonadism (LOH)

In women, age-related hormonal changes are well recognized, generally with a rapid onset and progression, leading to the characteristic menopausal symptoms. In males, the changes in the hypothalamic–pituitary–gonadal axis in general have an insidious onset and a slow progression, do not have clinical manifestations in all men, have a great variability from man to man—with the clinical picture of hypogonadism being mild or even nonexistent in many of them [159].

The clinical signs and symptoms of LOH can be [2,157] (Table 18.1):
- Decreased libido (sexual desire)
- Erectile dysfunction (diminished quality of the rigidity, intercourse frequency and nocturnal erections)
- Decrease in lean body mass, muscle volume and strength
- Decrease in BMD, resulting in osteopenia, osteoporosis and increased risk of bone fractures
- Increase in visceral fat
- Changes in mood, with concomitant decreases in intellectual activity, cognitive functions, spatial orientation ability, fatigue, depressed mood and irritability
- Decrease in body hair
- Skin alterations
- Gynecomastia
- Anemia

Hypogonadism is also prevalent in men with insulin resistance [160], especially in those with type 2 diabetes and metabolic syndrome, which are frequent in aging men [161].

These symptoms, though, can also be present in many medical conditions and also may be manifested in the normal process of aging. In conjunction with a complete anamnesis and physical examination, aging men with one or more of these complaints or conditions should be investigated when biochemical hypoandrogenism is suspected. Some screening questionnaires were developed to facilitate the clinical diagnosis of LOH [157,162,163]. Although not extensively used, they can be useful as an initial screening that could lead to a biochemical assessment. The ADAM questionnaire is a simple and sensitive questionnaire, but performs marginally on specificity, particularly in the elderly [162]. The AMS questionnaire from Heineman has also been validated in most languages [163], but has also a rather low specificity. On their introduction, these instruments promised to offer a versatile tool to identify men with LOH in large-scale communities. However, Beutel *et al.* recently demonstrated that the ADAM score is unrelated to T levels and only moderately associated with age. The AMS is unrelated both to T level and age. They conclude that, based on their high correlations with depression, both seem to measure symptoms associated with depression rather than symptoms of LOH [164]. In conclusion neither of these questionnaires replaces a proper history and clinical examination, and better instruments need to be developed.

Biochemical diagnosis

What hormone should be measured?

The laboratory reference values of T and FT show a wider range than those for most other hormones (for instance, thyroid hormones), which makes it difficult to establish whether measured values of T in patients are normal or abnormal. Is a patient whose plasma levels of T fall from the upper to the lower range of normal T levels (a drop of as much as 50%), T deficient? T levels may well remain within the reference range but may be inappropriately low for that particular individual or his particular age. In thyroid pathophysiology, plasma thyroid-stimulating hormone (TSH) proves to be a better criterion of thyroid hyper/hypofunction than plasma T4 or T3, but it is uncertain whether plasma LH is a reliable indicator of male hypogonadism in the elderly man. With aging there are reductions in LH pulse frequency and amplitude. Several studies have found that LH levels are elevated in response to the decline of T levels with aging, but less so than is observed in younger men with similarly reductions in T levels [75]. This may be due to a shift in the setpoint of the negative feedback of T on the hypothalamic pituitary unit, resulting in an enhanced negative feedback action, which consequently leads to a relatively lower LH output in response to lowered circulating levels of T. Another factor is the fact that a number of aging men have chronic illnesses that may cause secondary hypogonadism.

Another variable that might be significant to assess the androgen status in old age is plasma levels of SHBG. Its levels increase even with healthy aging, possibly due to a decrease in growth hormone (GH) production and an increase of the ratio of free estradiol over FT [75]. Vermeulen and co-workers could demonstrate that the FT value calculated by TT/SHBG (according to a second-degree equation following the mass action law) as determined by immunoassay appears to be a rapid, simple, and reliable indicator of BT and FT, comparable to FT values obtained by equilibrium dialysis [165]. An easy-to-use free calculator of calculated FT and BT can be found on www.issam.ch. So, determination of values of T and SHBG might provide a reasonable index of the androgen status in an aging person. BT is also a rather reliable index, but it should be mentioned that direct FT assays using a T analog do not yield a reliable estimate of FT [165].

What is a low T level?

The above has outlined the many unresolved questions as to the verification of deficiencies in the biologic action of androgens in old age, and has shown that there is no generally accepted lower limit of normal. Consequently, a pragmatic approach to this issue must be taken in order to let aging androgen-deficient men benefit from replacement therapy, while the above theoretical but important questions are resolved by clinical investigations. Vermeulen argues that, in the absence of convincing evidence for an altered androgen requirement in elderly men, he considers the normal range of T levels in young males also valid for elderly men [81,165]. There is now general agreement (official recommendations of ISSAM, ISA, and EAU) that TT levels above 12 nmol/L (3.46 ng/mL), or FT above 250 pmol/L (72 pg/mL) do not require substitution [2]. Similarly, based on the data

Table 18.2 Most often cited normal values for sex steroid levels in serum.

Parameter	Male reference ranges		Female reference ranges		Conversion factor
	Conv. units	SI units	Conv. units	SI units	
Testosterone (total)	3–10 ng/mL	10.4–34.6 nmol/L	<0.6 ng/mL	<2.1 nmol/L	3.46
Testosterone (free)	9–47 pg/mL	31–163 pmol/L	0.7–3.6 pg/mL	2.4–12.5 pmol/L	3.46
DHT	16–108 ng/dL	55–372 nmol/L	<20 ng/dL	<69 nmol/L	3.44
Androstenedione	0.57–2.65 ng/mL	1.99–9.25 nmol/L	0.47–2.68 ng/mL <1.0 ng/mL*	1.64–9.35 nmol/L <3.49 nmol/L*	3.49
DHEA-S	2.0–5.0 µg/mL	5.4–13.5 µmol/L	1.1–4.4 µg/mL <1.2 µg/mL*	2.97–11.88 µmol/L <3.24 µmol/L*	2.71
17ß-estradiol	10–50 pg/mL	36–183 pmol/L	30–300 pg/mL[1] 300–400 pg/mL[2] >130 pg/mL[3] <20 pg/mL*	110–1100 pmol/L[1] 1100–1468 pmol/L[2] >477 pmol/L[3] <73 pmol/mL*	3.67
Progesterone	0.1–1.0 ng/mL	0.32–3.2 nmol/L	<1.5 ng/mL[1] >12.0 ng/mL[2] 7.4–196 ng/mL[4] <0.8 ng/mL*	<4.8 nmol/L[1] >38.4 nmol/L[2] 23.7–627 nmol/L[4] <2.6 nmol/L*	3.2
Prolactin	2–14.5 ng/mL	40–290 mIU/L	<10.0 ng/mL[1] <16.0 ng/mL[2] <8.0 ng/mL*	<200 mLU/L[1] <320 mLU/L[2] <160 mLU/L*	20
SHBG		13–55 nmol/L		30–95 nmol/L	

Reference values for women: * postmenopause; [1] follicular phase; [2] ovulation phase; [3] luteal phase; [4] during pregnancy.
DHEA-S, dehydroepiandrosterone sulfate; DHT, dihydrotestosterone; SHBG, sex hormone-binding globulin.

of younger men, there is consensus that serum TT below 8 nmol/L (2.31 ng/mL) or FT below 180 pmol/L (52 pg/mL) require substitution [2]. Since symptoms of T deficiency become manifest between 12 and 8 nmol/L, trial of treatment can be considered in those in whom alternative causes of these symptoms have been excluded. Lastly since there are variations in the reagents and normal ranges among laboratories, the cutoff values given for serum TT and FT may have to be adjusted depending on the reference values given by each laboratory [2].

Precautions

To avoid a false diagnosis of hypogonadism, measurement of T has traditionally been recommend to take place before 11 am in view of the diurnal rhythm of plasma T. This should remain mandatory for men younger than 40, but the diurnal rhythm of T is less clearcut in elderly men compared to young men, but it is usually not absent [6,7], and the risk of falsely diagnosing hypogonadism when determining T after this time seems minimal in men over 40 [7].

The consequences of lower-than-normal value of T may have great impact, such as T-replacement. If indeed plasma T values /cBT/cFT are so low that T-therapy is considered, the measurement has to be repeated a couple of weeks later, together with an assessment of LH and prolactin. Many physical or psychologic stresses of daily living may temporarily depress T secretion. Otherwise, serial measurements of T in (elderly) men are fairly stable [166,167].

Table 18.2 lists some normal biochemical values. These ranges are only examples. They depend in fact on the determination methods used by the

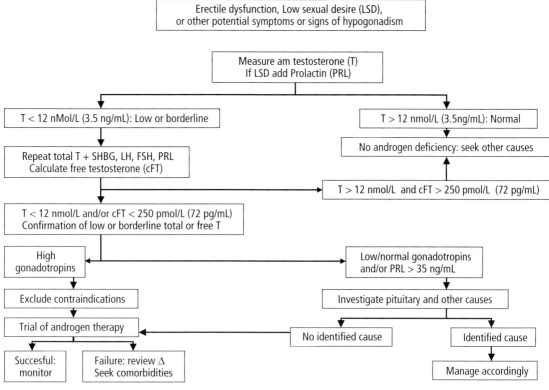

Fig. 18.3 Algorithm for the diagnosis of suspected hypogonadism.

laboratory. Each laboratory should provide its correspondents wih reference ranges established in the laboratory; it is better to select laboratories most experienced in hormone determinations.

Accuracy
Commercial radio-immunoassays and non-radioactive immunoassay kits, as well as automated platform immunoassays that mostly use chemiluminescence detection are widely available and provide fairly accurate measurements of TT between 10 and 35 nmol/L. Below 10 nmol/L their accuracy is considerably less. However, reference values vary significantly from laboratory to laboratory, and from measurement method to method. Consequently, it is advisable that every laboratory establishes its own "normal range" of T in men [168,169].

Searching for the etiology
In cases of secondary hypogonadism (normal or low serum LH), several etiologies involving risks for

health must be looked for: in any case hyperprolactinemia by determining serum prolactin, possibly hemochromatosis, by determining serum iron and ferritin, and in case of marked secondary hypogonadism a pituitary tumor searched for with magnetic resonance imaging (MRI), even in the absence of hyperprolactinemia.

The diagnostic approach is summarized in Fig. 18.3, the algorithm for suspected hypogonadism.

Androgen therapy
Androgen therapy has a number of benefits.

Benefits of androgen therapy
Testosterone monotherapy
Clinical studies examining T monotherapy for the treatment of ED have yielded varying results. Meta-analysis, including trials in young organic hypogonadal patients, has shown a 57% response rate for T therapy in patients with ED, ranging from 64% for primary hypogonadism to 44% for

secondary hypogonadism [14]. Morales *et al.* showed that T therapy is an effective treatment for hypogonadal impotence, with improvement in sexual attitudes and performance in 61% of patients [56]. In another study, T monotherapy has been observed to improve erectile function in only 36% of the hypogonadal patients consulting for ED [18] (see also pp. 203–2).

T therapy may have more significant effects on libido than on erectile function [170]. In one study, normalization of serum T levels in hypogonadal men with ED resulted in only short-term improvement (one month) in erectile function and sexual satisfaction, while improvement of sexual desire was statistically significant for the six months of the study, making the use of T therapy alone questionable in this population [74]. However, T monotherapy did improve sexual performance, desire, and motivation in men with hypogonadism, in clinical trials with transdermal T-gel formulation. Maximal improvement occurred on day 30 and continued for the six-month duration of the study [30].

There is a lack of data suggesting the efficacy of T therapy in older men who do not meet the clinical definition of hypogonadism. There is no convincing evidence that androgen therapy is either effective or safe for older men, unless a formal diagnosis of hypogonadism exists [161]. The US Institute of Medicine (IOM) has recommended additional clinical research focusing on the benefits of T therapy in older men as compared with placebo controls, followed by larger-scale and longer-term trials to assess risks and benefits [171].

Combination therapy
PDE5i are the first line of therapy in men who do not have potentially reversible causes of ED, such as hypogonadism [170]. Nonetheless, 23% to 50% of patients do not respond to PDE5i alone [73,172]. Given the role of T in the NO pathway central to proper erectile function, interest in PDE5i–testosterone combination therapy has risen in recent years [157]. As reported on p. 232, the most robust arguments supporting the validity of such a combination come from a randomized, placebo-controlled study of hypogonadal men with ED, non-responders to sildenafil [73]. In addition to improving erectile function,

T therapy improved orgasmic function [73]. In another randomized, placebo-controlled study, short-term transdermal T administration improved the erectile response to sildenafil by increasing arterial inflow to the penis during sexual stimulation [52]. T was also shown to improve arterial flow and subsequent response to tadalafil treatment, with a greater response after 10 weeks, compared to four weeks of pretreatment with T [172]. Lastly, in a recent RCT, sildenafil improved sleep-related erections even in hypogonadal men, but combined therapy with T had greater effects than the sum of the two compounds alone, proving synergy [69].

Other uncontrolled studies have reported beneficial effects of combination therapy in patients with co-morbid conditions. Administration of intramuscular T and sildenafil was found to be efficacious in renal transplant patients and in patients on renal dialysis [173]. Oral T has been reported to reverse ED associated with type 2 diabetes in patients failing on sildenafil therapy alone [71]. In conclusion, T combination therapy with PDE5i may improve the response to PDEi in patients with ED and hypogonadism.

Risks of androgen therapy
Recent reports suggesting increased risks associated with hormone replacement in women [174,175] have aroused concern that men receiving hormone replacement may also be vulnerable to increased health risks. However, no large-scale, long-term studies have yet been initiated to assess the benefits and risks of T therapy in men.

Benign prostatic hyperplasia
It is well recognized that the development of benign prostatic hyperplasia requires the presence of androgens and that the marked reduction in serum T caused by chemical or surgical castration reduces prostate volume. However, multiple studies [176] have failed to demonstrate exacerbation of voiding symptoms attributable to benign prostatic hyperplasia during T therapy, and complications such as urinary retention have not occurred at higher rates than in controls receiving placebo.

The literature on the effect on prostate volume with exogenous T in middle-aged and older men with clinical features of symptomatic LOH (SLOH) is controversial. Pechersky *et al.* found that prostate growth can be retarded or even reversed with androgen therapy [177]. Others found that prostate volume, as determined by ultrasonography, increases significantly during T therapy, mainly during the first six months, to a level equivalent to that of men without hypogonadism. However, urine flow rates, post-voiding residual urine volumes, and prostate voiding symptoms did not change significantly in these studies. This apparent paradox is explained by the poor correlation between prostate volume and urinary symptoms. Clinicians should nevertheless be aware that individual men with hypogonadism may occasionally have increased voiding symptoms with T therapy.

Prostate cancer

Prospective studies have demonstrated a low frequency of prostate cancer in association with T therapy. A compilation of published prospective studies of T therapy (http://content.nejm.org/cgi/content/full/350/5/482 - R6) revealed only five cases of prostate cancer among 461 men (1.1%) followed for six to 36 months, a prevalence rate similar to that in the general population. Some studies call for caution to administer T to elderly men. One recent study left its mark on minds by describing that in 20 patients prostate cancer was diagnosed within two years after initiation of T-replacement therapy, with 45 % in the Gleason 7–9 category, implying a poor prognosis [178]. The authors concluded that prostate cancer may become clinically apparent within months to a few years after the initiation of T treatment. However the methodology of this study was very poor, the authors were unable to find how many total patients were really at risk, and nearly half of these 20 men did not have a digital rectal examination prior to T therapy initiation that was done by primary care physicians. This study however-er emphasizes the necessity of systematic and careful screening for prostate cancer before any T therapy.

Men with low T levels are eligible for T administration. But it is of some concern that the underlying prevalence of occult prostate cancer in men with low T levels appears to be substantial. Morgentaler

et al. found prostate cancer on sextant prostate biopsy in 14% of men (median age 64 years) with hypogonadism who had normal prostate serum antigen (PSA) levels and normal results on digital rectal examinations before receiving T therapy [179]. In a separate, retrospective study of men with known prostate cancer, high-grade prostate cancers were associated with low FT levels [180]. Low pre-operative T values in patients with prostate cancer were associated with advanced pathological stage [181], and with extraprostatic disease in patients with localized prostate cancer [182]. These findings may be explained in part by the observation that the levels of T, LH, and FSH all increase after radical prostatectomy, suggesting that prostate cancer itself, or possibly even normal prostate tissue, may have an inhibitory effect on serum androgen levels [183,184].

Despite decades of research, there is no compelling evidence that T has a causative role in prostate cancer [177–189]. For example, studies using stored frozen plasma samples failed to show a difference in T levels between men in whom prostate cancer developed seven to 25 years later and those in whom it did not. In 2001, Hsing reviewed the 12 available prospective studies that examined the relation between serum androgen levels and prostate cancer. Only one case-control study (the Physicians' Health Study) suggested any significant relation between higher T levels and prostate cancer. However, this study found no significant difference in mean T levels between patients with prostate cancer and control subjects, and no significant difference in the risk of cancer between men in the highest and lowest quartiles for serum T. An increased risk of prostate cancer with higher T levels was observed only after simultaneous adjustment for four other hormones [190].

Thus, there appears to be no compelling evidence at present to suggest that men with higher T levels are at greater risk of prostate cancer, or that treating men who have hypogonadism with exogenous androgens increases this risk [81,191]. In fact, it should be recognized that prostate cancer becomes more prevalent exactly at the time of a man's life when T levels decline.

In conclusion, proper monitoring with PSA and

digital rectal examination (DRE) should promote the early diagnosis, and thus potential cure, of most "unmasked" prostate cancers identified during T therapy. Certainly, all men presenting for possible T therapy who are found to have an abnormal PSA level or abnormal DRE should first undergo prostate biopsy, and there should also be a low threshold for biopsy if the PSA level rises substantially or if there is a change on DRE, such as the development of a nodule, asymmetry, or areas of increased firmness. Although a history of prostate cancer has been considered an absolute contraindication to T therapy, this point is now under active debate for men who are deemed cured.

In follow-up studies of tens of thousands of men it appears that the risk of having prostate cancer is also high in the PSA range of 2–4 ng/mL, which implies that the commonly accepted cut-off value of PSA of 4 ng/mL as safe may not be valid [192]. Meanwhile the majority of the prostate cancer experts agree that, rather than the absolute value of PSA, its velocity during the observational period is of importance, and that an increase of PSA of more than 0.5 ng/mL/year over two following years is an indication for a prostate biopsy and withdrawal from T-replacement therapy [193]. The present recommendations are as follows: biopsy is recommended if the PSA velocity exceeds 0.2–0.5 ng/mL/year in men with a total PSA level less than 2.5 ng/mL/year, or if the PSA velocity is greater than 0.75 ng/mL/year and the total PSA is above 4 ng/mL [194]. A strict adherence to these guidelines is essential.

Lipids

Available data regarding the relation of T-replacement therapy to lipid profiles are inconsistent. Supraphysiologic doses of androgens, particularly oral non-aromatizable androgenic steroids, appear to lower HDL levels [195]. However, numerous controlled studies using physiologic doses of T have shown no change, or only a minimal reduction, in HDL, often accompanied by a reduction in total cholesterol. Whitsel *et al.* performed a meta-analysis of the effects of intramuscular T esters on serum lipids in men with hypogonadism, and reported that HDL levels were reduced in three studies and unchanged in 15 [196]. Total cholesterol levels were reduced in five studies, increased in two, and unchanged in 12. LDL levels were unchanged or reduced in 14 of the 15 studies in which they were measured. Thus, the limited information available would suggest a neutral effect of T therapy on lipid profiles. A double-blind, placebo-controlled study involving 108 healthy men receiving transdermal T failed to show any significant difference between groups in serum levels of lipids and apolipoprotein during 36 months of treatment [197]. In a 24-week, multicenter, randomized, parallel-group study, Dobs *et al.* [198] compared transdermal and intramuscular administration of androgens in 58 men and did not detect any significant difference in HDL levels or in the ratio of total cholesterol to HDL in either group, regardless of the mode of therapy. We have already cited on p. 234 the results of the meta-analysis by Isidori *et al.* [88], which concluded there was a significant decrease of serum total cholesterol on T therapy in aging men, whatever the T level, while no significant effect could be demonstrated on LDL cholesterol, and a significant decrease in HDL cholesterol was observed only in the aging men with baseline serum T >10 nmol/L.

Thus, the present data, taken together, suggest that T therapy within the physiologic range is not associated with significant worsening of the lipid profile.

Cardiovascular risk

The belief that T is a risk factor for cardiac disease is based on the observation that men have both a higher incidence of cardiovascular events and higher T levels than women. However, few, if any, data support a causal relation between higher T levels and heart disease [199–202]. Indeed, several studies suggest that higher T levels may actually have a favorable effect on the risk of cardiovascular disease [203,204].

Evidence that T therapy may be beneficial for men with cardiac disease was provided by English *et al.*, who found that 22 men with chronic stable angina who were treated with transdermal T therapy had greater angina-free exercise tolerance than 24 placebo-treated controls [205]. However, it is unknown how this observation may relate to cardiovascular risk during long-term T supplementation. In a study of 32 men treated for 52 weeks with 200 mg of intramuscular T enanthate weekly, Anderson *et al.* showed decreases in prothrombotic factors, pro-thrombinase activity, and proteins C and S to be counterbalanced by increases in antithrombin III activity and fibrinolytic activity. There was no effect on platelet activity [206]. The issues related to the possible impact of T therapy on cardiovascular function have also been extensively discussed on pp. 236–8.

Studies of T therapy have not demonstrated an increased incidence of cardiovascular disease or events such as myocardial infarction, stroke, or angina [207]. Although the data appear reassuring, definitive assessment of the long-term effects of T therapy on cardiovascular health will require prospective, large-scale, placebo-controlled studies [125].

Polycythemia

Testosterone is a physiologic stimulus for erythropoiesis. Men with hypogonadism have lower hemoglobin levels than age-matched controls, and T therapy can restore their hemoglobin levels to the normal range. The mild anemia prevalent in elderly men has been postulated to be due to declining T levels [208]. Although a rise in the hematocrit is generally beneficial for patients with anemia, elevation above the normal range may have grave consequences, particularly in the elderly [209]. The risk of hemoconcentration and of resulting thrombosis is greater if the patient also has a condition that may itself be associated with an increase in the hematocrit, such as smokers, men with chronic obstructive pulmonary disease, and congestive heart failure. Some cases of thrombosis of various arteries have been reported in literature. T injections appear to be associated with a greater risk of polycythemia than topical preparations. Dobs *et al.* [198] compared a transdermal non-scrotal T patch with intramuscular injections of T enanthate and observed that 15.4% and 43.8% of patients, respectively, had at least one documented elevated hematocrit value (defined as over 52%) during the course of the study.

Although untoward events are unlikely with mild erythrocytosis of relatively short duration, the hematocrit or hemoglobin level should be monitored in men receiving T therapy so that appropriate measures may be instituted if polycythemia develops.

Infertility

All delivery methods for T therapy share a common shortcoming. Some suppression of the hypothalamic–pituitary–gonadal axis is inevitable via a negative feedback mechanism [210]: the low LHRH levels decrease LH and FSH production by the pituitary gland; the low LH levels translate to low T production by the Leydig cells in the testes; and the reduction in FSH results in suppression of spermatogenesis [211]. Young men with hypogonadotropic hypogonadism who are interested in fathering children may avoid T therapy and seek treatment with agents that stimulate the internal production of T, such as hCG or in mild cases—clomiphene citrate.

Contraindications

The absolute contraindication for T therapy is the suspected or documented presence of prostate cancer or breast cancer [212]. Although there is no evidence that T or any other androgen initiates prostate cancer, it is generally accepted that T therapy may accelerate an already existing prostate cancer. Relative contraindications and cautions include severe congestive heart failure for concern of fluid retention, and polycythemia, severe sleep apnea, severe lower urinary tract symptoms, gynecomastia, and male infertility [157].

Candidates for androgen therapy

It is generally accepted in clinical practice that any male with any form of classical hypogonadism and inadequately low T for his age will require androgen therapy if hypogonadism occurred before the age of 50 [213]. Even in men who have proceeded normally through puberty, and who experience no or only minor symptoms (e.g. fatigue, reduced libido), T therapy may be recommended, to prevent long-term sequelae such as osteoporosis [1]. Conversely, there is much debate concerning the validity of this therapy in men with sexual dysfunction and low normal T levels, those with chronic illness and low T, and those with LOH, even if the decline in BT may be partially responsible for the frailty syndrome seen in the aging male [214]. The recommendation common to

ISSAM, ISA, and EAU is that a clear indication, based on a clinical picture together with biochemical evidence of low serum T (see Table 18.2, p. 242), should exist prior to the initiation of T substitution [2].

When screening for candidates for androgen therapy, it is essential to realize that:
• Good biologic markers of androgen action are lacking.
• The interpretation of serum TT levels in the low-normal range is difficult due to the complexities of circadian and pulsatile rhythms, and the binding proteins.
• Current screening questionnaires for androgen deficiency are inaccurate.
• T therapy is only one among other possibilities to reduce physical and affective complaints in the aging male, and/or limit the effects of aging. Actually reducing or stopping tobacco and alcohol, observing a hypolipidemic diet, and, even more, exercising regularly, are the first actions to be taken.

Interest of the "androgen test"
In case of minimal clinical signs of androgen deficiency, or of minimal or borderline serum T decrease, the final decision may rely on the results of a two or, better, three months' trial of androgen therapy [2], assessed with questionnaires such as AMS and IIEF administered both before and at the end of the trial.

Initiation of treatment and follow-up

Appropriate investigations to rule out contraindications before starting T therapy are DRE, determination of PSA, and possibly transrectal ultrasonography. If, after 3–6 months, the signs and symptoms causing the initiation of therapy do not improve, androgen administration should be reconsidered.

The second annual Andropause consensus meeting recommended performing DRE and serum PSA before treatment, at three and six months, and yearly thereafter [215]. In addition to that recommendation, a PSA level could be obtained one month after initiation of therapy to capture the patient with a previously undiagnosed prostate cancer that may be behaving in a very aggressive fashion following T-replacement. ISSAM and WHO guidelines also recommend periodic hematologic assessment, i.e.

before treatment, quarterly for one year, and then annually, to detect possible iatrogenic polycythemia [2,168]. It may also be useful to monitor serum T, especially when under- or overdosing is suspected. Blood has then to be sampled at appropriate times, depending on the T preparation that is used, and its specific pharmacokinetics.

Available preparations

Injectable, transdermal, buccal, and oral T formulations are available for clinical use (Table 18.3). These forms of treatment differ in several key areas, including their risk profiles.

Oral testosterone
Testosterone undecanoate is well absorbed after its oral administration but is quickly degraded during its passage through the liver. Therefore, it is not possible to achieve sustained blood levels of T after oral administration of crystalline T. 17α alkylated derivatives of T (especially methyltestosterone) are relatively resistant to hepatic degradation and can be given orally; however, because of the potential for, and history of, hepatotoxicity, these formulations are not recommended for clinical use.

Long-acting injectable testosterone
The esterification of the T molecule at the 17-β-hydroxy position makes the molecule hydrophobic and extends its duration of action. De-esterification of T is not a limiting factor in determining its duration of action. It is the slow release of the hydrophobic T ester from its oily depot in the muscle that accounts for its extended duration. The longer the side chain, the greater the hydrophobicity of the ester and the greater the duration of action. Thus, T enanthate and cypionate with longer side chains have longer duration of action than T propionate.

T enanthate and T cypionate are supplied as esterified oil-soluble preparations for injection. Their pharmacokinetics are identical as far as half-lives and peak levels. Serum levels of estradiol and DHT (metabolites that are derived by conversion from T) may be excessive in case of overdosing. A typical dose is 100 mg per week, or 200–300 mg every two to three weeks. Peak serum levels occur two to five days after injection, and a return to baseline is

Table 18.3 Available testosterone formulations.

Route	Formulation	Dose	Dosing frequency
Injectable	T propionate in oil	10–25 mg	Twice a week
	T cypionate in oil	50–250 mg	Every 2–4 weeks
	T enanthate in oil	50–250 mg	Every 2–4 weeks
	T undecanoate in oil	1000 mg	Every 10–14 weeks
Oral	T undecanoate*	40–80 mg	2–3 times a day
	T undecanoate caps**	40–80 mg	Twice a day
	Mesterolone	75–150 mg	Once a day
Buccal	T buccal system***	30 mg (1 system)	Twice a day
Transdermal	T patch	5 mg (1 patch)	Once or twice a day
	T gel	50–100 mg	Once a day
Subcutaneous	Crystalline T pellet	600 mg	Every 16–26 weeks

* in oleic acid; ** in a mixture of castor oil and propylene glycol laureate; *** to be stuck to gum.
Source: [75].

usually observed 10 to 14 days after injection. A regimen of T enanthate or cypionate results in highs and lows in serum T levels that are attended by similar changes in the patient's mood, sexual desire and activity, and energy level. The advantages of this form of therapy include low cost and high peak serum levels of T. The disadvantages include the pain of injection and the need for frequent medical visits for administration of the injections.

A new parenteral T preparation, T undecanoate, enables elimination of most of the shortcomings of these old preparations. It has the advantage that the serum T levels resulting from each injection are much more stable and physiologic. T undecanoate has been extensively investigated in hypogonadal men. After two loading doses of 1000 mg T undecanoate at 0 and 6 weeks, repeated injections at 12-week intervals are sufficient to maintain T levels in the reference range in the vast majority of eugonadal men, with intervals of up to 14 weeks in some men [216,217].

Transdermal T is available in either a skin patch and more recently as gel preparations. Daily application is required for each of these. They are designed to deliver 5–10 mg of T per day. The advantages include ease of use and maintenance of relatively uniform serum T levels over time [218,219]. Skin

irritation is a frequent adverse effect of T patches but is uncommon with gel preparations [30,220]. Inadequate absorption through the skin may limit the value of transdermal preparations in some persons, or may require a doubling of the daily dose.

Table 18.4 provides a summary of T therapy.

Alternatives to testosterone therapy

Oral clomiphene
Another potential method of the treatment of hypogonadism is the use of agents that increase the endogenous production of T in men with hypogonadotropic hypogonadism. Shabsigh *et al.* reported on a study on 36 men with hypogonadism defined as serum T level less than 3 ng/mL. Each patient was treated with a daily dose of 25 mg clomiphene citrate, and followed prospectively. The mean age was 39 years with the mean pretreatment T and estrogen levels of 2.47 ± 0.39 ng/mL and 32.3 ± 10.9 pg/mL, respectively. By the first follow-up visit (four to six weeks), the mean T level rose to 6.1 ± 1.78 ng/mL ($P < 0.00001$). Moreover, the T/E ratio improved from 8.7 to 14.2 ($P < 0.001$). This therapy may represent an alternative to T therapy by stimulating the endogenous androgen production pathway [211], and allowed Guay *et al.* to improve T secretion

Table 18.4 Synopsis of testosterone therapy.

Indications for testosterone supplementation

Clinical symptoms

Psychologic symptoms:	Irritability, depression, nervousness, anxiety, discouragement, lack of energy
Somatovegetative symptoms:	Joint/muscle complaints, sweating, hot flushes, sleep disturbances, increased need for sleep, deterioration in well-being, weakness, fatigue, exhaustion
Sexual symptoms:	Erectile dysfunction, decreased libido, decreased ejaculate volume, decreased orgasmic intensity

Laboratory tests

Total testosterone:	<2.3 ng/mL (<8 nml/L): T therapy mandatory. Between this level and 3.5 ng/mL or 12 nmol/L a trial of T therapy is also justified
Calculated free testosterone:	<52 pg/mL (<180 pml/L): T therapy mandatory. Between this level and 72 pg/mL or 180 pmol/L a trial is also justified
Bioavailable testosterone:	<0.75 ng/mL
SHBG	>50–60 nmol/L may be associated with a decrease in bioavailable testosterone

Contraindications

- History of prostate or breast cancer
- PSA elevation (>4 ng/mL). Warning: hypogonadal men with PSA levels of 2.5 to 4 ng/mL may also be at risk for prostate cancer!
- PSA increase >0.50 ng/mL/year for at least 2 years
- Symptomatic benign prostate hyperplasia with severe clinical symptoms
- Polycythemia/polyglobulism, hypercoagulability
- Sleep apnea syndrome
- Severe left cardiac insufficiency
- Poorly controlled severe hypertension
- Uncontrolled hyperprolactinemia

Possible benefits of T therapy

(marked in less than 40 years old hypogonal males, less constant and ample over 40)

Body composition:	↑ Muscle mass, ↓ fat mass, especially abdominal and visceral fat
Bone:	↑ Bone mineral density, prevention of osteoporosis
Blood:	↑ Red blood cell count, ↓ anemia and resulting fatigue
Physical functions:	↑ Muscle strength, ↑ energy, ↓ weakness, ↓ fatigue
Psychic functions:	↑ Spatial cognition and memory, ↑ energy, ↓ irritability and depression
Sexuality:	↑ Sexual desire, arousal, erections, volume of ejaculate

Possible side effects of T therapy

Prostate:	PSA increase but mostly within normal range
	Prostate enlargement but mostly within normal range
	Rarely prostate cancer
Metabolic and cardiovascular:	Possible ↓ HDL cholesterol
	In case of overdosing:
	Polycythemia with ↑ hematocrit and risk of thrombosis
	Fluid retention with risk of:
	Reinforcement of high blood pressure
	Decompensation of cardiac insufficiency
Sleep disturbances:	↑ Sleep apnea syndrome with possible reinforcement of ↑ hematocrit, ↑ blood viscosity and risk of thrombosis
Testes, fertility:	↓ Testes volume, ↓ spermatogenesis and fertility, till azoospermia
Psychic functions:	In case of overdosing aggression, excessive excitement
Stimulation of diseases sensitive to estrogens (due to aromatization into estradiol):	↑ Size of prolactinoma with possible headache, visual complications, and hypopituitarism
	Stimulation of breast cancer
	Gynecomastia

HDL, high density lipoprotein; PSA, prostate specific antigen; SHBG, sex hormone-binding globulin.

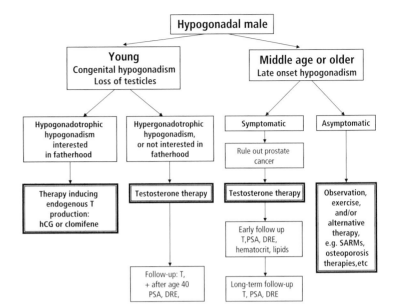

Fig. 18.4 Algorithm for androgen therapy in a man presenting with low testosterone. DRE, digital rectal examination; hCG, human chorionic gonadotropin; PSA, prostate-specific antigen; SARM, selective androgen recepor modulator; T, testosterone.

and erectile function in hypogonadal ED patients [221].

Human chorionic gonadotropin
Human chorionic gonadotropin (hCG) has the same biologic activity as LH, but a longer half-life. One injection of 5000 IU stimulates T secretion for three to five days on condition that the Leydig cells are responsive.

Summary of recommendations
Recommendations for screening and therapy
Currently there is no basis for androgen therapy in older men, unless they have overt androgen deficiency with symptoms and low testosterone [2].

Testosterone levels needed for normal sexual function may vary between individuals. Some men may have normal sexual function even if their T levels fall into the age-adjusted lower normal range [221]. However, *in patients with ED and/or hypoactive sexual desire, T testing is recommended to screen for hypogonadism. T therapy is appropriate when clinical indications and biochemical evidence of hypogonadism exist* [168,222]. In men with ED, determining T levels only in case of either low sexual desire or abnormal physical examination overlooks many patients with

low T who do not have these symptoms but may benefit from androgen therapy [18]. Testosterone monotherapy may correct sexual dysfunction caused by hypogonadism, but absence of an adequate response after appropriate therapy may require further evaluation to exclude associated co-morbidities, such as those causing vasculogenic or neurogenic ED [222].

Populations for combination therapy and screening
Testosterone efficacy as monotherapy for ED is limited, because of the multifactorial nature of the pathophysiology of ED. Combination therapy with T and other ED treatments, such as PDE5i, may be valuable in certain subpopulations of patients. *There is increasing evidence that combination therapy is effective in treating ED in patients where treatment failed with testosterone or PDE5i alone.* Combination therapy may be particularly useful in men with type 2 diabetes and metabolic syndrome, who frequently have hypogonadism. Additional studies are required to assess full utilization of combination therapy.

Two algorithms are proposed regarding androgen therapy: in a man presenting with low T (Fig. 18.4), and in a man presenting with ED as potential symptom of hypogonadism (Fig. 18.5).

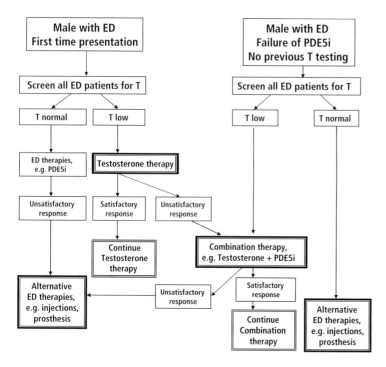

Fig. 18.5 Algorithm for androgen therapy in a man presenting with erectile dysfunction. ED, erectile dysfunction; PDE5i, phosphodiesterase 5 inhibitor; T, testosterone.

Future therapies

Selective androgen receptor modulators

The discovery and development of selective androgen receptor modulators (SARMs) provides the opportunity to design molecules that are not only orally active, but that target androgen receptors in different tissues to elicit the specific desired activity [223]. The desired activity profile of novel SARMs is described in Table 18.5. An ideal SARM for the treatment of primary or secondary male hypogonadism would have the following profile: orally active, with a pharmacokinetic profile consistent with once a day administration; capable or incapable of stimulating the prostate, seminal vesicles, and other sex accessory tissues at doses equipotent to those needed to provide increases in muscle mass and strength along with fat-free mass; support bone growth; and maintain/restore erectile function, libido, virilization, and male habitus. Unlike testosterone, these SARMs are not substrates for 5α-reductase activity. Other activities that are considered undesirable should be diminished or eliminated, such as potential liver toxicity, blood pressure effects, and fluid retention,

induction of gynecomastia, infertility, and overstimulation of erythropoiesis. On the other hand, use of SARMs for selected indications provides the rationale for developing molecules with distinct tissue specificity. For example, if the target is bone growth in elderly men with osteopenia or osteoporosis, but with no overt signs of hypogonadism, a more anabolic SARM with clear effects on bone and muscle, but lesser activity on prostate or other sex accessory tissues, would be more desirable.

The compound 7α-methyl-19-nortestosterone (MENT) has a biopotency per molecule 10 times greater than T [224] and it does not undergo 5α-reduction, which may or may not be an advantage for its effects on the prostate. It retains, however, its capacity to be aromatized to estradiol [225]. It cannot be regarded as a SARM since there is no tissue selectivity based on receptor mechanisms, but it is potentially prostate-sparing. The effects of MENT on the prostate are two to three times as potent as those of T, but studies with MENT given in a dose sufficient to sustain gonadotropin suppression and anabolism (1/10 of the amount of T) showed a 50% loss in

Table 18.5 Desired profile of activity of new selective androgen receptor modulators (SARMs): male applications.

	Indications	
Tissue/parameter	Hypogonadism	Selected indications*
Prostate/sex accessory tissues	Stimulatory, but less than DHT	Weak or neutral
Libido	Stimulatory	Stimulatory/neutral
Inhibition of gonadotropins	Present	Absent/reduced
Hair growth	Stimulatory	Neutral
Bone growth	Stimulatory	Stimulatory
Muscle mass/strength	Stimulatory	Stimulatory
Fat-free mass	Increase	Increase
Lipids/cardiovascular risk factors	Neutral	Neutral/beneficial
Blood pressure/fluid retention	Neutral	Neutral
Erythropoiesis	Weakly stimulatory	Stimulatory
Liver function (enzyme elevation)	Neutral	Neutral
Breast (gynecomastia)	Neutral	Neutral

* Selected indications may include glucocorticoid-induced osteoporosis, androgen replacement in eldery men, HIV-wasting, cancer cachexia, certain anemias, muscular dystrophies, and male contraception. DHT, dihydrotestosterone.
With permission of Negro-Villar A. *J Clin Endocrin Metab* 1999;**84**:3459–3462 [224].

prostate volume. MENT is capable of restoring and maintaining sexual behavior in the human male with plasma levels in the order of 15–20% of normal T levels [226]. The pharmacokinetics of MENT administered as MENT acetate subdermal implants has shown that serum MENT levels remain at a steady state level during the four weeks of implant use and are clearly dose-dependent [227].

Hyperprolactinemia

Prolactin (PRL) is a large polypeptide mainly responsible for the regulation of lactation and involved in over 300 other functions. The release of PRL from the pituitary lactotropic cells is under tonic inhibitory control by the hypothalamus, primarily by the neurotransmitter dopamine. The secretion of PRL is stimulated by estrogens, and therefore, indirectly, by aromatizable androgens such as T.

PRL has no known role in the physiologic control of human sexual behavior, except a possible contribution of the PRL secretion induced by orgasm in the sexual-satiation mechanisms [228]. All types of hyperprolactinemia (HPRL), however, can inhibit many aspects of male sexual behavior. Although HPRL is a rare condition, it should be known as a possible cause of male sexual dysfunctions, and should not be missed since many cases result from pituitary tumors (mostly PRL-secreting macro-adenomas or macroprolactinomas, >10 mm in diameter, sometimes micro-prolactinomas, <10 mm). Macro-adenomas are likely to result in serious endocrinological (hypopituitarism), visual and tumoral complications, due to the tumor's growth.

Sexual dysfunctions of hyperprolactinemic men

A literature review encompassing more than 300 men with HPRL [229] found sexual dysfunctions in 88%, including ED in almost every case. The most typical pattern associates ED with a reduced sexual desire. Delayed or absent orgasm are also associated in some cases, but virtually never isolated. Several cases of retrograde ejaculation, sometimes cured by dopamine-agonist therapy, were also reported [230]. Other clinical symptoms of HPRL are uncommon: reduced body hair in 40% of the cases, gynecomastia in 21%, galactorrhea in 13%.

Reports on nocturnal erections for HPRL men are inconsistent. Following recordings for three consecutive nights, De Rosa *et al.* considered that nocturnal erections were abnormal in every one of 41 patients with macroadenoma, and in 8/10 patients with microadenoma, with respect to a control group of normal men [231]. Conversely, in six men with PRL >300 ng/mL, Carani *et al.* found no difference with respect to their normal control group as concerns both the nocturnal erections and the erections induced by audiovisual stimulation [232].

Mechanisms of sexual dysfunction in hyperprolactinemic men

HPRL impairs the pulsatile release of LH, which results in a decrease of T secretion. It is often believed that this is the main cause of ED [233]. In fact it may not explain every case. Serum T is in the (low) normal range in nearly half of the ED patients with marked HPRL (for example in 17 of the 41 patients with prolactinoma of De Rosa *et al.* [231], who observed a highly significant inverse relationship between nocturnal erections and PRL, but not T). Moreover, during treatment of men with HPRL with the PRL-lowering agent bromocriptine, sexual improvement correlates better with the PRL decrease than with the T increase [229,231]. Erections can return prior to any increase in T.

The other mechanisms may include a decrease in the 5α-reduction of T into DHT observed in HPRL men. DHT seems the main metabolite accountable for the effects of T upon the primate brain centers. However the main T-independent mechanisms probably depend on PRL interactions with neurotransmitter systems: possibly downregulation of the brain receptors to dopamine, a neurotransmitter that stimulates sexual behavior of most animal species, because PRL increases the synthesis, turnover and release of central dopamine; interaction of PRL with the opioid and serotoninergic systems, both involved in the adjustment of sexual behavior. Studies in rats confirm a central inhibition of the penile reflexes by experimental HPRL [234]. However two experimental studies in dogs also suggest the possibility of a peripheral effect, with prolactin locally inhibiting the capacity to relax of the cavernous smooth muscle cells [235] and contract-

ing the corpus cavernosum by a direct effect in the case of local perfusion [236].

Prevalence and responsibility of hyperprolactinemia in erectile dysfunction
Prevalence

Routine determinations of serum PRL found HPRL in 1–5% of ED patients. Compiling the 10 largest series of literature leads to a prevalence of marked HPRL (serum PRL >35 ng/mL) at 0.62% and of pituitary adenomas at 0.38% of 8707 ED patients [238]. Though low, these figures are higher than the corresponding prevalences found in two studies of unselected Asiatic populations totaling over 13 000 men (HPRL in respectively 0.17 and 0.29%, and pituitary tumors in 0.036 and 0.06%) [239,240]. In addition some ED patients were found to have mild HPRL (serum PRL 20–35 ng/mL), for a 1.5% prevalence [238].

Responsibility

It is unlikely that such mild HPRLs were the real cause of ED, since very few cases had a low T level or pituitary tumors [238]. However two microadenomas were found in such cases by Johri *et al.* [241]. In addition, only 40% of such patients improved as regards their erectile function following treatment with bromocriptine [18]. This rate approximates the placebo effect and the 40% success rate reported with bromocriptine in normoprolactinemic ED patients [242]. Conversely bromocriptine restored normal erectile function in eight of 12 ED cases (67%) with serum PRL >35 ng/ml [18], which suggests a causative effect of HPRL in this category. Every one of the four other patients, although still unable to penetrate their partners after restoration of normal PRL levels, reported improved libido and morning erections. Two of them subsequently recovered normal erectile capacity following additional sexual counseling.

The macroprolactin problem

When evaluating the association between HPRL and sexual dysfunction, it should also be considered that biologically inactive or biologically inert variants of PRL may be assayed by immunological assays. It is especially the case of the "big" and "big–big" PRLs that have high molecular weights [243]. With immunological assays, excessive secretion of "macroprolactins" resembles a classical HPRL, while it has in fact generally no pathological consequence. Macroprolactinemias account for 10% [244] to 22% [245] of all HPRLs and are typically observed in otherwise normal individuals, mostly women with normal reproductive function despite high PRL levels, but also some ED patients in whom they seem coincidental [246,247]. Many of these cases suffered from psychogenic impotence. In such cases serum T is usually normal, as are computerized tomography (CT) scans and magnetic resonance imaging (MRI) of the hypothalamic–pituitary area. PRL-lowering agents are ineffective in improving sexual function, although the PRL level can be normalized. Such a discrepancy should lead to PRL chromatographic analysis, or precipitation of the macromolecules with polyethylene glycol, in a laboratory which specializes in endocrinology, allowing identification of the macroprolactin. However a diagnosis of macroprolactinemia in an ED patient should preclude neither MRI testing, since some cases are associated with pituitary adenomas, nor a trial of a PRL-lowering agent, since a biologic activity of the macroprolactin has been demonstrated at least in some women, including reversal of amenorrhea and infertility on dopamine-agonist therapy [221].

Prevalence of hyperprolactinemia in other sexual dysfunctions

Routine determination of serum PRL in men consecutively seen for hypoactive sexual desire without ED (n = 53), anorgasmia/retarded ejaculation (n = 74), and premature ejaculation (n = 124) [210,249] found no HPRL in the two former sexual dysfunctions. However Schwartz *et al.* [250] reported on some male HPRLs revealed by isolated hypoactive sexual desire or anorgasmia. In contrast, serum PRL was mildly elevated (20–35 ng/mL) in 13 men with premature ejaculation (10%). This was not the cause of sexual dysfunction since bromocriptine failed in every case to prolong the time to ejaculation. In addition serum T was normal in every case and no pituitary adenoma was detected in any patient.

Diagnosis of hyperprolactinemia in men with sexual dysfunction

Some precautions are critical to avoid false HPRLs resulting from stress (especially from venepuncture) and meals. Blood sampling must be performed fasting, following a 20-minute rest in a quiet place. Any elevated PRL level must be checked again, if possible following catheter insertion 20 minutes before sampling, and after discontinuation of any drug likely to increase PRL (Table 18.6). In case of discrepancy between high serum PRL and a pattern of non-endocrine sexual dysfunction, the patient may be referred to an endocrinologist who will decide about the usefulness of a PRL chromatography. As already discussed, the responsibility of mild HPRLs (20–35 ng/mL) in sexual dysfunction is questionable. In this respect, the threshold of significant HPRL is probably in the region of 35 ng/mL or 550 µU/mL (1 ng/mL = 21 µU/mL).

Etiologic diagnosis

Drug-induced HPRL is the first etiology to consider. It is responsible for a significant proportion of HPRLs in men. Many drugs may increase PRL (Table 18.6). The most common are antipsychotic agents. Other medications include antidepressants, some antihypertensive agents, and drugs that increase bowel motility [251]. HPRL may also be secondary to hypothyroidism, renal insufficiency, cirrhosis, and chest injury (mild or moderate in all four conditions), and to any process compressing or interrupting the hypothalamic–pituitary dopaminergic transmission. This includes many types of hypothalamic and pituitary tumors. Primary HPRL results from a primary defect of the dopaminergic inhibitory control of PRL secretion. It may be idiopathic, but in many cases it is associated with PRL-secreting pituitary adenomas. These, as the other types of hypothalamic or pituitary tumors, are likely to result in tumoral complications (visual disturbances or even blindness due to compression of the optic chiasma, and hypopituitarism, which may become life-threatening if decompensated).

Consequently, any man with non-drug-induced HPRL, confirmed by a repeat PRL determination after blood sampling in appropriate conditions, must benefit from morphologic investigations of the

Table 18.6 Drugs likely to increase serum prolactin (in most cases due to their anti-dopaminergic activity).

Opiates
  Methadone

Psychotropic drugs
  Neuroleptics
    Benzamides (+++): Amisulpride, Sulpiride, Sultopride,
      Tiapride
    Phenothiazines: Chlorpromazine, Cyamemazin,
      Fluphenazine, Levomepromazine, Perphenazine,
      Pipotiazine, Propericiazin, Thioridazine
    Butyrophenones: Droperidol, Haloperidol,
      Pipamperone, Flupentixol, Loxapine, Olanzapine,
      Pimozide, Risperidone, Zuclopenthixol
  Tricyclic antidepressants
    Amitriptyline, Amoxapine, Chlorimipramine,
      Desipramine, Dosulepine, Doxepin, Imipramine,
      Maprotiline, Trimipramine

Anti-emetics
  Metoclopramide (++), Metopimazine

Anti-ulcerous
  Cimetidine (only at high dose)

Anti-hypertensives
  Reserpinics, α-methy-DOPA

Estrogens

hypothalamic–pituitary area (if possible MRI) for detecting a possible tumor. This is especially mandatory in case of serum PRL >35 ng/mL. Bodie *et al.* [19] found adenomas in 57% of their patients with PRL over 50 ng/mL. A recent publication reported an unusually high rate of 86% of presumed pituitary adenomas, according to high resolution MRI, in a series of 29 men, with serum PRL at least twice over 15 ng/mL. Most of them had ED, and a serum T level <3.5 ng/mL [252]. Also unusual was the fact that half of these HPRLs were ≤30 ng/mL and that all these pituitary tumors were micro-adenomas (mean diameter 5.3 mm). Indeed macro-adenomas are the most frequent tumors (41 versus 10 micro-adenomas in the series of De Rosa *et al.*) [232]. They require a complete assessment of all pituitary functions, generally carried out by an endocrinologist, in order to detect possible hypopituitarism resulting from compression of the pituitary's stalk, or destruction of the pituitary itself by the tumor. De Rosa *et al.* [232] found

10 hypothyroidisms and three hypoadrenalisms of central origin among 41 ED patients with macro-prolactinomas.

Routine or selective serum PRL determination?

According to many authors, the very low prevalence of significant HPRL can hardly justify routine determination of PRL in ED patients, due to the frequency of this condition and the cost of the determination [234]. Most recommend determination of serum PRL only in case of low T level, or low sexual desire. However many ED patients with normal serum T despite marked HPRL have been reported, including some with pituitary tumors, therefore unlikely to be macroprolactinemias [230]. In one study, determining serum PRL only in case of low T would have led to neglect of six of 12 marked HPRL and three of seven pituitary tumors [18]. Likewise sexual desire may be normal, or seem normal to the patient, in ED patients with HPRL [241]. Buvat *et al.* [249] found that by restricting the determination to those men with low sexual desire, gynecomastia, or serum T <4 ng/mL (low and low–normal values), they would have saved more than half of determinations while overlooking only one of 10 marked HPRLs, and none of six pituitary tumors.

There is therefore no consensus with regard to serum PRL determination in ED patients: should it be systematic or restricted to men selected according to clinical (low sexual desire), and/or endocrine (low serum T) criteria? That first depends on local resources. Measurement of PRL should be performed in cases of isolated hypoactive sexual desire and retarded or absent orgasm.

Treatment of men with sexual dysfunction and hyperprolactinemia

The literature contains some observations of marked improvement of sexual dysfunctions associated with HPRL following non-specific treatments such as psycho- or sex-therapy [250] or, as concerns ED, sildenafil [241,253]. However, PRL-lowering dopamine-agonists (bromocriptine, lisuride, quinagolide, and cabergolide, the latter one being effective following a single administration per week) [254] most often not only normalize all aspects of sexual function, but also shrink the possible pituitary adenoma, or at least prevent its growth [18,230]. In addition, unlike PDE5-I, PRL-lowering agents allow return of sexual desire, and in the case of ED—spontaneous erections, and avoid the necessity to plan sexual intercourse. Therefore dopamine-agonists should be the first choice treatment. This therapy may not be definitive. If PRL returns within the normal range, while there is no macro-adenoma, it may be stopped every year, or every other year, for several weeks before determining the PRL level. In 20% of the cases, HPRL does not return after a number of years [255].

In the case of macro-adenoma, the patient should be referred both to an endocrinologist and to an ophthalmologist for thorough investigation of pituitary function, possible optic chiasma compression, and possible indications for its removal. This would protect the patient against tumoral complications. In case of micro-adenoma, surgical removal may be performed via the transphenoidal route, which is less damaging and may definitely cure both the tumor and the HPRL [254]. Wolfsberger *et al.* [256] reported on such a definitive cure in seven of 11 men with micro-adenomas. Today, however, medical therapy is more often chosen as first-line treatment [254].

In some cases, hypogonadism persists despite return to a normal PRL level, due to definitive interruption of the hypothalamic–pituitary connections or destruction of the pituitary gonadotrophs by the tumor or its surgical removal. Such patients require T substitution in addition to dopamine-agonist therapy. However, T administration may stimulate the growth of a pituitary tumor through its aromatization into estradiol if HPRL is not completely controlled by dopamine-agonist therapy, and even, more exceptionally, if it is so.

Finally, certain patients may need additional sexual counseling or therapy, especially in case of lifelong sexual dysfunction [234].

Role of other Hormonal Alterations in Sexual Dysfunctions and Men's Health

Estradiol

Estradiol, the most important biologically active estrogen, has important functions in men [257]. One of the most critical is its role in bone metabolism.

Men with aromatase deficiency or inactive estrogen receptor α develop severe osteoporosis. Most of the effects of T on bone depend on its aromatization into estradiol. Estradiol is also supposed to be the main active metabolite of T concerning its effects on the brain, though no significant sexual dysfunction was observed in men affected by congenital estrogen deficiency [258–260]. However in two men with aromatase deficiency, Carani *et al.* observed a synergistic effect of estradiol and T on sexual behavior

In men about 20% of estradiol is formed in the Leydig cells, and the rest in peripheral tissues, especially fat cells, from aromatization of androgens—mainly T but also adrenal androstenedione [1]. As a result, the estradiol level is higher in men with increased BMI, as well as in diabetic patients, while aromatization seems decreased by physical exercise [257]. According to the studies there is no or only a slight decrease of serum estradiol with age, resulting in an increase in the estradiol/T ratio. However serum levels of free estradiol decrease because concentrations of SHBG, which binds estradiol, increase with age.

Animal experiments from Adaikan and co-workers show that any estrogen increase results in a reduction of circulating T levels (probably due to inhibition of the gonadotropic axis at the hypothalamic level, where estradiol is the active metabolite of T for its negative feedback action) and that the resulting estrogen/T imbalance precipitates ED in both rats [262] and rabbits [263] by reducing intracavenosal pressure response to nerve stimulation, reducing relaxant response to acetylcholine and nitrergic transmission, and potentiating norepinephrine-induced anti-erectile contraction of corpora cavernosa [263]. Trichrome staining highlighted cavernosal connective tissue hyperplasia in the long-term study groups [262]. These effects were observed following both estradiol and phytoestrogen administrations [263] leading to conjecture about the impact of exposure to environmental estrogens on male sexual function. One study of ED patients reported a high prevalence of exposure to pesticides, some of which have estrogenic or anti-androgenic properties, and an association between such an exposure and the severity of ED based on flat nocturnal erectile pattern was made [264]. Mancini *et al.* also observed increased estradiol levels in a small group of ED

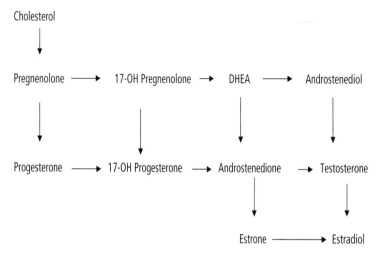

Fig. 18.6 The standard scheme of sex steroid production. Adapted from Grumach MM, Conte FA. Disorders of sex differentiation. In Wilson, Foster, Kronenberg, Larsen, eds. *Williams Textbook of Endocrinology*, 9th edition. WB Saunders (1998) [218]. DHEA, dehydroepiandrosterone.

patients with pure veno-occlusive dysfunction compared with patients with other etiologies [265]. More data are however requested to determine if hypo- or hyperestrogenism may be deleterious for sexual function in men. Presently there is no need for routine estradiol determination in male sexual dysfunctions, unless breast symptoms or signs are present.

Dehydroepiandrosterone
Biosynthesis of adrenal androgens
Dehydroepiandrosterone (DHEA) is synthesized in the zona reticularis of the adrenal gland partly in response to serum levels of the pituitary, adreno-corticotropic hormone (ACTH). DHEA is sulfated in the adrenal gland via the enzyme sulfo-transferase into DHEA-sulfate (DHEA-S), which is thought to be the storage form of DHEA. However, this concept has recently been challenged and thus so has the idea of DHEA-S reflecting the bioavailability of DHEA in the tissues. The current thinking has been that there is free interconversion between DHEA and DHEA-S, but recently the reverse conversion of DHEA-S to DHEA has been shown not to occur, at least in liver cells, although the study has been challenged on methodologic grounds [266,267].

DHEA and DHEA-S production follow an age-dependent pattern: high levels after birth due to increased synthesis by the fetal adrenal gland, a second

surge at the time of adrenarche (between the sixth and tenth years of life), maximum levels during the third decade of life, and a gradual decline to about 10–20% of maximum values by the seventh or eighth decade of life [268,269]. While serum DHEA-S concentration does not vary throughout the day, DHEA secretion follows a diurnal pattern similar to that of cortisol [270,271].

Figure 18.6 depicts the synthesis and metabolism of DHEA. DHEA itself is synthesized from 17-OH pregnenolone via conversion by the 17–20 lyase portion of the enzyme P450c17. Subsequently, DHEA is converted to androstenedione by the enzyme 3β-hydroxysteroid dehydrogenase (3β-HSD). Finally, androstenedione is converted to T by the enzyme 17β-OH hydroxysteroid dehydrogenase (17β-HSD), and subsequently to estrogen by the enzyme aromatase [233–235,270–272]. An important requirement for DHEA action is the ability of DHEA and DHEA-S to continuously interconvert, via the enzyme sulfotransferase, as only unsulfated DHEA can undergo downstream conversion to the biochemically-active hormone testosterone [270,272].

Mechanisms of action
Sex steroid activity
It has been well described that the physiologic effects of DHEA are related to its peripheral conversion to the downstream sex steroid hormones, which then act on nuclear steroid receptors to exert their effects

[270,273,274]. The ability for the conversion of active hormones in the peripheral tissues, where the hormone will be active, is called intracrinology. This phenomenon has been outlined for sex steroids very well by the work of Labrie [275,276]. Different peripheral tissues are able to selectively make androgens or estrogens. This is possible because of numerous different 17β-hydroxysteroid dehydrogenase enzymes that are able to selectively control the correct intracellular concentration of the correct sex steroid [277].

Non-sex steroid-related activity

The sex steroid activity of DHEA requires it to penetrate the cell and become converted to the active downstream sex steroids. Recently, a putative receptor specific for DHEA has been identified on endothelial cell plasma membranes with which structurally related steroids failed to compete for binding [278]. These receptors are coupled to eNOS activity through G proteins, and it has been shown that physiologic concentrations of DHEA acutely increase NO release from intact vascular endothelial cells, by a plasma membrane-initiated mechanism [279].

These effects on the vascular wall may be both genomic and non-genomic, and both effects are independent of other steroid hormone receptors [280]. These findings have possible implications for DHEA as an anti-atherogenic compound, as DHEA may inhibit human vascular smooth muscle cell proliferation independent of androgen or estrogen receptor activity [281].

DHEA has also been shown to increase endothelial proliferation and improve endothelial function in vitro using endothelial cells, as well as in vivo measured by flow-mediated dilatation of the brachial artery, by a mechanism independent of either androgen or estrogen receptor activity [281]. Iwasaki *et al.* demonstrated that DHEA and DHEA-S both had possible anti-inflammatory and immunomodulatory effects by inhibiting proinflammatory cytokine-induced transcription, an effect that neither estradiol nor T could duplicate [282].

Pathophysiology of DHEA deficiency

DHEA deficiency can be seen in several disease states. Regardless of the etiology, patients with pri-mary adrenal insufficiency manifest signs and symptoms associated with a deficiency or absence of all adrenal cortical hormones including cortisol, DHEA, and aldosterone [283,284]. Women with pan-hypopituitarism have severe androgen deficiency due to a lack of both ovarian and adrenal androgen production [248]. Pituitary insufficiency can lead to a deficit of DHEA as the zona reticularis of the adrenal gland produces DHEA in response to stimulation by pituitary ACTH, similar to the stimulation of DHEA in the Leydig cell by LH [286].

Low DHEA levels have also been described in a variety of non-endocrine medical conditions. The age-related decline in circulating DHEA levels may correlate with many age-related phenomena such as diabetes and states of insulin resistance, hypertension, atherosclerosis, coronary artery disease, decreased bone mineral density, cancer, and dementia [287–291]. Low levels of DHEA have also been described in correlation with various conditions unrelated to aging, including obesity, depression, and other mood disorders, eating disorders, autoimmune disorders, immune deficiency states, and chronic stress states [287–289,292,293]. In the Massachusetts Male Aging Study (MMAS) DHEA-S was the only hormone which showed a strong (negative) correlation with the prevalence of ED among 17 investigated hormones, including T and estradiol [294].

Various drugs can contribute to decreased circulating levels of DHEA. Exogenous corticosteroids can decrease adrenal DHEA synthesis via negative feedback to the hypothalamus and pituitary gland, decreasing corticotropin-releasing hormone (CRH) and ACTH secretion, respectively. Both adrenolytic drugs, such as mitotane, and inhibitors of corticosteroid synthesis, such as ketoconazole, can reduce adrenal production of DHEA along with cortisol [295,296].

More recently, a DHEA deficiency state has been reported in young, healthy, regularly menstruating premenopausal women presenting with decreased libido [297]. The regular menstrual periods support normal cyclical ovarian function and ovarian testosterone production. However, since adrenal DHEA contributes to almost half of a premenopausal woman's circulating androgens, such a deficiency can manifest with symptoms of sexual dysfunction. The clinical manifestations of such a DHEA deficiency become more evident when ovarian function is diminished (use of hormonal contraceptives or ovarian failure), as DHEA is also produced by the ovaries.

Measurement of DHEA

Measuring DHEA blood levels is generally not recommended because of variable secretion during the day and its short terminal half-life of approximately 4.5 hours [298]. DHEA also manifests a circadian rhythm and varies throughout the menstrual cycle. The measurement of DHEA-S is preferred over that of DHEA because of more stable levels in the blood due to DHEA-S's longer half-life of approximately 24 hours. The measurement of DHEA-S can be performed at any time during the day as there is no diurnal variation, or any time during the menstrual cycle, as there is no midcycle rise as is seen with androstenedione or testosterone. Two different reliable and reproducible assays for DHEA-S have been performed for many years.

DHEA therapy

DHEA replacement in adrenal insufficiency and pan-hypopituitarism

Traditionally, adrenal insufficiency, resulting from Addison's disease, has been treated with glucocorticoids and mineralocorticoids, while secondary adrenal insufficiency, resulting from pan-hypopituitarism, has been treated with glucocorticoids alone, as aldosterone production is regulated separately by the renin–angiotensin system [298]. However, management of the adrenal androgen deficiency associated with both conditions with DHEA replacement is still not considered to be the standard of care.

It has been shown that despite stable and long-standing conventional therapy with glucocorticoids with or without mineralocorticoids, many patients with adrenal insufficiency display a highly significant impairment of health-related quality of life [299]. Such patients have reported a reduced general health perception, decreased vitality, increased fatigue, reduced physical function, and sexual dysfunction [284,299,300].

DHEA replacement in women with adrenal insufficiency has been shown to have numerous beneficial effects including improved overall well-being, improved mood, and improved sexual functioning in the majority of the studies [284,286,298,301]. Conflicting reports have arisen concerning some of the metabolic effects of DHEA replacement in hypoadrenal patients. DHEA replacement has been shown by some investigators to improve insulin sensitivity and lipid profiles [298,302]. However, other studies did not confirm these effects [284,286,298,303]. DHEA replacement also has been shown to have little to no effect on body composition, body mass index, or exercise capacity in patients with adrenal insufficiency [303].

DHEA therapy in healthy aging subjects

The age-related decline in DHEA production has prompted study of the effects of DHEA administration in healthy elderly adults. One of the first studies looking at beneficial effects of DHEA supplementation in aging subjects found an improved overall sense of well-being in male and female subjects taking DHEA compared with placebo, but was based on rather poor methodology [304]. Several subsequent studies failed to find any benefit regarding overall well-being, mood, or cognition with DHEA supplementation [305–308]. The same negative findings extended to muscle strength and in muscle and fat cross-sectional areas [309]. Regarding improvement in sexual function, the effects of DHEA administration have been conflicting, demonstrating benefits in women over 70 years old, after more than six months of chronic administration, but no benefits in aging men [308,310,311]. The authors of a randomized, placebo-controlled trial in 40 ED patients claimed to have obtained a significant improvement of erectile function on 50 mg DHEA administered for six months, but objective data establishing this were lacking [312].

Metabolic effects of DHEA therapy in euadrenal subjects

Much controversy exists as to whether or not the DHEA-deficient state may contribute to a dysregulation of metabolism and hence may be associated with conditions such as diabetes and states of insulin resistance, atherosclerosis, and eventual vascular complications. Therefore, there has been great interest in studying the metabolic effects of DHEA supplementation in euadrenal subjects. Once again, study results have been inconsistent and conflicting.

A recent review of the effects of endogenous and exogenous DHEA on cardiovascular disease risks reiterates the inconsistencies regarding the metabolic effects of DHEA supplementation, discusses the shortcomings of several studies, and suggests that the effects of DHEA on cardiovascular disease risk (either favorable or unfavorable) should be considered more modest than previously believed [313].

Other proposed uses for DHEA therapy
In addition to theoretical anti-aging effects and potentially beneficial metabolic effects of DHEA supplementation, the effects of exogenous DHEA administration have been studied in other conditions. Beneficial effects on mood have been observed while using DHEA as treatment for depression and dysthymia [314,315]. DHEA supplementation in Alzheimer disease has been shown to cause only minor and transient improvements in cognitive performance [316]. In terms of bone health, the beneficial effects of DHEA supplementation are felt to be minor and limited to women [314]. DHEA supplementation has been shown to reduce the frequency of flares, and to decrease steroid dose requirements, in women with systemic lupus erythematosus [314,316]. DHEA has also been studied as a potential chemopreventive, anticarcinogenic agent [317]. The potential for immunoregulatory effects of DHEA has been demonstrated by the presence of specific binding found in murine T cells [318]. Specific binding of DHEA on muscle cells suggests the possibility of DHEA therapy in muscular disorders [319].

Availability of DHEA
DHEA had previously been banned by the Food and Drug Administration (FDA) in the USA until the passage of the Dietary and Supplemental Health and Education Act of 1994. Since then, it has been available over-the-counter in pharmacies and health food stores in most countries, including America. DHEA is classified as a food supplement and its production and distribution is not regulated by the FDA or any other agency. There is no pharmaceutical grade DHEA product and, therefore, no guaranteed consistency in DHEA content between brands, and even among different batches of the same brand of DHEA. As of the time of this writing, newer legislation is being introduced in an attempt to eliminate this loophole. The main objection is that estrogens are produced from DHEA and there are no warnings that this might not be in the best interest of women who have had estrogen-receptor positive breast cancer. Also, if women of reproductive age take DHEA while pregnant, it does cross the placenta and can potentially harm the reproductive development of the fetus.

Conclusions
DHEA is one of the most abundant circulating hormones. DHEA has been shown to exert its effects via downstream conversion to the steroid sex hormones, neuromodulation, improvement in endothelial function, and perhaps by means of action on a cell membrane-bound receptor. DHEA deficiency has been correlated with various endocrine, age-related, and other non-hormonal medical conditions. DHEA supplementation has been shown to be beneficial in patients with primary and secondary adrenal insufficiency. However, studies looking at the effects of DHEA supplementation on well-being, metabolism, and sexual function, in euadrenal subjects (including premenopausal and postmenopausal women with androgen insufficiency) have been inconsistent to date. Further research, in the form of randomized, blinded, placebo-controlled studies, is needed to better elucidate the efficacy and safety of DHEA supplementation for the treatment of androgen insufficiency in women.

Melatonin
Melatonin is a methoxyindole generated by enzymatic conversion of serotonin. It is synthesized and secreted principally by the pineal gland. Light is able to suppress or synchronize melatonin production. This explains the diurnal rhythm of melatonin secretion with a maximum during night time hours (02:00–04:00 h) [320,321]. Melatonin receptors are present in different organs and involved in multiple physiologic functions [322]. The primary function of

melatonin is to convey information concerning the daily cycle of light and darkness to body physiology. This information is used for the organization of the seasonal rythms, as well as of circadian rhythms that melatonin seems to stabilize and strengthen, especially as concerns core temperature and sleep–wake rhythms. The circadian organization of other physiologic functions, for instance immune, antioxidative defenses, hemostasis, and glucose regulation could also depend on the melatonin signal [320,321].

Melatonin levels gradually decline over the life span, which may be related to lowered sleep efficacy, very often associated with advancing age, as well as to deterioration of many circadian rhythms. This decline has thus been invoked in the aging process. Melatonin exhibits intracrine and paracrine immunomodulatory properties [323] with high levels promoting, and low levels suppressing, a number of immune system parameters, while melatonin receptors have been detected in various lymphoid organs and in lymphocytes [324]. A suppressed immunocompetence has been implicated in the acceleration of the aging process. Finally because melatonin is a potent free radical scavenger, its deficiency may result in reduced antioxidant protection in the elderly, which may have significance not only for aging per se, but also may contribute to the incidence or severity of some age-related diseases, including cancers, since an oncostatic action of melatonin was demonstrated in several types of cancer [324,325].

The best-known effects of melatonin administration are those on sleep. Exogenous melatonin reportedly induces drowsiness and sleep, and may ameliorate sleep disturbances, including the awakenings associated with old age [326]. Existing studies have been highly heterogeneous but a meta-analysis of 17 double-blind, placebo-controlled studies, involving 284 subjects, confirmed that melatonin treatment significantly reduced sleep onset latency, and increased sleep efficiency and total sleep duration [326]. These sleep-promoting effects of melatonin are distinctly different from those of common hypnotics and are not associated with alterations in sleep architecture [322,326]. They are mediated via specific melatonin receptors and physiologic doses of the hormone [322]. Aging reduces responsiveness to melatonin treatment, and in animals this correlates

with reduced functional potency of melatonin receptors [322].

Decreased melatonin concentrations were found in some, but not all, patients suffering from Alzheimer disease [325]. In vitro studies suggest that the antioxidative effects of melatonin may reduce the neurotoxicity of the amyloid beta, and open trials reported a beneficial effect of melatonin on sleep and progression of cognitive impairment in Alzheimer patients [325]. However a multicenter placebo-controlled trial failed to prove that melatonin has a clinically significant effect on objective measures of sleep in patients suffering from Alzheimer disease [327].

The preceding meta-analysis implies that exogenous melatonin may have some use in treating insomnia, particularly that associated with nocturnal melatonin deficiency in aged individuals [325] or with an abnormal pattern of melatonin secretion: blind people, jetlag (confirmed by a meta-analysis) [328], with an overall 50% reduction in subjective assessment of symptoms using 5 mg fast-release melatonin and specific instructions for timing of the treatment [321], shiftwork, delayed sleep phase syndrome, and the elderly [321]. Physiologically relevant doses of 0.5–5 mg orally and administration at bedtime are generally recommended [322]. However the optimal dose and time of administration need further delineation. In addition, although melatonin treatment seems to be safe because of its very low toxicity and absence of any significant side effects [325], no data on long-term follow-up is available.

No effect on sexual function or dysfunction has been reported. Presently, available data do not allow us to conclude that melatonin may have a role in extending normal longevity, or is a "rejuvenating" agent. However some of its actions may be beneficial for the aging process, especially its sleep-promoting effects. More extensive studies are needed to confirm whether it may improve the quality of life in old age. Presently there is no recommendation for routine melatonin replacement in the elderly.

Thyroid hormones

The prevalence of hypothyroidism increases with age due to autoimmune thyroid diseases, and may reach up to 20% in the elderly. Thyroid hormones have no known direct role in the control of sexual function but hypothyroidism may impede many vital functions. In addition, by increasing the level of SHBG, hyperthyroidism decreases the level of FT, which could impact sexual function.

Few studies have reported on the prevalence of sexual dysfunction in men presenting with thyroid dysfunction. Veronelli *et al.* [329], using the IIEF-5, found that prevalence and severity of ED were significantly higher in men with both hyperthyroidism (10/13, 77%, including two severe and two moderate cases) and hypothyroidism (30/55, 55%, including four severe and 11 moderate cases), than in 109 control men of the same age (33/109, 30%, including no severe and only three moderate cases). In 48 men with hypo- or hyperthyroidism, Isidori *et al.* [330] found ED in 64% and 15%, respectively (associated with hypoactive sexual desire and retarded ejaculation in most of the hypothyroid patients), and premature ejaculation in 7% and 50%, respectively. After return to normal levels of serum thyroid hormones for eight to 12 weeks, the prevalence of premature ejaculation fell from 50 to 15% in the hyperthyroid patients, while that of retarded ejaculation was reduced by half in those with hypothyroidism. The mean ejaculation latency time doubled in the former and significantly decreased in the latter, suggesting the possibility of a direct involvement of thyroid hormones in the physiology of ejaculation. In 38 patients referred for ED and found to be hypothyroid, Baskin [331] reported that erectile function returned in "the majority" following thyroid hormone substitution. Conversely Wortsman *et al.* [332] did not observe any sexual improvement following thyroxin treatment in a short series of ED patients with primary hypothyroidism. In conclusion, a majority of the patients with thyroid dysfunction have some form of sexual dysfunction, which may improve following normalization of the thyroid hormones.

Some studies have reported on the prevalence of thyroid dysfunction in men presenting with ED. Among 600 ED patients preselected (since sent to endocrinologists by urologists who suspected an endocrine cause), Baskin found hypothyroidism in 6% [331]. Earle and Stuckey [20] found only two patients with hypothyroidism in 1455 men consulting for ED (no benefit of hormone therapy on sexual function). The prevalence was somewhat higher in the series of Bodie *et al.* [19], but the 2240 otherwise unselected ED patients were all more than 50 years old (hypothyroidism in 3.9% and hyperthyroidism in 1%, based on serum TSH values; no indication of the effects of specific endocrine therapies on sexual function). In another Italian study of men with ED, plasma TSH concentrations were significantly lower in men who also had premature ejaculation, and premature ejaculation was two-fold more frequent in men with ED and suppressed plasma TSH, again suggesting a possible relationship with hyperthyroidism [333]. However Waldinger *et al.* did not find any relationship between premature ejaculation and thyroid dysfunction in a cohort of 620 men with premature ejaculation [334]. In conclusion, although few objective data is available, the prevalence of thyroid dysfunctions does not seem clearly increased in the patients consulting for sexual dysfunction, and routine determination of thyroid hormones is not justified in this population unless symptoms of thyroid disease are present.

Growth hormone

It is difficult to distinguish the signs and symptoms of androgen deficiency from GH deficiency as they are quite similar [168]. Both androgens and GH decrease with age, making evaluation of cause and effect difficult if the cause may be due to a pituitary problem. Also, GH replacement reverses the same symptoms as does T-replacement [335]. The biologic effects of GH and androgens are mutually interdependent and synergistic [336]. But in boys with micropenis and GH and T defiiciency, treatment with GH alone resulted in a normal penis size [337]. Most biologic effects of GH are not mediated by itself but by insulin-like growth factor (IGF)-1 which is synthesized in the liver cells following stimulation by GH, or locally in target tissues of GH, and is released into the bloodstream from there.

In acromegaly—the state of GH excess—sexual dysfunction is noted, but these tumors are large and there is often extensive destruction of the pituitary gland, frequently causing hypogonadism and causing confusion as to the etiology of the symptoms. Hypogonadism may also occur in the 40% of patients with acromegaly who also hypersecrete prolactin—another cause of secondary hypogonadism [338].

Evaluating GH deficiency is also difficult because the various conditions that may cause it may also cause T deficiency at the same time. Most cases of pan-hypopituitarism are caused by destruction of the gland from a large pituitary adenoma or else by autoimmune destruction that is also rather devastating to the entire pituitary gland [339]. Lymphocytic hypophysitis, once thought to be found exclusively in women, is now being reported more in men, and has even been shown to present with ED [340]. Even metastatic carcinoma to the pituitary gland, although rare, has been reported to cause pituitary destruction and present with sexual dysfunction [341].

Little data is available relative to growth hormone therapy alone for sexual function, but Brill *et al.* gave physiologic doses of GH and testosterone to older men for one month, without no effect on sexual function and mood whether the GH was given alone or in combination with testosterone. The lack of response might have been due to the short duration of therapy or due to the fact that the men were not severely growth hormone-deficient to begin with [342]. When GH has been given to GH-deficient men over a long period of time, a positive effect was noted on peripheral circulation—needed for sexual function, and on positive mood [343]. It has to be mentioned that during erection a 90% intracavernosal increase of GH concentrations was observed in a study of 35 voluntary potent men, and recombinant human GH elicited dose-dependent relaxation of human corpus cavernosum strips in vitro [334]. This relaxant potency of recombinant human GH was accompanied by an elevation of the intracellular cGMP concentrations. A recent study on isolated human corpus cavernosum strips provided evidence that GH may influence corpus cavernosum smooth muscle cells by an NO-independent effect on guanylyl cyclase activity [345]. This new data should stimulate further research in this area. On the other hand, any good effects have to be balanced against possible side effects. GH therapy has been shown to possibly induce peripheral edema, arthralgias, carpal tunnel syndrome, gynecomastia, and mild glucose intolerance. There is also the possibility that patients who have excess GH may develop abnormal cell proliferation, as various tumors and cancers have a higher prevalence in acromegaly [347,348].

In conclusion, except in the rare condition of acromegaly, abnormal GH secretion does not seem involved in sexual dysfunctions and there is no need for routine determination of this hormone unless other symptoms of this condition are present.

Metabolic Diseases and Sexual Dysfunctions

Diabetes

Diabetes mellitus is of increasing importance in the area of sexual dysfunction as the prevalence of diabetes has been increasing, related perhaps to the increase in obesity and to intermarriages into families with this condition.

Epidemiology

In clinics that treat ED, the prevalence of diabetes as a risk factor has remained similar at 20–25%, irrespective of whether the clinic is endocrine-based [349] or urology-based [350]. The importance of abnormalities of glucose metabolism in the relationship with ED may be seen by a closer look at specific risk factors. One study of risk factors in 154 consecutive consultations for ED revealed the presence of diabetes in 22%, glucose intolerance in 12%, and impaired fasting glucose (FBS of >100 mg/dL) in 51% [351].

If we look at the corollary, the prevalence of ED in patients with diabetes, we will find that in a review by Braunstein the prevalence of ED in patients with diabetes was 40%, with a range of 27.5% to 75% [352]. The Massachusetts Male Aging Study found that diabetic men were three times more likely to have ED than non-diabetic men [353]. A large number of patients were evaluated by Giuliano *et al.* from patients who sought medical care for hypertension and/or diabetes [354]. Of 7689 patients, 3906 had hypertension alone and ED was present in 67%, according to the IIEF-5 and defined as a score of <21/25, and 2377 men had diabetes alone and ED was present in 71%. Both diabetes and hypertension were present in 1186 men, and the prevalence of ED rose to 77%. The authors also found that 80% of the men with ED were distressed by it, an important component of the evaluation. Equally important is the fact that in 65% of the men with ED, their condition had gone untreated.

The largest study of the prevalence of ED in men with diabetes was undertaken by Fedele *et al.*, who performed a cross-sectional study of 9868 Italian men [355]. The patients ranged in age from 20 to 69 years. The overall prevalence of ED was 35.8%, and increased with age, such that it was 4.6% in men in their 20s and 45.5% in men older than 60 years. This study is also important because it showed that there was an increased prevalence of ED with duration of diabetes, control of the diabetes, obesity, complications of diabetes, and cigarette smoking.

Pathophysiology

The main pathophysiologic factors related to ED in diabetes revolve around the main abnormalities of the disease—that is, vascular and neuropathic factors. ED, however, has both psychologic and organic factors associated with it, and this is also true in diabetes. Buvat *et al.* found that the psychologic factors were additive to the vascular and neuropathic factors that are prevalent in diabetes [356]. Veves *et al.* studied 110 men with diabetes, and found that psychogenic factors were the only cause for ED in 11% of patients, the main cause in 24%, and was a minor part in 17% [357].

Vascular factor

It is well established that decreased circulation is foremost in diabetes, and the penis is no exception. Wang *et al.* found that 87.2% of men with diabetes had moderate to severe cavernous arterial insufficiency, as measured by corpus cavernosum duplex ultrasound [358]. It is interesting that this increased to 100% if hypertension or alcohol abuse were added to the risk factors.

Endothelial factor

The endothelium is critical to blood flow and defects related to it are at the core of the pathophysiologic causes of ED. Sowers studied the abnormalities in diabetic women related to the endothelium and found an enhanced expression of endothelin-1, decreased nitric oxide activity, decreased prostacycline release, increased adhesion molecule expression, increased platelet adhesion and procoagulant activity, and increased advanced glycosylated end products [359]. This is also true of men, and the importance of the endothelium was highlighted by the Atherosclerosis Risk in Communities Study that followed 1675 people with diabetes but no coronary disease [360]. They found that endothelial dysfunction was the main predictor of future cardiovascular disease. Sáenz de Tejada found that diabetic men had impairment of endothelial-dependent penile mechanisms [361].

Endothelin

Endothelin is an extremely powerful vasoconstrictor emanating from the endothelial cell. Sullivan *et al.* found an increase in one type on endothelin receptor sites in rabbits with diabetes [362]. Francavilla found elevated levels of endothelin-1 in the blood of diabetic men, versus a control group [363]. The issue, however, is not clear, as Christ *et al.* looked at isolated corpus cavernosal tissue strips and found no difference in the response of endothelin on contraction of smooth muscle in the diabetic versus the non-diabetic corporeal tissue [364].

Insulin resistance

Adult-onset diabetic patients are by definition insulin resistant. Insulin is a vasodilator and acts via a nitric oxide-dependent mechanism [365]. Insulin-mediated dilatation is impaired in states of insulin resistance, such as diabetes and obesity, as a result of endothelial dysfunction. Metro and Broderick evaluated men with type 1 and type 2 diabetes, and found that insulin dependency increased the severity of the vascular insufficiency by increasing the insulin resistance [366]. Insulin resistance is increased from other co-factors in the diabetic patient, such as obesity and elevated cholesterol, especially small-particle LDL cholesterol [367]. Recently, impaired NOS activity has been thought to play an important role in the insulin resistance of type 2 diabetic individuals. Kashyap *et al.* studied NOS activity in skeletal muscle of well-controlled type 2 diabetic patients (A1C = 6.8%) and controls [368]. The basal and insulin-stimulated muscle NOS activity was impaired in well-controlled type 2 diabetic subjects, and the defect in insulin-stimulated NOS activity correlated closely with the severity of the insulin resistance.

Peripheral and autonomic neuropathy

Neuropathy is equal to vascular insufficiency in the pathogenesis of ED in diabetes. This is especially pertinent because of the nonA-nonB nerve fibers that are necessary in the penis to produce neuronal NO for initiation of rigidity. Nijhawan *et al.* studied men with type 1 diabetes [369]. They found that 60% had cardiac autonomic neuropathy and 80% had signs of peripheral neuropathy, but that the most common symptom was ED (44%) rather than postural hypotension (28%). Bemelmans *et al.* found that somatic and autonomic neurologic testing showed a higher incidence of more severe peripheral and autonomic neuropathy in men with diabetes who had ED [370]. They also found that 85% of the men with diabetes and ED had some form of neuropathy, confirming neuropathy as an important pathophysiologic factor in diabetic ED.

Hypogonadism

The earlier literature was inconclusive as to whether diabetes lowered T levels, but this was predominantly using the total T assay. Murray showed that T levels were lower in diabetic men when the more accurate FT method was used [371]. He also showed that T therapy improved the ED, but only in those men who did not have severe vascular disease. Some feel that diabetes will lower T more than other chronic conditions. Guay *et al.* studied T in a population of 990 men with ED, 229 of whom had diabetes [372]. Other chronic illnesses in the group included hypertension, coronary artery disease, hyperlipidemia, and obesity. No difference was seen in the incidence of primary and secondary hypogonadism in diabetes versus the rest of the ED population, suggesting that many chronic illnesses may be related to the development of hypogonadism. In this population, 6% of the men had primary hypogonadism and 30% had secondary hypogonadism. The Rancho Bernardo Study followed 985 men and reported on 110 of the men with diabetes [373]. The incidence of diabetic men with hypogonadism was 21% whereas the incidence in a general population was 13%. Dhindsa *et al.* found that the prevalence of secondary hypogonadism in a cohort of men with type 2 diabetes was 33% [374].

Hyperglycemia

Hyperglycemia has been noted to affect penile physiology. Sobrevia and Mann, in an extensive review of the literature, noted that elevated blood sugar may cause regional hemodynamic changes and that endothelial-dependent relaxation is impaired [375]. Protein kinase C is activated and oxygen radicals are generated, which inactivate NO and cause injury to the endothelial cells. Bagg *et al.* studied poorly controlled diabetic patients [376]. Those patients whose HbA1C levels decreased from 10.2% to 8.2% noted a non-significant improvement over the short term in endothelial activation and fibrinolysis. Christ *et al.* found that hyperglycemia induced significant levels of free oxygen radicals [377]. This result was completely blocked by removal of the endothelium, proving that the source of the free radicals was abnormal endothelial function. At the clinical level, Romeo *et al.* found that elevated HbA1C levels were an independent predictor of ED [378]. Previously, Cartledge *et al.* had noted that the HbA1C molecule itself interfered with NO, by impairment of acetylcholine-stimulated smooth muscle relaxation, in a dose-dependent fashion [379]. This effect was reversed by a NO donor and by adding a superoxide anion scavenger. The conclusion reached was that HbA1C-generated superoxide anions decrease the production and bioavailability of endothelial and neuronal NO, which might help to explain why ED is worse in men with poor diabetic control.

Hypertension

The presence of other risk factors will increase the likelihood and severity of ED in diabetic men. In the literature, the prevalence of hypertension in diabetes varies from 40% to 60%, depending on the population studied. Lipson found the prevalence of hypertension at 68% in African-Americans with diabetes, and that it was two to three times that found in the same population without diabetes [380]. In men with both hypertension and diabetes he found the prevalence of sexual dysfunction to be 60% in African-Americans and 56% in Caucasians. Giuliano found the higher prevalence of ED at 77% in men with both hypertension and diabetes, but 20 years had passed since Lipson's report, and the techniques for diagnosis of ED have been refined greatly [354].

Cigarette smoking

Although the incidence of cigarette smoking has decreased in certain parts of the world, it still involves a quarter of the population in the Western world. Tobacco abuse is an independent risk factor for ED [381]. Bortolotti *et al.* studied smoking in type 1 and 2 diabetic men, and found that smoking increased the already large risk for ED [382]. Correcting for age and the diabetes, the odds ratio of ED for smokers was 1.4 versus never smokers and surprisingly similar at 1.5 for former smokers. The duration of the smoking and the amount of cigarettes smoked increased the risk of ED.

Disorder of collagen metabolism

The decrease in collagen tissue and the increase in corporeal fibrosis are factors of aging, and these effects are exaggerated and occur at an earlier age in diabetic men [383]. These changes are associated with an increase in penile venous efflux and early detumescence. Seftel *et al.* studied the mechanism of these changes in diabetic human corporeal tissue and found an upregulation of p53, known to be related to tissue hypoxia, and also an upregulation of hypoxia-inducible factor-1 alpha [384]. A clinical correlation is seen in men with diabetic nephropathy, especially those undergoing dialysis.

Treatment

Risk factor modification

Controlling the blood sugar is the essential first step. Decreasing the blood sugar by itself will correct certain metabolic abnormalities, but the use of insulin sensitizers will further increase blood flow by decreasing insulin resistance. Then comes the treatment of the related factors, such as hypertension, obesity, and any diabetic complications. The treatment of diabetic ED should begin with a review of potential risk factors in the patient, but also in the partner and the relationship [385]. Egede and Zheng studied 9496 adults with diabetes and found that the incidence of modifiable risk factors was higher in the population with diabetes versus the population

without: hypertension (56% vs. 22%), hyperlipidemia (41% vs. 20%), and obesity (78% vs. 57%) [386]. Beckman *et al.* in reviewing the literature from 1976 to 2001, proved the point that modifying risk factors in diabetes decreased cardiovascular events [343]. Since the common pathophysiologic factor between ED and cardiovascular disease is endothelial dysfunction, steps that can improve endothelial function may also improve both conditions. Cessation of smoking rapidly reverses ED, suggesting that biochemical parameters were being manipulated rather than a vascular obstruction [388].

Hypertension is significantly correlated with abnormal glucose metabolism and overall risk of cardiovascular mortality, so it is important to fully evaluate the patient [389]. The use of an angiotensin converting enzyme inhibitor (ACE-I) has been shown to increase blood flow in diabetics [390]. Other ACE-I, especially ramipril, as well as aminoguanidine, have been shown to positively affect the endothelial cell in diabetes, by decreasing the formation of harmful metabolic products in addition to increasing blood flow [391].

Treatment of the hypogonadism that is often seen in diabetes may correct many of the symptoms of androgen deficiency, and may improve ED, depending, of course, on how many other medical co-factors there are. Boyanov *et al.* treated hypogonadism in diabetic men with T undecanoate, 120 mg per day for three months [392]. The androgen replacement had a positive effect on visceral obesity, with a significant reduction in body weight, waist–hip ratio, and body fat. It significantly improved metabolic control, by decreasing blood glucose levels as mean as HbA1C levels from 10.4% to 8.6%. There was a reversal in the symptoms of androgen deficiency, including ED.

Phosphodiesterase inhibitors, type 5

The introduction of PDE5i agents in 1998 changed the treatment of ED for everyone, including men with diabetes. These drugs decrease the breakdown of cyclic GMP to GMP, thereby increasing the levels of the former to continue the action of vasodilatation. The cyclic GMP is produced from NO, which is turn is produced from the endothelium (eNO) and from the nonA-nonC nerve fibers (nNO). Diabetic men often have clinical or subclinical neuropathy and their production of nNO will be decreased. This is why the results of the PDE5i are not as positive in men with diabetes than with other risk factors for ED, such as hypertension alone, or hyperlipidemia. According to Costabile, no one PDE5i is more beneficial in diabetes than any other, although no head-to-head trials have been done to date in this population [393]. Rendell *et al.* showed good results with sildenafil versus placebo in men with diabetes, but not as good as the pivotal trials in a general population [394].

Sildenafil was found to be more efficacious in men whose diabetes was under better glycemic control. In a study the men with diabetes had a 64% success rate when their HbA1C levels were < 9.0%, and of 44% when the HbA1C was >9.0% [70]. Additionally, neuropathy, in diabetic men with good sugar control, also reduced the success rate to 50%.

Goldstein *et al.* studied 452 men with diabetes who took vardenafil for ED [395]. Patients with diabetic neuropathy and retinopathy were included in the study, but previous sildenafil failures were excluded. Although not quite as good as in their pivotal studies, 64% of the men were able to penetrate their partners, and 54% to complete intercourse versus 36% and 23%, respectively, for the placebo group. Sáenz de Tejada *et al.* evaluated the effect of tadalafil in 191 men with diabetes and ED, mainly moderate to severe, and including men with neuropathy and retinopathy [396]. Here also the results fell short of the pivotal trials for tadalafil in a general population, but were significantly higher than placebo. Their results were reported as percentage improvement over baseline, such that the ability to penetrate intravaginally increased 22.6% versus 4% for placebo. Fonseca *et al.* pooled several trials using tadalafil in diabetic men, for a total of 637 men with diabetes versus 1681 men without diabetes [397]. The baseline IIEF erectile function domain scores showed that the diabetic men had more severe ED—12.6 for the diabetic men and 15.0 for the non-diabetic men. The men who received tadalafil had a mean improvement of their IIEF score of 7.4 versus 0.9 for the placebo group. It is also interesting that the baseline IIEF scores correlated inversely with the HbA1C levels, showing that control of the diabetes correlates with the sever-

ity of the ED. It is also interesting that the responses to tadalafil were similar regardless of levels of baseline glycemic control, diabetic therapy received, or previous use of sildenafil.

Other treatments
Other therapies of ED and sexual dysfunctions in men with diabetes may be administered per the indications and guidelines of the use of such therapies. These may include intraurethral alprostadil, penile self-injection therapy, vacuum constriction devices, and penile prosthesis. Self-injection therapy is the most often used second-line treatment in this difficult-to-treat population, all the more that it is better accepted by the patients who are already familiarized with self-injections of insulin. In men with hypogonadism, T therapy may be indicated as a monotherapy or in combination with other ED therapies.

Metabolic syndrome

The metabolic syndrome comprises a group of risk factors that consist of endothelial dysfunction and atherosclerosis, which can lead to cardiovascular disease [398]. Although the definition of the various components of the metabolic syndrome has varied somewhat, there is now good consensus using the NCEP/ATP-III criteria [399]. The criteria are:

1 Triglyceride level >150 mg/dL
2 HDL cholesterol <40 mg/dL
3 Blood pressure >130/85
4 Fasting blood sugar >100 mg/dL
5 Waist circumference >40 inches (102 cm) in men, or BMI > 28.8

Any three of the five factors comprises an individual with the metabolic syndrome. These risk factors for cardiovascular disease are the same risks associated with ED [400,401], and this has been verified by a most recent consensus conference [402]. It was recognized that endothelial dysfunction is a common link between ED and cardiovascular disease. Endothelial dysfunction is predictive of future cardiovascular events, and is an integral part of the component risk factors inherent in the metabolic syndrome [403].

Roumeguere *et al.* outlined the relationship between ED and various components of cardiovascular risk [404]. We know that the various components of metabolic syndrome, such as blood pressure elevation, hyperlipidemia, obesity, and/or elevated blood sugar take time to extract its metabolic toll on the body. Montorsi *et al.* documented that ED symptoms were present several years before manifest coronary disease [405]. This was predicted a number of years before when Pritzker performed cardiac stress tests on 50 men with ED, but no history or symptoms of heart disease, and was surprised to find that 56% of the men failed the stress test because of silent ischemia [406]. He postulated that ED might be the early factor that could predict heart disease, and that pursuing this vigorously might enable physicians to practice primary cardiac prevention.

There is a high percentage of men with cardiovascular risks in clinics that treat ED, and the prevalence of the two most important risk factors, diabetes mellitus and hypertension, is amazingly similar whether the number is 150 in a single clinic [407] or several hundred thousand men from managed care statistics [408].

Although opinions have been mixed, there seems to be more data that indicates a certain relationship between T and the metabolic syndrome. The TT assay is the one most commonly used in clinical practice and the level is significantly affected by SHBG. Laaksonen *et al.* followed 702 middle-aged men participating in a population-based cohort study [409]. After 11 years 147 men developed the metabolic syndrome and 57 men developed diabetes. Men with TT, calculated FT, and SHBG levels in the lower fourth had a several-fold increased risk of developing the metabolic syndrome and diabetes. This has been confirmed in a recent analysis of the MMAS data [129]. The conclusion was that hypogonadism was an early marker for insulin and glucose metabolism. Kalme *et al.* confirmed the known fact that increased insulin downregulates SHBG production, which in turn decreases total T levels [410]. They followed 1711 men longitudinally. They found that low SHBG and IGF-binding protein-1 were both associated with an increased prevalence of abnormal glucose tolerance and the metabolic syndrome, and that SHBG alone was a better indicator of increased cardiovascular mortality. All of these factors, of course, are related to risks of ED. Conversely, Muller *et al.* have shown that higher T and SHBG levels in aging

men are independently associated with a higher insulin sensitivity and a reduced risk of the metabolic syndrome [411]. Their findings were independent of BMI and insulin levels, suggesting that androgens may protect against the development of the metabolic syndrome.

Few studies have looked at the incidence of the metabolic syndrome in an ED population, by looking at the specific NCEP/ATPIII criteria themselves. Bansal *et al.* evaluated the specific criteria in 154 consecutive consultations for ED [412]. Three of the five criteria for metabolic syndrome were present in 43% of the men with ED, as compared to a reported 24% in a general and similar population that is predominantly Caucasian. It is also interesting that metabolic syndrome correlated positively and moderately with increasing severity of ED. Looking at the converse, Esposito *et al.* looked at the prevalence of ED in men with the metabolic syndrome [413]. They evaluated 100 men with metabolic syndrome and an age and BMI matched control group. They found an increased prevalence of erectile dysfunction of 26.7% in the group with metabolic syndrome versus 13% in the control group. They also showed that the prevalence of ED increased as did the number of components of the metabolic syndrome. This is not surprising as the pathophysiologic common denominator for metabolic syndrome, ED, and cardiovascular disease is endothelial dysfunction [414]. Shabsigh *et al.* looked at ED as a predictor for the metabolic syndrome in a longitudinal study in an aging male population [415]. The longitudinal analysis of the MMAS data has shown that ED is predictive of incident metabolic syndrome, but that this association is modified by BMI. ED is associated with a two-fold increase in risk of metabolic syndrome in men with BMI <25, but not > 25.

Obesity

The prevalence of obesity is ever increasing, especially in developed countries. Increased weight (BMI 25.0–29.9) and obesity (BMI ≥30.0) are seen as risk factors in as many as 85% of men with ED [416]. This is quite pertinent to ED because the insulin resistance that accompanies excess weight is a cause of decreased blood flow [417]. The observation that insulin receptor numbers can be restored to normal if insulin levels are decreased in obese patients suggests that the changes in receptor numbers are secondary to the insulin resistance, and not a primary causal factor [418].

Elevated weight and obesity are now considered as independent and direct risks of heart disease [419], and not just because increased weight causes a higher prevalence of other known risks of heart disease, such as diabetes mellitus, hypertension, and hyperlipidemia. Suwaidi *et al.* showed decreased endothelial-related blood flow, which directly correlated with increasing weight [420]. The authors felt that the progressive decrease in endothelial function with increasing weight was related to insulin resistance. It is commonly held that the common pathophysiologic factor in the majority of risk factors for ED is endothelial dysfunction and it is also felt that insulin resistance, which is related to decreased blood flow, also has its basis in endothelial dysfunction [421].

It is not surprising, therefore, that the overweight state and frank obesity are important components in the pathophysiology of ED, as well as in the pathophysiology of cardiovascular disease. The treatment of excess weight may also be considered an important part of the treatment of ED, via the treatment modality of modification of risk factors. This has been confirmed by the randomized study of 110 obese men without any other metabolic disorder or vascular risk factor by Esposito *et al.* [422]. At two years' follow-up, the 55 men in the intensive intervention group (diet plus increased physical activity) had lost weight, improved their markers of inflammation and endothelial dysfunction, and improved their mean IIEF score from 13.9 to 17.0; while in the "control" group the mean score remained stable at around 13.5. Seventeen men in the intervention group, compared with only three controls, scored 22 or higher on the IIEF at follow-up.

References

1 Jockenhövel F. *Male hypogonadism.* Bremen, Germany: UNIMED-Verlag AG, 2004, Vol. 1.

2 Nieschlag E, Swerdloff R, Behre HM, Gooren LJ, Kaufman JM, Legros JJ, Lunenfeld B, Morley JE, Schulman C, Wang C, Weidner W, Wu FC. Investigation, treatment and monitoring of late-onset hypogonadism in males. ISA, ISSAM, and EAU recommendations. *Eur Urol* 2005;**48**:1–4.

3 Gennari L, Merlotti D, Martini G, Gonnelli S, Franci B, Campagna S, Lucani B, Dal Canto N, Valenti R, Gennari C, Nuti R. Longitudinal association between sex hormone levels, bone loss, and bone turnover in elderly men. *J Clin Endocrinol Metab* 2003;**88**:5327–5333.

4 Rochira V, Balestrieri A, Madeo B, Spaggiari A, Carani C. Congenital estrogen deficiency in men: a new syndrome with different phenotypes; clinical and therapeutic implications in men. *Mol Cell Endocrinol* 2002;**193**:19–28.

5 de Ronde W, van der Schouw YT, Pierik FH, Pols HA, Muller M, Grobbee DE, Gooren LJ, Weber RF, de Jong FH. Serum levels of sex hormone-binding globulin (SHBG) are not associated with lower levels of non-SHBG-bound testosterone in male newborns and healthy adult men. *Clin Endocrinol (Oxf)* 2005; **62**:498–503.

6 Luboshitzky R, Shen-Orr Z, Herer P. Middle-aged men secrete less testosterone at night than young healthy men. *J Clin Endocrinol Metab* 2003;**88**:3160–3166.

7 Morgentaler A, Barquawi A, O'Donnel C, Lynch J, Petrylak D, Crawford ED. Is it necessary to obtain a serum testosterone test in the morning? Cross-sectional analysis of diurnal serum testosterone variation in aging male from a large national screening program. *J Sex Med* 2006;**3**(suppl 1):47, abstr. 106.

8 Bhasin S, Woodhouse L, Casaburi R, Singh AB, Bhasin D, Berman N, Chen X, Yarasheski KE, Magliano L, Dzekov C, Dzekov J, Bross R, Phillips J, Sinha-Hikim I, Shen R, Storer TW. Testosterone dose-response relationships in healthy young men. *Am J Physiol Endocrinol Metab* 2001;**281**:E1172–1181.

9 Buena F, Swerdloff RS, Steiner BS, Lutchmansingh P, Peterson MA, Pandian MR, Galmarini M, Bhasin S. Sexual function does not change when serum testosterone levels are pharmacologically varied within the normal male range. *Fertil Steril* 1993;**59**:1118–1123.

10 Gooren LJ. Androgen levels and sex functions in testosterone-treated hypogonadal men. *Arch Sex Behav* 1987;**16**:463–473.

11 Schiavi RC, Rehman J. Sexuality and aging. *Urol Clin North Am* 1995;**22**:711–726.

12 Gray PB, Singh AB, Woodhouse LJ, Storer TW, Casaburi R, Dzekov J, Dzekov C, Sinha-Hikim I, Bhasin S. Dose-dependent effects of testosterone on sexual function, mood, and visuospatial cognition in older men. *J Clin Endocrinol Metab* 2005;**90**: 3838–3846.

13 Steidle C, Schwartz S, Jacoby K, Sebree T, Smith T, Bachand R. AA2500 testosterone gel normalizes androgen levels in aging males with improvements in body composition and sexual function. *J Clin Endocrinol Metab* 2003;**88**:2673–2681.

14 Jain P, Rademaker AW, McVary KT. Testosterone supplementation for erectile dysfunction: results of a meta-analysis. *J Urol* 2000;**164**:371–375.

15 Zitzmann M, Nieschlag E. The CAG repeat polymorphism within the androgen receptor gene and maleness. *Int J Androl* 2003;**26**:76–83.

16 Harkonen K, Huhtaniemi I, Makinen J, Hubler D, Irjala K, Koskenvuo M, Oettel M, Raitakari O, Saad F, Pollanen P. The polymorphic androgen receptor gene CAG repeat, pituitary-testicular function and andropausal symptoms in ageing men. *Int J Androl* 2003;**26**:187–194.

17 Catuogno C, Romano G. Androstanolone treatment for congenital penile curvature. *Eur Urol* 2001; **39**(suppl 2):28–32.

18 Buvat J, Lemaire A. Endocrine screening in 1022 men with erectile dysfunction: clinical significance and cost-effective strategy. *J Urol* 1997;**158**:764–767.

19 Bodie J, Lewis J, Schow D, Monga M. Laboratory evaluations of erectile dysfunction: an evidence based approach. *J Urol* 2003;**169**(6):2262–2264.

20 Earle CM, Stuckey BG. Biochemical screening in the assessment of erectile dysfunction: what tests decide future therapy? *Urology* 2003;**62**(4):727–731.

21 Maatman TJ, Montague DK. Routine endocrine screening in impotence. *Urology* 1986;**27**:499–502.

22 Buvat-Herbaut M, Buvat J, Dancoine F, Lemaire A, Marcolin G, Fourlinnie JC. More than 30% of the impotent patients with normal values of serum total testosterone have low values of free, and even more of bioavailable serum testosterone. Serono symposia review, IV International Congress of Andrology, Fiorenza, Italy, 1989;suppl I:196.

23 Buvat J, Lemaire A, Ratasczyk J. Rôle des hormones dans les dysfonctions sexuelles, l'homosexualité, le transsexualisme et les comportements sexuels déviants: Conséquences diagnostiques et thérapeutiques. *Contraception-Fertilité-Sexualité* 1996;**24** 834–846 [in French].

24 Kim YC, Buvat J, Carson CC, Gooren LJ, Jarow J, Rajfer J, Vermeulen A. Endocrine and metabolic aspects including treatment. In: *Erectile Dysfunction*. Jardin A, Wagner G, Khoury S, Giuliano F, Padma-Nathan H, Rosen R, Paris, Plymbridge, Plymouth, UK: Proceedings of the First International Consultation on Erectile Dysfunction, July 1–3, 1999, pp. 205–240.

25 Jannini EA, Screponi E, Carosa E, *et al.* Lack of sexual activity from erectile dysfunction is associated with a reversible reduction in serum testosterone. *Int J Androl* 1999;**22**:385–392.

26 Carosa E, Martini P, Brandetti F, *et al.* Type V phosphodiesterase inhibitor treatments for erectile dysfunction increase testosterone levels. *Clin Endocrinol (Oxf)* 2004;**61**:382–386.

27 O'Carroll R, Bancroft J. Testosterone therapy for low sexual interest and erectile dysfunction in men: a controlled study. *Br J Psych* 1984;**145**:146–151.

28 Beutel ME, Witlinck J, Hauck EW, Auch D, Behre HM, Brähler E, Weidner W. Correlations between hormones, physical and affective parameters in aging urological patients. *Eur Urol* 2005;**47**:749–755.

29 O'Carrol R, Shapiro C, Bancroft J. Androgens, behaviour and nocturnal erection in hypogonadal men: the effects of varying the replacement dose. *Clin Endocrinol* 1985;**23**:527–538.

30 Wang C, Swerdloff RS, Iranmanesh A, Dobs A, Snyder PJ, Cunningham G, Matsumoto AM, Weber T, Berman N, and the testosterone gel study group. Transdermal testosterone gel improves sexual function, mood, muscle strength, and body composition parameters in hypogonadal men. *J Clin Endocrinol Metab* 2000;**85**: 839–853.

31 Salmimies P, Kockott G, Pirke KM, Vogt HJ, Schill WB. Effects of testosterone replacement on sexual behavior in hypogonadal men. *Arch Sex Behav* 1982;**11**:345–353.

32 Kwan M, Greenleaf WJ, Mann J, Crapo L, Davidson JM. The nature of androgen action on male sexuality: a combined laboratory-self-report study on hypogonadal men. *J Clin Endocrinol Metab* 1983;**57**:557–562.

33 Bancroft J, Wu FCW. Changes in erectile responsiveness during androgen therapy. *Arch Sex Behav* 1983;**12**:59–66.

34 Carani C, Granata AR, Fustini MF, Marrama P. Prolactin and testosterone: their role in male sexual function. *Int J Androl* 1996;**19**:48–54.

35 Burris AS, Banks SM, Carter CS, Davidson JM, Sherins RJ. A long-term, prospective study of the physiologic and behavioral effects of hormone replacement in untreated hypogonadal men. *J Androl* 1992;**13**:297–304.

36 Kelleher S, Conway AJ, Handelsman DJ. Blood testosterone threshold for androgen deficiency symptoms. *J Clin Endocrinol Metab* 2004;**89**:3813–3817.

37 Seftel AD, Mack RJ, Secrest AR, Smith TM. Restorative increases in serum testosterone levels are significantly correlated to improvements in sexual functioning. *J Androl* 2004;**25**:963–972.

38 Carani C, Bancroft J, Granata A, Del Rio G, Marrama P. Testosterone and erectile function, nocturnal penile tumescence and rigidity, and erectile response to visual erotic stimuli in hypogonadal and eugonadal men. *Psychoneuroendocrinology* 1992;**17**:647–654.

39 WHO: Task force on psychosocial research in family planning. Hormonal contraception for men: acceptability and effects on sexuality. *Stud Family Planning* 1982;**13**:328–342.

40 Anderson RA, Bancroft J, Wu FCW. The effects of exogenous testosterone on sexuality and mood of normal men. *J Clin Endocrinol Metab* 1992;**75**:1503–1507.

41 Carani C, Granata AR, Bancroft J, Marrama P. The effects of testosterone replacement on nocturnal penile tumescence and rigidity and erectile response to visual erotic stimuli in hypogonadal men. *Psychoneuroendocrinology* 1995;**20**:743–753.

42 O'Connor DB, Archer J, Wu FCW. Effects of testosterone on mood, aggression and sexual behaviour in young men: a double blind, placebo controlled, cross over study. *J Clin Endrocinol Metab* 2004;**89**:2837–2845.

43 Park KH, Kim SW, Kim KD, Paick JS. Effects of androgens on the expression of nitric oxide synthase mRNAs in rat corpus cavernosum. *BJU Int* 1999;**83**:327–333.

44 Baba K, Yajima M, Carrier S, Morgan DM, Nunes L, Lue TF, *et al*. Delayed testosterone replacement restores nitric oxide synthase-containing nerve fibres and the erectile response in rat penis. *BJU Int* 2000;**85**:953–958.

45 Traish AM, Kim N. The physiological role of androgens in penile erection: regulation of corpus cavernosum and structure. *J Sex Med* 2005;**2**:759–770.

46 Rogers RS. Graziottin TM. Lin CM. Kan YW, Lue T. Intracavernosal vascular endothelial growth factor (VEGF) injection and adeno-associated virus-mediated VEGF gene therapy prevent and reverse venogenic erectile dysfunction in rats. *Int J Impot Res* 2003;**15**:26–37.

47 Stoleru S, Redoute J, Costes N, Lavenne F, Le Bars D, Dechaud H, Forest MG, Pugeat M, Cinotti L, Pujol JF. Brain processing of visual sexual stimuli in men with hypoactive sexual desire disorder. *Psychiatry Research: Neuroimaging* 2003;**124**:67–86.

48 Redoute J, Stoleru S, Pugeat M, Costes N, Lavenne F, Le Bars D, Dechaud H, Cinotti L, Pujol JF. Brain processing of visual sexual stimuli in treated and untreated hypogonadal patients. *Psychoneuroendocrinology* 2005;**30**:461–482.

49 Schultheiss D, Badalyan R, Pilatz A, Gabouev AI, Schlote N, Wefer J, von Wasielewski R, Mertsching H, Sohn M, Stief CG, Jonas U. Androgen and estrogen receptors in the human corpus cavernosum penis: immunohistochemical and cell culture results. *World J Urol* 2003;**21**:320–324.

50 Foresta C, Caretta N, Rossato M, Garolla A, Ferlin A. Role of androgens in erectile function. *J Urol* 2004;**171**:2358–2362.

51 Aversa A, Isidori AM, De Martino MU, Caprio M, Fabbrini E, Rocchietti-March M, *et al*. Androgens and penile erection: evidence for a direct relationship between free testosterone and cavernous vasodilation in men with erectile dysfunction. *Clin Endocrinol (Oxf)* 2000;**53**:517–522.

52 Aversa A, Isidori AM, Spera G, Lenzi A, Fabbri A. Androgens improve cavernous vasodilation and response to sildenafil in patients with erectile dysfunction. *Clin Endocrinol (Oxf)* 2003;**58**:632–638.

53 Isidori AM, Gianetta E, Gianfrilli D, Greco EA, Bonifacio V, Aversa A, Isidori A, Fabbri A, Lenzi A. Effects of testosterone on sexual function in men: results of a meta-analysis. *Clin Endocrinol (Oxf)* 2005;**63**:381–394.

54 Kropman RF, Verdijk R, Lycklama A, Nijohlt AAB, Roefsema F. Routine endocrine screening in impotence: significance and cest effectiveness. *Int J Impot Res* 1991;**3**:87–94.

55 Morales A, Johnson B, Heaton JW, Clark A. Oral androgens in the treatment of hypogonadal impotent men. *J Urol* 1994;**152**:1115–1118.

56 Morales A, Johnston B, Heaton JPW, Lundie M. Testosterone supplementation for hypogonadal impotence: assessment of biochemical measures and therapeutic outcomes. *J Urol* 1997;**157**:849–854.

57 Rakic Z, Starcevic V, Starcevic VP, Marinkovic J. Testosterone treatment in men with erectile disorder and low levels of testosterone in serum. *Arch Sex Behav* 1997;**26**(5):495–504.

58 Wylie K, Davies-South D. A study of treatment choices in men with erectile dysfunction and reduced androgen levels. *J Sex Mar Ther* 2004;**30**:107–114.

59 Greenstein A, Mabjeesh NJ, Sofer M, Kaver I, Matzkin H, Chen J. Does sildenafil combined with testosterone gel improve erectile dysfunction in hypogonadal men in whom testosterone supplement therapy alone failed? *J Urol* 2005;**173**:530–532.

60 Buvat J, Lemaire A, Alexandre B, Ratasczyk J. Effects of androgen therapy in 38 patients with low total, free, and/or bioavailable testosterone. *Int J Impot Res* 2002;**14**(suppl 3):S36.

61 Purvis K, Landgren B, Cekan Z, Diczfaluzy E. Endocrine effects of masturbation. *J Endocrinol* 1976;**70**:439–444.

62 Christiansen K, Knussman R, Couwenbergs C. Sex hormones and stress in the human male. *Horm Behav* 1985;**19**:426–440.

63 Christiansen K, Hars O. Effects of stress anticipation and stress coping strategies on salivary testosterone levels. *J Psychophysiol* 1995;**3**:264–269.

64 Carosa E, Benvenga S, Trimarchi F, *et al*. Sexual inactivity results in reversible reduction of LH bioavailability. *Int J Impot Res* 2002;**14**:93–99.

65 Traish AM, Park K, Dhir V, Kim NN, Moreland RB, Goldstein I. Effects of castration and androgen replacement on erectile function in a rabbit model. *Endocrinology* 1999;**140**:1861–1868.

66 Morelli A, Filippi S, Mancina R, Luconi M, Vignozzi L, Marini M, Orlando C, Vannelli GB, Aversa A, Natali A, Forti G, Giorgi M, Jannini EA, Ledda F, Maggi M. Androgens regulate phosphodiesterase type 5 expression and functional activity in corpora cavernosa. *Endocrinology* 2004;**145**:2253–2263.

67 Zhang XH, Morelli A, Luconi M, Vignozzi L, Filippi S, Marini M, Vannelli GB, Mancina R, Forti G, Maggi M. Testosterone regulates PDE5 expression and in vivo responsiveness to tadalafil in rat corpus cavernosum. *Eur Urol* 2005;**47**:409–416.

68 Traish AM, Munarriz R, O'Connell L, *et al*. Effects of medical or surgical castration on erectile function in an animal model. *J Androl* 2003;**24**:381–387.

69 Rochira V, Balestrieri A, Madeo B, Granata ARM, Carani C. Sildenafil improves sleep-related erections in hypogonadal men: evidence from a randomized, placebo-controlled, cross-over study of a synergistic role of both testosterone and sildenafil on penile erections. *J Androl* 2006;**27**:165–175.

70 Guay AT, Perez JB, Jacobson J, Newton RA. Efficacy and safety of Sildenafil citrate for treatment of erectile dysfunction in a population with associated organic risk factors. *J Androl* 2001;**22**:793–797.

71 Kalinchenko SY, Kozlov GI, Gontcharov NP, Katsiya GV. Oral testosterone undecanoate reverses erectile dysfunction associated with diabetes mellitus in patients failing on sildenafil citrate therapy alone. *Aging Male* 2003;**6**:94–99.

72 Shamloul R, Ghanem H, Fahmy I, El-Meleigy A, Ashoor S, Elnashaar A, Kamel I. Testosterone therapy can enhance erectile function response to Sildenafil in patients with PADAM: a pilot study. *J Sex Med* 2005;**2**:559–564.

73 Shabsigh R, Kaufman JM, Steidle C, Padma-Nathan H. Randomized study of testosterone gel as adjunctive therapy to sildenafil in hypogonadal men with erectile dysfunction who do not respond to sildenafil alone. *J Urol* 2004;**172**:658–663.

74 Mulhall JP, Valenzuela R, Aviv N, Parker M. Effect of testosterone supplementation on sexual function in hypogonadal men with erectile dysfunction. *Urology* 2004;**63**:348–352; discussion 352–353.

75 Kaufman JM, Vermeulen A. The decline of androgen levels in elderly men and its clinical and therapeutic implications. *Endocr Rev* 2005;**26**:833–876.

76 Moffat SD, Zonderman AB, Metter EJ, Blackman MR, Harman SM, Resnick SM. Longitudinal assessment of serum free testosterone concentration predicts memory performance and cognitive status in elderly men. *J Clin Endocrinol Metab* 2002;**87**:5001–5007.

77 Morley JE, Kaiser FE, Perry HM, 3rd, Patrick P, Morley PM, Stauber PM, Vellas B, Baumgartner RN, Garry PJ. Longitudinal changes in testosterone, luteinizing hormone, and follicle-stimulating hormone in healthy older men. *Metabolism* 1997;**46**:410–413.

78 Araujo AB, O'Donnell AB, Brambilla DJ, Simpson WB, Longcope C, Matsumoto AM, McKinlay JB. Prevalence and incidence of androgen deficiency in middle-aged and older men: estimates from the Massachusetts Male Aging Study. *J Clin Endocrinol Metab* 2004;**89**:5920–5926.

79 Meikle AW, Bishop DT, Stringham JD, West DW. Quantitating genetic and nongenetic factors that determine plasma sex steroid variation in normal male twins. *Metabolism* 1986;**35**:1090–1095.

80 Handelsman DJ. Testicular dysfunction in systemic disease. *Endocrinol Metab Clin North Am* 1994;**23**:839–856.

81 Vermeulen A. Androgen replacement therapy in the aging male: a critical evaluation. *J Clin Endocrinol Metab* 2001;**86**:2380–2390.

82 Vermeulen A, Goemaere S, Kaufman JM. Sex hormones, body composition and aging. *Aging Male* 1999;**2**:8–15.

83 Seidell JC, Bjorntorp P, Sjostrom L, Kvist H, Sannerstedt R. Visceral fat accumulation in men is positively associated with insulin, glucose, and C-peptide levels, but negatively with testosterone levels. *Metabolism* 1990;**39**:897–901.

84 Tchernof A, Labrie F, Belanger A, Prud'homme D, Bouchard C, Tremblay A, *et al*. Relationships between endogenous steroid hormone, sex hormone-binding globulin and lipoprotein levels in men: contribution of visceral obesity, insulin levels and other metabolic variables. *Atherosclerosis* 1997;**133**:235–244.

85 Kannel WB, Cupples LA, Ramaswami R, Stokes J, III, Kreger BE, Higgins M. Regional obesity and risk of

cardiovascular disease: the Framingham Study. *J Clin Epidemiol* 1991;**44**:183–190.

86 Björntorp P. Visceral obesity: a civilisation syndrome. *Obes Res* 1993;**1**:206–222.

87 Buvat J, Boujadoue G. Testosterone replacement therapy in the ageing man. *J Men's Health & Gender* 2005;**2**:396–399.

88 Isidori AM, Gianetta E, Greco E, Gianfrilli D, Bonifacio V, Isidori A, Lenzi A, Fabbri A. Effects of testosterone on body composition, bone metabolism and serum lipid profile in middle-aged men: a meta-analysis. *Clin Endocrinol (Oxf)* 2005;**63**:280–293.

89 Larsson L. Histochemical characteristics of human skeletal muscle during aging. *Acta Physiol Scand* 1983;**117**:469–471.

90 Frontera WR, Hughes VA, Fielding RA, Fiatarone MA, Evans WJ, Roubenoff R. Aging of skeletal muscle: a 12-yr longitudinal study. *J Appl Physiol* 2000;**88**: 1321–1326.

91 Reed RL, Pearlmutter L, Yochum K, Meredith KE, Mooradian AD. The relationship between muscle mass and muscle strength in the elderly. *J Am Geriatr Soc* 1991;**39**:555–561.

92 Van den Beld AW, de Jong FH, Grobbee DE, Pols HA, Lamberts SW. Measures of bioavailable serum testosterone and estradiol and their relationships with muscle strength, bone density, and body composition in elderly men. *J Clin Endocrinol Metab* 2000;**85**: 3276–3282.

93 Abbasi AA, Drinka PJ, Mattson DE, Rudman D. Low circulating levels of insulin-like growth factors and testosterone in chronically institutionalized elderly men. *J Am Geriatr Soc* 1993;**41**:975–982.

94 Baumgartner RN, Waters DL, Gallagher D, Morley JE, Garry PJ. Predictors of skeletal muscle mass in elderly men and women. *Mech Ageing Dev* 1999;**107**:123–136.

95 Verhaar HJJ, Samson MM, Aleman A, de Vries WR, de Vreede PL, Koppeschaar HPF. The relationship between indices of muscle function and circulating anabolic hormones in healthy. *Aging Male* 2000;**3**:75–80.

96 Orwoll ES, Klein RF. Osteoporosis in men. *Endocr Rev* 1995;**16**:87–116.

97 Foresta C, Ruzza G, Mioni R, Guarneri G, Gribaldo R, Meneghello A, *et al.* Osteoporosis and decline of gonadal function in the elderly male. *Horm Res* 1984;**19**:18–22.

98 Center JR, Nguyen TV, Sambrook PN, Eisman JA. Hormonal and biochemical parameters in the determination of osteoporosis in elderly men. *J Clin Endocrinol Metab* 1999;**84**:3626–3635.

99 Rudman D, Drinka PJ, Wilson CR, Mattson DE, Scherman F, Cuisinier MC, *et al.* Relations of endogenous anabolic hormones and physical activity to bone mineral density and lean body mass in elderly men. *Clin Endocrinol (Oxf)* 1994;**40**:653–661.

100 Murphy S, Khaw KT, Cassidy A, Compston JE. Sex hormones and bone mineral density in elderly men. *Bone Miner* 1993;**20**:133–40.

101 Kaufman JM. Androgens, bone metabolism and osteoporosis. In Oddens B, Vermeulen A, eds. *Androgens and the aging male.* Parthenon Publ. Group, 1996; 39–60.

102 Drinka PJ, Olson J, Bauwens S, Voeks SK, Carlson I, Wilson M. Lack of association between free testosterone and bone density separate from age in elderly males. *Calcif Tissue Int* 1993;**52**:67–69.

103 Meier DE, Orwoll ES, Keenan EJ, Fagerstrom RM. Marked decline in trabecular bone mineral content in healthy men with age: lack of association with sex steroid levels. *J Am Geriatr Soc* 1987;**35**:189–197.

104 Clarke BL, Ebeling PR, Jones JD, Wahner HW, O'Fallon WM, Riggs BL, *et al.* Changes in quantitative bone histomorphometry in aging healthy men. *J Clin Endocrinol Metab* 1996;**81**:2264–2270.

105 Greendale GA, Edelstein S, Barrett-Connor E. Endogenous sex steroids and bone mineral density in older women and men: the Rancho Bernardo Study. *J Bone Miner Res* 1997;**12**:1833–1843.

106 Khosla S, Melton LJ, III, Atkinson EJ, O'Fallon WM, Klee GG, Riggs BL. Relationship of serum sex steroid levels and bone turnover markers with bone mineral density in men and women: a key role for bioavailable estrogen. *J Clin Endocrinol Metab* 1998;**83**:2266–2274.

107 Wang C, Cunningham G, Dobs A, Iranmanesh A, Matsumoto AM, Snyder PJ, Weber T, Berman N, Hull L, Swerdloff RS. Long term testosterone gel (AndroGel) treatment maintains beneficial effects on sexual function and mood, lean and fat mass, and bone mineral density in hypogonadal men. *J Clin Endocrinol Metab* 2004;**89**:2085–2098.

108 Carani C, Qin K, Simoni M, Faustini-Fustini M, Serpente S, Boyd J, *et al.* Effect of testosterone and estradiol in a man with aromatase deficiency. *N Engl J Med* 1997;**337**:91–95.

109 Barrett-Connor E, Mueller JE, von Muhlen DG, Laughlin GA, Schneider DL, Sartoris DJ. Low levels of estradiol are associated with vertebral fractures in older men, but not women: the Rancho Bernardo Study. *J Clin Endocrinol Metab* 2000;**85**:219–223.

110 Kirkland RT, Keenan BS, Probstfield JL, Patsch W, Lin TL, Clayton GW, *et al.* Decrease in plasma high-density lipoprotein cholesterol levels at puberty in boys with

delayed adolescence. Correlation with plasma testosterone levels. *JAMA* 1987;**257**:502–507.

111 Barrett-Connor EL. Testosterone and risk factors for cardiovascular disease in men. *Diabete Metab* 1995;**21**:156–161.

112 Bagatell CJ, Bremner WJ. Androgen and progestagen effects on plasma lipids. *Prog Cardiovasc Dis* 1995;**38**:255–271.

113 Haffner JM. Androgens in relation to cardiovascular disease and insulin resistance in aging male. In Oddens B, Vermeulen A, eds. *Androgens and the aging male*, Parthenon Publ.Group, 1996; pp. 65–84.

114 Caron P, Bennet A, Camare R, Louvet JP, Boneu B, Sie P. Plasminogen activator inhibitor in plasma is related to testosterone in men. *Metabolism* 1989;**38**:1010–1015.

115 Phillips GB, Pinkernell BH, Jing TY. The association of hypotestosteronemia with coronary artery disease in men. *Arterioscler Thromb* 1994;**14**:701–706.

116 Swartz CM, Young MA. Low serum testosterone and myocardial infarction in geriatric male inpatients. *J Am Geriatr Soc* 1987;**35**:39–44.

117 Haffner JE, Moss SE, Klein BEK, Klein R. Sex hormones and DHEASO4 in relation to ischemic heart disease in diabetic subjects. The WESDR Study. *Diabetes Care* 1996;**19**:1045–1050.

118 Barrett-Connor E, Khaw KT. Endogenous sex hormones and cardiovascular disease in men. A prospective population-based study. *Circulation* 1988;**78**:539–545.

119 Cauley JA, Gutai JP, Kuller LH, Dai WS. Usefulness of sex steroid hormone levels in predicting coronary artery disease in men. *Am J Cardiol* 1987;**60**:771–777.

120 Polderman KH, Stehouwer CD, van Kamp GJ, Dekker GA, Verheugt FW, Gooren LJ. Influence of sex hormones on plasma endothelin levels. *Ann Intern Med* 1993;**118**:429–432.

121 Ajayi AA, Mathur R, Halushka PV. Testosterone increases human platelet thromboxane A2 receptor density and aggregation responses. *Circulation* 1995;**91**:2742–2747.

122 Barrett-Connor E. Lower endogenous androgen levels and dyslipidemia in men with non-insulin-dependent diabetes mellitus. *Ann Intern Med* 1992;**117**:807–811.

123 Makhsida N, Shah J, Yan G, Fisch H, Shabsigh R. Hypogonadism and metabolic syndrome: implications for testosterone therapy. *J Urol* 2005;**174**:827–34.

124 Liu PY, Death AK, Handelsman DJ. Androgens and cardiovascular disease. *Endocr Rev* 2003;**24**:313–340.

125 Shabsigh R, Katz M, Yan G, Makhsida N. Cardiovascular issues in hypogonadism and testosterone therapy. *Am J Cardiol* 2005;**96**:67M–72M.

126 Wu FCW, vonEckardstein A. Androgens and coronary artery disease. *Endocr Rev* 2003;**24**:183–217.

127 Gruenewald DA, Matsumoto AM. Testosterone supplementation therapy for older men: potential benefits and risks. *J Am Geriatr* 2003;**51**:101–115.

128 Schiavi RC. Androgens and sexual function in men. In Oddens B, Vermeulen A, eds. *Androgens and the aging male*, Parthenon Publish. Group, 1996; pp. 111–128.

129 Travison TG, Kupelian V, Page ST, Araujo AB, Bremner WJ, Mc Kinlay JB. The relationship between hormones and the Metabolic Syndrome. *Aging Male* 2006;**9**:62.

130 Tenover JS. Effects of testosterone supplementation in the aging male. *J Clin Endocrinol Metab* 1992;**75**:1092–1098.

131 Morley JE, Perry HM, III, Kaiser FE, Kraenzle D, Jensen J, Houston K, *et al.* Effects of testosterone replacement therapy in old hypogonadal males: a preliminary study. *J Am Geriatr Soc* 1993;**41**:149–152.

132 Barrett-Connor E, Goodman-Gruen D, Patay B. Endogenous sex hormones and cognitive function in older men. *J Clin Endocrinol Metab* 1999;**84**:3681–3685.

133 Janowsky JS, Oviatt SK, Orwoll ES. Testosterone influences spatial cognition in older men. *Behav Neurosci* 1994;**108**:325–332.

134 McKeever WF, Deyo A. Testosterone, dihydrotestosterone and spatial task performance of males. *Bull Psychonomic Soc* 1990;**28**:305–306.

135 Christiansen K, Knussmann R. Sex hormones and cognitive functioning in men. *Neuropsychobiology* 1987;**18**:27–36.

136 Fonda S, Bertrand R, O'Donnell A, Longcope C, McKinley JB. Age, Hormones and Cognitive Functioning among Middle-Aged and Elderly Men: Cross-Sectional Evidence frome the Massachusetts Male Aging Study. *J Gerontology* 2005;**60A**:385–390.

137 Moffat SD, Zonderman AB, Metter EJ, Blackman MR, Harman SM, Resnick SM. Longitudinal assessment of serum free testosterone concentration predicts memory performance and cognitive status in elderly men. *J Clin Endocrinol Metab* 2002;**87**:5001–5007.

138 Kaufman JM, Vermeulen A. The decline of androgen levels in elderly men and its clinical and therapeutic implications. *Endocr Rev* 2005;**26**:833–876.

139 Araujo AB, Durante R, Feldman HA, *et al.* The relationship between depressive symptoms and male erectile dysfunction: cross-sectional results from the Massachusetts Male Aging Study. *Psychosom Med* 1998;**60**:458–465.

140 Seidman SN, Walsh BT. Testosterone and depression in aging men. *Am J Geriatr Psychiatry* 1999;**7**:18–33.

141 Shores MM, Moceri VM, Sloan KL, Matsumoto AM, Kivlahan DR. Low testosterone levels predict incident depressive illness in older men: effects of age and medical morbidity. *J Clin Psychiatry* 2005;**66**:7–14.

142 Seidman SN, Araujo AB, Roose SP, Mc Kinlay JB. Testosterone level, androgen receptor polymorphism, and depressive symptoms in middle-aged men. *Biol Psychiatry* 2001;**50**:371–376.

143 Pope HG, Cohane GH, Kanayama G, Siegel AJ, Hudson JL. Testosterone gel supplementation for men with refractory depression. A randomized, placebo-controlled trial. *Am J Psychiatry* 2003;**160**:105–111.

144 Gooren LJ. Human male sexual functions do not require aromatization of testosterone: a study using tamoxifen, testolactone, and dihydrotestosterone. *Arch Sex Behav* 1985;**14**:539–548.

145 Carani C, Rochira V, Faustini-Fustini M, *et al.* Role of oestrogen in male sexual behaviour: insights from the natural model of aromatase deficiency. *Clin Endocrinol (Oxf)* 1999;**51**:517–524.

146 McEwen BS, Alves SE. Estrogen actions in the central nervous system. *Endocr Rev* 1999;**20**:279–307.

147 Schumacher M. Rapid membrane effects of steroid hormones: an emerging concept in neuroendocrinology. *Trends Neurosci* 1990;**13**:359–362.

148 Sherwin BB. Estrogen and cognitive functioning in women. *Endocr Rev* 2003;**24**:133–151.

149 Shumaker SA, Legault C, Rapp SR, *et al.* Estrogen plus progestin and the incidence of dementia and mild cognitive impairment in postmenopausal women: the Women's Health Initiative Memory Study: a randomized controlled trial. *JAMA* 2003;**289**:2651–2662.

150 Nilsen J, Brinton RD. Impact of progestins on estrogen-induced neuroprotection: synergy by progesterone and 19-norprogesterone and antagonism by medroxyprogesterone acetate. *Endocrinology* 2002;**143**:205–212.

151 Gouras GK, Xu H, Gross RS, *et al.* Testosterone reduces neuronal secretion of alzheimer's beta-amyloid peptides. *Proc Natl Acad Sci USA* 2000;**97**:1202–1205.

152 Wolf OT, Kirschbaum C. Endogenous estradiol and testosterone levels are associated with cognitive performance in older women and men. *Horm Behav* 2002;**41**:259–266.

153 Yaffe K, Lui LY, Zmuda J, *et al.* Sex hormones and cognitive function in older men. *J Am Geriatr Soc* 2002;**50**:707–712.

154 Lathe R. Hormones and the hippocampus. *J Endocrinol* 2001;**169**:205–231.

155 Carlson LE, Sherwin BB. Higher levels of plasma estradiol and testosterone in healthy elderly men compared with age-matched women may protect aspects of explicit memory. *Menopause* 2000;**7**:168–177.

156 Traish AM, Guay AT. Are androgens critical for penile erections in humans? Examining the clinical and preclinical evidence. *J Sex Med* 2006;**3**:382–407.

157 Morales A, Buvat J, Gooren LJ, Guay AT, Kaufman JM, Kim YC, Tan HM, Torres LO. Endocrine aspects of men sexual dysfunctions. In: Lue TF, Basson R, Rosen R, Giuliano F, Khoury S, Montorsi F, eds. *Sexual Medicine, sexual dysfunctions in men and women.* Paris, France: Health Publications; 2004: pp. 345–382.

158 Zlotta AR, Teillac P, Raynaud JP, Schulman CC. Evaluation of male sexual function in patients with lower urinary tract symptoms (LUTS) associated with benign prostatic hyperplasia treated with a phytotherapeutic agent (Permixon), Tamsulosin or Finasteride. *Eur Urol* 2005;**48**:269–276.

159 Lunenfeld B, Saad F, Hoesl CE. ISA, ISSAM and EAU recommendations for the investigation, treatment and monitoring of late-onset hypogonadism in males: scientific background and rationale. *Aging Male* 2005; **8**(2):59–74.

160 Pitteloud N, Hardin M, Dwyer AA, Valassi E, Yialamas M, Elahi D, Hayes F. Increasing insulin resistance is associated with a decrease in Leydig cell testosterone secretion in men. *J Clin Endocrinol Metab* 2005;**90**: 2636–2641.

161 Handelsman DJ, Zajac JD. Androgen deficiency and replacement therapy in men. *Med JAust* 2004;**180**: 529–535.

162 Morley JE. Clinical diagnosis of age-related testosterone deficiency. *Aging Male* 2000;**3**(suppl 1):195.

163 Heinemann LA, Saad F, Thiele K *et al.* The aging male's symptom rating scale: cultural and linguistic validation into English. *Aging Male* 2001;**4**:14.

164 Beutel ME, Schneider H, Weidner W. Symptoms or complaints in the aging male: which questionnaires are available? *Urologe A* 2004;**43**:1069–1075.

165 Vermeulen A, Verdonck L, Kaufman JM. A critical evaluation of simple methods for the estimation of free testosterone in serum. *J Clin Endocrinol Metab* 1999;**84**: 3666–3672.

166 Vermeulen A, Verdonck G. Representativeness of a single point plasma testosterone level for the long term hormonal milieu in men. *J Clin Endocrinol Metab* 1992;**74**:939–942.

167 Tancredi A, Reginster JY, Luyckx F, Legros JJ. No major month to month variation in free testosterone

levels in aging males. Minor impact on the biological diagnosis of "andropause." *Psychoneuroendocrinology* 2005;**30**:638–646.

168 Wang C, Catlin DH, Demers LM, Starcevic B, Swerdloff RS. Measurement of total serum testosterone in adult men: comparison of current laboratory methods versus liquid chromatography-tandem mass spectrometry. *J Clin Endocrinol Metab* 2004;**89**: 534–543.

169 Matsumoto AM, Bremner WJ. Serum testosterone assays: accuracy matters. *J Clin Endocrinol Metab* 2004; **89**:520–524.

170 Shabsigh R. Hypogonadism and erectile dysfunction: the role for testosterone therapy. *Int J Impot Res* 2003;**15**(suppl 4):S9–S13.

171 Liverman CT, Blazer DG, eds. *Testosterone and Aging: Clinical Research Directions*. Committee on Assessing the Need for Clinical Trials of Testosterone Replacement Therapy. Washington, DC: The National Academies Press, 2004, pp. 1–9. Available at: http://www.nap.edu. Accessed January 12, 2005.

172 Yassin AA, Saad F, Diede HE. Combination therapy with testosterone and tadalafil in hypogonadal patients with erectile dysfunction who do not respond to tadalafil as monotherapy [in German]. *Blickpunkt der Mann* 2003;**2**:37–39.

173 Chatterjee R, Wood S, McGarrigle HH, Lees WR, Ralph DJ, Neild GH. A novel therapy with testosterone and sildenafil for erectile dysfunction in patients on renal dialysis or after renal transplantation. *J Fam Plann Reprod Health Care* 2004;**30**:88–90.

174 Rossouw JE, Anderson GL, Prentice RL, *et al*. Risks and benefits of estrogen plus progestin in healthy postmenopausal women: principal results from the Women's Health Initiative randomized controlled trial. *JAMA* 2002;**288**:321–333.

175 Manson JE, Hsia J, Johnson KC, *et al*. Estrogen plus progestin and the rise of coronary heart disease. *N Engl J Med* 2003;**349**:523–534.

176 Kenny AM, Prestwood KM, Gruman CA, Marcello KM, Raisz LG. Effects of transdermal testosterone on bone and muscle in older men with low bioavailable testosterone levels. *J Gerontol A Biol Sci Med Sci* 2001;**56**:M266–M272.

177 Pechersky AV, Mazurov VI, Semiglazov VF, Karpischenko AI, Mikhailichenko VV, Udintsev AV. Androgen administration in middle-aged and ageing men: effects of oral testosterone undecanoate on dihydrotestosterone, oestradiol and prostate volume. *Int J Androl* 2002;**25**:119–125.

178 Gaylis FD, Lin DW, Ignatoff JM, Amling CL, Tutrone RF, Cosgrove DJ. Prostate cancer in men using testosterone supplementation. *J Urol* 2005;**174**:534–538.

179 Morgentaler A, Bruning CO III, DeWolf WC. Occult prostate cancer in men with low serum testosterone levels. *JAMA* 1996;**276**:1904–1906.

180 Hoffman MA, DeWolf WC, Morgentaler A. Is low serum free testosterone a marker for high grade prostate cancer? *J Urol* 2000;**163**:824–827.

181 Isom-Batz G, Bianco FJ, Kattan MW, Mulhall JP, Lilja H, Eastham JA. Testosterone as a predictor of pathological stage in clinically localized prostate cancer. *J Urol* 2005;**173**:1935–1937.

182 Massengill JC, Sun L, Moul JW, Wu H, Mc Leod DG, Amling C, Lance R, Foley J, Sexton W, Kusuda L, Chung A, Soderdahl D, Donahue T. Pretreatment total testosterone level predicts pathological stage in patients with localized prostate cancer treated with radical prostatectomy. *J Urol* 2003;**169**: 1670–1675.

183 Miller LR, Partin AW, Chan DW, *et al*. Influence of radical prostatectomy on serum hormone levels. *J Urol* 1998;**160**:449–453.

184 Madersbacher S, Schatzl G, Bieglmayer C, *et al*. Impact of radical prostatectomy and TURP on the hypothalamic-pituitary-gonadal hormone axis. *Urology* 2002; **60**:869–874.

185 Krieg M, Nass R, Tunn S. Effect of aging on endogenous level of 5 alpha-dihydrotestosterone, testosterone, estradiol, and estrone in epithelium and stroma of normal and hyperplastic human prostate. *J Clin Endocrinol Metab* 1993;**77**:375–381.

186 Slater S, Oliver RTD. Testosterone: its role in development of prostate cancer and potential risk from use as hormone replacement therapy. *Drugs Aging* 2000;**17**: 431–439.

187 Carter HB, Pearson JD, Metter EJ, *et al*. Longitudinal evaluation of serum androgen levels in men with and without prostate cancer. *Prostate* 1995;**27**:25–31.

188 Heikkila R, Aho K, Heliovaara M, *et al*. Serum testosterone and sex hormone-binding globulin concentrations and the risk of prostate carcinoma: a longitudinal study. *Cancer* 1999;**86**:312–315.

189 Hsing AW. Hormones and prostate cancer: what's next? *Epidemiol Rev* 2001;**23**:42–58.

190 Gann PH, Hennekens CH, Ma J, Longcope C, Stampfer MJ. Prospective study of sex hormone levels and risk of prostate cancer. *J Natl Cancer Inst* 1996;**88**:1118–1126.

191 Gustafsson O, Norming U, Gustafsson S, Eneroth P, Astrom G, Nyman CR. Dihydrotestosterone and testosterone levels in men screened for prostate

cancer: a study of a randomized population. *Br J Urol* 1996;**77**:433–440.

192 Thompson IM, Pauler DK, Goodman PJ, Tangen CM, Lucia MS, Parnes HL, Minasian LM, Ford LG, Lippman SM, Crawford ED, Crowley JJ, Coltman CA Jr. Prevalence of prostate cancer among men with a prostate-specific antigen level ≤4.0 ng per milliliter. *N Engl J Med* 2004;**350**:2239–2246.

193 Kundu SB, Grubb RL, Roehl KA, Antenor JA, Han M, Catalona WJ. Delays in cancer detection using 2 and 4-year screening intervals for prostate cancer screening with initial prostate specific antigen less than 2 ng/ml. *J Urol* 2005;**173**:1116–1120.

194 Catalona WJ, Loeb S. The PSA era is not over for prostate cancer. *Eur Urol* 2005;**48**:541–545.

195 Singh AB, Hsia S, Alaupovic P, *et al.* The effects of varying doses of T on insulin sensitivity, plasma lipids, apolipoproteins, and C-reactive protein in healthy young men. *J Clin Endocrinol Metab* 2002;**87**:136–143.

196 Whitsel EA, Boyko EJ, Matsumoto AM, Anawalt BD, Siscovick DS. Intramuscular testosterone esters and plasma lipids in hypogonadal men: a meta-analysis. *Am J Med* 2001;**111**:261–269.

197 Snyder PJ, Peachey H, Berlin JA, *et al.* Effects of transdermal testosterone treatment on serum lipid and apolipoprotein levels in men more than 65 years of age. *Am J Med* 2001;**111**:255–260.

198 Dobs AS, Meikle AW, Arver S, Sanders SW, Caramelli KE, Mazer NA. Pharmacokinetics, efficacy, and safety of a permeation-enhanced testosterone transdermal system in comparison with bi-weekly injections of testosterone enanthate for the treatment of hypogonadal men. *J Clin Endocrinol Metab* 1999;**84**:3469–3478.

199 Zmuda JM, Cauley JÁ, Kriska A, Glynn NW, Guptai JP, Kuller LH. Longitudinal relation between endogenous testosterone and cardiovascular disease risk factors in middle-aged men: a 13-year follow-up of former Multiple Factor Intervention Trial participants. *Am J Epidemiol* 1997;**146**:609–617.

200 Kabakci G, Yildirir A, Can I, Unsal I, Erbas B. Relationship between endogenous sex hormone levels, lipoproteins and coronary atherosclerosis in men undergoing coronary angiography. *Cardiology* 1999;**92**:221–225.

201 Gooren LI. The age-related decline of androgen levels in men: clinically significant? *Br J Urol* 1996;**78**:763–768.

202 Gyllenborg J, Rasmussen SL, Borch-Johnsen K, Heitmann BL, Skakkebaek NE, Juul A. Cardiovascular risk factors in men: the role of gonadal steroids and sex hormone-binding globulin. *Metabolism* 2001;**50**:882–888.

203 English KM, Mandour O, Steeds RP, Diver MJ, Jones TH, Channer KS. Men with coronary artery disease have lower levels of androgens than men with normal coronary angiograms. *Eur Heart J* 2000;**21**:890–894.

204 Hak AE, Witteman JCM, de Jong FH, Geerlings MI, Hofman A, Pols HAP. Low levels of endogenous androgens increase the risk of atherosclerosis in elderly men: the Rotterdam Study. *J Clin Endocrinol Metab* 2002;**87**:3632–3639.

205 English KM, Steeds RP, Jones TH, Diver MJ, Channer KS. Low-dose transdermal testosterone therapy improves angina threshold in men with chronic stable angina: a randomized, double-blind, placebo-controlled study. *Circulation* 2000;**102**:1906–1911.

206 Anderson RA, Ludlam CA, Wu FC. Haemostatic effects of supraphysiological levels of testosterone in normal men. *Thromb Haemost* 1995;**74**:693–697.

207 Hajjar RR, Kaiser FE, Morley JE. Outcomes of long-term testosterone replacement in older hypogonadal males: a retrospective analysis. *J Clin Endocrinol Metab* 1997;**82**:3793–3796.

208 Basaria S, Dobs AS. Risks versus benefits of testosterone therapy in elderly men. *Drugs Aging* 1999;**15**:131–142.

209 The Endocrine Society. Clinical bulletins in andropause: benefits and risks of treating hypogonadism in the aging male. *Endocr Rep* 2002;**2**:1–6.

210 Morales A, Heaton JP, Carson CC 3rd. Andropause: a misnomer for a true clinical entity. *J Urol* 2000;**163**:705–712.

211 Shabsigh A, Kang Y, Shabsigh R, *et al.* Clomiphene citrate effects on testosterone/estrogen ratio in male hypogonadism. *J Sex Med* 2005;**2**:716–721.

212 Morales A. Androgen replacement therapy and prostate safety. *Eur Urol* 2002;**41**:113–120.

213 Jockenhoevel F. Testosterone therapy, what, when and to whom? *Aging Male* 2004;**7**:319–324.

214 Bhasin S, Bremner WJ. Emerging issues in androgen replacement therapy. *J Clin Endocrinol Metab* 1997;**82**:3–8.

215 Stas SN, Anastasiadis AG, Fisch H, Benson MC, Shabsigh R. Urologic aspects of andropause. *Urol* 2003;**61**:261–266.

216 Schubert M, Minnemann T, *et al.* Intramuscular testosterone undecanoate: pharmacokinetic aspects of a novel testosterone formulation during long-term treatment of men with hypogonadism. *J Clin Endocrinol Metab* 2004;**89**:5429–5434.

217 Harle L, Basaria S, *et al.* Nebido: a long-acting injectable testosterone for the treatment of male hypogonadism. *Expert Opin Pharmacother* 2005;**6**: 1751–1759.

218 Nieschlag E. If testosterone, which testosterone? Which androgen regimen should be used for supplementation in older men? Formulation, dosing, and monitoring issues. *J Clin Endocrinol Metab* 1998;**83**: 3443–3445.

219 Comhaire FH. Andropause: hormone replacement therapy in the aging male. *Eur Urol* 2000;**38**:655–662.

220 McNicholas TA, Dean JD, Mulder H, Carnegie C, Jones NA. A novel testosterone gel formulation normalizes androgen levels in hypogonadal men, with improvements in body composition and sexual function. *BJU Int* 2003;**91**:69–74.

221 Guay AT, Jacobson J, Perez JB, Hodge MB, Velasquez E. Clomiphene increases free testosterone levels in men with both secondary hypogonadism and erectile dysfunction: who does and does not benefit? *Int J Impot Res* 2003;**15**:156–165.

222 AACE Male Sexual Dysfunction Task Force. American Association of Clinical Endocrinologists medical guidelines for clinical practice for the evaluation and treatment of male sexual dysfunction: a couple's problem—2003 update. *Endocr Pract* 2003;**9**: 77–94.

223 Morales A, Buvat J, Gooren LJ, *et al.* Endocrine aspects of sexual dysfunction in men. *J Sex Med* 2004;**1**:69–81.

224 Negro-Villar A. Selective androgen receptor modulators: a novel approach to androgen therapy in the new millennium. *J Clin Endocrin Metab* 1999;**84**:3459–3462.

225 Kumar N, Didolkar AK, Monder C *et al.* The biological activity of 7 alpha-methyl-19-nortestosterone is not amplified in male reproductive tract as is that of testosterone. *Endocrinology* 1992;**130**:3677–3683.

226 Cummings DE, Kumar N, Bardin CW, *et al.* Prostate-sparing effects in primates of the potent androgen 7alpha-methyl-19-nortestosterone: a potential alternative to testosterone for androgen replacement and male contraception. *J Clin Endocrinol Metab* 1998;**83**: 4212–4219.

227 Anderson RA, Martin CW, Kung AW, *et al.* 7Alpha-methyl-19-nortestosterone maintains sexual behavior and mood in hypogonadal men. *J Clin Endocrinol Metab* 1999;**84**:3556–3562.

228 Suvvisaari J, Moo-Young AJ, Juhakoski A, *et al.* Pharmacokinetics of 7 alpha-methyl-19-nortestosterone (MENT) delivery using subdermal implants in healthy men. *Contraception* 1999;**60**:299–303.

229 Haake P, Exton MS, Haverkamp J, *et al.* Absence of orgasm-induced prolactin secretion in a healthy multi-orgasmic male subject. *Int J Impot Res* 2002;**14**: 133–135.

230 Buvat J, Lemaire A, Buvat Herbaut M, Fourlinnie JC, Racadot A, Fossati P. Hyperprolactinemia and sexual function in men. *Hormone Res* 1985;**22**:196–203.

231 Ishikawa H, Kaneko S, Ohashi M, Nakagawa K, Hata M. Retrograde ejaculation accompanying hyperprolactinemia. *Arch Andrology* 1993;**30**:153–155.

232 De Rosa M, Zarrilli S, Vitale G, *et al.* Six months of treatment with Cabergoline restores sexual potency in hyperprolactinemic males: an open longitudinal study monitoring nocturnal penile tumescence. *J Clin Endocrin Metab* 2004;**89**:621–625.

233 Carani C, Zini D, Baldini A, Della Casa L, Ghizzani A, Marrama P. Testosterone and prolactin: behavioral and psychophysiological approaches in men. In: Bancroft, ed. *The Pharmacology of Sexual Function and Dysfunction.* Esteve Foundation Symposia, Vol. 6. Excerpta Medica; Elsevier Science: Amsterdam, 1995, pp. 145–150.

234 Buvat J. Hyperprolactinemia and sexual function in men: a short review. *Int J Impot Res* 2003;**15**: 373–377.

235 Rehman J, Christ G, Alyskewycz M, Kerr E, Melman A. Experimental hyperprolactinemia in a rat model: alteration in centrally mediated neuroerectile mechanism. *Int J Impot Res* 2000;**12**:23–32.

236 Aoki H, Fujioka T, Matsuzaka J, *et al.* Suppression by prolactin of the electrically induced erectile response through its direct effect on the corpus cavernosum penis in the dog. *J Urol* 1995;**154**:595–600.

237 Ra S, Aoki H, Fujioka T, *et al.* In vitro contraction of the canine corpus cavernosum penis by direct perfusion with prolactin or growth hormone. *J Urol* 1996; **156**:522–525.

238 Buvat J, Bou Jaoudé G. Hyperprolactinemie et fonction sexuelle chez l'homme. *Andrologie* 2005;**15**: 366–373.

239 Miyai K, Ichihara K, Kondo K, Mori S. Asymptomatic hyperprolactinemia and prolactinoma in the general population: mass screening by paired assays of serum prolactin. *Clin Endocrinol* 1986;**25**:549–554.

240 Miyake A, Ikegami M, Chen CF, Arita N, Aono T, Tanizawa O, Yowhikawa T. Mass screening for hyperprolatinemia and hyperprolactinemia and hyperprolactinemia in men. *J Endocrinol Invest* 1988;**11**: 373–384.

241 Johri AM, Heaton JPW, Morales A. Severe erectile dysfunction is a marker for hyperprolactinemia. *Int J Impot Res* 2001;**13**:176–182.

242 Ambrosi B, Bara R, Travaglini P, *et al.* Studies of the effects of bromocriptine on sexual impotence. *Clin Endocrinol (Oxf)* 1987;**7**:417–420.

243 Sinha YN. Structural variants of prolactin: occurrence and physiological significance. *Endocr Rev* 1995;**16**: 354–369.

244 Vallette-Kasic S, Morange-Ramos I, Selim A, *et al.* Macroprolactinemia revisited: a study on 106 patients. *J Clin Endocrinol Metab* 2002;**87**:581–588.

245 Gibney J, Smith TP, McKenna TJ. The impact on clinical practice of routine screening for macroprolactin. *J Clin Endocrinol Metab* 2005;**90**:3927–3932.

246 Lemaire C, Lemaire A, Dewailly D, Fossati P. Hyperprolactinemia with an excess of high molecular weight prolactin in men. *Int J Impot Res* 1994;**6**(suppl 1):P79.

247 Guay AT, Sabharwal P, Varma S, Malarkey WB. Delayed diagnosis of psychological erectile dysfunction because of the presence of macroprolactinemia. *J Clin Endocr Metab* 1996;**81**:2515–2514.

248 Tritos NA, Guay AT, Malarkey WB. Asymptomatic "big" hyperprolactinemia in two men with pituitary adenomas. *Eur J Endocrinol* 1998;**138**:82–85.

249 Buvat J, Lemaire A, Buvat-Herbaut M, Marcolin G. Dosage de la prolactine chez les impuissants. *Presse Med* 1989;**18**:1167.

250 Schwartz MF, Bauman JE, Masters WH. Hyperprolactinemia and sexual disorders in men. *Biol Psychiat* 1982;**17**:861–876.

251 Molitch ME. Medication-induced hyperprolactinemia. *Mayo Clin Proc* 2005;**82**:1050–1057.

252 Porst H, Broemel T. Hyperprolactinemia in men with sexual dysfunctions. Still a diagnostic challenge. *J Sex Med* 2006;**3**(suppl 1):53.

253 Garg RK, Khaishgi A, Dandona P. Is management with Sildenafil changing clinical practice? *Lancet* 1999;**353**: 375–376.

254 De Rosa M, Zarrilli S, Di Sarno A, *et al.* Hyperprolactinemia in men. *Endocrine* 2003;**20**:75–82.

255 Passos VQ, Souza JJS, Musolino NRC, Bronstein MD. Long-term follow-up of prolactinomas: normoprolactinemia after bromocriptine withdrawal. *J Clin Endocrinol Metab* 2002;**87**:3578–3582.

256 Wolfsberger S, Czech T, Vierhapper H, Benavente R, Knosp E. Microprolactinomas in males treated by transsphenoidal surgery. *Acta Neurochir* 2003;**145**: 935–941.

257 Oettel M. Is there a role for estrogens in the maintenance of men's health? *Aging Male* 2002;**5**:248–257.

258 Smith EP, Boyd J, Frank RG, Takahashi H, Cohen RM, Specker B *et al.* Estrogen resistance caused by a mutation in the estrogen-receptor gene in a man. *N Eng J Med* 1994;**16**:1056–1061.

259 Morishima A, Grumbach MM, Simpson ER, Fisher C, Qin K. Aromatase deficiency in male and female siblings caused by a novel mutation and the physiological role of estrogens. *J Clin Endocrinol Metab* 1995;**80**: 3689–3699.

260 Carani C, Rochira V, Faustini-Fustini M, Balastrieri A, Granata ARM. Role of estrogen in male sexual behavior: insights from the natural model of aromatase deficiency. *Clin Endocrinol* 1999;**51**:517–525.

261 Carani C, Granata ARM, Rochira V, Caffagni G, Aranda C, Antunez P, Maffei LE. Sex steroids and sexual desire in a man with a novel mutation of aromatase gene and hypogonadism. *Psychoneuroendocrinology* 2005;**30**:413–417.

262 Adaikan PG, Srilatha B. Oestrogen-mediated hormonal imbalance precipitates erectile dysfunction. *Int J Impot Res* 2003;**15**:38–43.

263 Srilatha B, Adaikan PG. Estrogen and phytoestrogen predispose to erectile dysfunction: do ER-α and ER-β in the cavernosum play a role? *Urology* 2004;**63**: 382–386.

264 Oliva A, Giami A, Multigner L. Environmental agents and erectile dysfunction: a study in a consulting population. *J Androl* 2002;**23**:546–550.

265 Mancini A, Milardi D, Bianchi A, Summaria V, De Marinis L. Increased estradiol levels in venous occlusive disorder: a possible functional mechanism of venous leakage. *Int J Impot Res* 2005;**17**:329–342.

266 Hammer F, Subtil S, Lux P, Maser-Gluth C, Stewart P, Allolio B, Arlt W. No evidence for hepatic conversion of dehydroepiandrosterone (DHEA) sulfate to DHEA: in vivo and in vitro studies. *J Clin Endocrinol Metab* 2005;**90**:3600–3605.

267 Siiteri P. Editorial: The continuing saga of dehydroepiandrosterone (DHEA). *J Clin Endocrinol Metab* 2005;**90**:3795–3796.

268 Orentreich N, Brind J, Rizer R, Vogelman J. Age changes and sex differences in serum dehydroepiandrosterone sulfate concentrations throughout adulthood. *J Clin Endocrinol Metab* 1984;**59**:551–555.

269 Sulcova J, Hill M, Hampl R, Starka L. Age and sex related differences in serum levels of unconjugated dehydroepiandrosterone and its sulfate in normal subjects. *J Endocrinol* 1997;**154**:57–62.

270 Arlt W. Dehydroepiandrosterone and ageing. *Best Prac Res Clin Endocrinol Metab* 2004;**18**:363–380.

271 Hornsby P. Biosynthesis of DHEAS by the human adrenal cortex and its age-related decline. *Ann NY Acad Sci* 1995;**774**:29–46.

272 Legrain S, Massien C, Lahlou N, Roger M, Debuire B, Diquet B, Chatellier G, Azizi M, Faucounau V, Porchet H, Forette F, Baulieu E. Dehydroepiandrosterone replacement administration: pharmacokinetic and pharmacodynamic studies in healthy elderly subjects. *J Clin Endocrinol Metab* 2000;**85**:3208–3217.

273 Hayashi T, Esaki T, Muto E, Kano H, Asai Y, Thakur N, *et al*. Dehydroepiandrosterone retards atherosclerosis formation through its conversion to estrogen: the possible role of nitric oxide. *Arterioscler Thromb Vasc Biol* 2000;**20**:782–792.

274 Nawata H, Yanase T, Goto K, Okabe T, Ashida K. Mechanism of action of anti-aging DHEA-S and the replacement of DHEA-S. *Mech Ageing Dev* 2002;**123**:1101–1106.

275 Labrie F. Intracrinology. *Mol Cell Endocrinol* 1991;**78**:C113–118.

276 Labrie F, Belanger A, Van LT, Labrie C, Simard J, Cusan L. DHEA and the intracrine function of androgens and estrogens in peripheral target tissue: its role during aging. *Steroids* 1998;**63**:322–328.

277 Labrie F, Luu-The V, Lin SX, Simard J, Labrie C, El-Alfy M, Pelletier G, Belanger A. Intracrinology: role of the family of 17β-hydroxysteroid dehydrogenases in human physiology and disease. *J Mol Endocrin* 2000;**25**:1–16.

278 Liu D, Dillon J. Dehydroepiandrosterone activates endothelial cell nitric-oxide synthase by a specific plasma membrane receptor coupled to $G\alpha_{i2,3}$. *J Biol Chem* 2002;**277**:21379–21388.

279 Liu D, Dillon J. Dehydroepiandrosterone stimulates nitric oxide release in vascular endothelial cells: evidence for a cell surface receptor. *Steroids* 2004;**69**:279–289.

280 Simoncini T, Mannella P, Fornari L, Varone G, Caruso A, Genazzani A. Dehydroepiandrosterone modulates endothelial nitric oxide synthesis via direct genomic and nongenomic mechanisms. *Endocrinology* 2003;**144**:3449–3455.

281 Williams M, Ling S, Dawood T, Hashimura K, Dai A, Li H, Liu J, Funder J, Sudhir K, Komesaroff P. Dehydroepiandrosterone inhibits human vascular smooth muscle cell proliferation independent of androgen and estrogen receptors. *J Clin Endocrinol Metab* 2002;**87**:176–181.

282 Iwasaki Y, Asai M, Yoshida M, Nigawara T, Kambayashi M, Nakashima N. Dehydroepiandrosterone-sulfate inhibits nuclear factor-kB-dependent transcription in hepatocytes, possibly though antioxidant effect. *J Clin Endocrinol Metab* 2004;**89**:3449–3454.

283 Ten S, New M, Maclaren N. Clinical Review 130: Addison's Disease 2001. *J Clin Endocrinol Metab* 2001;**86**:2909–2922.

284 Arlt W. Quality of life in Addison's disease: the case for DHEA replacement. *Clin Endocrinol* 2002;**56**:573–574.

285 Miller K, Sesmilo G, Schiller A, Schoenfeld D, Burton S, Klibanski A. Androgen deficiency in women with hypopituitarism. *J Clin Endocrinol Metab* 2001;**86**:561–567.

286 Johannsson G, Burman P, Wiren L, Engstrom B, Nilsson A, Ottosson M, Jonsson B, Bengtsson B, Karlsson F. Low dose dehydroepiandrosterone affects behavior in hypopituitary androgen-deficient women: a placebo-controlled trial. *J Clin Endocrinol Metab* 2002;**87**(5):2046–2052.

287 Herrington D. DHEA: a biologic conundrum. *J Lab Clin Med* 1998;**131**:292–294.

288 Buvat J. Androgen therapy with dehydroepiandrosterone. *World J Urol* 2003;**21**:346–355.

289 Shealy C. *DHEA the Youth and Health Hormone.* New Canaan, CT: Keats Publishing, Inc.; 1996.

290 Wolkowitz O, Kramer J, Resus V, Costa M, Yaffe K, Walton P, Raskind M, Peskind E, Newhouse P, Sack D, De Souza E, Sadowsky C, Roberts E; DHEA-Alzheimer's Disease Collaborative Research. DHEA treatment of Alzheimer's disease: a randomized, double-blind, placebo-controlled study. *Neurology* 2003;**60**:1071–1076.

291 Szathmári M, Treszi A, Vásárhelyi B. Left ventricular mass index and ventricular septum thickness are associated with serum dehydroepiandrosterone-sulfate levels in hypertensive women. *Clin Endocrinol* 2003;**59**:110–114.

292 Bloch M, Schmidt P, Danaceau M, Adams L, Rubinow D. Dehydroepiandrosterone treatment of midlife dysthymia. *Biol Psychiatry* 1999;**45**:1533–1541.

293 Gordon C, Grace E, Emans S, Feldman H, Goodman E, Becker K, Rosen C, Gundberg C, LeBoff M. Effects of oral dehydroepiandrosterone on bone density in young women with anorexia nervosa: a randomized trial. *J Clin Endocrinol Metab* 2002;**87**:4935–4941.

294 Feldman HA, Goldstein I, Hatzichristou DG, *et al*. Impotence and its medical and psychosocial correlates: results of the Massachussets Male Aging Study. *J Urol* 1994;**151**:54–61.

295 Seki M, Nomura K, Kanazawa M, Sawada T, Takaski K, Demura H. Changes in neoplastic cell features and sensitivity to mitotane during mitotane-induced remission in a patient with recurrent, metastatic adrenocortical carcinoma. *Endocr Relat Cancer* 1999;**6**:529–533.

296 Deuschle M, Lecei O, Stalla G, Landgraf R, Hamann B, Lederbogen F, Uhr M, Luppa P, Maras A, Colla M, Heuser I. Steroid synthesis inhibition with ketoconazole and its effect upon the regulation of the hypothalamus-pituitary-adrenal system in healthy humans. *Neurospsychopharmacology* 2003;**28**:379–383.

297 Guay A. Decreased testosterone in regularly menstruating women with decreased libido: a clinical observation. *J Sex Marital Therap* 2001;**27**:513–519.

298 Gebre-Medhin G, Husebye E, Mallmin H, Helström L, Berne C, Karlsson F, Kämpe O. Oral dehydroepiandrosterone (DHEA) replacement therapy in women with Addison's disease. *Clin Endocrinol* 2000; **52**:775–780.

299 Lovås K, Loge J, Husebye E. Subjective health status in Norwegian patients with Addison's disease. *Clin Endocrinol* 2002;**56**:581–588.

300 Miller K, Sesmilo G, Schiller A, Schoenfeld D, Burton S, Klibanski A. Androgen deficiency in women with hypopituitarism. *J Clin Endocrinol Metab* 2001; **86**:561–567.

301 Achermann J, Silverman B. Dehydroepiandrosterone replacement for patients with adrenal insufficiency. Commentary. *Lancet* 2001;**357**:1381–1382.

302 Dhatariya K, Bigelow M, Nair K. Effect of dehydroepiandrosterone replacement on insulin sensitivity and lipids in hypoadrenal women. *Diabetes* 2005;**54**:765–769.

303 Callies F, Fassnacht M, Van Vlijmen J, Koehler I, Huebler D, Seibel M, Arlt W, Allolio B. Dehydroepiandrosterone replacement in women with adrenal insufficiency: effects on body composition, serum leptin, bone turnover, and exercise capacity. *J Clin Endocrinol Metab* 2001;**86**:1968–1972.

304 Morales A, Nolan J, Nelson C, Yen S. Effects of replacement doses of dehydroepiandrosterone in men and women of advancing age. *J Clin Endocrinol Metab* 1994;**78**:1360–1367.

305 Wolf O, Neumann O, Hellhammer D, *et al.* Effects of a two-week physiological dehydroepiandrosterone substitution on cognitive performance and well-being in healthy elderly men and women. *J Clin Endocrinol Metab* 1997;**82**:2363–2367.

306 Arlt W, Callies F, Koehler I, *et al.* Dehydroepiandrosterone supplementation in healthy men with an age-related decline of dehydroepiandrosterone secretion. *J Clin Endocrinol Metab* 2001;**86**:4686–4692.

307 Van Niekerk J, Huppert F, Herbert J. Salivary cortisol and DHEA: association with measures of cognition and well-being in normal older men, and effects of three months of DHEA supplementation. *Psychoneuroendocrinology* 2001;**26**:591–612.

308 Baulieu E, Thomas G, Legrain S, Lahou N, Roger M, Debuire B, Faucounau V, Girard L, Hervy M, Latour F, Leaud M, Mokrane A, Pitti-Ferrandi H, Trivalle C, deLacharriere O, Nouveau S, Rakoto-Arison B, Souberbielle J, Raison J, LeBouc Y, Raynaud A, Girerd X, Forette F. Dehydroepiandrosterone (DHEA), DHEA sulfate, and aging: contribution of the DHEAge study to a sociobiomedical issue. *Proc Natl Acad Sci USA* 2000;**97**:4279–4284.

309 Percheron G, Hogrel J, Denot-Ledunois S, Fayet G, Forette F, Baulieu E, Fardeau M, Marini J. Effect of 1-year oral administration of dehydroepiandrosterone to 60 to 80 year-old individuals on muscle function and cross-sectional area: a double-blind placebo-controlled trial. *Arch Int Med* 2003;**163**:720–727.

310 Barnhart K, Freeman E, Grisso J, Rader D, Sammel M, Kapoor S, Nestler J. The effect of dehydroepiandrosterone supplementation to symptomatic perimenopausal women on serum endocrine profiles, lipid perameters, and health-related quality of life. *J Clin Endocrinol Metab* 1999;**84**:3896–3902.

311 Lasco A, Frisina N, Morabito N, Gaudio A, Morini E, Trifiletti A, Basile G, Nicita-Mauro V, Cucinotta D. Metabolic effects of dehydroepiandrosterone replacement therapy in postmenopausal women. *Eur J Endocrinol* 2001;**145**:457–461.

312 Reiter WJ, Pycha A, Schatzl G, *et al.* Dehydroepiandrosterone in the treatment of erectile dysfunction: a prospective, double-blind, randomized, placebo-controlled study. *Urology* 1999;**53**:590–594.

313 Tchernof A, Labrie F. Dehydroepiandrosterone, obesity, and cardiovascular disease risk: a review of human studies. *Eur J Endocrinol* 2004;**151**:1–14.

314 Schmidt P, Daly R, Bloch M, Smith M, Danaceau M, St. Clair L, Murphy J, Haq N, Rubinow D. Dehydroepiandrosterone monotherapy in midlife-onset of major and minor depression. *Arch Gen Psychiatr* 2005;**62**(2):154–162.

315 Block M, Schmidt P, Danaceau M, Adams L, Rubinow D. Dehydroepiandrosterone treatment of midlife dysthymia. *Biol Psychiatry* 1999;**45**:1533–1541.

316 Chang D, Lan J, Lin H, Luo S. Dehydroepiandrosterone treatment of women with mild-to-moderate systemic lupus erythematosus: a multicenter randomized, double-blind, placebo-controlled trial. *Arthr Rheumatol* 2002;**46**:2924–2927.

317 Aoki K, Nakajima A, Mukasa K, Osawa E, Mori Y, Sekihara H. Prevention of diabetes, hepatic injury, and

colon cancer with dehydroepiandrosterone. *J Ster Biochem Mol Biol* 2003;**85**:469–472.

318 Meikle A, Dorchuk R, Araneo B, Stringham J, Evans T, Spruance S, Daynes R. The presence of a dehydroepiandrosterone-specific receptor binding complex in murine T cells. *J Ster Biochem Mol Biol* 1992; **42**:293–304.

319 Tsuji K, Furutama D, Tagami M, Oshawa N. Specific binding and effects of dehydroepiandrosterone sulfate (DHEA-S) on skeletal muscle cells: possible implication for DHEA-S replacement therapy in patients with myotonic dystrophy. *Life Sci* 1999;**65**:17–26.

320 Claustrat B, Brun J, Chazot G. The basic and pathophysiogy of melatonin. *Sleep Med Rev* 2005;**9**:11–24.

321 Arendt J, Skene DJ. Melatonin as a chronobiotic. *Sleep Med Rev* 2005;**9**:25–39.

322 Zhdanova IV. Melatonin as a hypnotic: pro. *Sleep Med Rev* 2005;**9**:51–65.

323 Arlt W, Hewison M. Hormones and immune function: implications of aging. *Aging Cell* 2004;**3**:209–216.

324 Macchi MM, Bruce JN. Human pineal physiology and functional significance of melatonin. *Front Neuroendocrinol* 2004;**25**:177–195.

325 Karazek M. Melatonin, human aging, and age related diseases. *Exp Gerontol* 2004;**39**:1723–1729.

326 Brzezinski A, Vangel MG, Wurtman RJ, Norrie G, Zdhanova I, Ben-Shushan A, Ford I. Effects of exogenous melatonin on sleep: a meta-analysis. *Sleep Med* 2005;**9**:41–50.

327 Singer C, Tractenbergh RE, Kaye J, Schafer K, Garmst A, Grundman M, Thomas R, Thal LJ. A multicenter, placebo-controlled trial of melatonin for sleep disturbance in Alzheimer's disease. *Sleep* 2003;**26**:893–901.

328 Herxheimer A, Petrie KJ. Melatonin for the prevention and treatment of jet lag (review). In: *The Cochrane database of systematic reviews*. The Cochrane Library; 2002.

329 Veronelli A, Masu A, Ranieri R, Rognoni C, Laneri M, Pontiroli AE. Prevalence of erectile dysfunction in thyroid disorders: comparison with control subjects and with obese and diabetic patients. *Int J Impot Res* 2006;**18**:111–114.

330 Isidori AM, Carani C, Granata A, Carosa E, Maggi M, Lenzi A, Jannini E. Multicenter study on the prevalence of sexual symptoms in male hypo and hyperthyroid patients. *J Sex Med* 2006; Suppl1: 21.

331 Baskin HJ. Endocrinologic evaluation of impotence. *South Med J* 1989;**82**:446–449.

332 Wortsman J, Rosner W, Dufau ML. Abnormal testicular function in men with primary hypothyroidism. *Am J Med* 1987;**82**:207–212.

333 Corana G, Petrone L, Mannuci E, Jannini EA, Mansani R, Magini A, Giomini E, Forti G, Maggi M. Psychobiological correlates of rapid ejaculation in patients attending an andrology unit for sexual dysfunctions. *Eur J Urol* 2004;**46**:615–622.

334 Waldinger DH. Thyroid stimulation hormone assessments in a Dutch cohort of 620 men with premature ejaculation without erectile dysfunction. *J Sex Med* 2005;**2**:865–870.

335 Murray RD, Shalet SM. Adult growth hormone replacement: lessons learnt and future direction. *J Clin Endocrinol Metab* 2002;**87**:4427–4434.

336 Gibney J, Wolthers T, Johannsson G, Umpleby AM, Ho KK. Growth hormone and testosterone interact positively to enhance protein and energy metabolism in hypopituitary men. *Am J Physiol Endocrinol Metab* 2005;289:E266–271.

337 Levy JB, Husmann DA. Micropenis secondary to growth hormone deficiency: does treatment with growth hormone alone result in adequate penile growth? *J Urol* 1996;**156**:214–216.

338 Fradkin JE, Eastman RC, Lesniac MA. Specificity spillover at the hormone receptor: exploring its role on human disease (review). *N Engl J Med* 1989;**370**: 640–645.

339 Muir A, Maclaren NK. Autoimmune diseases of the adrenal glands, parathyroid glands, gonads, and hypothalamic-pituitary axis. *Endocrinol Metab Clin North Amer* 1991;**20**:619–644.

340 Guay AT, Agnello V, Tronic BC, Gresham DG, Freidberg SR. Lymphocytic hypophysitis in a man. *J Clin Endocrinol Metab* 1987;**64**:631–634.

341 Weiss RE, Corvalan AH, Dillon RW. Metastatic renal carcinoma presenting as impotence. *J Urol* 1993; **149**:821–823.

342 Brill KT, Weltman AL, Gentili A, Patrie JT, Fryburg DA, Hanks JB, Urban RJ, Veldhuis JD. Single and combined effects of growth hormone and testosterone administration on measures of body composition, physical performance, mood, sexual function, bone turnover, and muscle gene expression in healthy older men. *J Clin Endocrinol Metab* 2002;**87**:5649–5657.

343 Gibney J, Wallace JD, Spinks T, Schnorr L, Ranicar R, Cuneo RC, Lockhart S, Burnard KG, Salomons P, Sonksen PH, Rusell-Jones D. The effect of 10 years of recombinant human GH in adult GH-deficient patients. *J Clin Endocrinol Metab* 1999;**84**:2596–2602.

344 Becker AJ, Ückert S, Stief CG, *et al.* Possible role of human growth hormone in penile erection. *J Urol* 2000;**164**:2138–2142.

345 Ückert S, Ness B, Becker A, *et al*. Mechanisms of action of human growth hormone (GH) on isolated human penile erectile tissue. *J Urol* 2005;**173**(suppl):291 abstr.1072.

346 Baum HB, Biller BM, Finkelstein JS, *et al*. Effects of physiologic growth hormone therapy on bone density and body composition in patients with adult onset growth hormone deficiency. A randomized, placebo-controlled trial (see comments). *Ann Int Med* 1996;**125**:883–890.

347 Rudman D, Feller AG, Nagraj HS, Gergans GA, Lalitha PY, Goldberg AF, Schenkler RA, Cohn L, Rudman IW, Mattson DE. Effects of human growth hormone in men over 60 years old. *N Engl J Med* 1990;**323**:1–6.

348 Marcus R, Butterfield G, Holloway L, Gilliland L, Baylink DJ, Hintz RL, Sherman BM. Effects of short term administration of recombinant human growth hormone to elderly people. *J Clin Endocrinol Metab* 1990;**70**:519–527.

349 Guay AT, Velasquez E, Perez JB. Characterization of patients in a medical endocrine-based center for male sexual dysfunction. *Endocr Pract* 1999;**5**:314–321.

350 Sairam K, Kulinskaya E, Boustead GB, Hanbury DC, McNicholas TA. Prevalence of undiagnosed diabetes mellitus in male erectile dysfunction. *BJU Int* 2001;**88**:68–71.

351 Bansal TC, Guay AT, Jacobson J, Woods BO, Nesto RW. Incidence of metabolic syndrome and insulin resistance in a population with organic erectile dysfunction. *J Sex Med* 2005;**2**:96–103.

352 Braunstein GD. Impotence in diabetic men. *Mt Sinai J Med* 1987;**54**:236–240.

353 Feldman HA, Goldstein I, Hatzichristou DG, Krane RJ, McKinlay JB. Impotence and its medical and psychological correlates: results of the Massachusetts Male Aging Study. *J Urol* 1994;**151**:54–61.

354 Giuliano FA, Leriche A, Jaudinot EO, Solesse de Gendre A. Prevalence of erectile dysfunction among 7689 patients with diabetes or hypertension or both. *Urology* 2004;**64**:1196–1201.

355 Fedele D, Coscelli C, Santeusanio F, Bortolotti A, Chatenoud L, Colli E, Landoni M, Parazzini F. Erectile dysfunction in diabetic subjects in Italy. *Diabetes Care* 1998;**21**:1973–1977.

356 Buvat J, Lemaire A, Buvat-Herbaut M, Guieu JD, Bailleul JP, Fossati P. Comparative investigations in 26 impotent and 26 nonimpotent diabetic patients. *J Urol* 1985;**133**:34–38.

357 Veves A, Webster L, Chen TF, Payne S, Boulton AJ. Aetiopathogenesis and management of impotence in diabetic males: four years experience from a combined clinic. *Diabetic Med* 1995;**12**:77–82.

358 Wang CJ, Shen SY, Wu CC, Huang CH, Chiang CP. Penile blood flow study in diabetic impotence. *Urol Int* 1993;**50**:209–212.

359 Sowers JR. Diabetes mellitus and cardiovascular disease in women. *Arch Intern Med* 1998;**158**:617–621.

360 Saito I, Folsom AR, Brancati FL, Duncan BB, Chambless LE, McGovern PG. Nontraditional risk factors for coronary heart disease incidence among persons with diabetes: the Atherosclerosis Risk in Communities (ARIC) Study. *Ann Int Med* 2000;**133**:81–91.

361 Sáenz de Tejada I, Goldstein I, Azadzoi K, Krane RJ, Cohen RA. Impaired neurogenic and endothelium-mediated relaxation of penile smooth muscle from diabetic men with impotence. *N Engl J Med* 1989;**320**:1025–1030.

362 Sullivan ME, Dashwood MR, Thompson CS, Mikhailidis DP, Morgon RJ. Alterations in endothelin B receptor sites in cavernosal tissue of diabetic rabbits: potential relevance to the pathogenesis of erectile dysfunction. *J Urol* 1997;**158**:1966–1972.

363 Francavilla S, Properzi G, Bellini C, Marino G, Ferri C, Santucci A. Endothelin-1 in diabetic and non-diabetic men with erectile dysfunction. *J Urol* 1997;**158**:1770–1774.

364 Christ GJ, Lerner SE, Kim DC, Melman A. Endothelin-1 as a putative modulator of erectile dysfunction: I. Characteristics of contraction of isolated corporeal tissue strips. *J Urol* 1995;**153**:1998–2003.

365 Baron AD. Insulin and the vasculature: old actors, new roles. *J Invest Med* 1996;**44**:P406–442.

366 Metro MJ, Broderick GA. Diabetes and vascular impotence: does insulin dependence increase the relative severity? *Int J Imp Res* 1999;**11**:87–88.

367 Friedlander Y, Kidron M, Caslake M, Lamb B, McConnell M, Baron H. Low density lipoprotein particle size and risk factors of insulin resistance syndrome. *Atherosclerosis* 2000;**148**:141–149.

368 Kashyap SR, Roman LJ, Lamont J, Masters BSS, Bejaj M, Suraamornkul S, Belfort R, Berria R, Kellogg DL, Liu Y, DeFronzo RA. Insulin resistance is associated with impaired nitric oxide synthase activity in skeletal muscle of type 2 diabetic subjects. *J Clin Endocrinol Metab* 2005;**90**:1100–1105.

369 Nijhawan S, Mathur A, Singh V, Bhandari VM. Autonomic and peripheral neuropathy in insulin dependent diabetics. *J Assoc Physicians India* 1993;**41**:565–566.

370 Bemelmans BL, Meuleman EJ, Doesburg WH, Notermens SL, Debruyne FM. Erectile dysfunction in

diabetic men: the neurological factor revisited. *J Urol* 1994;**151**:884–889.

371 Murray FT, Wyss HU, Thomas RG, Spevack M, Glaros AG. Gonadal dysfunction in diabetic men with organic impotence. *J Clin Endocrinol Metab* 1987;**65**:127–135.

372 Guay AT, Velasquez E, Perez JB. Characterization of patients in a medical endocrine-based center for male sexual dysfunction. *Endocr Pract* 1999;**5**:314–321.

373 Barrett-Connor E, Khaw KT, Yen SS. Endogenous sex hormone levels in older adult men with diabetes mellitus. *Am J Epidemiol* 1990;**132**:895–901.

374 Dhinsa S, Prabhakar S, Sethi M, Bandyopadhyay A, Chaudhuri A, Dandona P. Frequent occurrence of hypogonadotropic hypogonadism in type 2 diabetes. *J Clin Endocrinol Metab* 2004;**89**:5462–5468.

375 Sobrevia L, Mann GE. Dysfunction of the endothelial nitric oxide signaling pathway in diabetes and hyperglycemia. *Exp Physiol* 1997;**82**:423–452.

376 Bagg W, Ferri C, Desideri G, Gamble G, Okelford P, Braatvedt GD. The influences of obesity and glycemic control on endothelial activation in patients with type 2 diabetes. *J Clin Endocrinol Metab* 2001;**86**:5491–5497.

377 Christ M, Bauersachs J, Liebetrau C, Heck M, Gunter A, Wehling M. Glucose increases endothelial-dependent superoxide formation in coronary arteries by NAD(P)H oxidase activation: attenuation by the 3-hydroxy-3methylglutaryl coenzyme A reductase inhibitor atorvastatin. *Diabetes* 2002;**51**:2648–2652.

378 Romeo JH, Seftel AD, Madhun ZT, Aron DC. Sexual function in men with diabetes type2: association with glycemic control. *J Urol* 2000;**163**:788–791.

379 Cartledge JJ, Eardley I, Morrison JF. Impairment of corpus cavernosal smooth muscle relaxation by glycosated human haemoglobin. *BJU Int* 2000;**85**: 735–741.

380 Lipson LG. Special problems in the treatment of hypertension in the patient with diabetes mellitus. *Arch Int Med* 1984;**144**:1829–1831.

381 Mannino DM, Klevenes RM, Flanders WD. Cigarette smoking: an independent risk factor for impotence? *Am J Epidemiol* 1994;**140**:1003–1008.

382 Bortolotti A, Fedele D, Chatenoud L. Cigarette smoking: a risk factor for erectile dysfunction in diabetics. *Eur Urol* 2001;**40**:392–397.

383 Salama N, Kagawa S. Ultra-structural changes in collagen of penile tunica albuginea in aged and diabetic rats. *Int J Imp Res* 1999;**11**:99–105.

384 Seftel AD, Maclennan GT, Chen ZJ. Loss of TGF beta, apoptosis, and Bcl-2 in erectile dysfunction and upregulation of p53 and HIF-alpha-associated erectile dysfunction. *Mol Urol* 1999;**3**:103–107.

385 Guay AT. Treatment of erectile dysfunction in men with diabetes. *Diabetes Spectrum* 1998;**11**: 101–111.

386 Egede LE, Zheng D. Modifiable cardiovascular risk factors in adults with diabetes: prevalence and missed opportunities for physician counseling. *Arch Intern Med* 2002;**162**:427–433.

387 Beckman JA, Creager MA, Libbly P. Diabetes and atherosclerosis: epidemiology, pathophysiology, and management. *JAMA* 2002;**287**:2570–2581.

388 Guay AT, Perez JB, Heatley GJ. Cessation of smoking rapidly decreases erectile dysfunction. *Endocr Pract* 1998;**4**:23–26.

389 Henry P, Thomas F, Benetos A, Guize L. Impaired fasting glucose, blood pressure and cardiovascular disease mortality. *Hypertension* 2002;**40**:458–43.

390 Heart Outcomes Prevention Evaluation (HOPE) Study Investigators. Effects of ramipril on cardiovascular and microvascular outcomes in people with diabetes mellitus: results of the HOPE study and MICRO-HOPE substudy. *Lancet* 2000;**355**:253–25.

391 Forbes JM, Cooper ME, Thallas V. Reduction of the accumulation of advanced glycation end products by ACE inhibition in experimental diabetic nephropathy. *Diabetes* 2002;**51**:3274–3282.

392 Boyanov MA, Boneva Z, Christov VG. Testosterone supplementation in men with type 2 diabetes, visceral obesity and partial androgen deficiency. *Aging Male* 2003;**6**:1–7.

393 Costabile RA. Optimizing treatment for diabetes mellitus induced erectile dysfunction. *J Urol* 2003;**170**: S35–3.

394 Rendell MS, Rajfer J, Wicker PA, Smith MD. Sildenafil for treatment of erectile dysfunction in men with diaetes: a randomized controlled trial. *JAMA* 1999;**281**: 421–42.

395 Goldstein I, Young JM, Fischer J, Bangerter K, Segerson T, Taylor T, Vardenafil Diabetes Study Group. Vardenafil, a new phosphodiesterase type 5 inhibitor, in the treatment of erectile dysfunction in men with diabetes. *Diabetes Care* 2003;**26**:777–73.

396 Sáenz de Tejada I, Anglin G, Knight JR, Emmick J. Effects of tadalafil on erectile dysfunction in men with diabetes. *Diabetes Care* 2002;**25**:2159–2164.

397 Fonseca V, Seftel A, Denne J, Fredlund P. Impact of diabetes mellitus on the severity of erectile dysfunction and response to treatment: analysis of data from tadalafil clinical trials. *Diabetologia* 2004;**47**:1914–1923.

398 Lakka HM, Laaksonen DE, Lakka TA, Niskanen LK, Kumpusalo E, Tuomilehto JET. The metabolic

syndrome and total and cardiovascular disease mortality in middle-aged men. *JAMA* 2002;**288**:2709–2716.

399 Expert Panel on Detection, Evaluation, and Treatment of High Blood Cholesterol in Adults. Executive summary of the third report of the National Cholesterol Education Program (NCEP) Expert Panel on Detection, Evaluation, and Treatment of High Blood Cholesterol in Adults (Adult Treatment Panel III). *JAMA* 2001;**285**:2486–2497.

400 Billups KL, Bank AJ, Padma-Nathan H, Katz S, Williams R. Erectile dysfunction is a marker for cardiovascular disease: results of the Minority Health Institute Expert Advisory Panel. *J Sex Med* 2005;**2**:40–52.

401 Maas R, Schwedhelm E, Albsmeier J, Boger RH. The pathophysiology of erectile dysfunction related to endothelial dysfunction and mediators of vascular function. *Vasc Med* 2002;**7**:213–225.

402 Kostis JB, *et al*. Sexual dysfunction and cardiac risk (the Second Princeton Consensus Conference). *Am J Cardiol* 2005;**96**:313–321.

403 Hsueh WA, Lyon CJ, Quinones MJ. Insulin resistance and the endothelium. *Am J Med* 2004;**117**:109–117.

404 Roumeguere T, Wespes E, Carpentier Y, Hoffman P, Schulman CC. Erectile dysfunction is associated with a high prevalence of hyperlipidemia and coronary heart disease risk. *Eur Urol* 2003;**44**:355–359.

405 Montorsi F, Briganti A, Salonia A, Rigatti P, Margonato A, Macchi A. Erectile dysfunction prevalence, time of onset and association with risk factors in 300 consecutive patients with acute chest pain and angiographically documented coronary artery disease. *Eur Urol* 2003;**44**:360–364.

406 Pritzker MR. The penile stress test. A window to the hearts of man? (Abstract) *Circulation* 1999;**100**(S1): S375.

407 Walczak MK, Lokhandwala N, Hodge MB, Guay AT. Prevalence of cardiovascular risk factors in erectile dysfunction. *J Gender Specific Med* 2002;**5**:19–24.

408 Seftel AD, Sun P, Swindle R. The prevalence of hypertension, hyperlipidemia, diabetes mellitus and depression in men with erectile dysfunction. *J Urol* 2004;**171**:2341–2345.

409 Laaksonen DE, Niskanen L, Punnonen K, Nyyssonen K, Tuomainen TP, Valkonen VP, Salonen R, Salonen JT. Testosterone and sex hormone-binding globulin predict the metabolic syndrome and diabetes in middle-aged men. *Diabetes Care* 2004;**27**:1036–1041.

410 Kalme T, Seppala M, Qiao Q, Koistinen R, Nissinen A, Harrela M, Loukovaara M, Leinonen P, Tuomilehto J. Sex hormone-binding globulin and insulin-like growth factor-binding protein-1 as indicators of metabolic syndrome, cardiovascular risk, and mortality in elderly men. *J Clin Endocrinol Metab* 2005;**90**:1550–1556.

411 Muller M, Grobbee DE, den Tonkelaar I, Lamberts SWJ, van der Schouw Y. Endogenous sex hormones and metabolic syndrome in aging men. *J Clin Endocrinol Metab* 2005;**90**:2618–2623.

412 Bansal TC, Guay AT, Jacobson J, Woods BO, Nesto RW. Incidence of metabolic syndrome and insulin resistance in a population with organic erectile dysfunction. *J Sex Med* 2005;**2**:96–103.

413 Esposito K, Giugliano F, Martedi E, Feola G, Marfella R, D'Amiento M, Giugliano D. High proportions of erectile dysfunction in men with the metabolic syndrome. *Diabetes Care* 2005;**28**:1201–1203.

414 Bivalacqua TJ, Usta MF, Champion HC, Kadowitz PJ, Hellstrom WJG. Endothelial dysfunction in erectile dysfunction: role of the endothelium in erectile physiology and disease. *J Androl* 2003;**24**:S17–37.

415 Shabsigh R, Kupelian V, Araujo A, O'Donnell A, McKinlay J. Erectile dysfunction as a predictor for metabolic syndrome: results from the Massachusetts Male Aging Study (MMAS). (Abstract) American Urology Association. San Antonio, 2005.

416 Bansal TC, Guay AT, Jacobson J, Woods BO, Nesto RW. Incidence of metabolic syndrome and insulin resistance in a population with organic erectile dysfunction. *J Sex Med* 2005;**2**:96–103.

417 Rabinowitz D. Some endocrine and metabolic aspects of obesity. *Annu Rev Med* 1970;**21**:241–258.

418 Bar RS, Gorden P, Roth J. Fluctuations in the affinity and concentrations of insulin receptors on circulating monocytes of obese patients: effects of starvation, refeeding and dieting. *J Clin Invest* 1976;**58**:1123–1135.

419 Grundy SM. Obesity, metabolic syndrome, and cardiovascular disease. *J Clin Endocrinol Metab* 2004;**89**:2595–2600.

420 Suwaidi JA, Higano ST, Holmes DR, Lennon R, Lerman A. Obesity is independently associated with coronary endothelial dysfunction in patients with normal or mildly diseased coronary arteries. *J Am Coll Card* 2001;**37**:1523–1528.

421 Pinkney JH, Stehouwer CDA, Coppack SW, Yudkin JS. Endothelial dysfunction: cause of the insulin resistance syndrome. *Diabetes* 1997;**46**:S9–13.

422 Esposito K, Giugliano F, DiPalo C, *et al*. Weight loss and exercise improve sexual function in obese men with erectile dysfunction. *JAMA* 2004;**291**:2978–2984.

Introduction to Female Sexual Disorders

Alessandra Graziottin

The aim of this section is to offer to health care providers a constructive, easy to use, practical approach to address female sexual disorders (FSD), in a timely and effective manner.

Sexual issues are increasingly raised in the clinical setting. They may be discussed in a number of contexts, including obtaining background information about sexual function and sexual health, addressing possible consequences of illness, injury, procedures and/or medications or responding to a patient presenting with a sexual problem or question [1].

Public and health care agencies' awareness on the importance of sexuality as a core part of the quality of life of every human being increases the need for appropriate knowledge and training in this rapidly-growing field. The ultimate goal is to fulfill patients' expectations of a comprehensive understanding and treatment of the individual or couple's sexual concerns [2].

To help the reader, who is busy updating the domains of his/her specialty, a focused attention has been devoted to the critical questions that will help clinicians to optimize sexual history taking so that key biologic, psychosexual and contextual factors will be rapidly elicited and recorded.

The stress given to the importance of an accurate *physical* examination in any FSD complaint is needed in the clinical diagnosis of FSD [2,3]. For decades the prominent focus on psychosexual and relational issues has deprived women of the right to have a thorough medical evaluation of their sexual concerns. The appropriate evaluation of potential endocrinologic [4–7], vascular [8,9], dismetabolic [10], neurologic [11], neuroimmunologic [12] or iatrogenic factors [13–16], in addition to the neglected role of pelvic floor dysfunctions in contributing to and maintaining FSD [3,14,15], is essential to avoid both a systematic medical omission and a still persistent gender bias.

The past neglect of the biologic basis of FSD is demonstrated by the lack of objective research and clinical delay in the medical treatment of women's sexual complaints, in comparison to men.

For both genders, the challenge sexual medicine is facing today is the same: to blend together a "medicine without soul," which pays little attention to the emotions, concerns and affective dynamics associated with medical illnesses, and a "psychology without body," which still under appreciates the neurobiologic basis of any feeling, memory, emotion or thought.

The over-focus on the medical perspective in men and on the psychosexual/relational perspective in women is to be resolved in a balanced and integrated view aimed at a comprehensive approach for both genders. This is the ultimate goal of this book, and of this FSD section in particular.

Contemporary sexual medicine is focusing on this goal, with a refreshed attention to couple dynamics as well [1,7,17]. Every chapter on FSD is therefore aimed at maintaining this integrated perspective. This is why male factors and couple dynamics involved in FSD will be analyzed and discussed when indicated, to help the health care provider in building a structured diagnostic approach to each disorder [1,3,4–7,13–17].

Special effort has been given to maintain a limited length in each FSD chapter, to help the busy clinician, to distil the most relevant information in the shortest time.

A chapter on the iatrogenic and post-traumatic factors involved in FSD has been included to open a window on another critical and growing territory in the medical evaluation of women's sexual concerns [3,13–16].

Finally, as menopause is a key turning point in women's and couple's sexuality, a detailed chapter aimed at summarizing the current knowledge on the controversial arena of hormonal treatment has been included [17–20], as virtually every clinician may be asked to comment on risks, side-effects or contraindications of hormonal treatment, when prescribed to improve a sexual disorder.

The wish is that this section will significantly contribute to increase both the clinician's confidence in asking and listening to FSD concerns and his/her "clinical impact factor," i.e. his/her ability to appropriately diagnose and effectively treat FSD, or to refer to a sex therapist, in an increasing number of women—and couple's—who seek help in a difficult moment of their sexual life [2].

References

1 Plaut M, Graziottin A, Heaton J. *Sexual Dysfunction.* Health Press, Abingdon, Oxford (UK), 2004.

2 Graziottin A. Women's right to a better sexual life. In: Graziottin A. (Guest Ed.), Female Sexual Dysfunction: Clinical Approach. *Urodinamica* 2004;**14**(2):57–60.

3 Graziottin A. Treatment of sexual dysfunction. In: Bo K, Berghmans B, van Kampen M, Morkved S, eds. *Evidence Based Physiotherapy for the Pelvic Floor—Bridging Research and Clinical Practice*, Elsevier, Oxford, UK (2005, in press).

4 Bachmann G, Bancroft J, Braunstein G, *et al.* FAI: The Princeton consensus statement on definition, classification and assessment. *Fertil Steril* 2002;**77**:660–665.

5 Graziottin A. Libido: The biologic scenario. *Maturitas* 2000;**34**S.1:S9–S16.

6 Dennerstein L, Koochaki PE, Barton I, Graziottin A. Surgical menopause and female sexual functioning: a survey of Western European women. *Menopause* (2005, in press).

7 Graziottin A, Leiblum SR. Biological and psychosocial pathophysiology of female sexual dysfunction during the menopausal transition. *J Sex Med* 2005;Supp.3; 133–145.

8 Goldstein I, Berman J. Vasculogenic female sexual dysfunction: vaginal engorgement and clitoral erectile insufficiency syndrome. *Int J Impot Res* 1998;**10**:S84–S90.

9 Addis IB, Ireland CC, Vittinghoff *et al.* Sexual activity and function in postmenopausal women with heart disease. *Obstet Gynecol* 2005 Jul;**106**:121–7.

10 Rutherford D, Collins A. Sexual dysfunction in women with diabetes mellitus. *Gynecol Endocrinol* 2005 Oct;**21**:189–92.

11 Komisaruk BR, Whipple B. Brain activity imaging during sexual response in women with spinal cord injury. In Hyde J, ed. *Biological Substrates of Human Sexuality.* American Psychological Association: Washington, DC, 2005, pp. 109–146.

12 Bornstein J, Goldschmid N, Sabo E Hyperinnervation and mast cell activation may be used as a histopathologic diagnostic criteria for vulvar vestibulitis. *Gynecol Obstet Invest* 2004;**58**:171–178.

13 Graziottin A, Basson R. Sexual dysfunction in women with premature menopause. *Menopause* 2004;**11**(6 Pt 2):766–777.

14 Glazener CMA. Sexual function after childbirth: women's experiences, persistent morbidity and lack of professional recognition. *Br J Obstet Gynaecol* 1997;**104**:330–335.

15 Baessler K, Schuessler B. Pregnancy, childbirth and pelvic floor damage. In: Bourcier A, McGuire E, Abrams P, eds. *Pelvic Floor Disorders.* Elsevier Saunders, Philadelphia, 2004, pp. 33–42.

16 Seagraves RT Balon R. *Sexual Pharmacology: Fast facts.* WW Norton & Company, New York, 2003.

17 Leiblum SR, Rosen RC, eds. *Principles and Practice of Sex Therapy,* 3rd ed. New York: Guilford, 2000.

18 Writing Group of the International Menopause Society Executive Committee. Guidelines for the hormone treatment of women in the menopausal transition and beyond. *Climacteric* 2004;**7**:8–11.

19 The North American Menopause Society Position Statement. Recommendations for estrogen and progestogen use in peri and postmenopausal women. *Menopause* 2004;**11**:589–600.

20 Skouby SO and the EMAS Writing Group. Climacteric medicine: European Menopause and Andropause Society (EMAS) Position statements on postmenopausal hormonal therapy. *Maturitas* 2004;**48**:19–25.

Acknowledgments

Alessandra Graziottin (chairwoman of the FSD subcommittee) for writing the Introduction and Future Trends and Conclusions, and the chapters on Classification, Etiology and Key Issues in Female Sexual Disorders (FSD), Sexual Pain Disorders, Hormonal Therapy after Menopause, Iatrogenic and Post-Traumatic FSD, and co-authoring the chapters on Sexual Desire Disorders, Sexual Aversion Disorders, Sexual Arousal Disorders and Orgasmic Disorders.

Beverly Whipple for co-writing the chapter on Orgasmic Disorders, for editing all chapters in the section, and for providing pertinent comments for each chapter.

Lorraine Dennerstein for co-writing the chapter on Sexual Desire Disorders and for constructive comments and suggestions on each chapter.

Annamaria Giraldi for co-writing the chapters on Anatomy and Physiology of Womens' Sexual Function, and Sexual Arousal Disorders, and for her comments on other chapters.

Jeanne Alexander for her contribution to the chapter on Sexual Desire Disorders and for her comments on other FSD.

Linda Banner for her contribution to the chapter on Sexual Aversion Disorders and for her comments on the chapter on Iatrogenic and Post-traumatic FSD.

CHAPTER 19

Anatomy and Physiology of Women's Sexual Function

Alessandra Graziottin and Annamaria Giraldi

This chapter summarizes the anatomy and physiology of women's sexual response with a clinical perspective. The neurobiology of sexual function in women will be only briefly mentioned for conciseness. More attention will instead be given to the anatomy and physiology of the external genitalia and female organs, which will be summarized focusing on what clinicians should consider when examining the patient complaining of female sexual disorders (FSD).

The Sexual Brain

The limbic system and the neocortex

A normal sexual response requires the anatomic and functional integrity of the brain's entire limbic system, rather than a particular anatomic structure within it [1]. The limbic system is part of the so-called "paleo-cortex": a comprehensive network involving the hypothalamus and the thalamus (both within the diencephalon), the anterior cingulate gyrus, and many structures of the temporal lobes, including the amygdala, the mammillary bodies, the fornix, and the hippocampus, a phylogenetically ancient type of cortex [1–4].

Together with the prefrontal lobe, which has a predominantly inhibitory role over the basic instinctual drives, the limbic system is essential in both sexes for the initiation of sexual desire and related sexual phenomena [1,5–7]. Its function activates sexual fantasies, sexual daydreams, erotic dreams, mental sexual arousal, and the initiation of the cascade of neurovascular events triggering all the somatic and genital responses of sexual function as well as the

associated socially appropriate behaviors [7–9]. It is thought that the amygdala maintains a key role as the control center for the four "basic emotional command systems" described by Panksepp: the seeking appetitive/lust system, the anger/rage, the fear/anxiety, and the panic/separation distress system [5]. All these systems may interact to modulate the final perception of sexual desire and central arousal and correlated sexual behaviors. The disruption of any level of the limbic system may cause sexual dysfunction in both sexes, particularly in the domains of desire, central arousal, and socially appropriate sexual behavior [1,5,9–11].

The neocortex is increasingly involved in the sexual response in human, first as final target of sensory inputs which arrive from the different sensory organs. Different smells, tastes, words, sights, or touch stimuli may activate both the pertinent sensory cortex and the limbic sexual cortex when the signal is "coded" as sexual. Cognitive factors are also in play in evaluating the sexual stimulus and modulate the "judgment" of concomitant risks and wishes before engaging, or not, in a specific sexual behavior [1,10,12].

Neurotransmitters

In men and women, the sexual response is coordinated by the same neurotransmitters, with the most studied being monoamines (dopamine, norepinephrine, and serotonin), neuropeptides (opioid peptides), neurohormones (oxytocin and vasopressin) and neurotrophins (including the nerve growth factor, NGF, which increases in the brain and peripheral blood when people fall in love) [1,6,7,9,13].

Regional and quantitative differences in neurotransmitter activities reflect brain sexual dimorphism that is modulated by prenatal and postnatal endocrine milieus and their interactions with environmental factors [1,5,6,14].

Sexual dimorphisms

Many aspects of adult sexual life, both functional and dysfunctional, can claim their origins in the very earliest steps of "sexual dimorphism" [1,5,6,9,14]. The gene sequences of chromosomes have two functions: the ability to replicate, termed the "template" function, and the expression of genes, called "transcription." The process of activating and expressing genes results in the genotype becoming the phenotype; that is, the transformation of the potential, virtual DNA code into actual, functional tissue [1,5]. Interestingly, the "default" phenotypic expression for the human organism, including its brain, is female [1]. Unless a specific substance called testis-determining factor (TDF) is expressed by a short sequence of genes on the Y-chromosome during the maturation process of the fetus, every baby born would have a female brain and body structure [1,9].

The neurons of men and women share all the basic anatomic and functional characteristics. Similarly, neurotransmitters, neurohormones, neuropeptides, and neurotrophins have exactly the same structure and roles in both men and women, with some quantitative differences as well as some variability in regional distribution [1,5–7,9,14]. Even the potential for neuroplasticity—the ability to increase and modulate connections among neurons through neuronal sprouting and the creation of dendritic spines, and the morphologic correlate of psychoplasticity—is shared equally in both genders. It appears, then, that the major neurologic differences between men and women lie mainly in their respective degrees of brain dimorphism; that is, in the differences caused by the action of testosterone on the brain. Quite interestingly, many of the central nervous system effects of testosterone are mediated by estrogen, as a result of the aromatization of testosterone by the enzyme aromatase [1,5,6].

Sexually dimorphic variations in overall brain weight (which is higher, on average, in men) do not appear to be of importance in human sexuality.

Quality of brain functioning, sexual and non-sexual, depends on the complex pattern of connections between cells, their continuous plasticity, and the intensity by which they are stimulated through affective events, educational level, and environmental challenges (8–10).

Clinical relevance of brain dimorphism

Hemispheric asymmetry and brain dimorphism have manifest implications in male and female sexual function. For example, the most important sexual cues in women for increasing mental arousal—as well as the mental awareness of that arousal—typically involve verbal intimacy, such as having her partner's receptive and attentive ear, or having affectionate or erotic words spoken to her. Men, on the other hand, rely much more strongly on visual stimulation, either in reality or fantasy, for mental and genital arousal. Much disappointment and frustration results when these two primary sexual cues are polarized in a couple; the consequent mental dissatisfaction may then potentially contribute to sexual dysfunction and even to sexual avoidance [9,12,15].

Another main neuroanatomic difference between men and women lies in the medial preoptic area of the hypothalamus, the key center of the autonomic nervous system in both sexes [1,6]. Located within this region is a set of nuclei known as the interstitial nuclei of the anterior hypothalamus (INAH) that express their products in a "tonic" or relatively continuous secretory state in men, while they exhibit a "cyclic" pattern of secretion in fertile, ovulating women. This variability has many important consequences on brain function and sexual behavior as well as many other somatic effects. Notably, while the hypothalamic hormone oxytocin is the primary peptide in female sexual circuitry, the male sexual cycle is most represented by vasopressin [1,6,7,9].

"Need detectors" located within the hypothalamus are responsible for the activation of the four "basic emotional command systems" of the brain: seeking, rage, fear, and panic [1,5]. These hypothalamic detectors are typically switched on and off by different hypothalamic regions. Prefrontal connections also influence the hypothalamic detectors, typically to inhibit the basic drives [1,4,5,10,11]. Many additional cognitive and perceptual inputs and cues serve to regulate the basic emotional command systems, as well.

The hypothalamic dimorphisms correlates with gender-related reproductive and sexual behaviors. For example, male sexual behavior is typically stable over the entire adult male life span; this may potentially be explained by a typical male's lifelong production of testosterone at a relatively tonic, constant rate (notwithstanding the gradual decrease in serum levels that has been described from the second decade of life onwards). In contrast, the physiology of female sexuality is highly discontinuous, both during the regular menstrual cycle, as well as during major reproductive life events such as pregnancy, puerperium, abortion, and menopause [9,15,16–18].

Interestingly, it has also been shown that while receptivity to pheromones remains relatively stable over life in men, there is a peak in pheromone receptivity during ovulation in women, as well as an overall greater level of odor discrimination ability during the years of fertility. After menopause, odor discrimination ability in women decreases significantly and much resembles physiologic male levels [19]. Pheromones may be responsible for mediating interactions in the mid-cycle variations observed in women, which may in turn be triggered by the ovulatory androgen peak, promoting the atresia of non-dominant follicles in the ovary as well as a mental and physical peak in sexual desire, arousability and receptivity [20]. The biologic ramification of these relationships is to increase female sexual responsiveness when the likelihood of conception is at its highest. Human pheromones and their role in sexual attraction and reproduction have been recently reviewed [20].

Central nervous system dimorphisms may well represent the biologic basis for the differences in sexual desire, perception, and expression experienced by men and women, including the disparities in the frequency, content, and intensity of erotic fantasies, nocturnal erotic dreams, and sexual daydreams; the perception of central arousal; the quality and quantity of expression of the sexual response, and the likelihood and emotional resonance of orgasm [1,6–9,12,15–18,21–27].

A more dynamic understanding of the continuous interactions between the somatic body and the psychic mind and how these processes differ between men and women, will help to clarify the similarities that are neglected by the polarized focus on contextual factors in women and on biologic factors in men.

Neural pathways

At the level of the spine, the neural pathways of sympathetic and parasympathetic sexual responses in both genders follow the same anatomic distributions until their termination in different male and female target sexual organs [1–3,9,28]. These pathways involve the superior hypogastric plexus, the middle hypogastric plexus (which gives rise to the hypogastric nerves joining the testicular or ovarian plexus), the ureteric plexus, the internal iliac arterial plexus, the inferior hypogastric plexus (which receives mostly sympathetic afferent and efferent fibers from the hypogastric nerves, the postganglionic sympathetic fibers derived from the sacral splanchnic nerves, and the parasympathetic fibers derived from pelvic splanchnic nerves—the nervi erigentes in both sexes—that have their cell bodies in the S2, S3, and S4 segments of the spinal cord) [2,9,28].

The uterovaginal plexus is simply the terminal ramifications of the lower part of the inferior hypogastric plexus. In women, the uterovaginal plexus supplies the uterus, salpinges, ovaries, vagina, erectile tissue of the clitoris and vestibular bulbs (via the cavernous nerves of the clitoris), urethra, and greater vestibular glands [2,28].

In both genders, the perineum receives its primary somatic innervation from the pudendal nerve (derived from S2, S3, and S4) and its sympathetic innervation from the sacral portion of the sympathetic chain [2,28,30–32]. The anatomic pathway of the pudendal nerve is very similar in both men and women, forming a single trunk that runs approximately 1 cm posterior to the ischial spine through the greater sciatic foramen inferior to the piriformis muscle. It then re-enters the pelvic cavity through the lesser sciatic foramen and proceeds anteriorly through Alcock's canal, passing posterior to the junction between the ischial spine and sacrospinous ligament and anterior to the sacrotuberous ligament and medial to the internal pudendal vessels. At this point, the pudendal nerve branches into its three main pathways: the inferior hemorrhoidal nerve, the perineal nerve, and the dorsal nerve of the clitoris in women, or penis in men.

These similarities in neural pathways have important implications for oncologic surgeries, in which the sparing of the vesical nerve plexus fibers that accompany the vesical artery to the bladder may significantly reduce sexual and urinary morbidity in both men and women [9].

They may as well help explain the equal risks of numbness, reduced sensibility, and arousal difficulties of the external genitalia secondary to compression of the pudendal nerve, experienced by both men and women who ride bicycles for long periods of time without adequate protection or frequent position changes [29].

Finally, knowledge of similarities and differences between male and female basic anatomic structures and neurologic pathways may contribute to a parallel thinking of the pathophysiology of male and female sexual disorders, which could be useful in the clinical practice [2,9,28,30–32].

The External Female Genitalia

Accurate examination of the female external and internal genitalia is often disregarded in the sexual consultation, particularly when sexual disorders are complained of. On the contrary, the physical examination can be extremely informative not only on the close interaction between biologic and psychosexual factors, but also on the variety of critical information that a clinician can obtain.

The following paragraphs will therefore discuss the anatomy and physiology of women's genitalia with, a clinical perspective: what physicians should look for to complete their diagnosis on the reported female sexual disorder.

The **vulva** includes mons pubis, clitoris and labia majora and minora, which are the structures that are surrounding the urogenital cleft (the external genitals) [2,28].

The **mons pubis** is the hair-covered area over the pubis bone and forms the anterosuperior limit of the urogenital cleft with the labia majora on both sides, and ends posteriorly at the anterior margin of the perineal body.

Clinical relevance

1 A "male" hair distribution, towards the umbilicus, may suggest an excess of ovarian or adrenal production of androgens. It may be associated with acne, hypertrichosis (when excess hair maintain a female distribution) or hirsutism (when excess hair has a male distribution). These changes may be associated with body image concerns which may contribute to a feeling of sexual inadequacy, contributing to sexual disorders [15].

2 Loss of pubic hair may anticipate the menopausal changes; it may be perceived as a sign of inadequate sexual aging and may be associated with vulvar dystrophy, loss of sexual desire and/or of genital arousal [33].

The **labia majora** are the two prominent lateral fatty folds of the urogenital cleft. They meet anteriorly, creating the anterior commissure in front of the glans of the clitoris, and posteriorly, forming the posterior commissure. The internal surface has multiple sebaceous follicles, which keep the surface lubricated.

The **labia minora** are smaller, composed of supple elastic skin without subcutaneous fat, but rich in sebaceous glands. Anteriorly they form the clitoral prepuce and clitoral frenulum.

The **clitoris and the vestibular bulbs** form the erectile apparatus of the vulva. The clitoris is a 7–13 cm cylindric structure composed of glans clitoris, corpus clitoris (which is comprised of the paired corpora), and the crura, the deep extensions of the corpora, which diverge under the pubic arch [2,28,34]. The microscopic anatomy of the clitoris is consistent among different subjects. It consists of cavernous tissue with trabecular smooth muscle and collagen connective tissue [34,35], encircled by a thin fibrous capsule surrounded by large nerve trunks [36]. The vestibular bulbs are paired organs of erectile tissue structure located directly beneath the skin of the labia minora.

The **vulvar vestibule** includes the vulvar area comprised between the inferior part of the clitoris, the medial part of labia minora, and the fourchette. The central part includes the external side of the hymen, which marks the limit between the vagina, which has a mullerian origin, and the introitus, which has a cloacal origin.

Clinical relevance

1 The shape of external genitalia and clitoral dimension can vary, until the frank anomaly of the intersexual states that may contribute to sexual identity problems and body image concerns [37].

2 Clitoromegaly may be spontaneous or iatrogenic, as consequence of topical and/or systemic treatment with androgens, or with corticosteroids with androgenic activity. It may be associated with a number of clinical conditions, which include the above, plus avoidance of physical contact if the bigger size is perceived as a marker of pathology. When associated with spontaneous or iatrogenic hyperandrogenism, clitoromegaly may be associated with unwanted excess of genital arousal. Persistent, unwanted, intrusive congestion of the clitoris, not associated with increase of sexual desire, may be the objective correlate of the persistent sexual arousal disorder (PSAD) recently described (see Chapter 23) [38].

Priapism of the clitoris, when the glands and the shaft are engorged and painful, is a rare condition which should be considered in women complaining of "clitoralgia" [9]. Priapism may cause or be associated with pain in the clitoris in non-sexual conditions (i.e. it is spontaneous) and/or it can be provoked or worsened when the woman is aroused [9].

3 Atrophy of the clitoris is often associated with lichen sclerosus, an autoimmune pathology characterized by progressive involution of the external genitalia and of the corpora cavernosa [39]. In this condition, the labia minora may disappear and be conglutinated in a unique tissue involution (Fig. 19.1). The vulvar skin becomes thin, pale or white, with loss or the normal papillae, and/or with area of pathologic keratinization ("leukoplakia") [33].

Mistakenly considered as an "aging" condition, lichen sclerosus may be present in children, adolescents and young women as well (Fig. 19.2). It may be associated with lifelong or acquired genital arousal difficulties, orgasmic difficulties or anorgasmia, introital dyspareunia, and acquired loss of sexual desire. A disabling vulvar itching is another key symptom associated with vulvar dystrophy.

Attention to the trophism of the external genitalia is mandatory in all women complaining of acquired genital arousal disorders and/or acquired introital

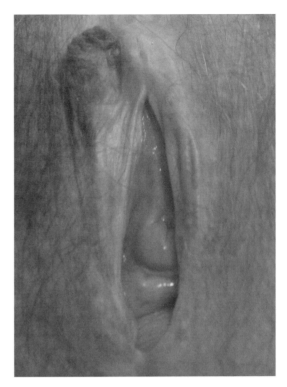

Fig. 19.1 Severe lichen sclerosus. The left labia minora is almost completely conglutinated, the clitoris is entrapped in the retracted tissue. Severe acquired genital arousal disorder, with acquired anorgasmia, may be the correlated female sexual disorder. Courtesy of A. Graziottin, 2006.

dyspareunia, particularly in the postmenopausal years (Fig. 19.3) [33].

4 The skin of the labia minora is covered by regularly distributed, soft micropapillae. Irregularly distributed papillae, with harder consistency, are suggestive of papillomavirus (HPV) infections (condylomata). Physiologic papillae should be differentiated from condylomata [40]. This sexually transmitted disease requires topically invasive physical and/or pharmacologic treatment and may be associated with acquired sexual dysfunctions (vulvodynia contributing to acquired dyspareunia).

5 Retracting scars from episiotomy/rraphy [41], vestibulectomy, or perineal surgery [42] may be associated with vaginal dryness, acquired genital arousal difficulties, and acquired introital dyspareunia, as pain is the strongest reflex inhibitor of vaginal lubrication.

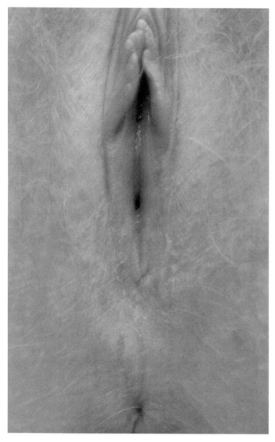

Fig. 19.2 Progressive lichen sclerosus in a 32-year-old woman complaining of lifelong hypoactive sexual desire disorders and anorgasmia. Courtesy of A. Graziottin, 2006.

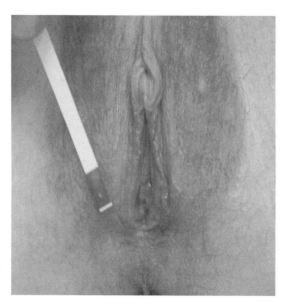

Fig. 19.3 Normal aging. Vulvar and vaginal aging in a 57-year-old postmenopausal woman, not using hormonal therapy. She complains of vaginal dryness, difficulty in getting aroused, introital dyspareunia and orgasmic difficulties. Courtesy of A. Graziottin, 2006.

6 The vulvar vestibule is increasingly involved in inflammatory states (vulvar vestibulitis, VV), with bacterial, mycotic, chemical, neurogenic, or allergic etiology [43]. Reddening of the vestibular area is associated with, but not pathognomonic of, vulvar vestibulitis (Figs 19.4 and 19.5). Exquisite tenderness at 5 o'clock and 7 o'clock of the vaginal introitus, on the external side of the hymen, at the exit of the Bartholin's duct, is a key symptom of VV, which is the leading etiology of chronic dyspareunia in the fertile age (see Chapter 25).

7 Reddening of the vulvar region, with edema, swelling of the labia, itching, and pain is caused by candida infection. It causes introital dyspareunia.

Recurrent candida is one of the precipitating etiologies of VV. For more details see Chapter 25).

8 Ritual female genital mutilation may be responsible for major changes in the vulvar anatomy (Fig. 19.6). However, after laser de-infibulation the underneath anatomy may appear more maintained than expected when observing the modified genitals (Fig. 19.7). This maintenance may concur with the reported persistence of a normal sexual response, in spite of gross anatomic changes (see Chapter 25), in many women who have undergone genital mutilation.

The **vagina** extends from the vestibule to the uterine cervix and posterior fornix and connects the uterus with the external genitals. It has four walls and is composed of mucosa (stratified squamous epithelium), lamina propria, and the muscularis, which is composed of an outer longitudinal and an inner circular layer of smooth muscle fibers [2,28].

The **hymen vaginae** is a thin fold of mucous membrane, seen just within the vaginal orifice, that varies greatly in appearance. It may be absent, may

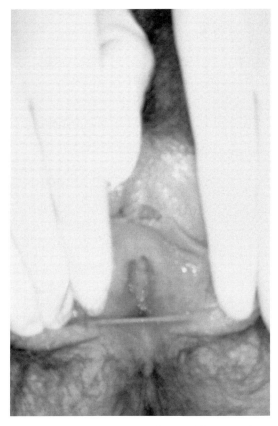

Fig. 19.4 Vulvar vestibulitis: reddening of the introital mucosa is visible at 5 and 7, when looking at the vaginal entry as a clock-face. Courtesy of A. Graziottin, 2006.

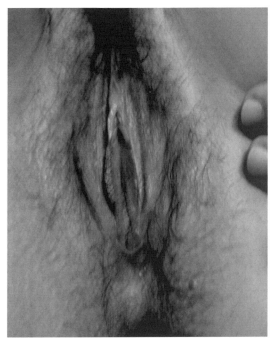

Fig. 19.5 Vulvitis and vulvar vestibulitis: diffuse reddening of the introital mucosa is clearly visible, as the inflammation covers all the area of the vestibule. It extends to the fourchette and part of the centrum tendineum, thus indicating a larger vulvar involvement. Courtesy of A. Graziottin, 2006.

Fig. 19.6 Female genital mutilation. The vulvar anatomy is disrupted. The labia have been fused, the glands of the clitoris is no longer visible, a tiny opening indicates the vaginal entrance, sufficient only for the menstrual blood to flow. Courtesy of Dr Lucrezia Catania, 2005.

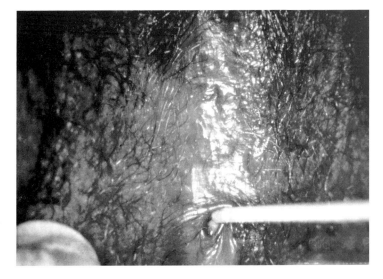

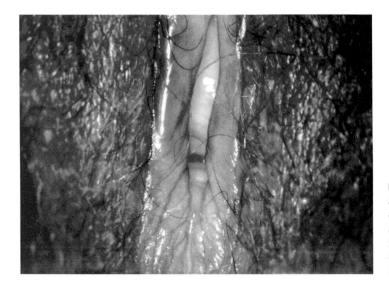

Fig. 19.7 Female genital mutilation, after laser de-infibulation. After excision, the vaginal mucosa shows a normal appearance and allows intercourse without pain. Coital orgasm is reported. Courtesy of Dr Lucrezia Catania, 2005.

or may not rupture with sexual activity, or be particularly fibrous and thick, thus contributing to introital dyspareunia. Its remnants after rupture are small round "carunculae hymenales" [2,28,34].

The **greater vestibular (Bartholin's) glands** lie deep to the cavernosal bulbs, between those structures and the lateral or outer aspect of the distal vaginal wall [2,28,34].

For descriptive purposes, reproductive organs lying within the body cavity such as ovaries, uterus and fallopian tubes are grouped as **internal genitalia**. The uterus may be involved in the orgasmic response. However, the research on the effect of hysterectomy on female sexual functioning is not conclusive.

During sexual quiescence, the vagina is a potential space with an H-shaped transverse cross-section and an elongated S-shaped longitudinal section. Grafenberg described the G (Grafenberg) spot of the anterior vagina along the urethra, and reported that stimulation of this spot gave special sexual pleasure and orgasm for women [44]. Perry and Whipple [45,46] named this sensitive area the Grafenberg, or G spot, in honour of Dr. Grafenberg. Other investigators could not locate a spot, but found, rather than a spot, a general excitable area along the whole length of the urethra running along the anterior vaginal wall [47]. Type 5 phosphodiesterase is expressed in

the anterior wall of the human vagina [36,48]. For more details see Chapter 24.

Clinical relevance

The vagina is the key organ of women's physical receptivity. The quality of vaginal trophism is mediated by the level of tissue estrogens [33], which determine: (1) the mucosal trophism; (2) the vaginal wall elasticity and resistance to coital microtraumas; (3) the responsiveness of perivaginal vessels as mediator of the genital arousal, with vaginal congestion and lubrication [22,49,50]; (4) the vaginal ecosystem, with the leading Doderlein bacilli, responsible for the maintenance of vaginal acidity at pH around 4, which contributes to the biologic defense of the vagina against invasive germs, mostly saprophytic pathogens of colonic origin [33].

The clinical evaluation of vaginal pH (see Figs 19.1 and 19.3) may help the clinician to diagnose tissue hypoestrogenism and altered ecosystem [33]. The former may contribute to genital arousal disorder (see Chapter 23), the latter to dyspareunia (see Chapter 25).

The urogenital triangle and pelvic floor muscles

The pelvic floor muscles in both men and women have the same composition: the pubococcygeous and the coccygeous muscles form the muscular diaphragm that supports the pelvic viscera and opposes the downward thrust produced by increases in intra-abdominal pressure. In both genders, the urogenital region consists of superficial and deep spaces created by the bulbospongiosus, ischiocavernosus, sphincter urethrae, and the transversus perinei superficialis and profundus [2,28,30–32].

In women, the bulbospongiosus surrounds the orifice of the vagina, covering the lateral parts of the vestibular bulb. Anteriorly, it becomes attached to the body of the clitoris and similarly compresses the female deep dorsal vein, enabling erection of the clitoral tissue.

The ischiocavernosus is typically smaller in women, and covers the unattached surface of the crura clitoridis, compressing these and retarding the outflow of venous blood during sexual arousal to assist in maintaining clitoral erection. Similarly, the transversus perinei profundus and the sphincter urethrae perform identical functions in both genders [2,28,30–32].

Clinical relevance

The integrity of the pelvic floor muscles is important in both sexes [18,28,30–32]. Co-morbidity of urologic, proctologic, and pelvic floor-related conditions adversely influences sexual function in men and women [51]. However, the vulnerability to anatomic and functional damages is higher in women as the result of reproductive events [30–32,41,42]. Lesion of the medial fiber of the pubococcygeus at delivery may cause an impairment of vaginal sensitivity during thrusting, and contribute to postpartum orgasmic difficulties, besides contributing to stress incontinence [30–32,41,42,52]. Defects of the hiatus are responsible for many pathologic entities such as cystocele, rectocele (Fig. 19.8), uterine prolaps which may all cause sexual problems for the woman [30–32,41,42,52].

At the opposite end of the spectrum, hyperactivity of the pelvic floor muscles is associated with vaginismus, dyspareunia, and vulvar vestibulitis, and to postcoital bladder irritative symptoms such as frequency, urgency, and the elusive "urethral syndrome" [42,43]. Co-morbidity between lower urinary tract symptoms and dyspareunia is a fre-

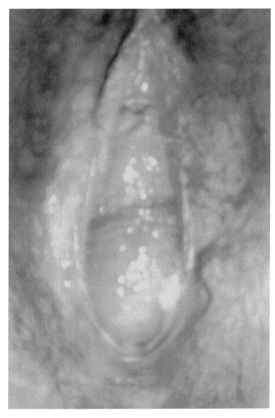

Fig. 19.8 Cystocele and rectocele in a 65-year-old woman complaining of vaginal dryness, lack of vaginal sensations, and anorgasmia. Severe hypotonus of the levator ani is present, with co-morbid moderate stress incontinence. Courtesy of A.Graziottin, 2006.

quent and still neglected clinical association, with an odds ratio of 7.62, according to Laumann *et al.* [53]. It is likely that hyperactivity of the pelvic floor is one of the key factors contributing to this co-morbidity [54] (see Chapter 25).

Observation and clinical examination of the external genitalia may indicate the tonus of the elevator ani [54]:

1 Hyperactivity of the muscle is associated with a retraction of the area between the fourchette and the anus, and is suggestive of vaginismus or acquired dyspareunia and coital orgasmic difficulties.

2 Hypotonicity of the muscle is associated with cystocele and or rectocele (Fig. 19.8).

Genital Vascular Anatomy

The genitals have a rich artery blood supply [2,28]. The labia are supplied from the inferior perineal and posterior labial branches of the internal pudendal artery as well as from superficial branches from the femoral artery. The clitoris is supplied form the ileohypogastric pudendal arterial bed. After the internal iliac artery has given off its last anterior branch, it transverses Alcock's canal and terminates as the common clitoral artery, which gives off the clitoral cavernosal arteries and the dorsal clitoral artery. The proximal (middle) part of the vagina is supplied by the vaginal branches of the uterine artery and the hypogastric artery. The distal part of the vagina is supplied by the middle hemorrhoidal and clitoral arteries (Fig. 19.9) [2,28,49,50].

Clinical relevance

The integrity and dynamic responsiveness of vaginal vessels to sexual stimuli, mediated through the neurovascular pathways, is a key contributor of genital arousal response. Factors—such as smoking, cardiovascular diseases, hypertension, diabetes, atherosclerosis—affecting the integrity of vessels may contribute to FSD, especially to genital arousal disorders [55–57] (see also Chapter 23).

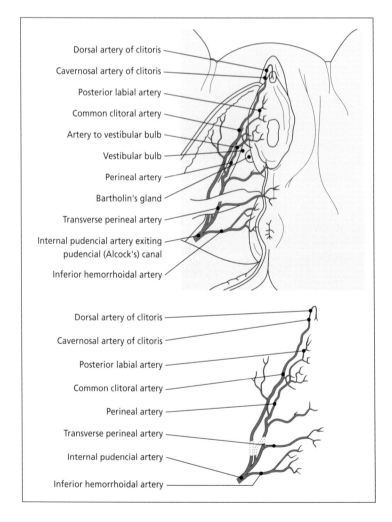

Fig. 19.9 Arterial inflow to the external female genitalia. Redrawn with permission from [63].

Peripheral Neurophysiology

There is limited understanding of the precise location of the autonomic neurovascular structures related to the uterus, cervix, and vagina. Uterine nerves arise from the inferior hypogastric plexus formed by the union of the hypogastric nerves (sympathetic T10–L1) and the splanchnic fibers (parasympathetic S2–S4). This plexus has three portions: vesical plexus, the rectal plexus, and the uterovaginal plexus, which lies at the base of the broad ligament, dorsal to the uterine vessels and lateral to the uterosacral and cardinal ligament. This plexus provides innervation via the cardial ligament and uterosacral ligaments to the cervix, upper vagina, urethra, vestibular bulbs, and clitoris. At the cervix, sympathetic and parasympathetic nerves form the paracervical ganglia. The larger one is called the uterine cervical ganglion. It is at this level that injury to the autonomic fibers of the vagina, labia, and cervix may occur during hysterectomy. The pudendal nerve (S2–S4) reaches the perineum through Alcock's canal and provides sensory and motor innervation to the genitalia (Figs 19.10 and 19.11).

As such, the anatomic structures involved in the female genital sexual response are innervated by autonomic and somatic nerves: (1) the pelvic nerve issuing from level S2–S4 of the spinal cord (parasympathetic); (2) the hypogastric and lumbosacral chain issuing from level (T12–L2) of the spinal cord (sympathetic); (3) the pudendal nerve (somatic) with cell bodies of the motoneurons located in the Onuf's nucleus (S2–S4); and (4) the vagus nerve issuing from the nucleus tractus solitaries. For review see [58].

Sensory stimuli relevant to sexual function are conveyed by afferent pathways consisting of pudendal, pelvic and hypogastric nerves and the lumbosacral sympathetic chain. They relay information to the dorsal horn, medial central and lateral gray matter of the lumbosacral spinal cord, and the vagal afferent fibers convey sensory information from the genital apparatus to the nucleus tractus solitarus (NTS) [58].

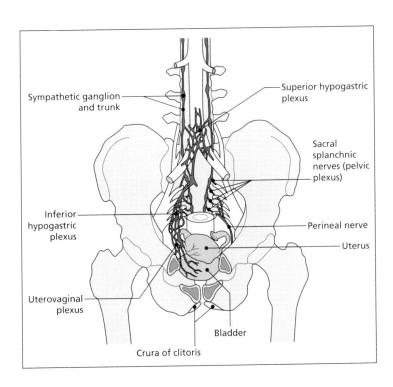

Fig. 19.10 Autonomic and somatic innervation of the female genitals. Redrawn with permission from [63].

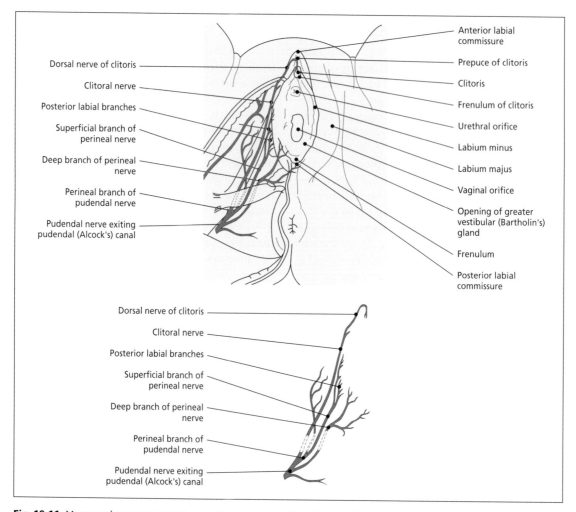

Fig. 19.11 Motor and sensory nerves innervating the external female genitalia. Redrawn with permission from [63].

Genital Physiological Response During Sexual Arousal

During female sexual arousal the blood flow to the genitals is increased in the clitoris, the labia, and the vagina leading to vasocongestion, engorgement, and lubrication [22,49,50,58–61]. Furthermore orgasm may involve rhythmic contractions of the pelvic striated circumvaginal musculature, often with concomitant uterine and anal contractions [58]. For more details see Chapter 24.

Vaginal lubrication is a consequence of the increased blood flow. During the non-aroused state the anterior and posterior walls are normally collapsed and touch each other. Nevertheless, they do not adhere as they are covered with a thin layer of basal fluid, allowing them to separate easily. As such, the fluid is a mixture of secretions from the whole genital tract. This is mainly a vaginal plasma transudate mixed with desquamated cervical and vaginal cells and cervical secretion. No glandular elements have ever been identified in the normal human vagina

[22,49,50]. The vaginal transudate is formed from the blood, slowly circulating through the capillaries supplying the vaginal epithelium. A plasma filtrate from the blood leaks out of the capillaries into the interstitial tissue space. In the vagina the fluid then passes through the epithelium. In the sexually unstimulated state the vaginal fluid has a higher K^+ and lower Na^+ concentration throughout the phases of the menstrual cycle [50]. In the non-sexually stimulated state there is a slow passage through the epithelium in balance with reabsorption; this leads to the just-moist vagina, but not moistened enough to allow penetration without pain. The slow blood circulation also results in a hypoxic lumen with low oxygen tension [22,49,50]. During sexual arousal, the blood flow to the vaginal epithelium is rapidly increased as a consequence of neural innervation via the sacral anterior nerves (the parasympathetic pathway (pelvic nerve) [62]. The increased blood flow results in an increased volume of ultrafiltrate percolating between the vaginal epithelial cells, saturating the reabsorption capacity and thereby the excess of fluid accumulates at the vaginal surface as a clear, slippery and smooth lubricant, moistening the vagina so that painless penetration and thrusting is possible. Despite many inaccurate accounts in physiology textbooks, vaginal lubrication during sexual arousal does not occur from increased secretion of vaginal glands.

Activation of the sympathetic nervous system occurs during the later stages of arousal and orgasm and is responsible for the increase in heart rate and blood pressure in women [58].

During the arousal response there is a relaxation of the trabecular smooth muscle in the clitoris and the clitoral blood flow increases. This leads to a rise in intraclitoral pressure, with increased tumescence and engorgement [22,58–62]. As the tunica of the clitoris is elastic, no veno-occlusive mechanism occurs such as that seen in the penis.

Neurotransmitters of importance for the arousal response

Several adrenergic, cholinergic, and nonadrenergic-noncholinergic (NANC) neurotransmitters/mediators have been identified in the female genital tract (epinephrine, acetylcholine, vasoactive intestinal polypeptide, nitric oxide synthase, neuropeptide Y, calcitonin gene-related peptide, substance P, pituitary adenylate cyclase-activating polypeptide, helospectine, and peptide histidine methionine) [22,49,50]. There remains a lack of knowledge of which mediators are crucial in the regulation of female genital arousal response [50]. Vasoactive intestinal polypeptide (VIP) has traditionally been considered the most important neurotransmitter in the regulation of vaginal blood flow [22], but nitric oxide (NO) has also been identified as an important mediator of increased blood flow to the female genitals during arousal, based on human and animal studies [36,48]. However, the exact roles of these and other neurotransmitters/mediators in the physiologic and pathophysiologic arousal response require need further investigation.

In summary, during sexual stimulation, the genital female sexual arousal response is elicited by sensory stimulation as well as central nervous system activation. This culminates in a series of vasocongestive as well as neuromuscular events leading to physiologic changes—vaginal lubrication, increased length and width of the clitoris, engorgement of the labia as well as increased sensitivity of the genitalia—representing the physiologic genital arousal response in women.

Conclusion

The re-reading of women's anatomy and physiology with the clinical perspective of an updated sexual medicine is a necessary prerequisite for a better understanding of biologic contributors in women's sexual function and dysfunction. However, for the sake of conciseness, the description in this chapter covers only some of the aspects of anatomy and physiology of importance for sexual function in women.

The potential clinical relevance of the physical examination has been stressed with the aim of stimulating a closer examination of the biologic conditions potentially associated with female sexual disorders.

This is of special relevance when genital arousal disorders, dyspareunia, and vaginismus are complained of. However, the clinical examination should be performed in any female sexual disorder, as anatomic and/or genital dysfunctional problems may contribute to lifelong or acquired desire and/or orgasmic disorders.

References

1 Solms M, Turnbull O. *The Brain and the Inner World*. London: Karnac Books, 2002.

2 Gray H. Clemente CD, eds. *Gray's Anatomy of the Human Body*. 30th edn. Philadelphia, PA: Lea & Febiger, 1985.

3 Netter FH. *Nervous System: Anatomy and Physiology*. The Ciba Collection of Medical Illustrations. 1983.

4 LeVay S. *The Sexual Brain*. Cambridge, MA: MIT Press, 1994.

5 Panksepp J. *Affective Neuroscience: The Foundations of Human and Animal Emotions* (Series in Affective Science). New York: Oxford University Press, 1998.

6 Bloom FE, Kupfer D, eds. *Psychopharmacology: The Fourth Generation of Progress*. New York: Raven Press, 1995.

7 Pfaus JG, Everitt BJ. The psychopharmacology of sexual behaviour. In: FE Bloom, D Kupfer, eds. *Psychopharmacology: The Fourth Generation of Progress*. New York: Raven Press, 1995, pp. 743–758.

8 Meston CM, Frohlich PF. The neurobiology of sexual function. *Arch Gen Psychiatry* 2000;**57**:1012–1030.

9 Graziottin A. Similarities and differences between male and female sexual dysfunctions. In Kandeel F, Lue T, Pryor J, Swerdloff R, eds. *Male Sexual Dysfunction: Pathophysiology and Treatment*. New York: Marcel Dekker, 2006 (in press).

10 Anderson SW, Bechara A, Damasio H, Tranel D, Damasio AR. Impairment of social and moral behavior related to early damage in human prefrontal cortex. *Nat Neurosci* 1999;**2**(11):1032–1037.

11 Kafka MP. Hypersexual desire in males: an operational definition and clinical implications for males with paraphylias and paraphylia-related disorders. *Arch Sex Behav* 1997;**26**(5):505–526.

12 Levine SB. The nature of sexual desire: a clinician's perspective. *Arch Sex Behav* 2003;**32**(3):279–285.

13 Emanuele E, Politi P, Bianchi M *et al.* Raised plasma nerve growth factor levels associated with early-stage romantic love. *Psychoneuroendocrinology* 2006;**31**(3): 288–294.

14 Springer PS, Deutsch G. *Left Brain, Right Brain: Perspectives from Cognitive Neuroscience*. New York: WH Freeman, 1988.

15 Graziottin A. Libido: the biologic scenario. *Maturitas* 2000;**34**(suppl 1):S9–S16.

16 Basson R. Women's desire deficiencies and avoidance. In: Levine SB, Risen CB, Althof SE, eds. *Handbook of Clinical Sexuality for Mental Health Professionals*. New York: Brunner Routledge, 2003, pp. 111–130.

17 Basson R, Leiblum S, Brotto L, Derogatis L, Fourcroy J, Fugl-Meyer K, Graziottin A, Heiman JR, Laan E, Meston C, Schover L, van Lankveld J, Schultz WW. Definitions of women's sexual dysfunction reconsidered: advocating expansion and revision. *J Psychosom Obstet Gynaecol* 2003;**24**:221–229.

18 Plaut M, Graziottin A, Heaton J. *Sexual Dysfunctions*. Fast Fact Series. Oxford: Health Press, 2004.

19 Arimondi C, Vannelli GB, Balboni GC. Importance of olfaction in sexual life: morpho-functional and psychological studies in man. *Biomed Res (India)* 1993;**4**:43–52.

20 Grammer K, Fink B, Neave N. Human pheromones and sexual attraction. *Eur J Obst Gynecol* 2005;**118**:135–142.

21 Komisaruk B, Whipple B. Brain activity imaging during sexual response in women with spinal cord injury. In: Hyde J, ed. *Biological Substrates of Human Sexuality*. Washington, DC: American Psychological Association, 2005, pp. 109–146.

22 Levin RJ. The physiology of sexual arousal in the human female: a recreational and procreational synthesis *Arch Sex Behav* 2002;**31**(5):405–411.

23 Mah K, Binik YM. The nature of human orgasm: a critical review of major trends. *Clin Psychol Rev* 2001;**21**(6): 823–856.

24 Meston CM, Hull E, Levin RJ, Sipski M. Disorders of orgasm in women *J Sex Med* 2004;**1**(1):66–68.

25 LeDoux J. *The Emotional Brain*. London: Weidenfeld & Nicolson, 1996.

26 Bradford C. Meston CM. The impact of anxiety on sexual arousal in women. *Behav Res Ther* 2005;**4**:206–209.

27 Hamann S. Sex differences in the responses of the human amygdala. *Neuroscientist* 2005;**11**(4):288–93. Review.

28 Netter FH. *The Ciba Collection of Medical Illustrations: Reproductive System*. Vol 2. Summit, NJ: Ciba Pharmaceuticals, 1979, pp. 89–123.

29 Andersen KV, Bovim G. Impotence and nerve entrapment in long distance amateur cyclists. *Acta Neurol Scand* 1997;**95**(4):233–240.

30 Bourcier AP, McGuire EJ, Abrams P. *Pelvic Floor Disorders*. Philadephia, PA: Elsevier Saunders, 2004.

31 Raz S. *Female Urology*. Philadelphia, PA: WB Saunders, 1983.

32 Kursh ED, McGuire EJ. *Female Urology*. Philadelphia, PA: JB Lippincott, 1994.

33 Graziottin A. Sexuality in postmenopause and senium. In: Lauritzen C, Studd J, eds. *Current Management of the Menopause*. London: Martin Dunitz, 2003, pp. 185–203.

34 O'Connell HE, Sanjeevan KV. Anatomy of female genitalia. In: Goldstein I, Meston C, Davis SR, Traish A, eds. *Women's Sexual Function and Dysfunction: Study, Diagnosis and Treatment*. London: Taylor & Francis, 2006, pp. 105–112.

35 Tarcan T, Park K, Goldstein I, Maio G, Fassina A, Krane RJ, Azadzoi KM. Histomorphometric analysis of age-related structural changes in human clitoral cavernosal tissue. *J Urol* 1999;**161**(3):940–944.

36 Jannini EA, D'Amati G, Lenzi A. Histology and immunohistochemical studies of female genital tissue. In: Goldstein, I., Meston, C., Davis, S. R, Traish, A, eds. *Women's Sexual Function and Dysfunction: Study, Diagnosis and Treatment*. London: Taylor & Francis, 2006, pp. 125–148.

37 Al-Bassam A, Gado A. Feminizing genital reconstruction: experience with 52 cases of ambiguous genitalia. *Eur J Pediatr Surg* 2004;**14**(3):172–178.

38 Leiblum SR, Nathan S. Persistent sexual arousal syndrome in women: a not uncommon but little recognized complaint. *Sex Relat Ther* 2002;**17**(2):191–198.

39 Val I, Almeida G. An overview of lichen sclerosus. *Clin Obstet Gynecol* 2005;**48**(4):808–817. Review.

40 Dupin N. Genital warts. *Clin Dermatol* 2004;**22**(6): 481–486. Review.

41 Glazener C. Sexual function after childbirth: women's experiences, persistent morbidity and lack of professional recognition. *Br J Obstet Gynaecol* 1997;**104**:330–335.

42 Graziottin A. Etiology and diagnosis of coital pain. *J Endocrinol Invest* 2003;**26**(suppl 3):115–121.

43 Graziottin A, Brotto LA. Vulvar vestibulitis syndrome: a clinical approach. *J Sex Marital Ther* 2004;**30**:125–139.

44 Grafenberg, E. The role of urethra in the female orgasm. *Int J Sexology* 1950;**3**:145–148.

45 Perry JD, Whipple B. Pelvic muscle strength of female ejaculators: evidence in support of a new theory of orgasm. *J Sex Res* 1981;**17**:22–39.

46 Perry JD, Whipple B. Multiple components of the female orgasm. In Graber B. (ed.) *Circumvaginal Musculature and Sexual Function*. New York: S. Karger, 1982, pp. 101–114.

47 Meston C, Hull E, Levin RJ, Sipski M. Women's orgasm. Lue TF, Basson R, Rosen R, Giuliano F, Khoury S, Montorsi F. *Sexual Medicine: Sexual Dysfunctions in Men and Women*. 2nd edn. Paris: Health Publications, 2004, pp. 783–850.

48 D'Amati G, di Gioia CR, Bologna M *et al.* Type 5 phosphodiesterase expression in the human vagina. *Urology* 2002;**60**(1):191–195.

49 Levin RJ. The ins and outs of vaginal lubrication. *Sex Relat Ther* 2003;**18**(4):509–513.

50 Giraldi A, Levin RJ. Vascular physiology of female sexual function. In: Goldstein I, Meston C, Davis SR, Traish A, eds. *Women's Sexual Function and Dysfunction: Study, Diagnosis and Treatment*. London: Taylor & Francis, 2006, pp. 174–180.

51 Wesselmann U, Burnett AL, Heinberg LJ. The urogenital and rectal pain syndromes. *Pain* 1997;**73**(3):269–294.

52 Kegel AH. Sexual functions of the pubococcygeus muscle. *West J Surg Obstet Gynecol* 1952;**60**(10):521–524.

53 Laumann EO, Paik A, Rosen RC. Sexual dysfunction in the United States: prevalence and predictors. *JAMA* 1999;**281**(6):537–544.

54 Graziottin A. Female sexual dysfunction. In: Bo K, Berghmans B, van Kampen M, Morkved S, eds. *Evidence Based Physiotherapy For The Pelvic Floor: Bridging Research and Clinical Practice*. Oxford: Elsevier, 2006 (in press)

55 Goldstein I, Berman JR. Vasculogenic female sexual dysfunction: vaginal engorement and clitoral erectile insufficiency syndromes. *Int J Impot Res* 1998;**10**(suppl 2):S84–S90.

56 Addis IB, Ireland CC, Vittinghoff *et al.* Sexual activity and function in postmenopausal women with heart disease. *Obstet Gynecol* 2005;**106**:121–127.

57 Rutherford D, Collins A. Sexual dysfunction in women with diabetes mellitus. *Gynecol Endocrinol* 2005;**21**:189–192.

58 Giuliano F, Julia-Guilloteau V. Neurophysiology of female genital sexual response. In: Goldstein I, Meston C, Davis SR, Traish A, eds. *Women's Sexual Function and Dysfunction: Study, Diagnosis and Treatment*. London: Taylor & Francis, 2006, pp. 168–173.

59 Berman JR, Berman LA, Werbin TJ, Flaherty EE, Leahy NM, Goldstein I. Clinical evaluation of female sexual function: effects of age and estrogen status on subjective and physiologic sexual responses. *Int J Impot Res* 1999;**11**(suppl 1):S31–S38.

60 Deliganis AV, Maravilla KR, Heiman JR, Carter WO, Garland PA, Peterson BT, Hackbert L, Cao Y, Weisskoff RM. Female genitalia: dynamic MR imaging with use of MS-325 initial experiences evaluating female sexual response. *Radiology* 2002;**225**(3):791–799.

61 Maravilla KR, Cao Y, Heiman JR, Garland PA, Peterson BT, Carter WO, Weisskoff RM. Serial MR imaging with

MS-325 for evaluating female sexual arousal response: determination of intrasubject reproducibility. *J Magn Reson Imaging* 2003;**18**(2):216–224.

62 Giuliano F, Rampin O, Allard J. Neurophysiology and pharmacology of female genital sexual response. *J Sex Marital Ther* 2002;**28**(suppl 1):101–121.

63 Goldstein I, Heiman J, Johannes C, Laan E, Levin RL, McKenna KE. Female sexual dysfunction. In: Jardin A, Wagner G, Khoury S, Giuliano F, Padma-Nathan H, Rosen R, eds. *Erectile Dysfunction. 1st International Consultation on Erectile Dysfunction.* 1st edn. Plymouth: Plymbridge Distributors Ltd, 2000, pp. 507–556.

CHAPTER 20

Classification, Etiology, and Key Issues in Female Sexual Disorders

Alessandra Graziottin, Lorraine Dennerstein, Jeanne L. Alexander, Annamaria Giraldi, and Beverly Whipple

This chapter will summarize the leading characteristics of women's sexuality, to give a comprehensive view of the key factors in sexual health [1,12]. The most updated classification will be presented, with a focus on descriptors essential to qualify the disorders with a few questions [3]. Two concise paragraphs on ethical, legal, and moral issues [1,4–6], and on optimal referral will be presented [4,7].

Leading Characteristics of Women's Sexuality

Women's sexuality is *multifactorial*, rooted in biologic, psychosexual, and context-related factors [1,3,4,7–16]. The latter include couple dynamics, family and sociocultural issues and developmental factors, including sexual abuse [17–19].

Sexuality is also multisystemic: in men and women, a physiologic response requires the integrity of the hormonal, vascular, nervous, muscular, connective, and immune systems—a fact too often overlooked in women, until recently [7,15,16,20–25].

Three major dimensions—*female sexual identity, sexual function and sexual relationship*—interact to define women's sexual health [7,15,22]. Women's sexuality varies over the life cycle and is dependent on biologic (reproductive events) as well as personal, current contextual, and relationship variables [13,26]. Female sexual problems are age related, progressive, and highly prevalent, affecting up to 43% of women [27–31]. More importantly, a third to half of women who were defined as having a prob-

lem regarded the problem as distressing [30,32]. These sexual problems appear to increase with both menopause and with age [33–37]. Sexual disorder, among both men and women, has been associated with poor quality of life, lower perception of well-being, lower self-esteem, poor self-image, poor relationship quality, and depression and anxiety [38–40].

Female sexual problems may occur along a continuum from *dissatisfaction* (with potential integrity of the physiologic response but emotional/affective frustration), to *dysfunction* (with or without pathological modifications), to *severe pathology*, biologically rooted [26,41]. *Pelvic floor disorders* are among the most important and yet neglected medical contributors to women's sexual disorders [42–44].

Sexual dissatisfaction, disinterest and even dysfunction may occur in conjunction with male sexual disorders or in the context of an abusive relationship. Female sexual problems should not all be labelled per se as "diseases" or dysfunctions requiring medical treatment [30]. Low levels of female sexual function may occur with or without significant personal (and interpersonal) *distress* [9,30,45]. For example, although female sexual function declines with age and incrementally with menopause [46], women become less distressed about low sexual function with age [47].

Sociocultural factors may further modulate the perception, expression, and complaining modality—that is, the "wording"—of a sexual disorder. The *meaning* of sexual intimacy is a strong modulator of sexual response and of the quality of satisfaction the woman experiences, in addition to physical response [4,19,48–50]. The quality of feelings for the partner, change in relationship status, and length of the relationship, also significantly affect female sexual function [9,51].

Sexual problems reported by women are not discrete and often co-occur, *co-morbidity* being one of the leading characteristics of female sexual disorders [13,26]. Co-morbidity between *female sexual disorder and medical conditions*—urologic, gynecologic, proctologic, dysmetabolic, cardiovascular and nervous diseases, to mention a few—is beginning to be recognized [15,22,44,52,53]. For example, latent classes analysis of sexual dysfunctions by risk factors in women indicate that urinary tract symptoms have a RR = 4.02 (2.75–5.89) of being associated with arousal disorders, and a RR = 7.61 (4.06–14.26) of being associated with sexual pain disorders, according to the epidemiologic survey of Laumann and colleagues [27]. The attention dedicated to FSD-related co-morbidities—both between FSD subtypes and between FSD and medical conditions—in this document reflects the clinical relevance of this association, especially in the urogynecologic and proctologic domains.

Psychiatric co-morbidity impacts sexual function to different degrees in each individual, with past sexual trauma, eating disorders, or histrionic personality disorder [54–58] having some impact on sexual function. As many as 70% of patients with depression report a decline in libido [59]. The greater prevalence of anxiety disorders (30.5% to 19.2%) and depressive disorders (21% to 13%) in women in comparison to men increases the importance of evaluating and treating psychiatric co-morbidity [60].

Classification of Female Sexual Disorders

Over the last decades, classification of FSD has undergone intense scrutiny and revisions, which mirrors the new understanding of its complex etiology. Until a decade ago, the classification of FSD, which constitutes the frame of reference for an appropriate diagnosis, was focused almost entirely on its psychologic and relational components. Indeed, FSD were included in the broader manual of "psychiatric" disorders [61,62]. The first and second consensus conferences on FSD [3,13] set out to define women's sexual disorders, with special attention given to bringing together the current level of evidence with definitions fitting women's wording and experiences. The latest classification is reported in Table 20.1.

Clinical History

For a more comprehensive account of sexual concerns or complaints, healthcare providers should also investigate the so-called "descriptors" of the disorders, as defined by the International Consensus Conferences held in 1998 and 2003 [3,13]. They include:

1 The etiology of the disorder, further detailed in predisposing, precipitating, and maintaining factors (Tables 20.2a, 20.2b, and 20.2c) [15,63–65]. Each category includes biologic, psychosexual, and contextual causes.

  (a) Biologic descriptors include hormonal factors, pelvic floor disorders [43,44], cardiovascular problems, neurologic conditions (particularly pain related) [14,66], metabolic disorders (diabetes, adrenal, and thyroid dysfunction), affective disorders, and anxiety. All the medical conditions that may directly or indirectly affect sexuality, through their multisystemic impact and/or the consequences of pharmacologic, surgical, and/or radiotherapeutic treatment, should be considered in the differential diagnosis of potential contributors to reported FSD. Decline in sex steroids, consequent to natural or iatrogenic menopause, is a major contributor to FSD [9,47,65].

  (b) Psychosexual descriptors refer to emotional/affective/psychic factors such as negative upbringing/losses/trauma (physical, sexual, emotional) [67,68], body image issues [69], eating disorders affecting self-esteem and self-confidence, and attachment dynamics (secure, avoidant, anxious) [17] that may also modulate the level of trust in the relationship and the intensity of the commitment, and the confidence in loving and longstanding attitudes toward affective and erotic intimacy.

Table 20.1 Classification of female sexual disorders.

Women's sexual interest/desire disorder

There are absent or diminished feelings of sexual interest or desire, absent sexual thoughts or fantasies and a lack of responsive desire. Motivations (here defined as reasons/incentives), for attempting to become sexually aroused are scarce or absent. The lack of interest is considered to be more than that due to a normative lessening with the life cycle and length of a relationship.

Sexual aversion disorder

Extreme anxiety and/or disgust at the anticipation of/or attempt to have any sexual activity.

Subjective sexual arousal disorder

Absence of, or markedly diminished cognitive sexual arousal and sexual pleasure from any type of sexual stimulation. Vaginal lubrication or other signs of physical response still occur.

Genital sexual arousal disorder

Complaints of absent or impaired genital sexual arousal. Self-report may include minimal vulval swelling or vaginal lubrication from any type of sexual stimulation and reduced sexual sensations from caressing genitalia. Subjective sexual excitement still occurs from non-genital sexual stimuli.

Combined genital and subjective arousal disorder

Absence of, or markedly diminished subjective sexual excitement and awareness of sexual pleasure from any type of sexual stimulation, as well as complaints of absent or impaired genital sexual arousal (vulval swelling, lubrication).

Persistent sexual arousal disorder

Spontaneous, intrusive and unwanted genital arousal (e.g. tingling, throbbing, pulsating) in the absence of sexual interest and desire. Any awareness of subjective arousal is typically but not invariably unpleasant. The arousal is unrelieved by one or more orgasms and the feelings of arousal persist for hours or days.

Women's orgasmic disorder

Despite the self-report of high sexual arousal/excitement, there is either lack of orgasm, markedly diminished intensity of orgasmic sensations or marked delay of orgasm from any kind of stimulation.

Dyspareunia

Persistent or recurrent pain with attempted or complete vaginal entry and/or penile vaginal intercourse.

Vaginismus

The persistent or recurrent difficulties of the woman to allow vaginal entry of a penis, a finger, and/or any object, despite the woman's expressed wish to do so. There is often (phobic) avoidance and anticipation/fear/experience of pain, along with variable involuntary pelvic muscle contraction. Structural or other physical abnormalities must be ruled out/addressed.

From Basson *et al.* (2004) [3].

(c) Contextual descriptors include past and current significant relationships [1,68], cultural/religious restrictions [13,26], current interpersonal difficulties [19,70], partner's general health issues and/or sexual dysfunctions, inadequate stimulation, and unsatisfactory sexual and emotional contexts [50].

2 The disorder being generalized (with every partner and in every situation) or situational, specifically precipitated by partner-related or contextual factors, which should be specified [13,26]. Situational problems usually rule out medical factors that tend to affect the sexual response with a more generalized effect [53,71].

3 The disorder being lifelong (from the very first sexual experience) or acquired after months or years of satisfying sexual interaction. To ask the woman what in *her* opinion is causing the current FSD may offer useful insights into the etiology of the disorder, particularly when it is acquired [4].

4 The level of distress, which indicates a mild, moderate or severe impact of the FSD on personal life.

Table 20.2a Predisposing factors contributing to female sexual dysfunction.

Biologic
- Endocrine disorders (hypo androgenism, hypoestrogenism, hyperprolactinemia, adrenal dysfunction, thyroid dysfunction, diabetes)
- Recurrent vulvovaginitis and/or cystitis
- Pelvic floor disorders: lifelong or acquired
- Drug treatments affecting biovailability of sex steroids or neurotransmitter levels
- Chronic diseases (cardiovascular, neurologic or psychiatric diseases, and so on)
- Benign diseases (e.g. endometriosis) predisposing to iatrogenic menopause and dyspareunia
- Persistent residual conditions (e.g. dyspareunia/chronic pain associated with endometriosis)

Psychosexual
- Inadequate/delayed psychosexual development
- Borderline personality traits
- Previous negative sexual experiences: sexual coercion, violence, or abuse
- Body image issues/concerns
- Affective disorders (dysthymia, depression, mania) and anxiety disorders
- Inadequate coping strategies
- Inadequate sexual education

Contextual
- Ethnic/religious/cultural messages, expectations, and constraints regarding sexuality
- Social ambivalence towards sexual activity, when separated from reproduction or marriage
- Negative social attitudes towards female contraception
- Low socioeconomic status/reduced access to medical care and facilities
- Support network

Modified from Graziottin (2005) [75].

Table 20.2b Precipitating factors contributing to female sexual disorder.

Biologic
- Negative reproductive events (unwanted pregnancies, abortion, traumatic delivery with damage of the pelvic floor, child problems, infertility)
- Postpartum depression
- Vulvovaginitis/sexually transmitted diseases
- Sexual pain disorders
- Age at menopause
  - Premature ovarian failure (POF)—menopause before age 40
  - Premature menopause—menopause between age 40 and 45
- Biologic vs. surgical menopause (especially for premature menopause)
- Surgical menopause
  - Androgen (besides estrogen) loss
  - Associated disorder/disease
- Extent and severity of menopausal symptoms and impact on well-being
- Current disorders
- Current pharmacologic treatment
- Substance abuse (mainly alcohol and opiates)

Psychosexual
- Loss of loving feelings toward partner
- Unpleasant/humiliating sexual encounters or experiences
- Affective and anxiety disorders
- Relationship of fertility loss to fulfillment of life goals

Contextual
- Relationship discord
- Life-stage stressors (e.g. child's diseases, divorce, separation, partner infidelity)
- Loss or death of close friends or family members
- Lack of access to medical/psychosocial treatment and facilities
- Economic difficulties

Modified from Graziottin (2005) [75].

Sexual distress should be distinguished from non-sexual distress and from depression. The degree of reported distress may have implications for the woman's motivation for therapy and for prognosis.

Physical Examination

An accurate *physical* examination in any FSD complaint is important. The appropriate evaluation of potential medical factors, endocrinologic, vascular, dysmetabolic, neurologic, neuroimmunologic or iatrogenic factors, as well as the neglected role of pelvic floor disorders in contributing to and maintaining FSD, is essential to avoid both a systematic medical omission and a gender bias [1–7,12,17,72–76]. What to look for while examining the patient and the key potential findings and associated co-morbidities

Table 20.2c Maintaining factors contributing to female sexual disorder.

Biologic
- Diagnostic omissions: unaddressed predisposing/precipitating biologic etiologies
- Untreated or inadequately treated co-morbidities:
  - Physical: pelvic floor disorders
  - Urologic: incontinence, lower urinary tract symptoms, urogenital prolapse
  - Proctologic: constipation, rhagades
  - Metabolic: diabetes
  - Psychiatric: depression, anxiety, phobias
- Pharmacologic treatments
- Substance abuse
- Multisystemic changes associated with chronic disease or secondary to menopause
  - Hormonal
  - Vascular
  - Muscular
  - Neurologic
  - Immunologic
- Contraindications to hormone therapy (HT)
- Inadequacy of HT in ameliorating menopause-associated biologic symptoms

Psychosexual
- Low or loss of sexual self-confidence
- Performance anxiety
- Distress (personal, emotional, occupational, sexual)
- Diminished affection for, or attraction to, partner
- Unaddressed affective disorders (depression and/or anxiety)
- Negative perception of menopause-associated changes
- Body image concerns and increased body changes (wrinkles, body shape/weight, muscle tone)

Contextual
- Omission of FSD investigation from provider's diagnostic and therapeutic approach
- Lack of access to adequate care
- Partner's general health or sexual problems or concerns
- Ongoing interpersonal conflict (with partner or others)
- Environmental constraints (lack of privacy, lack of time)

Modified from Graziottin (2005) [75].

will be detailed in each subchapter related to women's sexual problems. In addition, there is information concerning addressing FSD in both Chapters 26 and 27.

Key point

An interdisciplinary team is a valuable resource for a patient-centered approach, both for diagnostic accuracy and tailored treatment. Disciplines that may take part in such a team of professional figures, or be available for referral, include medical sexologist, gynecologist, urologist, psychiatrist, endocrinologist, psychologist, anethesiologist, neurologist, proctologist, dermatologist, psychotherapist (individual and couple), sex therapist, and physical therapist. This latter professional is emerging as a key resource in addressing pelvic floor disorders. Clearly not all are needed in any team or for a particular consultation.

Ethical, Legal, and Counseling-Related Considerations

All patients may have sexual interests or concerns, including the elderly, those with a disability, and those with chronic illnesses. Wrong assumptions about disinterest about sex in the patient who is consulting for whatever medical reason would prevent the possibility of an open, frank, constructive, and comforting conversation in the intimate area of sexuality and sexual health.

Basic training in human sexuality, focused continuing education, and practice in counseling will give the clinician increasing confidence in dealing with sexual issues [4,76].

A positive, proactive, empathic approach to the patient's sexual life needs to convey an attitude of availability and acceptance. This requires an honest self-awareness of the healthcare provider's areas of comfort and discomfort with sexual issues. It is easy to avoid asking important questions in an area in which the clinician may feel uncomfortable. It is important to be sure to address such issues in a way that is comfortable for both the clinician and the patient and yet effective in securing the necessary information [4,76].

Healthcare providers should refrain from projecting their own values and attitudes onto those of the patient, either verbally or non-verbally. Doing so may reduce the patient's comfort and feeling of acceptance, and introduce inappropriate assumptions into the history [1,4,5].

Wording is important to ease communication: for example, one might ask "How comfortable are you with masturbation?" rather than "Have you ever masturbated?". This subject may be addressed with an opening statement such as: "Research has demonstrated that x% of people have masturbated at some point in their lives." Or, when addressing the emotionally loaded area of sexual abuse, it might be better to ask "Have you ever had an unwanted sexual experience?" rather than "Have you ever been sexually abused?" [1,4].

The healthcare provider should be aware that the topic of sexuality requires special attention to confidentiality and informed consent, depending on the profession of the clinician and on any local laws that place limits on confidentiality, such as in the reporting of sexual abuse [1,4,76].

While the discussion of sexual matters is often an appropriate part of medical evaluation and treatment, it is also important not to sexualize the clinical setting when it is not necessary. Patients may be confused or embarrassed by comments about their attractiveness, disclosure of intimate personal information by the clinician, or by sex-related questions that are not clinically relevant and justifiable. It is essential to maintain appropriate boundaries with the patient [4–6].

The modesty of the patient should be respected in touching, disrobing, and draping procedures [4]. Key aspects of appropriate counseling attitudes are summarized in Table 20.3.

Key point

Information on the quality of sexual life should be recorded *before* any medical or surgical intervention, especially when systemic diseases are diagnosed. This will have two relevant consequences—giving the patient the feeling that the clinician cares about this aspect of their life, but also preventing further litigation in the case of an undiagnosed, neglected FSD, which could then be attributed to the clinician's negligence or malpractice, after whatever medical or

Table 20.3 Talking with women patients about sexual issues.

- Be empathic and matter-of-fact
- Use simple terms
- Be sensitive to the optimal time to ask the most emotionally-charged questions
- Look for and respond to non-verbal cues that may signal discomfort or concern
- Be sensitive to the impact of emotionally charged words (e.g. "rape", "abortion")
- If you are not sure of the patient's sexual orientation, use gender-neutral language in referring to his or her partner
- Explain and justify your questions and procedures
- Teach and reassure as you examine
- Clearly explain how to relax the pelvic floor *before* any pelvic examination (urologic, gynecologic, proctologic) or exam (cystoscopy, speculum examination, colposcopy, anoscopy)
- Intervene to the extent that you are qualified and comfortable; refer to qualified medical or mental health specialists as necessary

Adapted from Plaut *et al.* (2004) [4].

surgical intervention, including assistance to operative delivery (see also Chapter 26).

Optimal Referral

Biologic, psychosexual, and couple issues may be differently relevant in the individual case and should be appropriately investigated in a careful history taking. Sexual disorders need a multidisciplinary approach, given the heterogeneity of etiologic factors and the variety of co-morbidity, both in the medical and psychosexual domain [1–4,7,72–76].

One individual clinician could become skilled in all areas but often appropriate referral is required (see Table 20.4). If the first healthcare provider diagnosing FSD is a physician, before referral, he or she should establish that the woman has one or more treatable sexual disorders, has been educated about the disorder(s), and has tried a first-line hormonal or other pharmacologic approach, when indicated and

Table 20.4 Referral resources.

- Gynecologist with special interest in sexual dysfunction: when FSD requires specialized evaluation and/or treatment, especially hormonal
- Urologist or andrologist: when the partner has erectile or ejaculatory dysfunction that is assessed to require medical intervention
- Internist or family physician with special interest in sexual medicine: for sexual dysfunctions in either partner
- Oncologist: when HT is considered for cancer survivors with premature menopause
- Psychiatrist: when depression and anxiety are precipitated by or associated with FSD
- Certified sex therapist: to address the specific psychosexual component of the woman's complaint, situational erectile dysfunction, either partner's orgasmic difficulties, as well as loss of sexual motivation in either partner (www.aasect.org)
- Couple therapist: when relationship issues are a primary contributor to the sexual dysfunction
- Individual psychotherapist: when personal psychodynamic issues are inhibiting sexual function
- Physical therapist: when hyper- or hypotonicity of pelvic floor is contributory

Adapted from Plaut *et al.* (2004) [4].

if he/she feels competent in treating the potential biologic contributors of her sexual complaint.

Generally, the woman should not currently be undergoing other significant medical interventions, so as to not overburden an already demanding emotional and physical situation. Other medical, lifestyle, and relationship issues need to be addressed before specific sexual referral [4,7,75,76].

The sexual symptoms as described by the patient can be summarized in the referral letter, along with the provisional diagnoses. Other medical problems, medications, past relevant medical and surgical interventions, and important psychologic and relationship issues should be included, together with details of management to date, plus outcome. It is helpful to end with the expectations (treat, advise, educate, operate, and so on) of the specialist and of the patient.

Such transfer of information gives the patient or couple the feeling of coordinated caring and confirms the legitimacy of their sexual complaints [4,7].

Finally, it is well known that in the couple one member could be the symptom "carrier," that is, the person who actively discloses a personal sexual problem that could have been elicited by the partner's sexual problem. In this dynamic, the latter is the "symptom inducer." This is frequent in FSD reporting when the male partner primarily suffers from loss of desire, erectile deficits, and/or ejaculatory problems or general health issues [1,4,73,74]. Evaluation of those potential co-factors of FSD and appropriate referral to specialists in male sexual dysfunctions is an essential part of a comprehensive caring [1,4,7].

Conclusion

To address the complexity of FSD requires a balanced clinical perspective between biologic and psychosexual/relational factors. Different contributors should be appropriately investigated in a careful history taking. A systematic, accurate *physical* examination in any FSD complaint is the most innovative factor to be included in a comprehensive medical diagnosis of FSD.

Apart from counseling, when the issue of FSD is openly raised by the patient, the healthcare provider can contribute to improving the quality of (sexual) life of their patients, by routinely asking them, during the clinical history taking: "Are you happy with your sexual life?" or "How's your sex life?", thus offering an overture to current or future disclosure.

Clinicians can help patients to communicate their sexual problems and concerns effectively by creating an atmosphere of acceptance and by clarifying communication. As sexuality is most often expressed in the context of a relationship, whenever possible, clinicians should take into consideration the history, need, values, and preferences of *both* members of the couple. Appropriate referral is an integral part of a competent approach to FSD.

Finally, it should be acknowledged that for many women sex is motivated by love: attention to the quality of the couple's emotional intimacy is a key aspect of the clinical consultation when addressing FSD.

References

1 Leiblum S, Rosen R. *Principles and Practice of Sex Therapy.* New York: Guilford, 2000, pp. 181–202.

2 Dennerstein L, Koochaki P, Barton I, Graziottin A. Hypoactive sexual desire disorder in menopausal women: a survey of western European women. *J Sex Med* 2006;**3**:212–22.

3 Basson R, Leiblum S, Brotto L. Revised definitions of women's sexual dysfunction. *J Sex Med* 2004;**1**:40–48.

4 Plaut M, Graziottin A, Heaton J. *Sexual Dysfunction.* Oxford: Health Press, 2004.

5 Gabbard GO, Nadelson C. Professional boundaries in the physician—patient relationship. *JAMA* 1995;**273**: 1445–1449.

6 Plaut S. Understanding and managing professional—client boundaries. In: Levine SB, Althof SE, Risen CB, eds. *Handbook of Clinical Sexuality for Mental Health Professionals.* New York: Brunner Rutledge, 2003, pp. 407–424.

7 Graziottin A, Basson R. Sexual dysfunction in women with premature menopause. *Menopause* 2004;**11**:766–777.

8 Dennerstein L, Lehert P. Modeling mid-aged women's sexual functioning: a prospective, population-based study. *J Sex Marital Ther* 2004;**30**:173–183.

9 Dennerstein L, Lehert P, Burger H. The relative effects of hormones and relationship factors on sexual function of women through the natural menopausal transition. *Fertil Steril* 2005;**84**:174–180.

10 Dennerstein G. Dyspareunia and DSM: a gynecologist's opinion. *Arch Sex Behav* 2005;**34**:28:57–61; author reply 63–67.

11 Dennerstein G. Vaginal yeast colonization in nonpregnant women: a longitudinal study. *Obstet Gynecol* 2005; **105**:1493; author reply 1494.

12 Segraves R, Balon R. *Sexual Pharmacology: Fast facts.* New York: WW Norton & Co, 2003.

13 Basson R, Berman J, Burnett A, Derogatis L, Ferguson D, Fourcroy J, Goldstein I, Graziottin A, Heiman J, Laan E, Leiblum S, Padma-Nathan H, Rosen R, Segraves K, Segraves RT, Shabsigh R, Sipski M, Wagner G, Whipple B. Report of the International Consensus Development Conference on female sexual dysfunction: definitions and classifications. *J Urol* 2000;**163**:888–893.

14 Binik YM, Reissing E, Pukall C, Flory N, Payne KA, Khalife S. The female sexual pain disorders: genital pain

or sexual dysfunction? *Arch Sex Behav* 2002; **31**:425–429.

15 Graziottin A, Brotto LA. Vulvar vestibulitis syndrome: a clinical approach. *J Sex Marital Ther* 2004;**30**:125–139.

16 Levin R. The physiology of sexual arousal in the human female: a recreational and procreational synthesis. *Arch Sex Behav* 2002;**31**:405–411.

17 Clulow C. *Adult Attachment and Couple Psychotherapy.* Hove, UK: Brunner-Routledge, 2001.

18 Basson R. Introduction to special issue on women's sexuality and outline of assessment of sexual problems. *Menopause* 2004;**11**:709–713.

19 Klausmann D. Sexual motivation and the duration of the relationship. *Arch Sex Behav* 2002;**31**:275–287.

20 Goldstein I, Berman JR. Vasculogenic female sexual dysfunction: vaginal engorgement and clitoral erectile insufficiency syndromes. *Int J Impot Res* 1998;**10**(suppl 2):S84–90; discussion S98–101.

21 O'Connell HE, Hutson JM, Anderson CR, Plenter RJ. Anatomical relationship between urethra and clitoris. *J Urol* 1998;**159**:1892–1897.

22 Graziottin A. Libido: the biologic scenario. *Maturitas* 2000;**34**(suppl 1):S9–16.

23 Bachmann GA. The hypoandrogenic woman: pathophysiologic overview. *Fertil Steril* 2002;**77**(suppl 4): S72–76.

24 Pfaus J, Everitt B. The psychopharmacology of sexual behaviour. In: Bloom FE, Kupfer D, eds. *Psychopharmacology.* New York: Raven Press, 1995, pp. 743–758.

25 Meston CM, Frohlich PF. The neurobiology of sexual function. *Arch Gen Psychiatry* 2000;**57**:1012–1030.

26 Basson R. Recent advances in women's sexual function and dysfunction. *Menopause* 2004;**11**:714–725.

27 Laumann EO, Paik A, Rosen RC. Sexual dysfunction in the United States: prevalence and predictors. *JAMA* 1999;**281**:537–544.

28 Dunn KM, Croft PR, Hackett GI. Sexual problems: a study of the prevalence and need for health care in the general population. *Fam Pract* 1998;**15**:519–524.

29 Osborn M, Hawton K, Gath D. Sexual dysfunction among middle-aged women in the community. *Br Med J (Clin Res Ed)* 1988;**296**(6627):959–962.

30 Bancroft J, Loftus J, Long J. Distress about sex: a national survey of women in heterosexual relationships. *Arch Sex Behav* 2003;**32**:193–204.

31 Fugl-Meyer A, Fugl-Meyer K. Sexual disabilities, problems and satisfaction in 18–74 year old Swedes. *Scand J Sexology* 1999;**2**:79–105.

32 Bancroft J. Biological factors in human sexuality. *J Sex Res* 2002;**39**:15–21.

33 Hallstrom T. Sexuality in the climacteric. *Clin Obstet Gynaecol* 1977;**4**:227–239.

34 Hallstrom T, Samuelsson S. Changes in women's sexual desire in middle life: the longitudinal study of women in Gothenburg. *Arch Sex Behav* 1990;**19**:259–268.

35 Pfeiffer E, Davis GC. Determinants of sexual behavior in middle and old age. *J Am Geriatr Soc* 1972;**20**:151–158.

36 Dennerstein L, Alexander JL, Kotz K. The menopause and sexual functioning: a review of the population-based studies. *Annu Rev Sex Res* 2003;**14**:64–82.

37 Dennerstein L, Lehert P, Burger H, Dudley E. Biological and psychosocial factors affecting sexual functioning during the menopausal transition. In: Bellino F, ed. *Biology of Menopause.* New York: Springer-Verlag, 1999, pp. 211–222.

38 Laumann EO, Paik A, Rosen RC. The epidemiology of erectile dysfunction: results from the National Health and Social Life Survey. *Int J Impot Res* 1999;**11**(suppl 1):S60–64.

39 Dennerstein L, Randolph J, Taffe J, Dudley E, Burger H. Hormones, mood, sexuality, and the menopausal transition. *Fertil Steril* 2002;**77**(suppl 4):S42–48.

40 NIH Consensus Conference. Impotence. NIH Consensus Development Panel on Impotence. *JAMA* 1993;**270**:83–90.

41 Basson R. The female sexual response: a different model. *J Sex Marital Ther* 2000;**26**:51–65.

42 Graziottin A, Nicolosi A, Caliari I. Vulvar vestibulitis and dyspareunia: addressing the biological etiologic complexity. Poster presented at the International meeting of the Female Sexual Function Forum, 2001: Boston, MA.

43 Graziottin A. Sexual pain disorders in adolescents. In: *12th World Congress of Human Reproduction*, International Academy of Human Reproduction. 2005. Venice.

44 Graziottin A. Why deny dyspareunia its sexual meaning? *Arch Sex Behav* 2005;**34**:32–34, 57–61; author reply 63–67.

45 Graziottin A, Koochaki P. Self-reported distress associated with hypoactive sexual desire in women from four European countries. In: *Abstract book.* North American Menopause Society (NAMS) meeting, Miami, 2003.

46 Dennerstein L, Dudley E, Burger H. Are changes in sexual functioning during midlife due to aging or menopause? *Fertil Steril* 2001;**76**:456–460.

47 Hayes R, Dennerstein L. The impact of aging on sexual function and sexual dysfunction in women: a review of population-based studies. *J Sex Med* 2005;**2**:317–330.

48 Kaplan H. *Disorders of Sexual Desire.* New York: Simon & Schuster, 1979.

49 Basson R, Leiblum S, Brotto L, Derogatis L, Fourcroy J,

Fugl-Meyer K, Graziottin A, Heiman JR, Laan E, Meston C, Schover L, van Lankveld J, Schultz WW. Definitions of women's sexual dysfunction reconsidered: advocating expansion and revision. *J Psychosom Obstet Gynaecol* 2003;**24**:221–229.

50 Levine SB. The nature of sexual desire: a clinician's perspective. *Arch Sex Behav* 2003;**32**:279–285.

51 Dennerstein L, Lehert P. Women's sexual functioning, lifestyle, mid-age, and menopause in 12 European countries. *Menopause* 2004;**11**:778–785.

52 Wesselmann U, Burnett AL, Heinberg LJ. The urogenital and rectal pain syndromes. *Pain* 1997;**73**: 269–294.

53 Graziottin A, Bottanelli M, Bertolasi L. Vaginismus: a clinical and neurophysiological study. In: Graziottin A (guest ed.) "Female sexual dysfunction: clinical approach." *Urodinamica* 2004;**14**:117–121.

54 Pariser SF, Niedermier JA. Sex and the mature woman. *J Womens Health* 1998;**7**:849–859.

55 Reiter R. A profile of women with chronic pelvic pain. *Clin Obstet Gynecol* 1990;**33**:130–136.

56 Ryan ML, Dennerstein L, Pepperell R. Psychological aspects of hysterectomy: a prospective study. *Br J Psychiatry* 1989;**154**:516–522.

57 Walker EA, *et al.* Psychiatric diagnoses and sexual victimization in women with chronic pelvic pain. *Psychosomatics* 1995;**36**:531–540.

58 Lampe A, Solder E, Ennemoser A, Schubert C, Rumpold G, Sollner W. Chronic pelvic pain and previous sexual abuse. *Obstet Gynecol* 2000;**96**:929–933.

59 Morgan CD, Wiederman MW, Pryor TL. Sexual functioning and attitudes of eating-disordered women: a follow-up study. *J Sex Marital Ther* 1995;**21**:67–77.

60 Kessler RC, McGonagle KA, Swartz M, Blazer DG, Nelson CB. Sex and depression in the National Comorbidity Survey. I: Lifetime prevalence, chronicity and recurrence. *J Affect Disord* 1993;**29**:85–96.

61 *Diagnostic Statistic Manual of Mental Disorders.* Washington DC: The American Psychiatric Association Press, 1987.

62 *DSM IV TR.* Washington DC: The American Psychiatric Association Press, 2000.

63 Graziottin A. Etiology and diagnosis of coital pain. *J Endocrinol Invest* 2003;**26**(3 suppl):115–121.

64 Graziottin A. The challenge of sexual medicine for women: overcoming cultural and educational limits and gender biases. *J Endocrinol Invest* 2003;**26**(3 suppl):139–142.

65 Graziottin A, Leiblum S. Biological and psychosocial etiology of female sexual dysfunction during the menopausal transition. *J Sex Med* 2005;**2**(suppl 3):133–145.

66 Binik Y. Should dyspareunia be retained as a sexual dysfunction in DSM-V? A painful classification decision. *Arch Sex Behav* 2006;**34**:(1)11–21.

67 Edwards L, Mason M, Phillips M. Childhood sexual and physical abuse: incidence in patients with vulvodynia. *J Reprod Med* 1997;**42**:135–139.

68 Basson R. Women's desire deficiencies and avoidance. In: Levine SB, Risen CB & Althof SE, eds. *Handbook of Clinical Sexuality for Mental Health Professionals.* New York: Brunner Routledge, 2003, pp. 111–130.

69 Graziottin A. Breast cancer and its effects on women's self-image and sexual function. In: Goldstein I, Meston C, Davis S, Traish A, eds. *Women's Sexual Function and Dysfunction: Study, Diagnosis and Treatment.* London: Taylor & Francis, 2005.

70 Liu C. Does quality of marital sex decline with duration? *Arch Sex Behav* 2003;**32**:55–60.

71 Graziottin A, Giovannini N, Bertolasi L, *et al.* Vulvar vestibulitis: pathophysiology and management. *Current Sexual Health Report* 2004;**1**:151–156.

72 Komisaruk B, Whipple B. Brain activity imaging during sexual response in women with spinal cord injury. In: Hyde J, ed. *Biological Substrates of Human Sexuality.* Washington, DC: American Psychological Association, 2005, pp. 109–146.

73 Kaplan H. *Sexual Aversion, Sexual Phobia and Panic Disorders.* New York: Brunnel Mazel, 1987.

74 Bachmann G, Bancroft J, Braunstein G, Burger H, Davis S, Dennerstein L, Goldstein I, Guay A, Leiblum S, Lobo R, Notelovitz M, Rosen R, Sarrel P, Sherwin B, Simon J, Simpson E, Shifren J, Spark R, Traish A; Princeton. Female androgen insufficiency: the Princeton consensus statement on definition, classification, and assessment. *Fertil Steril* 2002;**77**:660–665.

75 Graziottin A. Treatment of sexual dysfunction. In: Bo K, Berghmans B, van Kampen M, Morkved S, eds. *Evidence Based Physiotherapy for the Pelvic Floor. Bridging Research and Clinical Practice.* Oxford: Elsevier, 2005.

76 Graziottin A. Women's right to a better sexual life. In: Graziottin A (guest ed) "Female sexual dysfunction: clinical approach." *Urodinamica* 2004;**14**:57–60.

CHAPTER 21

Sexual Desire Disorders in Women

Lorraine Dennerstein, Jeanne L. Alexander, and Alessandra Graziottin

Definition

Hypoactive sexual desire disorder is defined as absent or diminished feelings of sexual interest or desire, absent sexual thoughts or fantasies and a lack of responsive desire. Motivations (here defined as reasons/incentives) for attempting to become sexually aroused are scarce or absent. The lack of interest is considered to be more than that due to a normative lessening with the life cycle and length of a relationship [1].

The complaint of low desire becomes a clinically relevant sexual *disorder* when it causes significant personal *distress* to the woman.

The focus on "sexual fantasies/thoughts and/or desire" stresses the importance of a mental activity dedicated to anticipating and fantasizing about the sexual encounter. In women, this is more typical of the first months and years of a relationship. In stable, long-lasting relationships, many women report that the leading motivation to have sex is a need for intimacy that may then trigger a sexual response, with increased willingness to be receptive to the partner's initiative.

The "personal distress" criterion applied to desire disorders means that the woman herself has to be sufficiently motivated to seek treatment because she is personally disturbed by the problem. However, relationship distress caused by the loss of desire may also affect the perception of the problem and the motivation, or not, to seek treatment.

Prevalence

Population data indicate a prevalence of low desire in 32% of women between 18 and 59 years of age [2]. A recent European survey of 2467 women, in France, UK, Germany, and Italy, indicates that the percentage of women with low sexual desire is 16% in the age cohort from 20 to 49; 29% in the same age cohort, in women who experienced surgical menopause; 42% in postmenopausal women aged 50 to 70 with natural menopause; and 46% in the same age cohort after surgical menopause [3].

The percentage of women *distressed* by their loss of desire, having hypoactive sexual desire disorder (HSDD), was respectively: 7% in fertile women and 16% after surgical menopause, in the age cohort 20 to 49; 9% in women with natural menopause; and 12% in those with surgical menopause aged 50 to 70 [3]. The likelihood of low sexual desire increases with age, while the *distress* associated with the loss of desire is inversely correlated with age [4].

Surgical menopause, secondary to bilateral ovariectomy, has a specific damaging effect due to the loss of ovarian estrogens and androgens. Ovaries contribute more than 50% of total body androgens in the fertile age. The European survey found that surgically menopausal women were more likely to have HSDD than premenopausal or naturally menopausal women (OR = 2.1; CI = 1.4, 3.4; $p = 0.001$) [3]. Sexual desire scores and sexual arousal, orgasm and sexual pleasure, were highly correlated ($p < 0.001$) [3]. Women with HSDD were more likely to be dissatisfied with their sex life and their partner relationship than women with normal desire ($p < 0.001$) [3].

Pathophysiology

Sexual desire/interest, alternatively referred to as sexual appetite, drive, and sexual impulse, reflects the sexual appetitive feeling that motivates a person to obtain sex and focus her attention on that goal. It has three major dimensions: biologic, motivational, and cognitive.

Biologic

Basic instinctual (or physical) drive is rooted in the rhinencephalic and limbic brain, which is strongly hormone-dependent and is modulated by different mental states, especially mood, and is neurochemically driven. Dopamine is the key neurotransmitter of the seeking-appetitive-lust system, in the appetitive side; endorphins mediate the final consummatory/satisfactory feelings. This system interacts with, and is modulated by three other basic emotions command systems [5]: anger-rage, fear-anxiety, and panic-separation-distress. The final sexual behavior expresses the "net" result of this complex neurobiologic interplay between driving and inhibiting forces. Hormones, in their complex interplay, seem to control the intensity of libido and sexual behavior, rather than its direction, which is more dependent on motivational-affective and cognitive factors.

Estrogens contribute to the appearance and the maintenance of secondary sex characters and to central and peripheral aspects of female sexual function, including level of sexual interest [6–8]. Estrogens affect central sexual desire and central arousal (which are difficult to be differentiated from the research point of view [9], as perception of desire immediately translates into neuronal activation, registered as central sexual arousal).

Appropriate levels of androgens also affect sexual interest in women as in men. Whether androgens or estrogens are the primary modulators of female sexuality remains controversial [10]. Androgens also act as conditioners in the cavernosal bodies in both genders. Estrogens and androgens modulate the trophism of sensory organs, which are sexual targets and sexual determinants of libido. When all values of sexual hormones are converted to picograms/ml, androgens appear to be much more quantitatively present in the female body than estrogens [11]. Postmenopausal hormone-dependent involution of sensory organs may be an important and often ignored biologic contributor of loss of libido in aging women [12].

Prolactin, when supraphysiologic, may inhibit the cascade of events involved in the sexual response, in women as in men. Hypo- or hyperfunction of other endocrine organs (thyroid, adrenal) may also affect sexual desire.

Oxytocin is considered to be the most important neurochemical factor that links the affective and the erotic quality of bonding involved in libido itself, but its clinical usefulness in the diagnosis and treatment of FSD has not yet been adequately assessed.

Alcohol and substance abuse may contribute to sexual disorders, and their potential role should be investigated. Psychotropic drugs may further inhibit or excite sexual desire [13].

Quality of health and well-being, or severity of diseases, are powerful modulators of the vital energy that nourishes the intensity of sexual drive [14]. Other sexual disorders may cause a secondary loss of libido and increasing frustration and dissatisfaction. Co-morbidity between different FSD, as mentioned before, is frequent.

Motivational

Emotional and affective meanings and intimacy needs, which seem to be particularly relevant to women, may contribute to and modulate basic sex drive. In our species, motivation for sex may shift from the primary biologic goal—reproduction—to recreational sex, where the pursuit of pleasure is key, and/or to instrumental sex, where sex is performed as a means to obtain advantages and express motivations different from procreation and/or pleasure.

Cognitive

Wishes and risks to behave sexually are set against the former two contributing factors in ultimately determining sexual behavior. In recent years, research on sexual desire has grown to include a deeper understanding of its biologic roots—both endocrine and neurochemical, of the motivational and relational components and of its vulnerability to personal factors and context-dependent agents. A population-based longitudinal study found that relational factors, such as gaining or losing a partner and feelings toward the partner, had greater effects on sexual interest than did hormonal levels [8].

Clinical History

Loss of sexual desire is multifactorial; it might be caused by biologic, motivational-affective, and cognitive factors that may partly overlap, leading to a progressive decrease of sexual drive that usually parallels the process of aging, with further decline associated with natural or surgical menopause [3,4,7,15] (see also Chapter 20).

A few appropriate questions may help the clinician to better define the etiology of the complaint, to note the presence of co-morbidity with other FSD, and to determine the need for further information (see also Chapter 20). A more detailed clinical history is outlined here, as a paradigm for how to investigate different sexual disorders in the health practitioner's office.

When did you notice that there was a problem? Was it present since the very beginning of your sexual life ("lifelong") or not?
• If yes (as reported on average by 22–28% of women), check psychosexual factors first, hormonal only when clinically indicated.
• If not, and symptoms have appeared recently ("acquired"), ask what—in the patient's opinion—might have caused the problem.

If acquired, did sexual interest fade slowly?
• If yes, check for relationship problems or erotic dissatisfaction, partner sexual or general health problems, work stress, chronic problems with children or close relatives, chronic personal illness, natural menopause, and so on.
• If not, and sex drive disappeared with a rather sudden loss, check hormonal consequences of surgery (e.g. bilateral ovariectomy), recent and current use of drugs (e.g. antidepressants), relationship problems (e.g. discovery of an affair, severe marital crisis).

Is your loss of desire limited to a partner and/or or to a special context ("situational")?
• If yes, check relationship and context-dependent issues.
• If not, and the loss is present in every context and with every partner ("generalized"), check personal psychosexual issues and biologic factors.

What was the average frequency of sexual activity per week (or per month) in the last six months, including with self and/or a partner?
• If fairly regular activity is reported, were you pleased and responsive, with adequate arousal and orgasm? If yes, this might just be a fairly normal response in a stable couple, where the woman responds to satisfy her intimacy needs in the absence of a high sexual drive.

If sexual activity is reported, is your partner experiencing low libido or other sexual problems?
• If yes, the partner could be the "symptom inducer" and the woman the "symptom carrier." A sexual disorder in the male partner may result in a loss of interest in the female partner as well. If this is the case, it may be his problem that needs to be addressed. Ultimately, both members of the couple should be involved in treatment if they are willing to do so.
• If not, how do you explain this erotic silence on both sides?

Do you have erotic dreams, sexual daydreams or sexual fantasies?
• If yes, this usually indicates a good hormonal profile as well as a substantial integrity of the mental sexual processes. The motivational side should then be investigated more thoroughly, as the loss of interest might be more closely related to relationship or other psychologic problems.
• If not, this suggests that biologic as well as psychologic factors, such as depression, may be at play.

Do you experience any other sexual problems such as vaginal dryness, difficulty in lubrication or orgasmic difficulties, despite normal foreplay? Do you feel pain during intercourse? (Co-morbidity may be the case—understanding which is the leading disorder is a key to effective treatment.)
• If no other sexual disorder is reported, endocrine, vascular, neurologic and muscular problem (levator ani hypertonicity up to defensive vaginismus) can be reasonably excluded (although a careful physical examination is always to be recommended).

Is there autoerotic (masturbatory) activity, with orgasm?
• If yes, this indicates good libido, positive body image and lack of inhibition. The loss of libido might therefore be secondary to relationship problems or

an inability to have intercourse due to the partner's physical or sexual problems.

• If not, assuming that the patient's value system does not permit masturbation per se, sexual inhibition, religious concerns, guilty feelings, poor body image, low self-confidence may be the leading inhibitors of a lifelong desire.

Do you enjoy intercourse?

• If yes, this indicates receptiveness and erotic availability.

• If not, and the woman prefers sexual activity other than intercourse, check two possibilities: a phobic aversive attitude toward intercourse and/or sexual pain-related disorder that should be looked for (vestibulitis, vaginitis, vulvitis, vaginismus, postcoital cystitis, clitoralgia, either spontaneous or after arousal, and congestion) that may all cause secondary loss of libido. Sometimes sexual pain-related problems may have started years before the consultation and the patient does not recognize this etiologic correlation until an accurate medical diagnosis put events in the correct etiologic sequence. Some women enjoy other forms of sexual experiences, not intercourse. Some of these women may have same-sex preference.

What made you aware of your sexual desire disorder and led you to look for help (e.g. intolerable personal frustration, fear of losing the partner, partner's complaint, new hope for effective treatment, more self-confidence in reporting)? This final question may well address the real motivation for treatment.

Key point

The clinician should try to become comfortable with these quite intimate questions, choosing ways of asking them that he/she feels at ease with. With time, proper training and familiarity with this issue, this clinical history recording will be increasingly rewarding in terms of diagnostic accuracy, patient satisfaction, and improvement of clinician–patient relationship.

Clinical Evaluation

If the clinical history suggests a possible biologic etiology, the clinician should assess the following:

• *The patient's hormone levels* (total and free testosterone, dehydroepiandrosterone sulfate, prolactin, 17-beta estradiol, sex hormone binding globulin (SHBG), with a plasma sample at the 5th or 6th day from the beginning of menses in fertile women; thyroid-stimulating hormone (TSH) should be assessed when individually indicated).

• *The trophism of the pelvic floor structures* (that may cause secondary loss of libido), with an accurate gynecologic/sexologic examination, particularly when co-morbidity with arousal, orgasm and/or sexual pain disorders is reported.

• *Psychosexual factors and affective state.* The clinician should briefly investigate these issues, referring to a sex therapist or couples therapist for a comprehensive diagnosis, if indicated.

Treatment

Sexual desire disorders have the lowest success treatment rate among sexual disorders. Etiologic complexity, the importance of relationship issues, intimacy frustration, or low motivation to improve sexual relations with the current partner, may explain why the response to treatment is generally so disappointing, particularly in unmotivated patients. Better results may be possible in highly motivated patients, when hormonal loss is the leading etiology (as in surgical menopause) and appropriate hormonal therapy (HT) may restore libido and a satisfactory sexual response.

Based on the etiologic diagnosis, biologic, psychogenic/relational, or combined treatment by the healthcare provider may be required. Referral to, or collaboration with specialists may be indicated:

• HT, systemic or topical, with or without androgens.

• Hypoprolactinemic drug, if high prolactin was diagnosed.

• Thyroxine, if hypothyroidism was diagnosed.

• Low-dose antidepressant, if a mood disorder is a co-factor (bupropion seems to offer better results) [13].

• Better glycemic control, in diabetic women.

• Checking and modification of drugs potentially causing iatrogenic loss of libido, such as levosulpiride, because of its hyperprolactinemic effect.

- Lifestyle improvement: smoking and alcohol reduction, weight control and regular physical exercise to improve body image and mood, better diet, sleep improvement to restore vital energy.
- Appropriate counseling and medical support in all patients suffering from a persistent low sexual desire after a serious or chronic illness.
- Treatment of any FSD co-morbidity, particularly with aversion disorder, vaginismus and/or dyspareunia, with accurate address of pelvic-floor related issues, or orgasmic disorder that would maintain low or absent sexual motivation to intimacy unless appropriately treated.

Optimal referral includes:

- the uroandrologist, when the loss of desire appears to be secondary to a male sexual problem;
- the couple therapist when the desire disorder reflects relational problems;
- the psychiatrist: (1) if low desire reflects development traumas such as child abuse or parental loss. Women who have conflict with intimacy or about sexuality should be referred for psychotherapy; (2) if the woman is found to have an underlying psychiatric disorder such as major depressive disorder or generalized anxiety disorder.

References

1 Basson R, Althof S, Davis S, Fugl-Meyer K, Goldstein I, Leiblum S, Meston C, Rosen R, Wagner G. Summary of the recommendations of sexual dysfunction in women. *J Sex Med* 2004;**1**:24–39.

2 Laumann EO, Paik A, Rosen RC. Sexual dysfunction in the United States: prevalence and predictors. *JAMA* 1999;**281**:537–544 [published erratum appears in *JAMA* 1999;**281**(13):1174] [see comments].

3 Dennerstein L, Koochaki P, Barton I, Graziottin A. Hypoactive sexual desire disorder in menopausal women: a survey of western European women. *J Sex Med* 2006;**3**:212–222.

4 Hayes R, Dennerstein L. The impact of aging on sexual function and sexual dysfunction in women: a review of population-based studies. *J Sex Med* 2005;**2**:317–330.

5 Panksepp J. *Affective Neuroscience: The Foundations of Human and Animal Emotions*. New York: Oxford University Press, 1998.

6 Dennerstein L, Burrows GD, Hyman GJ, Sharpe K. Hormones and sexuality: effects of estrogen and progestogen. *Obstet Gynecol* 1980;**56**:316–322.

7 Dennerstein L, Randolph J, Taffe J, Dudley E, Burger H. Hormones, mood, sexuality and the menopausal transition. *Fertil Steril* 2002;**77**(suppl 4):S42–S48.

8 Dennerstein L, Lehert P, Burger H. The relative effects of hormones and relationship factors on sexual functioning of women through the natural menopausal transition. *Fertil Steril* 2005;**84**:174–180.

9 Dennerstein L, Lehert P. Modeling mid-aged women's sexual functioning: a prospective, population-based study. *J Sex Marital Ther* 2004;**30**:173–183.

10 Wallen K. Sex and context: hormones and primate sexual motivation. *Horm Behav* 2001;**40**:339–357.

11 Lobo RA. *Treatment of the Postmenopausal Woman: Basic and Clinical Aspects*. New York: Lippincott Williams & Wilkins, 1999.

12 Graziottin A. Libido: the biologic scenario. *Maturitas* 2000;**34**(suppl 1):S9–S16.

13 Segraves RT, Balon R. *Sexual Pharmacology Fast Facts*. New York: Norton & Co, 2003.

14 Dennerstein L, Lehert P, Burger H, Guthrie J. Sexuality. *Am J Med* 2005;**118**(12B):59S–63S.

15 Dennerstein L, Dudley E, Burger H. Are changes in sexual functioning during midlife due to aging or menopause? *Fertil Steril* 2001;**76**(3):456–460.

CHAPTER 22

Sexual Aversion Disorders in Women

Linda Banner, Beverly Whipple, and Alessandra Graziottin

Physical intimacy in a relationship is a dynamic process in which sexual motivation is the willingness to behave sexually with a partner [1]. This intimacy can be perceived as frightening, and can increase anxiety for some women to an overwhelming point of sexual avoidance [2]. Sexual desire and arousal is complex in women [3] and many factors can cause or contribute to sexual aversion disorder (SAD).

Sexual aversion may have a prominent *involuntary neurovegetative* basis, which is accompanied by symptoms and signs of anxiety-evoked sympathetic arousal. Or it may have a prevalent *cognitive, voluntary motivation*, when the woman perceives her exposure to sexual intimacy as frustrating and/or increasing her sense of sexual inadequacy.

Both components may be present in the individual woman. However, the term aversion is more pertinent to the phobic attitude, while avoidance better describes the voluntary motivation in the choice of non-exposing oneself to sexual intimacy. Although frequently used interchangeably, they are not completely overlapping in meaning, nor in underlying pathophysiology.

Personal and family history can influence a woman's ability to be intimate and to perceive this intimacy as a factor of vulnerability [1]. A family history of anxiety disorders and phobias is frequent [2]. Health conditions, such as diabetes mellitus, breast cancer, and hyperprolactinemia, to name a few [4–6], can also contribute to sexual avoidance, with different pathophysiologic mechanisms. Instances of female genital cutting or circumcision may cause women not to feel physical pleasure in sexual intimacy and thus to want to avoid it [7,8]. Religious and cultural expectations regarding women's sexuality can influence women to inhibit their sexual desire

and pleasure [9], and thus want to avoid physical intimacy. Aging and body image frequently play a significant role in women's ability to enjoy sexual pleasure [10,11]. The personal (and interpersonal) distress caused by this disorder can create a rift in the intimacy of the relationship and influence one member's decision to seek treatment. In the early days of sex therapy, women presenting with these symptoms and this disorder were referred to as "frigid" or "sexually unresponsive" [12].

Definition

Defined as "severe anxiety or disgust at the thought of sexual activity" [3, p.30], sexual aversion disorder has many, often interrelated, causes. Incest, molestation, rape, and psychologic abuse, are often factors resulting in a woman developing complete a avoidance of physical intimacy and revulsion at the thought of sexual touch [13]. This anxiety can be severe enough to result in phobic and fear responses associated with dramatic physiologic symptoms [14].

By definition, sexual aversion disorder (SAD) specifically describes the clinical picture that correlates with a neurobiologically-based neurovegetative arousal with phobic characteristics, focused on or elicited by a sexual stimulus or context, which causes personal distress. It is not uncommon to see patients suffering from SAD who over time may develop post-traumatic stress disorder (PTSD) symptoms, with hypervigilance, flashbacks, and panic attacks evoked by recurrent exposure to sexual stimuli. This co-morbidity can be emotionally disturbing and further distressing to the patient and her partner.

Prevalence

This disorder is frequently a component of other diagnostic disorders, especially anxiety-based disorders. Hutchings and Dutton [15] demonstrated that 75% of sexually abused women had anxiety disorders, versus 21% of non-abused women with anxiety disorders. Another study by Dinwiddie *et al.* [16] demonstrated that the incidence of twins—either one or both—being sexually abused and developing any psychopathology over their lifetime was significantly increased when compared to non-twins and their psychopathology. The incidence of increased panic disorder was one of the most strongly correlated psychopathologies to childhood trauma or sexual abuse [16–18]. This hypothesis was initially linked to sexual aversion disorder by Kaplan [2] when she discussed clinical perspectives of intimacy and panic disorders.

Pathophysiology

The neurobiology of sexual aversion disorder is quite similar to that of other anxiety-based disorders, whether phobic or not. The sympathetic system initiates the fight or flight response, causing the increase in epinephrine and norepinephrine to be released from the sympathetic nerve endings in the adrenal glands. This triggers a response in the brain to initiate neurotransmitter responses releasing hormones to respond to this anxious feeling; the sexual hormones, such as estrogen and adrenal androgens, are reduced due to increased stress [20].

From a psychosexual perspective, women avoiding sexual intimacy could be described as having "emotional claustrophobia" [2]. Panic attacks can cause the increase in anticipatory anxiety. This escalating anxiety could be the result of genetic predisposition or memory of a traumatic event [2]. For example, childhood trauma could cause the individual to have depersonalization/derealization or dissociative symptoms in panic disorders [18]. Also, the woman's sexual aversion disorder may not be disclosed or dealt with until her partner seeks treatment for his sexual dysfunction.

Co-morbidity with hypoactive sexual desire disorder (HSSD) is frequent in women with SAD. The pathophysiology of this co-morbidity is rooted in both the neurobiology of basic emotions contributing to and modulating sexual desire, and to psychosexual factors that may act as predisposing or precipitating factors for both conditions (see Chapter 21) [21].

Clinical History

Patient issues

Women with a history of sexual trauma, such as molestation, incest or rape, tend to develop inappropriate sexual behaviors [13]: some will act out with hypersexuality—the opposite of sexual aversion disorder, and others will act out with sexual aversion disorder. Many have post-traumatic stress disorder (PTSD) symptoms and sexual avoidance from the experience. Frequently, symptoms of PTSD include increased anxiety, hypervigilance, flashbacks, and avoidance of "cues" from the traumatic event [14]. *Clinicians should inquire about a woman's sex history, including childhood sexual exploration with such questions as "When was the first time you were aware of your body parts?" "Were you given any special names for your genital area?" "Did you ever play Dr with a family member or neighbor—what were your feelings about this experience?". It is best to address it "as if" they have already had this experience, because that is a more permission-giving and accepting method to discuss this delicate topic.*

Women experiencing genital cutting, whether infibulation or clitoral circumcision and excision, can also have traumatic memories associated with their sexuality. It can also cause them to have difficulty receiving any physical pleasure from sexual intimacy [7,8], and thus want to avoid sexual intimacy. This procedure of female genital cutting is done on female infants within the first year or in the peripuberal years as a "rite of passage" for young women [9] (see Chapter 26). *If a woman is from another culture, such as Africa, there is a strong likelihood that she may have either experienced genital cutting or witnessed it—which could also be traumatic for her. Again, address it as if it has happened and then she can correct your assumptions, rather than probing and waiting for her to offer this information.*

Health conditions can play a role in women's sexual avoidance due to physiologic changes with the disease, biochemical and neurologic changes due to the disease or treatment chosen, and psychologic or emotional changes due to the nature of the disease or disorder. Women who have treatment for breast cancer often report a decrease in sexual function [5], which can result in voluntary avoidance of sexual intimacy. Depending on the treatment choice this could be caused by a change in body image due to a mastectomy, to lymphedema, or due to lack of sensual response resulting from surgery, from the iatrogenic menopause secondary to chemotherapy, and or other treatment options [21] (see Chapter 26). Diabetes mellitus can cause women to have decreased genital sensation and lubrication and thus lead to female sexual disorders and eventually sexual avoidance. Neither age, duration of diabetes, glycemic control, nor complications, predict the extent of sexual disorders in women [4]. However, age is an independent predictor of sexual disorders. Psychotropic medications, especially the serotonin-specific reuptake inhibitors (SSRIs), tend to influence tactile sensation and decrease orgasmic response [19]. The decrease or even delay in orgasmic response can cause women to avoid sexual intimacy because it becomes unpredictable and requires a frustratingly longer sex-play. *Frequently, if the clinician is empathic and understanding of the woman's various health conditions, it is easier for her to talk about her loss of intimacy and closeness, and to open the hope and possibility of treatment.*

Religious beliefs can influence women's ability to enjoy sexual intimacy. Some religious doctrines do not allow women to experience their sexuality with pleasure and prefer to focus on rigid role expectations about sexual intimacy, which creates the "sex for procreation not recreation" mindset [9]. It is clear that if a woman has guilt about enjoying her sexual pleasure, which goes against her religious beliefs, she will also experience high levels of anxiety and this can cause unsatisfactory physical symptoms resulting in sexual avoidance.

Partner-related issues

Aging and body image can have an impact on sexual function and levels of sexual desire or avoidance. Many older adults may have rigid expectations about their sexuality. Some may experience problems with their partner's physical and psychologic state, their body image, health conditions, psychologic well-being and social, cultural or religious beliefs, as well as levels of personal hygiene [10]. These partner-related conditions can cause various degrees of sexual function and disorders, and can lead to sexual aversion or avoidance. For older women, the most significant influences on their levels of sexual desire were attitudes about sexuality, including age, importance of sex, and education [11]. It is common for women to cease sexual interest and intimacy when their partner is experiencing a sexual difficulty, such as erectile dysfunction [11]. The anxiety caused by the vulnerability of physical intimacy can make some women very uncomfortable with their sexuality due to real or perceived body image problems, especially due to aging, health treatments, or eating disorders. Some women see themselves as "physically unattractive" without their clothes on and thus avoid all aspects of sexual intimacy.

Sexual function and disorders are dynamic phenomena and reciprocal events. When women experience sexual aversion disorder, avoidance of physical intimacy can impact the quality of the relationship. With discrepancies of desire, one person in the relationship can get angry and act out against the other in non-sexual ways, creating a power struggle within the relationship. This can then set up the woman to use sex as her power in the relationship and to completely avoid physical contact with her partner. It is not uncommon for couples to learn about the power of sex in the relationship and how to use it in their favor or against their partner [1]. Frequently, people in a sexual relationship confuse emotional intimacy with physical intimacy. Within the power dynamics of an intimate relationship, sexual aversion disorder can be the result of some deep psychologic event or belief within the woman, a physical condition of the woman or her partner, or a perceptual problem within the relationship. Regardless of the etiology, it can create a wedge within the relationship and become a source of distress for the woman and/or her partner. *Clinicians need to address the sexual history with the couple together and separately. Frequently, one person may reveal perspectives and experiences that may not come out in the conjoint session. Especially, if one person is really not turned on by the other for many reasons, it may be difficult to address this in front of their partner and yet it may have a profound impact on the woman's ability to engage in physical intimacy.*

Clinical Evaluation

It is important to obtain a thorough history from the woman and her partner. She may need to have some of this information taken privately once she feels safe with the clinician. For trauma survivors, it may take some time for the patient to build a level of trust and safety, in order to disclose deep personal and often shameful memories. When a patient has a medical etiology for their sexual aversion disorder or avoidant attitude, it may be more straightforward. However, the clinician needs to be mindful of the potential for secondary gain for keeping the problem. The clinician needs to be empathic and supportive of the patient to build the therapeutic rapport. Physical examination may be indicated when body image-related issues and/or negatively perceived outcomes of breast or genital surgery contribute to sexual avoidance (see Chapters 20 and 26).

Treatment

Integrative treatment

When available it has been shown that working in a collaborative manner can provide the most effective treatment choice because it involves both members of the relationship, and a sexual health professional team, which may include a physician, psychologist, sex therapist, or physical therapist, all working together for the benefit of the patient and her partner.

Medical

Depending on the etiology of the sexual aversion disorder, the medical treatment could include using drugs that reduce the phobic arousal, or changing medications. Corrective surgery may be indicated when sexual avoidance is based on body image issues or is secondary to negative outcomes of surgery or genital mutilation. Women who have had genital cutting may experience many complications to their urogenital functioning and need corrective surgery. Women who have had a mastectomy may need breast reconstruction to restore the visual component of their body image. However, loss of breast tac-

tile and nipple erotic perception, which is total after mastectomy and partial after quadrantectomy, may remain a major issue in maintaining a breast-focused sexual avoidance [22].

Psychologic

Couples therapy including communication, relationship, and negotiation skills, cognitive-behavior sex therapy with systematic desensitization and relaxation skills as a focal component, and group therapy to teach sexual function skills, would be included.

References

1 Levine SB. *Sexual Life: A Clinician's Guide*. New York: Plenum Press, 1992.

2 Kaplan HS. Intimacy disorders and sexual panic states. *J Sex Marital Ther* 1988;**14**:3–12.

3 Basson R, Althof S, Davis, Fugl-Meyer K, Goldstein I, Leiblum S, Meston C, Rosen R, Wagner G. Summary of the recommendations of sexual dysfunctions. J Sex Med 2004;**1**:24–34.

4 Muniyappa R, Norton M, Dunn ME, Banerji MA. Diabetes and female sexual dysfunction: moving beyond "benign neglect." *Curr Diab Rep* 2005;**5**:230–236.

5 Bukovic D, Fajdic J, Hrgovic Z, Kaufmann M, Hojsak I, Stanceric T. Sexual dysfunction in breast cancer survivors. *Onkologie* 2005;**28**:29–34.

6 Kadioglu P, Yalin AS, Tirakioglu O, Gazioglu N, Oral G, Sanli O, Onem K, Kadioglu A. Sexual dysfunction in women with hyperprolactinemia: a pilot study *J Urol* 2005;**174**:1921–1925.

7 Campbell CC. Care of women with female circumcision. *J Midwife W Health* 2004;**49**:364–365.

8 Daley A. Caring for women who have undergone genital cutting *Nurs Times* 2005;**100**:32–35.

9 Tannahill R. *Sex in History*. London: Abacus, 1992.

10 Butler RN, Lewis MI, Sunderland T. *Aging and Mental Health: Positive Psychological and Biomedical Approaches*, 4th edn. New York: Macmillan, 1991.

11 Delamater JD, Sill M. Sexual desire in later life *J Sex Res* 2005;**42**:138–149.

12 Kaplan HS. *The Illustrated Manual of Sex Therapy*, 2nd edn. New York: Brunner-Mazel, 1987.

13 Maltz W, Holman, B. *Incest and Sexuality: A Guide to Understanding and Healing*. Lexington, VA: Lexington Books, 1987.

14 Shapiro F, Forrest MS. *EMDR: The Breakthrough Therapy for Overcoming Anxiety, Stress, and Trauma.* New York: Perseus Books, 1997.

15 Hutchings PS, Dutton MA. Symptom severity and diagnoses related to sexual assault history. *J Anx Dis* 1997;**11**:607–618.

16 Dinwiddie S, Heath AC, Dunne MP, Bucholz KK, Madden PA, Slutske WS, Bierut LJ, Statham DR, Martin NG. Early sexual abuse and lifetime psychopathology: a co-twin study. *Psychol Med* 2000;**30**:41–52.

17 Safren SA, Gershuny BS, Marzol P, Otto MW, Pollack MH. History of childhood abuse in panic disorder, social phobia and generalized anxiety disorder. *J Nerv Ment Dis* 2002;**190**:453–456.

18 Marshall RD, Schneider FR, Lin SH, Simpson B, Vermes D, Liebowitz M. Childhood trauma and dissociative symptoms in panic disorder *Am J Psychiatry* 2000;**157**:451–453.

19 Frohlich P, Meston CM. Fluoxetine-induced changes in tactile sensation and sexual functioning among clinically depressed women *J Sex Marital Ther* 2005;**31**:113–128.

20 Sapolsky RM. *Why Zebras Don't Get Ulcers.* New York: WH Freeman, 1998.

21 Panksepp J. *Affective Neuroscience: The Foundation of Human and Animal Emotions.* New York: Oxford University Press, 1998.

22 Graziottin A. Breast cancer and its effects on women's self-image and sexual function. In: Goldstein I, Meston C, Davis S, Traish A, eds. *Women's Sexual Function and Dysfunction: Study, Diagnosis and Treatment.* London: Taylor & Francis, 2005, pp. 276–281.

CHAPTER 23

Sexual Arousal Disorders in Women

Annamaria Giraldi and Alessandra Graziottin

Definitions

Arousal

Definitions of sexual arousal have in the past focused solely on the physiologic aspect of genital arousal, i.e. genital vasocongestion, lubrication, tingling, as well as erection of the nipples and flushing of the skin, as introduced by the largely phenomenologic and objective descriptions by Dickinson [1], Kinsey [2], and Masters and Johnson [3].

However, in the clinical setting, some women very often relate arousal to the subjective feeling of being "turned on" more than the physiologic response, including vaginal lubrication, genital tingling, and warmth. As such, there is a discrepancy between what has been defined as sexual arousal in many studies and what women may perceive as sexual arousal. In the clinical setting women with decreased lubrication will typically complain of vaginal dryness or discomfort with intercourse and, when referring to a lack of arousal, the complaints will more likely be about the lack of subjective excitement in her mind [4]. This discrepancy was emphasized in the Second International Consultation on Sexual Medicine (2003), which suggested a theoretic model including the genital response as well as the subjective response [5]. Studies are being conducted to provide more empirical evidence for the definitions proposed [6,7].

Arousal disorder

Definitions of female sexual arousal disorder (FSAD) have undergone significant changes. In the *Diagnostic and Statistical Manual of Mental Disorders* (DSM-IV) FSAD was defined as: "*Persistent or recurrent inability to attain, or to maintain until completion of the sexual activity, an adequate lubrication-swelling response to sexual*

excitement. The disturbance causes marked distress or interpersonal difficulty. The sexual dysfunction is not better accounted for by another AXIS I disorder (except another sexual dysfunction) and is not due to the direct physiological effects of substance abuse or a general medical condition" [8].

The consensus conference 2000 defined FSAD as "*the persistent or recurrent inability to attain or maintain sufficient sexual excitement, causing personal distress, which may be expressed as lack of subjective excitement, or genital (lubrication/swelling) or other somatic responses*" [9, p. 890].

The Second International Consultation on Sexual Medicine (2003) made considerable changes in the definition of FSAD based on the observation that subjective arousal does not always correlate strongly with genital congestion [10]. This resulted in a subdivision of FSAD into three categories: subjective, genital, and combined.

Subjective arousal disorder
"*Absence of or markedly diminished feelings of sexual arousal (sexual excitement and sexual pleasure) from any type of sexual stimulation. Vaginal lubrication or other signs of physical response still occur*" [11, p. 982].

Genital sexual arousal disorder
"*Complaints of absent or impaired genital sexual arousal. Self-report may include minimal vulval swelling or vaginal lubrication from any type of sexual stimulation and reduced sexual sensations from caressing genitalia. Subjective sexual excitement still occurs from non-genital sexual stimuli*" [11, p. 982].

Combined genital and subjective arousal disorder
"*Absence of or markedly diminished feelings of sexual arousal (sexual excitement and sexual pleasure) from*

any type of sexual stimulation as well as complaints of absent or impaired genital sexual arousal (vulval swelling, lubrication)" [11, p. 982].

Persistent sexual arousal disorder

With the 2003 consensus a new category of female arousal disorder was described and recommended for inclusion in the diagnostic system, namely persistent sexual arousal disorder (PSAD) [11]. It is defined as: *"Spontaneous, intrusive and unwanted genital arousal (e.g. tingling, throbbing, pulsating) in the absence of sexual interest and desire. Any awareness of subjective arousal is typically but not invariably unpleasant. The arousal is unrelieved by one ore more orgasms, and the feelings of arousal persist for hours or days"* [11, p. 982]. (PSAD will be discussed at the end of this chapter.)

For all definitions, FSAD can be divided into primary arousal problems, meaning that the woman has never experienced sufficient arousal despite sufficient desire and sexual stimulation, and secondary arousal disorder, in which the woman experiences decreased arousal but has previously been able to become aroused. The secondary arousal disorder can be generalized (it appears in all sexual situations) or situational (it only appears in some situations).

It is considered to be a disorder only if the woman is distressed by the problem [5], and assessment of relative distress is recommended as a part of the diagnosis. Furthermore, the degree of subjective distress may have implications for treatment motivation and, in the end, treatment outcome [12].

At the present time, the DSM-IV or the first consensus report are the most widely accepted classifications. The revised definitions remain recommendations as they have not been included into the DSM or World Health Organization's *International Classification of Disease* (ICD-10). There is an ongoing evolvement of definitions of sexual disorders based on research and clinical data. The revised definitions provide greater specificity and refinement of the variety of sexual arousal disorders. These more specific and detailed diagnoses may be included in future diagnostic systems. Clinical studies are being conducted to obtain more empirical evidence for the definitions proposed. In the meantime, it is hoped that the new definitions will be helpful in the clinical diagnosis and treatment of arousal disorders.

Prevalence

The prevalence of FSAD is based on the conventional definitions of arousal, namely genital measures—mostly lubrication. As such, most epidemiologic research has focused on the genital arousal disorder. Furthermore, many epidemiologic investigations have not included the distress factor in their investigations, making it difficult to give accurate estimates on how large the problem really is. The epidemiologic investigations of the prevalence of arousal problems show considerable differences between the different investigations, ranging overall from 6% up to 49% of the women who were asked, with a majority of prevalence ranging between 13% and 24% [13–19]. Two studies have demonstrated that the prevalence of FSAD is increased with increasing age, peaking after the age of 50 years [18,20]. In a Swedish study it was found that, in women aged 50 or more, approximately 25% complained of lubrication problems, while 6–11% of women aged 18–49 experienced lubrication problems [18].

Pathophysiology

Biologic factors

As described in Chapter 19, lubrication and genital congestion rely on intact nerve mediation and vascular function, as well as the hormonal milieu, which is crucial for a moistened vagina. Therefore, disruptions to any of these parameters may result in impaired genital arousal response.

An estrogenized milieu is strongly correlated with the ability to lubricate, and genital arousal disorders are therefore correlated to the menopausal transition [21–23]. Furthermore, genital arousal disorder may be associated with medical diseases (for example, neurologic conditions affecting the autonomic nervous system, diabetes mellitus with neuropathy and vascular complications) and medical therapies (for example, surgical procedures or radiation damaging tissue structures and autonomic nerves and vessels). Recurrent urinary tract infections also affect the arousal response as well as recurrent vaginal infections, which create irritation, pain, and decreased lubrication.

Table 23.1 Questions of importance when evaluating women with sexual arousal disorder.

1 *Can you describe your problem in your own words?*
  — When she describes the problems ask clarifying question in order to find out whether it is the primary problem or secondary to other sexual disorders. Arousal disorders are very often secondary to desire disorders.

2 *Has the problem always been there?*
  — If yes, check psychosexual and relational factors first and awareness/lack of awareness of signs of genital arousal.
  — If not, ask when it appeared and what—in the patient's opinion—might have triggered the problem. Did it come slowly or suddenly?

3 *Are you sexually active? With or without a partner?*
  — If she is regularly sexually active, is she pleased with the activity? Are there differences in her response?
  — Does she enjoy intercourse?
  — Does she masturbate? If yes, is the problem also present when she masturbates?

4 *Is the problem limited to your partner and/or to a special context or situation?*
  — If yes, check relational and contextual factors.
  — If no, and the problem is generalized, check personal psychosexual factors and biologic factors.

5 *Does your partner have a sexual problem?*
  — For example, erectile dysfunction, desire problem, orgasm problem, or rapid or delayed ejaculation? Be aware that she can be the "carrier" of the partner's sexual dysfunction.

6 *What does the problem mean to you?*
  — To estimate the degree of distress. Does it lead to frustration, guilt, shame or other feelings?

7 *What does the problem mean to your partner?*
  — What does it mean for the relationship?

Psychosocial and context-dependent factors

Many factors may influence a woman's arousal, both genital and subjective:
• Lack of desire.
• Sexual inhibition.
• Lack of awareness of genital responses.
• Anxiety, fear, lack of energy.
• Lack of intimacy or sufficient sexual stimulation.
• Partner's sexual problems.
• Contextual factor, which may be past, current, or medical (for example, life situation, negative upbringing, losses, trauma, risk of unwanted pregnancy or of STI, lack of privacy, the situation is inappropriate, time of day, interpersonal problems, substance abuse).

Clinical Approach

Loss of arousal is multifactorial and might be caused by biologic, motivational, relational, and cognitive factors. A thorough medical and sexologic history and a medical examination is therefore of great importance when evaluating the women (as described in Chapter 20). Focus should be on biologic, sexologic, psychologic, and relational factors, as well as predisposing, precipitating, and maintaining factors. Finally, the degree of distress should be evaluated. Table 23.1 contains suggestions for questions that can be helpful in initiating assessment of the problem.

Sexologic history

What type of arousal disorder does she have?
• Is she mentally sexual excited from, for example:
  — reading, viewing, hearing erotica?
  — stimulating the partner?
  — receiving sexual stimulation to non-genital and genital areas?
  — deliberate sexual fantasy or recall of sexual memories?

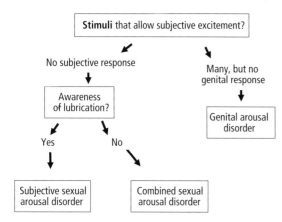

Fig. 23.1 Diagnostic algorithm for assessment of arousal disorder. Adapted with permission from [11].

- Direct awareness of genital congestion:
  — tingling, pulsing, throbbing in response to the above stimuli, vaginal lubrication?
- Indirect evidence of genital congestion:
  — progressively intense sexual sensation from direct massaging of vulval structures with her or partner's fingers, partner's body, oral stimulation, dildo, penile-vulval contact?
- Is there co-morbidity with other sexual disorders?
  — Is there a desire problem, a pain problem, or an orgasm problem?
  — What came first? Is the arousal problem secondary to other sexual problems or the primary problem?
- Is she distressed by the condition? [5]

Figure 23.1 is a diagnostic algorithm for sexual arousal disorders.

Psychologic and relational history

- Cognitive and affective evaluation:
  — Clarify her thoughts: is she feeling distracted, feeling tired, feeling sexually substandard, worried that the outcome would be negative, unsafe situation (pregnancy, STIs), feeling used, not being considered, unhappy about their sexual intimacy/practices?
  — Clarify her emotions: is there sadness, embarrassment, guilt, awkwardness, displeasure?
- Relational evaluation:

— Does the partner have a sexual dysfunction? (erectile dysfunction, low desire, rapid or delayed ejaculation or orgasmic disorders)
— Is she attracted to her partner? Are there relational problems? (e.g. Is she disturbed by inadequacy of his personal hygiene, is there conflict, aggressiveness, abuse, or limited privacy?) [5,24,25]

Medical and gynecologic history

- Menstrual cycle, menopause (natural or surgical), pregnancy/breastfeeding:
  — related to menstrual irregularities, breastfeeding, the menopause, or oral contraceptives?
  — gynecologic and obstetric history?
- Somatic problems: Does she have any disease known to predispose to lubrication problems?
  — diabetes, recurrent lower urinary tract infections, recurrent vaginal infections, neurologic diseases (multiple sclerosis, neuropathies, Sjögren's syndrome)?
- Iatrogenic causes:
  — surgical procedures in the genital area, the pelvis or lower abdomen with damage of the genitalia as well as vasculature or nerves, for example, hysterectomy, pelvic cancer, episiotomy/rraphy with retracted/painful scarring?
  — radiation therapy of the pelvic/genital area?
- Psychiatric diseases that may influence the arousal response:
  — phobias, anxiety, depression?
- Medication that may affect lubrication and/or desire? (see Chapter 26)

Physical examination

A general physical examination is highly recommended and can be directed by the medical history and its outcome. However, a gynecologic examination is always recommended. For women with genital arousal disorder, the information will be limited, as the genitalia are in the non-aroused state, but vaginal dystrophy suggesting estrogen deficiency or rarer conditions can be identified, as described below. For women with subjective or combined arousal disorders, there most likely will be no abnormality. Nevertheless a "normal" examination can be highly informative for the woman [5,26].

The gynecologic examination should focus on:

- Inspection of vulvar anatomy. Are there any changes or abnormalities?
  — For example, signs of inflammation, poor outcome of pelvic or perineal surgery, signs of lichen sclerosus or lichen planus, as well as involution or conglutination of the clitoris?
  — Skin colour and quality. Is the skin thin and dry, or pink, supple and elastic? Are there fissures, eczema, papules, pustules, vesicles, or ulcerations?
  — Does the vaginal mucosa appear estrogenized and moistened or does it appear atrophic with inflammation, fissures, erosions, and ulcers?
  — Does the speculum examination show signs of atrophy (e.g. petechiae or atrophy discharge)?
- Palpation:
  — Signs of myogenic or referred pain, or associated urogenital and rectal pain? If the woman experiences pain, the pain map should be identified as described in Chapter 25. Pain is a strong reflex inhibitor of lubrication and therefore an important point to investigate.
  — Pelvic floor trophism, muscular tone and strength?
  — Scarring?
- Sampling:
  — Determination of pH, which gives indirect evidence of tissue estrogen level and related vaginal ecosystems.
  — Sampling and culture of discharge when infection is suspected.

Laboratory tests

Laboratory tests may be directed by relevant symptoms or findings in the general medical assessment. If low desire is co-morbid or suspected as the reason for low arousal (genital as well as subjective or combined), measuring testosterone status is recommended (including free testosterone).

Plasma levels of estrogens can give information on the endocrine component of arousal disorder and the menopausal status (see also Chapter 27). However, plasma levels are not sufficient indicators of the experienced degree of vaginal dryness [27]. Prolactin levels should be checked if there is co-morbidity with marked oligomenorrhea or amenor-rhea, and/or if bilateral breast milky discharge is present (not related to lactation). If the clinical history or objective findings suggest hypothyroidism, TSH should be evaluated.

Investigational tests

Vaginal plethysmography may be used to quantify the hemodynamic changes with female sexual arousal. The everyday use of the method in clinical work is questionable. This is due to the lack of a true baseline, the limited number of studies comparing women with disorders and functional women, and the difficulties in drawing conclusions on findings from one measurement. Furthermore, several studies have not found a correlation between the subjective report of arousal and the objective measured by the method [6,28]. As such the method is at the present time mostly investigational.

Duplex doppler ultrasound can be used to measure changes in the clitoral, vaginal, labial, and urethral blood flow; for example, it can be measured before and after sexual stimulation. Use of this method as a standard part of the evaluation is uncertain as larger studies still need to be conducted to identify cut-off values, normative data, correlation between disorder and objective parameters, as well as correlation between subjective and objective data. In the future it may have a role in diagnosis, for example, in women with atherosclerotic changes leading to genital arousal problems [28–30].

Principles of Treatment of Sexual Arousal Disorder

If possible, treatment should be based on the etiologic diagnosis directed toward biologic, psychologic/relational or combined factors. In the clinical situation, arousal disorder is often combined with desire and/or orgasmic disorders, and a more integrative treatment will then focus on the other disorders that may lead to arousal disorder (see also Chapters 21, 24, and 25). Furthermore, different treatment modalities should be chosen depending upon the type of arousal disorder.

Women with subjective or combined arousal disorder may benefit from a treatment focusing on awareness of genital responses and becoming subjectively aroused. The techniques that can be used are cognitive-behavioral techniques and/or traditional sex-therapy with sensate focus or psychodynamic treatment. Women with genital arousal disorder may benefit from pharmacologic treatment enhancing genital congestion and lubrication.

Non-pharmacologic treatment of arousal disorder

There are no published outcome studies describing psychologic treatment of arousal disorders in women [5,7].

Pharmacologic treatment of arousal disorder

Pharmacologic treatment can be hormonal and non-hormonal.

Hormonal treatment

For women who are estrogen-deficient, several studies have shown that local or systemic estrogens may improve vaginal lubrication and decrease vaginal irritation and dryness.

A Cochrane review showed that local estrogen in women with vaginal atrophy had a positive effect on dryness and dyspareunia, no matter how the local estrogens were applied (creams, tablets, vaginal ring, or pessaries) compared to placebo when given regularly and continuously [31].

Systemic treatment with estrogens without or with progesterones has been shown to decrease vaginal dryness, irritation, and pain compared to placebo in surgical and natural postmenopausal women, although a large interpatient variability has been observed [32–34]. As discussed in Chapter 27, the latest knowledge on adverse events related to long-term hormone therapy (HT) after the menopause has changed the recommendations on how and for how long HT should be used. It is therefore important to individualize recommendations and treatment of women with arousal problems who may benefit from HT. If HT is recommended for sexual problems and there is no effect, it should also be considered whether it should be continued. For more discussion see Chapter 27.

Tibolone is a synthetic steroid with estrogen, progesterone, and some androgenic effect. In one large study it has been demonstrated to improve lubrication, but it is doubtful whether the effect on lubrication is better than estrogen substitution. However, as tibolone has a weak androgenic effect, it may be a choice for women with decreased desire and arousal, although larger-scale studies are still needed [35–37].

Non-hormonal treatment

At the time of writing (January 2006) there are no approved non-hormonal pharmacologic treatments for arousal disorders.

The success of vasoactive agents (PDE-5 inhibitors) in the treatment of male sexual arousal dysfunction (erectile dysfunction) has encouraged the search for vasoactive agents that enhance women's genital congestion and vaginal lubrication. However, the results until today are limited and are mainly on postmenopausal women. The explanation is most likely that there is a lack of recognition of the need to distinguish between genital arousal and subjective arousal; women may have impaired genital congestion that can be reversed by drugs, but they not necessarily identify this as decreased arousal.

Sildenafil has been investigated in several studies for treatment of female sexual problems. In a few studies of women identified with arousal disorder, benefit has been shown; however, in women with hypoactive desire disorder there is limited effect. As such, sildenafil (and other phosphodiesterase inhibitors) may be beneficial in specific groups of women with genital arousal disorder who recognize the effect on vasocongestion [6,38–40].

Local lubricants applied intravaginally can be useful for women with genital arousal disorder and are often used in the clinical setting. Oil-based lubricants should not be used with latex products that are being used for birth control (such as the male condom) or for safer sex (such as a dental dam or male condom). The latex will be destroyed by oil-based products and will not be effective.

The EROS-CTD device (clitoral therapy device) has been approved by the FDA as therapy for FSD. The EROS-CTD is a small, battery-powered device designed to enhance clitoral engorgement and increase blood flow to the clitoris and vascular response. Only a few, small, non-controlled studies exist on the effect and no data exist on the long-term effect [41–44].

Conclusion

Arousal disorders with impaired arousal response can be defined as genital, subjective, or combined arousal disorder. The prevalence varies and is increased with increasing age, especially at the time of menopause. Arousal disorders are often co-morbid with desire disorder or orgasm and pain disorders. In the evaluation, a thorough sexologic history as well as medical and gynecologic history and examination should be carried out. Treatment should be based on type of arousal disorder and clinical findings. PDE-5 inhibitors and HT may be of benefit if there is genital arousal disorder. Women with subjective or combined arousal disorder may benefit from a treatment focusing on awareness of genital responses and becoming subjectively aroused. The techniques that can be used are cognitive-behavioral techniques, traditional sex-therapy with sensate focus, or psychodynamic treatment and vaginal lubricants.

Persistent Sexual Arousal Disorder

PSAD is a poorly documented condition characterized by persistent genital arousal in the absence of conscious feeling of sexual desire, which has recently been included as a provisional diagnosis [10]. The literature on PSAD is limited and is mainly based on case reports.

Prevalence
The prevalence of PSAD is unknown.

Pathophysiology
To date the pathophysiology is unknown and no obvious hormonal, vascular, neurologic, or psychologic causes have been identified. However, the major etiologic hypothesis are: (1) central neurologic changes; (2) peripheral neurologic changes; (3) vascular changes; (4) mechanical pressure against genital structures; (5) medication-induced changes; (6) psychologic changes, or combinations of all five [45–47].

Clinical approach
As very little is known about the condition, it is difficult to give clear guidelines for the clinical approach. As women may be very embarrassed by the condition, it is important that the physician is aware of it and we recommend a medical and gynecologic history and examination, as described above for decreased arousal disorder. Many women may benefit from realizing that they are not alone with the symptoms and can be referred to a website (www.twshf.org).

If the condition is caused by abnormal clitoral blood flow, a duplex ultrasound may help identifying this [45].

Principle of treatment
As no single cause for PSAD has been identified and there is a lack of substantial experience with treatment, no single treatment can be recommended [48].

Conclusion
PSAD is a poorly documented condition with unknown prevalence and etiology. No accepted treatment can be recommended. In the clinical evaluation it is important to be aware of the condition, to perform a thorough medical and gynecologic examination, to help the woman to feel that she is not alone with this condition.

References

1 Dickinson RL. *Human Sex Anatomy*, 2nd edn. London: Balliere, Tindall & Cox, 1949.

2 Kinsey AC, Pomeroy WB, Martin CE, Gebhard PH. *Sexual Behavior in the Human Female*. Philadelphia, PA: WB Saunders, 1953.

3 Masters WH, Johnson VE. *Human Sexual Response*. Boston, MA: Little Brown, 1966.

4 Laan E, Everaerd W, van der Velde J, Geer JH. Determinants of subjective experience of sexual arousal in women: feedback from genital arousal and erotic stimulus content. *Psychophysiology* 1995;**32**(5):444–551.

5 Basson R, Weijmar Schultz WCM, Binik YM, Brotto LA, Eschenbach DA, Laan E, Utian WH, Wesselmann U, Van Lankveld J, Wyatt G, Leiblum S, Althof SE, Redmond G. Woman's sexual desire and arousal

disorders and sexual pain. In: Lue TF, Basson R, Rosen R, Giuliano F, Khoury S, Montorsi F, eds. *Sexual Medicine: Sexual Dysfunctions in Men and Women*, 2nd edn. Paris: Health Publications, 2004, pp. 851–990.

6 Basson R, Brotto LA. Sexual psychophysiology and effects of sildenafil citrate in oestrogenised women with acquired genital arousal disorder and impaired orgasm: a randomised controlled trial. *Br J Obst Gyn* 2003; **110**(11):1014–1024.

7 Brotto L. Psychological-based desire and arousal disorders: treatment strategies and outcome results. In: Goldstein I, Meston C, Davis SR, Traish A, eds. *Women's Sexual Function and Dysfunction: Study, Diagnosis and Treatment*, 1st edn. London: Taylor & Francis, 2006, pp. 441–448.

8 American Psychiatric Association. *DSM-1: Diagnostic and Statistical Manual of Mental Disorders*. Washington, DC: American Psychiatric Association, 2000.

9 Basson R, Berman J, Burnett A, Derogatis L, Ferguson D, Fourcroy J, Goldstein I, Graziottin A, Heiman J, Laan E, Leiblum S, Padma-Nathan H, Rosen R, Segraves K, Segraves RT, Shabsigh R, Sipski M, Wagner G, Whipple B. Report of the International Consensus Development Conference on Female Sexual Dysfunction: definitions and classifications. *J Urol* 2000; **163**(3): 888–893.

10 Basson R, Leiblum S, Brotto L, Derogatis L, Fourcroy J, Fugl-Meyer K, Graziottin A, Heiman J, Laan E, Meston C, Schover L, van Lankveld J, Weijmar Schultz W. Revised definitions of women's sexual dysfunction. *J Sex Med* 2004; **1**(1):40–48.

11 Basson R, Althof SE, Davis SR, Fugl-Meyer K, Goldstein I, Heiman J, Leiblum S, Meston C, Rosen R, Wagner G, Weijmar Schultz WCM. Summary of the recommendations on women's sexual dysfunctions. In: Lue TF, Basson R, Rosen R, Giuliano F, Khoury S, Montorsi F, eds. *Sexual Medicine: Sexual Dysfunctions in Men and Women*, 2nd edn. Paris: Health Publications, 2004, pp. 975–990.

12 Leiblum S. Classification and diagnosis of female sexual disorders. In: Goldstein I, Meston C, Davis SR, Traish A, eds. *Women's Sexual Function and Dysfunction: Study, Diagnosis and Treatment*, 1st edn. London: Taylor & Francis, 2006, pp. 323–330.

13 Lewis RW, Fugl-Meyer KS, Bosch R, Fugl-Meyer AR, Laumann EO, Lizza E, Martin-Morales A. Definitions, classification, and epidemiology of sexual dysfunction. In: Lue TF, Basson R, Rosen R, Giuliano F, Khoury S, Montorsi F, eds. *Sexual Medicine: Sexual Dysfunctions in Men and Women*, 2nd edn. Paris: Health Publications, 2004, pp. 37–72.

14 Fugl-Meyer AR, Fugl-Meyer KS. Prevalence data in Europe. In: Goldstein I, Meston C, Davis SR, Traish A, eds. *Women's Sexual Function and Dysfunction: Study, Diagnosis and Treatment*, 1st edn. London: Taylor & Francis, 2006, pp. 34–41.

15 Paik A, Laumann EO. Prevalence of women's sexual problems in the USA. In: Goldstein I, Meston C, Davis SR, Traish A, eds. *Women's Sexual Function and Dysfunction: Study, Diagnosis and Treatment*, 1st edn. London: Taylor & Francis, 2006, pp. 23–33.

16 Oberg K, Fugl-Meyer AR, Fugl-Meyer KS. On categorization and quantification of women's sexual dysfunctions: an epidemiological approach. *Int J Impot Res* 2004; **16**(3):261–269.

17 Dunn KM, Croft PR, Hackett GI. Sexual problems: a study of the prevalence and need for health care in the general population. *Fam Pract* 1998; **15**(6):519–524.

18 Fugl-Meyer AR, Fugl-Meyer KS. Sexual disabilities, problems and satisfaction in 18–74 year old Swedes. *Scand J Sexol* 1999; **2**(2):79–97.

19 Laumann EO, Paik A, Rosen RC. Sexual dysfunction in the United States: prevalence and predictors. *JAMA* 1999; **281**(6):537–544.

20 Dunn KM, Croft PR, Hackett GI. Sexual problems: a study of the prevalence and need for health care in the general population. *Fam Pract* 1998; **15**(6):519–524.

21 Hayes R, Dennerstein L. The impact of aging on sexual function and sexual dysfunction in women: a review of population-based studies. *J Sex Med* 2005; **2**(3):317–330.

22 Graziottin A, Leiblum S. Biological and psychosocial pathophysiology of female sexual dysfunction during the menopausal transition. *J Sex Med* 2005; **2**(suppl 3):133–145.

23 Dennerstein L, Hayes R. Confronting the challenges: epidemiological study of female sexual dysfunction and the menopause. *J Sex Med* 2005; **2**(suppl 3): 118–132.

24 Brandenburg U, Schwenkhagen A. Sexual history. In: Goldstein I, Meston C, Davis SR, Traish A, eds. *Women's Sexual Function and Dysfunction: Study, Diagnosis and Treatment*, 1st edn. London: Taylor & Francis, 2006, pp. 343–346.

25 Perelman MA. Psychosocial history. In: Goldstein I, Meston C, Davis SR, Traish A, eds. *Women's Sexual Function and Dysfunction: Study, Diagnosis and Treatment*, 1st edn. London: Taylor & Francis, 2006, pp. 336–342.

26 Stewart EG. Physical examination in female sexual dysfunction. In: Goldstein I, Meston C, Davis SR, Traish A, eds. *Women's Sexual Function and Dysfunction: Study,*

Diagnosis and Treatment, 1st edn. London: Taylor & Francis, 2006, pp. 347–355.

27 Sarrel PM. Effects of hormone replacement therapy on sexual psychophysiology and behavior in post-menopause. *J Womens Health Gend Based Med* 2000;**9**(suppl 1):S25–S32.

28 Heiman J, Guess MK, Connell K, Melman A, Hyde JS, Segraves T, Wyllie M. Standards for clinical trials in sexual dysfunctions of women: research designs and outcome assessment. In: Lue TF, Basson R, Rosen R, Giuliano F, Khoury S, Montorsi F, eds. *Sexual Medicine: Sexual Dysfunctions in Men and Women*, 2nd edn. Paris: Health Publications, 2004, pp. 631–681.

29 Berman JR, Berman LA, Werbin TJ, Flaherty EE, Leahy NM, Goldstein I. Clinical evaluation of female sexual function: effects of age and estrogen status on subjective and physiologic sexual responses. *Int J Impot Res* 1999;**11**(suppl 1):S31–S38.

30 Nader SG, Maitland SR, Munarriz R, Goldstein I. Blood flow: duplex Doppler ultrasound. In: Goldstein I, Meston C, Davis SR, Traish A, eds. *Women's Sexual Function and Dysfunction: Study, Diagnosis and Treatment*, 1st edn. London: Taylor & Francis, 2006, pp. 383–390.

31 Suckling J, Lethaby A, Kennedy R. Local oestrogen for vaginal atrophy in postmenopausal women. *Cochrane Database Syst Rev* 2003;(4):CD001500.

32 Dennerstein L, Burrows GD, Wood C, Hyman G. Hormones and sexuality: effect of estrogen and progestogen. *Obstet Gynecol* 1980;**56**(3):316–322.

33 Kovalevsky G. Female sexual dysfunction and use of hormone therapy in postmenopausal women. *Semin Reprod Med* 2005;**23**(2):180–187.

34 Nathorst-Boos J, Wiklund I, Mattsson LA, Sandin K, von Schoultz B. Is sexual life influenced by transdermal estrogen therapy? A double blind placebo controlled study in postmenopausal women. *Acta Obstet Gynecol Scand* 1993;**72**(8):656–660.

35 Wu MH, Pan HA, Wang ST, Hsu CC, Chang FM, Huang KE. Quality of life and sexuality changes in postmenopausal women receiving tibolone therapy. *Climacteric* 2001;**4**(4):314–319.

36 Kokcu A, Cetinkaya MB, Yanik F, Alper T, Malatyalioglu E. The comparison of effects of tibolone and conjugated estrogen-medroxyprogesterone acetate therapy on sexual performance in postmenopausal women. *Maturitas* 2000;**36**(1):75–80.

37 Nathorst-Boos J, Hammar M. Effect on sexual life: a comparison between tibolone and a continuous estradiol-norethisterone acetate regimen. *Maturitas* 1997;**26**(1):15–20.

38 Basson R, McInnes R, Smith MD, Hodgson G, Koppiker N. Efficacy and safety of sildenafil citrate in women with sexual dysfunction associated with female sexual arousal disorder. *J Womens Health Gend Based Med* 2002;**11**(4):367–377.

39 Berman JR, Berman LA, Toler SM, Gill J, Haughie S. Safety and efficacy of sildenafil citrate for the treatment of female sexual arousal disorder: a double-blind, placebo controlled study. *J Urol* 2003;**170**(6 Pt 1):2333–2338.

40 Caruso S, Intelisano G, Lupo L, Agnello C. Premenopausal women affected by sexual arousal disorder treated with sildenafil: a double-blind, cross-over, placebo-controlled study. *Br J Obst Gyn* 2001;**108**(6):623–628.

41 Billups KL, Berman L, Berman J, Metz ME, Glennon ME, Goldstein I. A new non-pharmacological vacuum therapy for female sexual dysfunction. *J Sex Marital Ther* 2001;**27**(5):435–441.

42 Billups KL. The role of mechanical devices in treating female sexual dysfunction and enhancing the female sexual response. *World J Urol* 2002;**20**(2):137–141.

43 Munarriz R, Maitland S, Garcia SP, Talakoub L, Goldstein I. A prospective duplex doppler ultrasonographic study in women with sexual arousal disorder to objectively assess genital engorgement induced by EROS therapy. *J Sex Marital Ther* 2003;**29**(suppl 1):85–94.

44 Schroder M, Mell LK, Hurteau JA, Collins YC, Rotmensch J, Waggoner SE, Yamada SD, Small W Jr, Mundt AJ. Clitoral therapy device for treatment of sexual dysfunction in irradiated cervical cancer patients. *Int J Radiat Oncol Biol Phys* 2005;**61**(4):1078–1086.

45 Goldstein I, De, EJB; Johnson JA. Persistent sexual arousal syndrome and clitoral priapism. In: Goldstein I, Meston C, Davis SR, Traish A, eds. *Women's Sexual Function and Dysfunction: Study, Diagnosis and Treatment*, 1st edn. London: Taylor & Francis, 2006, pp. 674–688.

46 Leiblum S, Nathan SG. Persistent sexual arousal syndrome: a newly discovered pattern of female sexuality. *J Sex Marital Ther* 2001;**27**(4):365–380.

47 Leiblum S, Brown C, Wan J, Rawlinson L. Persistent sexual arousal syndrome: a descriptive study. *J Sex Med* 2005;**2**(3):331–337.

48 Leiblum S. Arousal disorders in women: complaints and complexities. *Med J Austr* 2003;**178**(638):640.

CHAPTER 24

Orgasmic Disorders in Women

Beverly Whipple and Alessandra Graziottin

Definitions

Orgasm

There are many definitions of orgasm, from Ford and Beach [1], through Kinsey [2], Masters and Johnson [3,4], Kothari [5], and others, to the Second International Consultation on Sexual Medicine, held in Paris in July 2003. Most of these definitions address subjective sensations and pelvic muscle contractions. Members of the Paris consultation offer the following definition of women's orgasm: "*An orgasm in the human female is a variable, transient peak sensation of intense pleasure creating an altered state of consciousness usually with an initiation accompanied by involuntary, rhythmic contractions of the pelvic striated circumvaginal musculature often with concomitant uterine and anal contractions and mytonia that resolves the sexually-induced vasocongestion (sometimes only partially) and myotonia usually with an induction of well-being and contentment*" [6, p. 66].

None of these definitions account for the report of orgasms experienced from imagery alone, or in women with complete spinal cord injury. A more comprehensive definition of orgasm would be "*Orgasm is a peak intensity of excitement generated by: (a) afferent and re-afferent stimulation from visceral and/or somatic sensory receptors activated exogenously and/or endogenously, and/or (b) higher-order cognitive processes, followed by a release and resolution (decrease) of excitation*" [7, p. 71]. By this definition, orgasm is characteristic of, but not restricted to, the genital system.

Orgasmic disorder

The First International Consensus panel in 1998 defined orgasmic disorder as "*the persistent or recurrent difficulty, delay in or absence of attaining orgasm following sufficient sexual stimulation and arousal, which causes personal distress*" [8, p. 890]. We prefer to use the word "experiencing" orgasm rather than "attaining" orgasm, because experiencing does not connote sexual response in women as being linear or goal oriented.

In the *Diagnostic and Statistical Manual of Mental Disorders* (DSM-IV-TR), female orgasmic disorder is defined as: "*Persistent or recurrent delay in, or absence of, orgasm following a normal sexual excitement phase. Women exhibit wide variability in the type or intensity of stimulation that triggers orgasm. The diagnosis of Female Orgasmic Disorder should be based on the clinician's judgment that the woman's orgasmic capacity is less than would be reasonable for her age, sexual experience, and the adequacy of sexual stimulation she receives*" [9(302.73)].

The Second International Consultation on Sexual Medicine defined women's orgasmic disorder as "*Despite the self-report of high sexual arousal/excitement, there is either lack of orgasm, markedly diminished intensity of orgasmic sensations or marked delay of orgasm from any kind of stimulation*" [10, p. 10]. This panel developed the new definition because the old definitions ignored the criterion of high or adequate sexual arousal. This current definition incorporates the criterion that the woman has no problem becoming aroused. It is considered to be a disorder only if the woman is distressed by the problem [11].

Prevalence

Anorgasmia is a common problem that is reported to affect an estimated 24–37% of women [12]. In a review of 34 studies, the rates of anorgasmia, orgasmic difficulty, or orgasmic disorders ranged from below

20% to as high as 50% [13]. Findings from the National Social and Health Life Survey of 1749 US women suggest that orgasmic problems are the second most frequently reported sexual problem in women. In this random sample, 24% reported a lack of orgasm in the past year for at least several months or more [14].

With aging, orgasms may be shorter in duration and less intense than when a woman was younger [15]. If sexual arousal is high, none of the data indicate that problems experiencing orgasm increase with age [16].

Anorgasmia can be divided into primary orgasmic disorder, in which a woman has never experienced orgasm through any means of stimulation, and secondary orgasmic disorder, in which a woman is anorgasmic after having been orgasmic. Secondary anorgasmia can be classified as situational (e.g. when a woman can experience orgasm via masturbation but not with a partner) or generalized [11].

Pathophysiology

Biologic

Much of our information about orgasmic disorders comes from studies of the side effects of pharmacologic agents, endocrine studies in animal models, and neurophysiologic studies in laboratory animals. (See anatomic and physiologic basis of female sexual function, Chapter 19.) There is no definitive explanation as to what triggers orgasms in women.

The clitoris has been characterized as the "most densely innervated part of the human body" [17, p. 137]. Most women experience orgasm from stimulation of the clitoris [18], and it has been reported that all orgasms follow the same reflex pattern [19]. Sipski and colleagues reported the importance of an intact sacral reflex in order to experience orgasm [20].

However, the most recent studies have demonstrated that genital self-stimulated orgasm in women with complete spinal cord injury above the level of the known genital spinal nerves (pudendal, pelvic, and hypogastric nerves) activates the same regions of the brain as orgasm from genital self-stimulation in women without spinal cord injury. The brain regions that were activated, using fMRI during orgasm

experienced from vaginal-cervical self-stimulation, include the nucleus tractus solitarii (NTS), hypothalamic paraventricular nucleus, amygdala, hippocampus, cingulated cortex, insula, and nucleus accumbens [21]. During this study, as the women began vaginal-cervical self-stimulation there was no activation in any of the seven brain regions that were activated at orgasm. The amygdala and other regions of the basal ganglia were activated after at least two minutes of cervical self-stimulation, as were the cingulate cortex and insula. The basal ganglia showed intense activation during orgasm. The two brain regions that became activated during orgasm, but not before, were the paraventricular nucleus of the hypothalamus and the hippocampus [21]. (See Figs 24.1, 24.2, and 24.3.)

It is of interest that, in fMRI studies of the brain, the amygdala is not activated during imagery-induced orgasm, but is activated during genital-induced orgasm in the same subjects [22]. It is tempting to speculate, on the basis of this observation, that the amygdala is therefore closer to having a genital sensory role, while the hippocampus, accumbens, cingulate cortex, and paraventricular nucleus may have a more cognitive role in orgasm, since their activation during orgasm does not depend on physical genital sensory input.

Whipple and Komisaruk postulated the existence of a sensory pathway that bypassed the spinal cord, carrying sensory input from the vagina and cervix directly to the brain. They postulated this to be the vagus nerves, based on nerve transactions and tracer studies in laboratory rats [23]. In women, the sensory vagus nerves carry genital sensory input to the NTS in the medulla, as documented by PET and fMRI [21–23].

Orgasm is more than simply a reflex. While it may incorporate sensory-motor reflex components, it includes perception, which is not a necessary component of true reflexes. It may be triggered by a number of physical and mental stimuli. It does not even require direct genital stimulation. As stated above, mental (imagery-induced) orgasm has been demonstrated in laboratory conditions [24] and documented with fMRI of the brain [22].

A recent study reported some evidence of a genetic factor playing a minor but significant role in

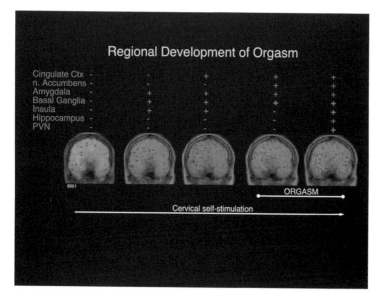

Fig. 24.1 Gradual increases in brain regions activated during cervical self-stimulation leading up to and during orgasm. Note that at the start of the stimulation, none of the seven brain regions showed activation, whereas at orgasm each of these seven areas was activated.

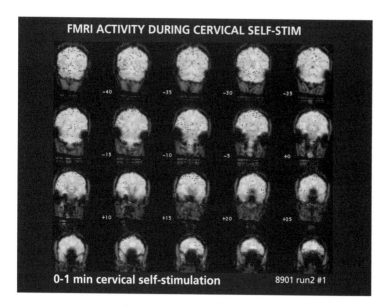

Fig. 24.2 Functional magnetic resonance imaging (fMRI) of serial "sections" through the brain during cervical self-stimulation.

orgasmic response. Based upon a questionnaire study of "sexual problems" in women in England who are twins, and comparing identical with fraternal twins, the authors concluded that there is a significant heritable component for, in their words, "difficulty reaching orgasm during intercourse." The underlying mechanism is unknown [25].

Psychosocial and context-dependent factors

A number of psychosocial factors have been discussed in relation to a woman's ability to experience orgasm. These include interpersonal and marital distress, psychologic distress, psychiatric disorders, the use of antidepressants, especially selective serotonin

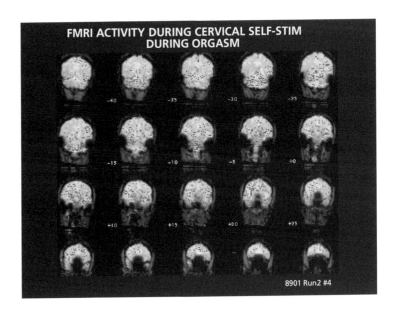

Fig. 24.3 Functional magnetic resonance imaging (fMRI) of the same brain "sections" as in Fig. 24.2, during orgasm induced by cervical self-stimulation.

reuptake inhibitors (SSRIs), age, education, social class, and religion [6,11]. However, there are no consistent empirical findings that psychosocial factors alone differentiate orgasmic from anorgasmic women [6].

What we do know about some psychosocial factors is that Laumann *et al.* found that 87% of women with an advanced degree reported always or usually experiencing orgasm during masturbation, compared with 42% of women with a high-school education [14]. There is no significant relation between education level and orgasmic ability with a partner [26]. Laumann and colleagues also found a negative relation between experiencing orgasm and high religiosity. That is, 79% of women with no religious affiliation reporting experiencing orgasm during masturbation, compared with 53–67% of those having an affiliation with religious groups [14].

In a review article, Mah and Binik reported that orgasm consistency, quality, and satisfaction in women have been related to relationship factors, such as marital satisfaction, marital adjustment, happiness, and stability [27].

Orgasm and orgasm through vaginal intercourse may be learned rather than a natural biologic act, and may have cross-cultural influences. There are cultures in which sexual pleasure has a high value

and women are taught to be orgasmic and often multi-orgasmic [28,29]. In some cultures, women are taught to experience female ejaculation, such as the Batoro of Uganda [30]. Other cultures assume that women have no pleasure from vaginal intercourse and that orgasm for women does not exist, such as the Arapesh. In this culture orgasm in women does not occur [31].

Therefore, many factors have to be considered when a woman reports orgasmic difficulties that cause personal distress. Usually orgasmic problems involve many factors and a multidisciplinary approach is usually most effective in treatment. It is important for the clinician to remember that each woman is unique and that women cannot be compartmentalized into one linear way of responding or be labeled with one sexual response pattern. Women need to be aware of what brings them pleasure and what helps them to experience orgasm and to feel good about the various ways that they can experience sensual and sexual pleasure and orgasm.

Clinical Approaches

In taking a sexual history in a woman who is experiencing personal distress due to either a lack of orgasm, markedly diminished intensity of orgasmic sensations, or marked delay of orgasm from any kind of stimulation, asking the following questions may be helpful.

• Do you feel pleasure and satisfaction without orgasm? Is not experiencing orgasm a concern for you? If it is a concern, the following questions are recommended.

• Is your orgasmic difficulty generalized (in every situation and independent of the partner) or is it situational? If generalized, it may suggest a biologic component, particularly if sex drive and arousal is maintained. There may also be nerve damage from surgery or an injury that must be assessed. If situational, there may be relationship issues to be addressed.

• Was the onset gradual or rapid? Gradual orgasmic difficulties are usually age-dependent and may be exacerbated by menopause. They are characterized by an increased length of time between sex-play and orgasm, more intense stimulation required, decreased quality and intensity of the orgasmic pleasure, and possibly diminished number of orgasmic contractions. Also co-morbidity must be considered in both gradual and rapid onset.

If rapid, the use of medications such as amphetamines and related anorexic drugs, antipsychotics, benzodiazepines, methyldopa, narcotics, tricyclic antidepressants, and SSRIs should be investigated. Other medications should also be investigated because of their effect on sexual response in women.

• What, in your opinion, is causing your orgasmic difficulty? Check the potential role of worsening incontinence, depression, pain, too rapid or absence of sex-play, loss of sexual drive and arousal, alcohol abuse, and relationship problems.

• Do you feel a selective loss in your clitoral sensitivity and pleasure ability and/or a reduction in your coital pleasure? If the complaint is focused on the clitoris, and vulvar involution or dystrophia is present, then topical androgen treatment may be useful. If it is coital, two further questions should be asked.

• Do you have a decreased coital sensation? This latter may suggest a hypotonia of the perivaginal muscles, which may be related to loss of estrogen due to menopause and/or loss of androgens associated with aging. Vaginal pleasure and sensitivity are physically dependent also on the tonus of perivaginal muscles. Biofeedback retraining of the pelvic floor muscles or teaching Kegel exercises may help. Many women experience female ejaculation, an expulsion of about 3–5 ml of fluid from the urethra, which is chemically different from urine and is perfectly normal. It comes from the female prostate gland (G spot), formerly called the paraurethral glands [32]. A differential diagnosis between urinary incontinence and female ejaculation must be made (see Table 24.1).

• Do you feel pain during intercourse? Coital pain of whatever origin must be investigated.

• Have you changed positions of intercourse to a position that does not stimulate the anterior vaginal wall (Grafenberg or G spot)?

Table 24.1 Differential diagnosis.

Incontinence at orgasm	Female ejaculation
Weak pelvic floor muscles	Strong pelvic floor muscles
Contains: urea, creatinine	Contains: glucose, fructose, prostatic specific androgen, prostatic acid phosphatase
Volume: >15 ml	Volume: 3–5 ml
Urine characteristics	Clear, pale white liquid with no urine
Associated with daily or night symptoms of incontinence	No symptoms of urgency and/or stress incontinence
Intensity of orgasm may be inhibited for fear of leaking	Is associated with intense pleasure at orgasm
Urodynamic examinations indicate detrusor instability	Urodynamic examination shows a continent bladder

Modified from Graziottin (1996) [40], Belzer *et al.* (1984) [41], Addiego *et al.* (1981) [42], Ladas *et al.* (2005) [30], and Zaviacic (1999) [32].

Based on the information emerging from the clinical history, the healthcare provider should look for:

- Hormonal balance.
- Signs and symptoms of vulvar dystrophia and, specifically, of clitoral and vaginal involution and traumatic consequences of ritual genital mutilation.
- Signs and symptoms of incontinence, or of either hypotonic or hypertonic pelvic floor, or female ejaculation (education and permission-giving is needed here).
- Iatrogenic influences, when potentially orgasmic-inhibiting drugs are prescribed.

Treatment Options

Psychosexual issues are more frequently a cause in life-long orgasmic difficulties, while biologic etiology should be considered with gradual or rapid onset of anorgasmia.

If the history and physical assessment has ruled out any hormonal, neurophysiologic, or pharmacologic-related causes, the treatment of orgasmic disorders should then focus on an assessment of knowledge. Teaching women and their partners about appropriate arousal techniques may be all that is needed.

In addition, sociocultural factors need to be considered; that is, there may be inhibitions about receiving pleasurable sexual stimuli (usually in generalized primary anorgasmia, but not always). Education can be given about how women become aroused, the amount of time needed for arousal, and the types of stimulation commonly needed for orgasm to be experienced. Information that most women are not able to experience orgasm from vaginal intercourse, and that extended clitoral or vaginal (G spot) stimulation may be needed, is also important information to disseminate [33,34]. Referral of the woman and/or couple to a certified sex therapist is helpful here (see www.aasect.org for a certified sex therapist in your geographic area).

The treatment of anorgasmia has been based on psychoanalytic, cognitive-behavioral, systems theory, and pharmacologic approaches [35]. According to Meston and colleagues, "cognitive behavioral therapy for anorgasmia focuses on promoting changes in attitudes and sexually-relevant thoughts, decreasing anxiety, and increasing orgasmic ability and satisfaction" [6, p. 67].

In the 1970s the small-group format was suggested and a number of books and videos were developed to give women permission to experience orgasm and to share ways in small pre-orgasmic groups that they found helpful to experience sensual and sexual pleasure [36].

Behavioral exercises include directed masturbation, with and without vibrators, which has been shown to be effective in groups and individually. If a woman is able to experience orgasm through masturbation, but not with a partner (if this is her desire), then couple therapy may be recommended, once issues of anxiety, communication, trust, and past history have been addressed. Another behavioral approach often suggested is Kegel exercises. Graber and Kline-Graber found a positive correlation between the strength of a woman's pelvic muscles and her orgasmic response. The women with very weak muscles were anorgasmic in their retrospective study [37]. Perry and Whipple found that women who experienced female ejaculation have significantly stronger pelvic muscles than women who did not experience this phenomenon [38,39]. Sensate focus exercises were developed by Masters and Johnson to reduce anxiety by using a series of body touching exercises, moving from sensual to increasingly sexual [4]. These exercises are used by many healthcare providers today, although Meston and colleagues note that there has been no reported substantial improvement in orgasmic ability with these exercises [6].

There are no pharmacologic agents that have been demonstrated to be effective for treating women with orgasmic disorders. However, a good history will determine if other medical conditions or medications taken may inhibit orgasmic response. A change of medication or taking bupropion with an SSRI, or in place of the SSRI, may help. More double-blind, placebo-controlled studies are needed here. There is an excellent review of psychosocial and pharmacologic treatments for orgasmic disorders in West *et al.* [13].

It may be that permission and education are the most important treatment modalities. And since orgasm is not always essential for sexual satisfaction, and the inability to orgasm during intercourse is not abnormal, when would an orgasm difficulty warrant therapy? If it is a problem for the woman and causes her personal distress. It is important for women to know that they are in charge of their own orgasms, that no one can give them an orgasm, and they are responsible for their pleasure and satisfaction.

It is also important to remember that each woman is unique, that each woman responds differently, and that we cannot put women into one linear way of responding sensually and sexually. Women need to be encouraged to feel good about what brings them pleasure, to be aware of this, to acknowledge it, and then to communicate it to a partner if they choose.

References

1 Ford CS, Beach FA. *Patterns of Sexual Behavior.* New York: Harper & Brothers, 1951.

2 Kinsey AC, Pomeroy WB, Martin CE. *Sexual Behavior in the Human Female.* Philadelphia, PA: WB Saunders Co, 1953.

3 Masters WH, Johnson VE. *Human Sexual Response.* Boston, MA: Little, Brown, 1966.

4 Masters WH, Johnson VE. *Human Sexual Inadequacy.* Boston, MA: Little, Brown, 1970.

5 Kothari P. *Orgasm: New Dimensions.* Bombay, India: VRP Publishers, 1989.

6 Meston CM, Hull E, Levin RJ, Sipski M. Disorders of orgasm in women. *J Sex Med* 2004;**1**:66–68.

7 Komisaruk BR, Whipple B. Physiological and perceptual correlates of orgasm produced by genital or non-genital stimulation. In: Kothari P, ed. *Proceedings of the First International Conference on Orgasm.* Bombay, India: VRP Publishers, 1991, pp. 69–73.

8 Basson R, Berman J, Burnett A, Degrogatis L, Ferguson D, Foucroy J, Goldstein I, Graziottin A, Heiman J, Laan E, Leiblum S, Padma-Nathan H, Rosen R, Segraves K, Segraves RT, Shabsigh R, Sipski M, Wagner G, Whipple B. Report of the international consensus development conference on female sexual dysfunction: definitions and classifications. *J Urol* 2000;**163**: 888–893.

9 American Psychiatric Association. *Diagnostic and Statistical Manual of Mental Disorders.* Washington, DC: American Psychiatric Association, 2000.

10 Basson R, Althof S, Davis S, Fugl-Meyer K, Goldstein I, Leiblum S, Meston C, Rosen R, Wagner G. Summary of the recommendations on sexual dysfunctions in women. *J Sex Med* 2004;**1**:24–39.

11 Jones KP, Kingsberg S, Whipple B. *Women's Sexual Health in Midlife and Beyond: Clinical Proceedings.* Washington, DC: Association of Reproductive Health Professionals, 2005.

12 Rosen RC. Prevalence and risk factors of sexual dysfunction in men and women. *Curr Psychiatry Rep* 2000;**2**:189–195.

13 West SL, Vinikoor LC, Zolnoun D. A systematic review of the literature on female sexual dysfunction prevalence and predictors. *Ann Rev Sex Res* 2004;**15**:40–172.

14 Laumann EO, Gagnon JH, Michael RT, Michaels S. The social organization of sexuality: sexual practices in the United States. Chicago, IL: University of Chicago Press, 1994.

15 Bachmann GA, Leiblum SR. The impact of hormones on menopausal sexuality: a literature review. *Menopause* 2004;**11**:120–130.

16 Avis NE, Stellato R, Crawford S, *et al.* Is there an association between menopause status and sexual functioning? *Menopause* 2000;**7**:297–309.

17 Crouch NS, Minto CL, Laio L-M, Woodhouse CRJ, Creighton SM. Genital sensation after feminizing genitoplasty for congenital adrenal hyperplasia: a pilot study. *BJU Int* 2004;**93**:135–138.

18 Oberg K, Fugl-Meyer KS. On Swedish women's distressing sexual dysfunctions: some concomitant conditions and life satisfaction. *J Sex Med* 2005;**2**: 169.

19 Masters WH, Johnson VE, Kolodny RC. *Human Sexuality.* Boston, MA: Little Brown & Co, 1982.

20 Sipski ML, Alexander CJ, Rosen RC. Sexual arousal and orgasm in women: effects of spinal cord injury. *Ann Neurol* 2001;**49**:35–44.

21 Komisaruk BR, Whipple B, Crawford A, Grimes S, Liu W-C, Kalin A, Mosier K. Brain activation during vaginocervical self-stimulation and orgasm in women with complete spinal cord injury: fMRI evidence of mediation by the vagus nerves. *Brain Res* 2004;**1024**: 77–88.

22 Komisaruk BR, Whipple B. Brain activity imaging during sexual response in women with spinal cord injury. In Hyde J. ed. *Biological Substrates of Human Sexuality.* Washington, DC: American Psychological Association, 2005, pp. 109–146.

23 Whipple B, Komisaruk BR. Brain (PET) responses to vaginal-cervical self-stimulation in women with complete spinal cord injury: preliminary findings. *J Sex Marital Ther* 2002;**28**:79–86.

24 Whipple B, Ogden G, Komisaruk BR. Physiological correlates of imagery induced orgasm in women. *Arch Sex Behav* 1992;**21**:121–133.

25 Dunn KM, Cherkas LF, Septor TD. Genetic influences on variation in female orgasmic function: a twin study. *Biol Lett* 2005;**1**:260–263.

26 Meston CM, Levin RJ, Sipski ML, Hull EM, Heiman JR. Women's orgasm. *Ann Rev Sex Res* 2004;**15**:173–257.

27 Mah K, Binik YM. The nature of human orgasm: a critical review of major trends. *Clin Psychol Rev* 2001;**21**: 823–856.

28 Marshall DS. Sexual behavior on Mangaia. In: Marshall DS, Suggs RC, eds. *Human Sexual Behavior: Variations in the Ethnographic Spectrum*. New York: Basic Books, 1971, pp. 103–162.

29 Mead M. *Male and Female: A Study of the Sexes in a Changing World*. New York: William Morrow, 1939.

30 Ladas AK, Whipple B, Perry JD. *The G Spot and Other Discoveries about Human Sexuality*. New York: Owl Books, 2005.

31 Bateson G, Mead M. *Balinese Character: A Photographic Analysis*. New York Academy of Sciences: New York, 1942.

32 Zaviacic M. *The human female prostate: From vestigial Skene's paraurethral glands and duct to woman's functional prostate*. Bratislava, Slovakia: Slovak Academic Press, 1999.

33 Whipple B, Brash-McGreer K. Management of female sexual dysfunction. In: Sipski ML, Alexander CJ, eds. *Sexual Function in People with Disability and Chronic Illness: A Health Professional's Guide*. Gaithersburg, MD: Aspen Publishers Inc, 1997, pp. 511–536.

34 Phillips NA. Female sexual dysfunction: evaluation and treatment. *Am Fam Physician* 2000;**62**:127–136, 141–142.

35 Heiman, JR. Orgasmic disorders in women. In Leiblum SR, Rosen RC, eds. Principles and Practice of Sex Therapy. New York: Guilford, 2000.

36 Barbach LG. *For Yourself: The Fulfillment of Female Sexuality*. New York: Doubleday, 1975.

37 Graber B, Kline-Graber G. Female orgasm: role of the pubococcygeus. *J Clin Psychiatry* 1979;**30**:34–39.

38 Perry JD, Whipple B. Pelvic muscle strength of female ejaculators: evidence in support of a new theory of orgasm. *J Sex Res* 1981;**17**:22–39.

39 Perry JD, Whipple B. Multiple components of the female orgasm. In: Graber B, ed. *Circumvaginal Musculature and Sexual Function*. New York: S. Karger, 1982, pp. 101–114.

40 Graziottin A. Implicazioni psicosessuali dell'incontinenza femminile (Psychosexual implications of female incontinence), Rivista Italiana di Colon-Proctologia 1996;**15**(4):249–252.

41 Belzer E, Whipple B, Moger W. On female ejaculation. *J Sex Res* 1984;**20**:403–406.

42 Addiego F, Belzer EG, Comolli J, Moger W, Perry JD, Whipple B. Female ejaculation: a case study. *J Sex Res* 1981;**17**:13–21.

CHAPTER 25

Sexual Pain Disorders: Dyspareunia and Vaginismus

Alessandra Graziottin

Introduction

Pain is almost never "psychogenic," except for pain from grieving. Pain has biologic basis; when it is the alerting signal of an impending or current tissue damage from which the body should withdraw, it is defined as "nociceptive" [1]. When pain becomes a disease per se, that is, generated within the nerves and nervous centers, it is called "neuropathic" [1–3]. It is a complex perceptive experience, involving psychologic and relational meanings, which may become increasingly important with the chronicity of pain [1–3].

Sexual pain disorders—dyspareunia and vaginismus—are very sensitive issues, as the pain involves emotionally charged behaviors: sexual intimacy and vaginal intercourse [4–6]. Most patients have been denied for years that their pain was real, and therefore feel enormously relieved when they finally meet a clinician who trusts their symptoms and commits him/herself to a thorough understanding of the complex etiology of their sexual pain.

Talking with patients about sexual pain disorders requires special attention to the sensitivity of the issue and an empathic attitude to the biologic "truth" of pain [7]. This is the basis of a very rewarding clinician–patient relationship and is the basis of an effective therapeutic alliance.

Definitions

Dyspareunia defines the persistent or recurrent pain with attempted or complete vaginal entry and/or penile vaginal intercourse [8].

Vaginismus indicates the persistent or recurrent difficulties of the woman to allow vaginal entry of a penis, a finger, and/or any object, despite the woman's expressed wish to do so. There is often (phobic) avoidance and anticipation, fear or experience of pain, along with variable involuntary pelvic muscle contraction. Structural or other physical abnormalities must be ruled out or addressed [8].

Although there is a longstanding tradition to distinguish female sexual pain disorders into vaginismus and (superficial) dyspareunia, recent research has demonstrated persistent problems with the sensitivity and specificity of the differential diagnosis of these two phenomena.

Both complaints may comprise, to a smaller or larger extent [5–7,9–10]:

1 Problems with muscle tension (voluntary, involuntary, limited to vaginal sphincter, or extending to pelvic floor, adductor muscles, back, jaws or entire body).

2 Pain upon genital touching: superficially located at the vaginal entry, the vulvar vestibulum and/or the perineum; either event-related, limited to the duration of genital touching or pressure, or more chronic, lasting for minutes/hours/days after termination of touching; ranging from unique association with genital touching during sexual activity to more general association with all types of vulvar/vaginal/pelvic pressure (e.g. sitting, riding horse or bicycle, wearing tight trousers).

3 Fear of sexual pain (either specifically associated with genital touching/intercourse or more generalized fear of pain, or fear of sex).

4 Propensity for behavioral approach or avoidance. Despite painful experiences with genital touching/ intercourse, a subgroup of women continues to be receptive to their sexual partner's initiatives or to self-initiate sexual interaction.

Table 25.1 Severity of vaginismus.

Grade I	Spasm of the elevator ani, which disappears on reassuring the patient
Grade II	Spasm of the elevator ani, which persists during the gynecologic/urologic/proctologic examination
Grade III	Spasm of the elevator ani and tension of buttocks at any tentative or gynecologic examination
Grade IV	Mild neurovegetative arousal, spasm of the elevator, dorsal arching, adduction of thighs, defense and retraction
Grade XO	Extreme defense neurovegetative arousal, with refusal of the gynecologic examination

Modified from Lamont (1978) [15].

However, as no consensus has been reached so far in unifying the two entities, they will be kept separate according to the latest classification [8].

Prevalence

Various degrees of dyspareunia are reported by 12–15% of coitally active women [11–13], and up to 45.3% of postmenopausal women [14]. Vaginismus may occur in 0.5–1% of fertile women, although precise estimates are lacking [7]. However, mild hyperactivity of the pelvic floor, that could coincide with grade I or II vaginismus, according to Lamont [15] (Table 25.1), may permit intercourse while causing coital pain [16,17].

Pathophysiology

Vaginal receptiveness is a prerequisite for intercourse, and requires anatomic and functional tissue integrity, both in resting and aroused states [16–19]. Normal trophism, both mucosal and cutaneous, adequate hormonal impregnation, lack of inflammation, particularly at the introitus, normal tonicity of the perivaginal muscles, vascular, connective and neurologic integrity, and normal immune response are all considered necessary to guarantee vaginal "habitability" [6,7,15–17]. Vaginal receptiveness

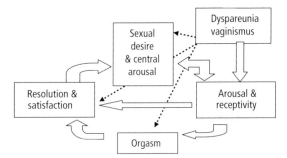

Fig. 25.1 Circular model of female sexual function and the interfering role of sexual pain disorders. This simplified circular model contributes to the understanding of: (1) frequent overlapping of sexual symptoms reported in clinical practice ("co-morbidity"), as different dimensions of sexual response are correlated from a pathophysiologic point of view; (2) potential negative or positive feedback mechanisms operating in sexual function; (3) the *direct* inhibiting effect of dyspareunia and/or vaginismus on genital arousal and vaginal receptivity and the *indirect* inhibiting effect they may have on coital orgasm, satisfaction, sexual desire, and central arousal, with close interplay between biologic and psychosexual factors. Pelvic floor disorders of the hyperactive type, causally related to sexual pain disorders as predisposing and/or maintaining factors (see Chapter 20), may inhibit all the sexual response. Modified from Graziottin (2003) [18].

may be further modulated by psychosexual, mental, and interpersonal factors, all of which may result in poor arousal with vaginal dryness [5,7,8–11].

Fear of penetration, and a general muscular arousal secondary to anxiety, may cause a defensive contraction of the perivaginal muscles, leading to vaginismus [7,9,10]. This disorder may also be the clinical correlate of a primary neurodystonia of the pelvic floor, as recently demonstrated with needle electromyography [20]. It may be so severe as to completely prevent penetration [15,16]. Vaginismus is the leading cause of unconsummated marriages in women. Co-morbidity between life-long vaginismus and dyspareunia, and other FSD is frequently reported (Fig. 25.1). The defensive pelvic floor contraction may also be secondary to genital pain, of whatever cause [21,22].

Dyspareunia is the common symptom of a variety of coital pain-causing disorders (Table 25.2).

Table 25.2 Etiology of dyspareunia: different causes may overlap or be associated with coital pain with complex and dynamic pathophysiologic interplay.

Biological

Superficial/introital and/or mid-vaginal dyspareunia
- infectious: vulvitis, vulvar vestibulitis, vaginitis, cystitis
- inflammatory: with upregulation of mast cells
- hormonal: vulvovaginal atrophy
- anatomic: fibrous hymen, vaginal agenesis, Rokitansky syndrome
- muscular: primary or secondary hyperactivity of levator ani muscle
- iatrogenic: poor outcome of genital or perineal surgery; pelvic radiotherapy
- neurologic, inclusive of neuropathic pain
- connective and immunitary: Sjögren's syndrome
- vascular

Deep dyspareunia
- endometriosis
- pelvic inflammatory disease (PID)
- pelvic varicocele
- chronic pelvic pain and referred pain
- outcome of pelvic or endovaginal radiotherapy
- abdominal cutaneous nerve entrapment syndrome (ACNES)

Psychosexual
- co-morbidity with desire and/or arousal disorders, or vaginismus
- past sexual harassment and/or abuse
- affective disorders: depression and anxiety
- catastrophism as leading psychologic coping modality

Context or couple related
- lack of emotional intimacy
- inadequate foreplay
- couple conflicts; verbally, physically, or sexually abusive partner
- poor anatomic compatibility (penis size and/or infantile female genitalia)
- sexual dissatisfaction and consequent inadequate arousal

Adapted from Graziottin (2003) [16].

Vulvar vestibulitis (VV), a subset of vulvodynia, is its leading cause in women of fertile age [6,7,11,12,16,17,23,24]. The diagnostic triad is: (1) severe pain upon vestibular touch or attempted vaginal entry; (2) exquisite tenderness to cotton-swab palpation of the introital area (mostly at the 5 o'clock and 7 o'clock positions); (3) dyspareunia [23].

From the pathophysiologic point of view, VV involves the upregulation of: (1) the immunologic system, ie of introital mast cells (with hyperproduction of both inflammatory molecules and nerve growth factors (NGF) [25–27]; (2) the pain system, with proliferation of local pain fibers induced by the NGF [27–28], which may contribute to the hyperalgesia and allodynia, associated with neuropathic pain, reported by VV patients [2,3,6]; (3) hyperactivity of the levator ani, which can be antecedent to VV and co-morbid with vaginismus of a mild degree [6,16,24], or secondary to the introital pain. In either case, addressing the muscle component is a key part of the treatment [28–30].

Hyperactivity of the pelvic floor may be triggered by non-genital, non-sexual causes, such as urologic factors (urge incontinence, when tightening the pelvic floor may be secondary to the aim of reinforcing the ability to control the bladder) [17], or anorectal problems (anismus, haemorrhoids, rhagades) [22].

Medical ("organic") factors, which are often under-evaluated in the clinical setting, may cause pain and they may combine with psychogenic (psychosexual) factors contributing to pain during intercourse. They include hormonal/dystrophic, inflammatory, muscular, iatrogenic, neurologic and/or post-traumatic, vascular, connective, and immunologic causes [6,7,9–11,16–22,27].

Co-morbidity with other sexual dysfunctions—loss of desire, arousal disorders, orgasmic difficulties, and/or sexual pain related disorders—is frequently reported with persisting or chronic dyspareunia [16]. The second leading etiology of dyspareunia in the fertile age is postpartum pain associated with poor episiorraphy outcome and vaginal dryness secondary to the hypoestrogenic state when the woman is breastfeeding [31].

Clinical Approach

In sexual pain disorders, the accurate clinical history and careful physical examination are essential for the diagnosis and prognosis. Location and characteristics of pain have been demonstrated to be the most significant predictors of the etiology of pain [16,18,19,21,32]. No instrumental examination has so far been demonstrated to be more informative than a carefully performed clinical examination.

Focusing on the presenting symptom—dyspareunia—and with the above-mentioned attention to the sensitivity of the issue, key questions to obtain the most relevant information can be summarized as follows [16–18,33]:

• Did you experience coital pain from the very beginning of your sexual life onwards (life-long) or did you experience it after a period of normal (painless) sexual intercourse (acquired disorder)? If life-long, were you afraid of feeling pain before your first intercourse? When life-long, dyspareunia might usually be caused by mild/moderate vaginismus (which allows a painful penetration) and/or coexisting, life-long low libido and arousal disorders.

• If acquired, do you remember the situation or what happened when it started? The answer can give information about the "natural history" of the current sexual complaint.

• *Where* does it hurt? At the beginning of the vagina, in the mid vagina or deep in the vagina? Location of the pain and its onset within an episode of intercourse is the strongest predictor of presence and type of organicity [32].

— Introital dyspareunia may be more frequently caused by poor arousal, mild vaginismus, vestibulitis, vulvar dystrophia, painful outcome of vulvar physical therapies, perineal surgery (episiorraphy, colporraphy, posterior perineorraphy), pudendal nerve entrapment syndrome and/or pudendal neuralgia, Sjogren syndrome [5–7,9–12,14–19] (see also Chapter 26).

— Mid vaginal pain, acutely evoked during physical examination by a gentle pressure on the sacrospinous insertion of the levator ani muscle, is more frequently due to levator ani myalgia, the most frequently overlooked biologic cause of dyspareunia [6,16,17,21].

— Deep vaginal pain may be caused more frequently by endometriosis or pelvic inflammatory disease (PID) or by outcomes of pelvic radiotherapy or vaginal radical surgery. Varicocele, adhesions, referred abdominal pain, and ab-

dominal cutaneous nerve entrapment syndrome (ACNES) are less frequent and still controversial causes of deep dyspareunia, which should nevertheless be considered in the differential diagnosis [16,17].

• *When* do you feel pain? Before, during or after intercourse?

— Pain before intercourse suggests a phobic attitude toward penetration, usually associated with vaginismus, and/or the presence of chronic VV, and/or vulvodynia [24,35].

— Pain during intercourse is more frequently reported. This information, combined with the previous—"where does it hurt?"—is the most predictive of the organicity of pain [5–7,9–12,14–19].

— Pain after intercourse indicates that mucosal damage was provoked during intercourse, possibly because of poor lubrication, concurring to vestibulitis, pain, and defensive contraction of the pelvic floor [6,16–17].

• Do you feel other accompanying symptoms, vaginal dryness, pain or paresthesias in the genitals and pelvic areas? Or do you suffer from cystitis 24–72 hours after intercourse?

— Vaginal dryness, either secondary to loss of estrogen and/or to poor genital arousal may coincide with or contribute to dyspareunia [6,16–19].

— Clitoralgia and/or vulvodynia, spontaneous and/or worsening during sexual arousal, may be associated with dyspareunia, hypertonic pelvic floor muscles, and/or neurogenic pain (pudendal nerve entrapment syndrome) [36].

— Postcoital cystitis should suggest a hypoestrogenic condition and/or the presence of hypertonic pelvic floor muscles: it should specifically be investigated in postmenopausal women who may benefit from topical estrogen treatment [37] and rehabilitation of the pelvic floor, aimed at relaxing the myalgic perivaginal muscles [28–30].

— Vulvar pruritus, vulvar dryness, and/or feeling of a burning vulva should be investigated, as they may suggest the presence of vulvar lichen sclerosus, which may worsen introital dyspareunia [19]. Neurogenic pain may cause not only dyspareunia but also clitoralgia. Eye and mouth dryness, when accompanying dyspareunia and vaginal dryness, should suggest Sjögren's syndrome, a connective and immunitary disease [16–19].

• How intense is the pain you feel? Focusing on the intensity and characteristics of pain is a relatively new approach in addressing dyspareunia [5–7,16,17]. A shift from nociceptive to neuropathic pain is typical of chronic dyspareunia, and treatment may require a systemic and local analgesic approach [3,6].

Key point

Suggest that the patient record a *diary of pain*, mirroring the menstrual cycle phases if the woman is in her fertile age (i.e. starting every page with the first day of her cycle, with the date on the x axis, and the 24 hours of the day in the y axis. Pain intensity could be reported using colours: zero = white; 1 to 3 = yellow; 4 to 7 = red, 8 to 10 = black).

This would: (1) improve the recording and understanding of pain flares before, during and/or after cycle, and the circadian rhythm of pain, to improve the diagnosis of etiology and contributors of pain; (2) suggest a better tailoring of the analgesic treatment; (3) make the recording of the impact of treatment of pain perception more accurate, with an easy to catch perspective [36]. Typically, nociceptive pain persists at night, while neuropathic pain is significantly reduced or absent during sleep.

Clinical Approach

The diagnostic work-up of dyspareunia should focus on:

• Accurate *physical* examination, to describe:
  — the "pain map", i.e. any site in the vulva, introitus, mid vagina, and deep vagina where pain can be elicited [16,18,19,40];
  — pelvic floor trophism (and vaginal pH), muscular tonus, strength, and performance and myogenic and referred pain [16,21];
  — signs of inflammation (primarily VV) [6,16,23];
  — poor outcome of pelvic [41] or perineal surgery (episiotomy/rraphy) [31];
  — associated urogenital and rectal pain syndromes [22];

— neuropathic pain, in vulvodynia or localized clitoralgia with no objective findings [3,5,7].
• Psychosexual factors, poor arousal and coexisting vaginismus [6,7,9,10,15,24].
• Relationship issues [7,42].
• Hormonal profile, if clinically indicated, when dyspareunia is associated with vaginal dryness [16–18].

In patients with vaginismus, the diagnosis and prognosis may be made based on three variables:
• Intensity of the phobic attitude (mild, moderate, severe) toward penetration [7,9,10,15,16];
• Intensity of the pelvic floor hypertonicity (in four degree, according to Lamont [15,28–30];
• Coexisting personal and/or relational psychosexual problems [6,7,9,10,15,24].

Principles of Treatment of Sexual Pain Disorders

Sexual co-morbidity is a key issue in sexual pain disorders. Dyspareunia and vaginismus, because of coital pain, directly inhibit genital arousal and vaginal receptivity. Indirectly, they may affect the (coital) orgasmic potential during the intercourse and impair physical and emotional satisfaction, causing loss of desire for and avoidance of sexual intimacy [16,18,19,21,26,40,42].

Dyspareunia may benefit from a well-tailored clinical approach, based on a clear understanding of the pathophysiology of coital pain the patient is complaining of, with attention to predisposing, precipitating, and maintaining factors in any of the systems potentially involved (Table 25.3).

Medical treatment
Multimodal therapy

VV should be treated with a combined, multimodal treatment aimed at reducing:

1 The upregulation of mast cells, both by reducing the agonist stimuli (such as Candida infections, microabrasions of the introital mucosa because of intercourse with a dry vagina and/or a contracted pelvic floor, chemicals, allergens, and so on) that cause degranulation leading to chronic tissue inflammation, and/or with antagonist modulation of

Table 25.3 Treatment of dyspareunia.

Medical
Inflammatory etiology (upregulation of mast cells)
- Pharmacologic modulation of mast cells' hyperreactivity
  - with antidepressants: amitriptyline
  - with aliamide topical gel
- Reduction of agonist factors causing hyperreactivity of mast cells
  - recurrent Candida or Gardnerella vaginitis
  - microabrasions of the introital mucosa: from intercourse with a dry vagina or from inappropriate lifestyles
  - allergens or chemical irritants
  - physical agents
  - neurogenic stimuli
Muscular etiology (upregulation of the muscular system)
- Self-massage and levator ani stretching
- Physical therapy of the levator ani
- Electromyografic biofeedback
- Type A botulin toxin
Neurologic etiology (upregulation of the pain system)
- Systemic analgesia
  - amitriptyline
  - gabapentin
  - pregabalin
- Local analgesia
  - electroanalgesia
  - ganglion impar block
- Surgical therapy: vestibulectomy (?)
Hormonal etiology
- Hormonal therapy
  - local: vaginal estrogens, or testosterone for the vulva
  - systemic: with hormonal replacement therapies

Psychosexual
- Behavioral cognitive group therapy
- Individual psychotherapy
- Couple psychotherapy

Modified from Graziottin (2005) [42].

its hyperreactivity, with amitriptyline or aliamide gel [6,42,44].

2 The upregulation of pain system secondary to both the proliferation of introital pain fibers [25–27] induced by NGF produced by the upregulated mast cells, and the lowered central pain threshold [45]. A thorough understanding of the pathophysiology of pain, in its nociceptive and neuropathic component, is essential. Anthalgic treatment should be prescribed: locally, with electroanalgesia [39] or, in severe cases, with the ganglion impar block [3]; systemically with tricyclic antidepressant, gabapentin or pregabalin in the most severe cases with a neuropathic component [3,6,38,43].

3 The upregulation of the muscular response, with hyperactivity of the pelvic floor, which may precede VV, when the predisposing factor is vaginismus [6,24], or be acquired in response to genital pain [6,20,33]. In controlled studies, electromyographic feedback [28–30] has been demonstrated to significantly reduce pain in VV patients. Self-massage, pelvic floor stretching, and physical therapy may also reduce the muscular component of coital pain [6,40,42]. When hyperactivity of the pelvic floor is elevated, treatment with type A botulin toxin has been proposed on the basis of its efficacy and safety profile in pelvic floor disorders of the hyperactive type [46,47].

Individually tailored combinations of this approach are useful to treat introital dyspareunia with etiologies different from VV.

Key point
Patients—and couples—should be required to abstain from vaginal intercourse and use other forms of sexual intimacy during VV treatment, until introital pain and burning feelings have disappeared. This is essential to prevent the introital microabrasion caused by penetration when there is vaginal dryness, overall poor genital arousal and/or tightened pelvic floor that would maintain the upregulation of mast cells, pelvic floor defensive hypertonus, and proliferation of peripheral pain fibers [6].

Deep dyspareunia, secondary to endometriosis, pelvic inflammatory disease (PID), chronic pelvic pain, and other less frequent etiologies requires specialist treatment that goes beyond the scope of this chapter.

Topical hormones
Vaginal estrogen treatment is the first choice (when no contraindications are present) when dyspareunia is associated with genital arousal disorders and hypoestrogenism [16–19,37] (see also Chapter 23).

This biologic contributor of dyspareunia in long-lasting hypothalamic amenorrhea, puerperium, and postmenopause, can be easily improved with this topical treatment [16–19,37]. Safety of such hormonal topical treatment is discussed in Chapter 27. Vulvar treatment with testosterone (1% or 2% in Vaseline, oil, or petrolatum) may be considered when vulvar dystrophy and/or lichen sclerosus contribute to introital dyspareunia.

Psychosexual treatment
Psychosexual and/or behavioural therapy
This is the first-line treatment of *life-long* dyspareunia associated with *vaginismus* [6,40,48]. It should be offered in parallel with a progressive rehabilitation of the pelvic floor and a pharmacologic treatment to modulate the intense systemic arousal in the subset of intensely phobic patients [33,40]. In this latter group, co-morbidity with sexual aversion disorder should be investigated and treated (see Chapter 22).

This contributes to the multimodal treatment of life-long dyspareunia, which is reported in one-third of VV patients [40]. Anxiety, fear of pain, and sexual avoidant behaviors should be addressed as well. The shift from pain to pleasure is key from the sexual point of view. Sensitive and committed psychosexual support of the woman and the couple are mandatory.

Vaginismus may as well be treated with a multimodal approach, given its complex neurobiologic, muscular, and psychosexual etiology.

Pharmacologic therapy
• Depending on the intensity of the phobic attitude, the general anxiety arousal may be reduced with pharmacologic treatment. [33,40].
• Botulin A toxin may be injected in the levator ani when the patient is able to accept the injection [46,47].

Psychosexual behavioral therapy
• Address underlying negative affects (fear, disgust, repulsion to touch, but also loss of self-esteem and self-confidence, body image concerns, fear of being abandoned by the partner) when reported [48].
• Teach how to command the pelvic floor muscles and to control the ability to do so with a mirror [40,49].
• Encourage self-contact, self-massage, self-awareness, through sexual education. If the woman has a current partner, encourage active sex-play, to maintain and/or increase desire, arousal and possibly clitoral orgasm, with specific prohibition of coital attempts until the pelvic floor is adequately relaxed and the woman is willing and able to accept intercourse [33,49].
• When good pelvic floor voluntary relaxation has been obtained, teach how to insert a dilator under pelvic floor relaxation [33,49].
• Discuss contraception, if the couple does not desire children at present [33].
• Encourage the sharing of control with the partner.
• Give permission for more intimate play, inserting of penis with the woman in control.
• Support the possible performance anxiety of the male partner with vasculogenic active drugs [33].
• Support the couple during the first attempts, as anxiety is frequent and may undermine the result if not adequately addressed, both emotionally and pharmacologically. Phosphodiesterase (PDE-5) inhibitors are useful when performance erectile dysfunction (ED) is reported [33].
• If possible, recommend concurrent psychotherapy, sex-therapy or couples therapy when significant psychodynamic or relationship issues are evident [33,48,49].

Conclusion

Pain is rarely purely psychogenic, and dyspareunia is no exception. Like all pain syndromes, it usually has one or more biologic etiologic factors. Hyperactive pelvic floor disorders are a constant feature and co-morbidity with urologic and/or proctologic disorders is a frequent and yet neglected area to be explored for comprehensive treatment. Psychosexual and relationship factors, generally life-long or acquired low sexual desire because of the persisting pain, and life-long or acquired arousal disorders due to the inhibitory effect of pain, should be addressed in parallel, in order to provide comprehensive, integrated, and effective treatment.

Vaginismus, which may contribute to life-long

dyspareunia when mild or moderate, and may prevent intercourse when severe, needs to be better understood in its complex neurobiologic, muscular, and psychosexual etiology, and to be addressed with a multimodal approach.

Couple issues should be diagnosed and appropriate referral considered when the male partner presents with a concomitant male sexual disorder.

References

1 Bonica J. Definitions and taxonomy of pain. In: Bonica J, ed. *The Management of Pain*. Philadelphia, PA: Lea & Febiger, 1990.

2 Woolf C. The pathophysiology of peripheral neuropathic pain: abnormal peripheral input and abnormal central processing. *Acta Neurochir* 1993;Suppl **58**:125–130.

3 Vincenti E, Graziottin A. Neuropathic pain in vulvar vestibulitis: diagnosis and treatment. In: Graziottin A (Guest, ed.) Female Sexual Dysfunction: Clinical Approach. *Urodinamica* 2004, pp. 112–116.

4 Foster D. Chronic vulval pain. In: MacLean AB, Stones RW, Thornton S, eds. *Pain in Obstetrics and Gynecology*. London: RCOG Press, 2001, pp. 198–208.

5 Binik Y. Should dyspareunia be retained as a sexual dysfunction in DSM-V? A painful classification decision. *Arch Sex Behav* 2006; **34**(1):11–21.

6 Graziottin A, Brotto LA. Vulvar vestibulitis syndrome: a clinical approach. *J Sex Marital Ther* 2004;**30**:125–139.

7 Pukall C, Lahaie M, Binik Y. Sexual pain disorders: etiologic factors. In: Goldstein I, Meston CM, Davis S, Traish A, eds. *Women's Sexual Function and Dysfunction: Study, Diagnosis and Treatment*. London: Taylor & Francis, 2005.

8 Basson R, Leiblum S, Brotto L. Revised definitions of women's sexual dysfunction. *J Sex Med* 2004;**1**:40–48.

9 Reissing E, Binik Y, Khalifé S. Does vaginismus exist? A critical review of the literature. *J Nerv Ment Dis* 1999;**187**:261–274.

10 Van der Velde J, Laan E, Everaerd W. Vaginismus, a component of a general defensive reaction: an investigation of pelvic floor muscle activity during exposure to emotion inducing film excerpts in women with and without vaginismus. *Int Urogynecol J Pelvic Floor Dysfunct* 2001;**12**:328–331.

11 Harlow B, Wise L, Stewart E. Prevalence and predictors of chronic lower genital tract discomfort. *Am J Obstet Gynecol* 2001;**185**:545–550.

12 Harlow B, Stewart B. A population-based assessment of chronic unexplained vulvar pain: have we underestimated the prevalence of vulvodynia? *J Am Med Womens Assoc* 2003;**58**:82–88.

13 Laumann EO, Paik A, Rosen RC. Sexual dysfunction in the United States: prevalence and predictors. *JAMA* 1999;**281**:537–544.

14 Oskai U, Baj N, Yalcin O. A study on urogenital complaints of postmenopausal women aged 50 and over. *Acta Obstet Gynecol Scand* 2005;**84**:72–78.

15 Lamont J. Vaginismus. *Am J Obstet Gynecol* 1978;**131**:632–636.

16 Graziottin A. Etiology and diagnosis of coital pain. *J Endocrinol Invest* 2003;**26**:115–121.

17 Graziottin A. Sexual pain disorders in adolescents. In: *12th World Congress of Human Reproduction*, International Academy of Human Reproduction. 2005. Venice.

18 Graziottin A. Dyspareunia: clinical approach in the perimenopause. In: Studd J, ed. *The Management of the Menopause*, 3rd edn. London: Parthenon Publishing Group, 2003, pp. 229–241.

19 Graziottin A. Sexuality in postmenopause and senium. In: Lauritzen C, Studd J, eds. *Current Management of the Menopause*, London: Martin Dunitz, 2004, pp. 185–203.

20 Graziottin A, Bottanelli M, Bertolasi L. Vaginismus: a clinical and neurophysiological study. In: Graziottin A (Guest, ed.) Female Sexual Dysfunction: Clinical Approach. *Urodinamica* 2004, pp. 117–121.

21 Alvarez D, Rockwell P. Trigger points: diagnosis and management. *Am Fam Physician* 2002;**65**:653–660.

22 Wesselmann U, Burnett AL, Heinberg LJ. The urogenital and rectal pain syndromes. *Pain* 1997;**73**:269–294.

23 Friedrich E. Vulvar vestibulitis syndrome. *J Reprod Med* 1987;**32**:110–114.

24 Abramov L, Wolman I, David M. Vaginismus: an important factor in the evaluation and management of vulvar vestibulitis syndrome. *Gynecol Obstet Invest* 1994;**38**:194–197.

25 Bohm-Starke N, Hilliges M, Falconer C. Neurochemical characterization of the vestibular nerves in women with vulvar vestibulitis syndrome. *Gynecol Obstet Invest* 1999;**48**:270–275.

26 Bohm-Starke N, Hilliges M, Blomgren B. Increased blood flow and erythema in posterior vestibular mucosa in vulvar vestibulitis. *Am J Obstet Gynecol* 2001;**98**:1067–1074.

27 Bornstein J, Goldschmid N, Sabo E. Hyperinnervation and mast cell activation may be used as a histopathologic diagnostic criteria for vulvar vestibulitis. *Gynecol Obstet Invest* 2004;**58**:171–178.

28 Glazer H, Rodke G, Swencionis C. Treatment of vulvar vestibulitis syndrome with electromyographic feed-

back of pelvic floor musculature. *J Reprod Med* 1995;**40**: 283–290.

29 Bergeron S, Khalife S, Pagidas K. A randomized comparison of group cognitive-behavioural therapy surface electromyographic biofeedback and vestibulectomy in the treatment of dyspareunia resulting from VVS. *Pain* 2001;**91**:297–306.

30 McKay E, Kaufman R, Doctor U. Treating vulvar vestibulitis with electromyographic biofeedback of pelvic floor musculature. *J Reprod Med* 2001;**46**: 337–342.

31 Glazener C. Sexual function after childbirth: women's experiences, persistent morbidity and lack of professional recognition. *Br J Obstet Gynaecol* 1997;**104**: 330–335.

32 Meana M, *et al.* Dyspareunia: sexual dysfunction or pain syndrome? *J Nerv Ment Dis* 1997;**185**:561–569.

33 Plaut M, Graziottin A, Heaton J. *Sexual Dysfunction*. Oxford: Health Press, 2004.

34 Ferrero S, Esposito F, Abbamonte L. Quality of sex life in women with endometriosis and deep dyspareunia. *Fertil Steril* 2005;**83**:573–579.

35 Graziottin A. Female sexual dysfunction. In: Bo K, Berghmans B, van Kampen M, Morkved S, eds. *Evidence Based Physiotherapy for the Pelvic Floor: Bridging Research and Clinical Practice*. Oxford: Elsevier, 2005.

36 Shafik A. Pudendal canal syndrome as a cause of vulvodynia and its treatment by pudendal nerve decompression. *Eur J Obstet Gynecol Reprod Biol* 1998;**80**: 215–220.

37 Simunic V, Banovic I, Ciglar S, Jeren L, Pavicic Baldani D, Sprem M. Local estrogen treatment in patients with urogenital symptoms. *Int J Gynecol Obstet* 2003;**82**: 187–197.

38 Edwards L, Mason M, Phillips M. Childhood sexual and physical abuse: incidence in patients with vulvodynia. *J Reprod Med* 1997;**42**:135–139.

39 Nappi RE, Ferdeghini F, Abbiati I, Vercesi C, Farina C, Polatti F. Electrical stimulation (ES) in the management of sexual pain disorders. *J Sex Marital Ther* 2003; **29**(suppl 1):103–110.

40 Graziottin A. Treatment of sexual dysfunction. In: Bo K, Berghmans B, van Kampen M, Morkved S, eds. *Evidence Based Physiotherapy for the Pelvic Floor: Bridging Research and Clinical Practice*. Oxford: Elsevier, 2005.

41 Graziottin A. Sexual function in women with gynecologic cancer: a review. *Ital J Gynec Obst* 2001;**2**:61–68.

42 Reissing E, Binik Y, Khalifé S. Etiological correlates of vaginismus: sexual and physical abuse, sexual knowledge, sexual self-schema, and relationship adjustment. *J Sex Marital Ther* 2003;**29**:47–59.

43 Shanker B, Mc Auley J. Pregabalin: a new neuromodulator with broad therapeutic indications. *Ann Pharmacother* 2005;**39**:2029–2037.

44 Mariani L. Vulvar vestibulitis sydrome: an overview of non-surgical treatment. *Eur J Obstet Gynecol Reprod Biol* 2002;**101**:109–112.

45 Pukall CF, Binik YM, Khalife S, Amsel R, Abbott FV. Vestibular tactile and pain thresholds in women with vulvar vestibulitis syndrome. *Pain* 2002;**96**:163–175.

46 Maria G, Cadeddu F, Brisinda D. Management of bladder, prostatic and pelvic floor disorders with botulinum neurotoxin. *Curr Med Chem* 2005;**12**:247–265.

47 Ghazizadah S, Nikzed M. Botulinum toxin in the treatment of refractory vaginismus. *Obstet Gynecol* 2004;**104**: 922–925.

48 Leiblum S. Vaginismus: a most perplexing problem. In: *Principles and Practice of Sex Therapy*, 3rd edn. New York: Guilford, 2000, pp. 181–204.

49 Katz D, Tabisel R. Management of vaginismus, vulvodynia and childhood sexual abuse. In: Bourcier AP, McGuire EJ, Abrams P, eds. *Pelvic Floor Disorders*. Philadephia, PA: Elsevier Saunders, 2004, pp. 360–369.

CHAPTER 26

Iatrogenic and Post-Traumatic Female Sexual Disorder

Alessandra Graziottin

Physicians and healthcare providers may contribute to sexual disorders, with a *predisposing* role, when they do not recognize and diagnose conditions that may prelude, precipitate, or maintain a female sexual disorder (FSD) [1–6]. They may act as *precipitating* factors, through the inappropriate prescription of medications that may negatively affect women's and couples' sexuality [1] (Table 26.1), or through the negative outcome of surgery, obstetrics, and/or chemotherapy, hormonotherapy, or radiotherapy [2–12]. A lack of respect for professional boundaries in the clinician–patient relationship is another neglected precipitating co-factor of FSD, especially for women who seek professional help at a vulnerable moment of their life [13,14] (see Chapter 20). They may behave as *maintaining* factors, through the most frequent mistake in the field of FSD: the *diagnostic omission*, which encompasses occasional or systematic diagnostic neglect, particularly in the area of biologic/medical etiology of FSD [2–6,10–12] and/or co-morbidity between medical conditions and FSD [1–6,11–12,15,16]. This chapter will discuss these three major areas of iatrogenic disorders, to open a mental window on the sexual scenario that we clinicians often do not consider.

The role of post-traumatic FSD will be briefly reviewed with a focus on spinal cord injuries [17–20] and ritual female genital mutilation (FGM) [21–24]. Sexual abuse, which may cause both physical and emotional trauma, may be related to post-traumatic stress disorder and long-term sexual disorders [25].

Iatrogenic Factors Predisposing to Female Sexual Disorder

It is difficult to provide an effective intervention, if there is no mention of a problem. The omission of a frank and respectful discussion about sexual issues may contribute to FSD with different dynamics, which will be briefly reviewed with a life-span perspective. With children, the systematic neglect of thinking about their sexuality, and/or about their being potential objects of sexual desire, may expose them to unrecognized abuses which may affect their sexuality throughout their life [16,25,26]. The neglect of urogenital and proctologic co-morbidities may prevent the early diagnosis of vulnerability factors that could have been appropriately addressed, if diagnosed in a timely manner [6,7,16,26–28]. During childhood or adolescence, invasive diagnostic or therapeutic maneuvers (urethral or vaginal swabs, cystoscopy, suturing of accidental genital traumas) without appropriate analgesia and care may be perceived as frank abuses by the frightened child. They are recalled as "the" only trauma predisposing to fear of penetration and dyspareunia in 5.8% of young women affected with vulvar vestibulitis and hyperactive pelvic floor [Graziottin, unpublished data].

In adolescents, a difficulty in using tampons for menstrual protection has been shown to be one of the first (neglected) signs of hyperactivity of the pelvic floor, predicting dyspareunia and vulvodynia [6,28,29]. The lack of attention, information, and support to adolescents, when adequate information about effective contraception and prevention of sexually transmitted infection is not given *before their first intercourse and during their first years of sexual activity*, may expose them to negative experiences, which may affect their sexuality [6]. Diagnosis of chlamydia, gonorrhea, and vaginitis is now possible in adolescents using urine testing and vaginal swabs obtained by the care provider or patient. However, a complete pelvic examination is necessary to

Table 26.1 Medications that can cause female sexual problems.

Medication		Desire disorder	Arousal disorders	Orgasm disorders
Psychotropics	Antipsychotics	+		+
	Barbiturates	+	+	+
	Benzodiazepines	+	+	
	Lithium	+	+	+
	SSRIs	+	+	+
	TCA	+	+	+
	MAO inhibitors			+
	Trazodone	+		
	Venlafaxin	+		
Cardiovascular and antihypertensive medications	Antilipid medications	+		
	Beta blockers	+		
	Clonidine	+	+	
	Digoxin	+		+
	Spironolactone	+		
	Methyldopa	+		
Hormonal preparations	Danazol	+		
	GnRh agonists	+		
	Hormonal contraceptives	+		
	Antiandrogens	+	+	+
	Tamoxifen	+	+	
	GnRh analogs	+	+	
	Ultralight contraceptive pills	+	+	
Other	Histamine H2-receptor blockers and pro-motility agents	+ +		
	Indomethacin	+		
	Ketoconazole	+		
	Phenytoin sodium	+		
	Aromatase inhibitors	+	+	
	Chemotherapeutic agents	+	+	
Anticholinergics			+	
Antihistamines			+	
Amphetamines and related anorexic drugs				+
Narcotics				+

SSRIs, selective serotonin reuptake inhibitors; TCA, tricyclic antidepressants; MAO inhibitors, monoamine oxidase inhibitors.
Adapted from ARHP Clinical Proceedings (2005), pp. 11 [51].

diagnose pelvic inflammatory disease (PID). It is thus important to identify patients who might have PID to assure complete gynecologic assessment of genitourinary and sexual symptoms. An observational study in adolescent and young adults indicated that lower abdominal pain was the most common symptom (90%) reported by these patients. All of the patients with PID reported either lower abdominal pain or dyspareunia in their medical history, compared with 56% of those without PID. The presence of lower abdominal pain and/or dyspareunia in the clinical history yielded a sensitivity of 100%, specificity of 44%, and positive and negative predictive value of 17% and 100%, respectively, for identifying patients given a diagnosis of PID [30]. To omit the physical examination could therefore lead to further PID complications and more severe deep dyspareunia. Other studies indicate that adolescents younger than 18, using hormonal contraception, have an OR of 4.0 of having dyspareunia and vulvodynia [6,28]. Use of hormonal contraception with a higher dosage of ethinyl estradiol seems to reduce this risk [6].

In the adult life, the omission of key questions such as "Are you sexually active? Are you happy with your sexual life?" may deprive the clinical picture of critical information that could modify the overall perception of the reported complaint. Anxiety and phobic disorders often have undiagnosed co-morbidity with performance anxiety (present in women as well) [16], with aversion disorders (see Chapter 22) and with vaginismus [6,27] (see Chapter 25). Lower urinary tract symptoms (LUTS) and dyspareunia, and LUTS and arousal disorders (with vaginal dryness) have a consistent co-morbidity, due to shared pathophysiology (see Chapter 25) [6,15,16,31–34].

Postpartum amenorrhea may be associated with low desire, vaginal dryness, and dyspareunia, which may be worsened by the lack of professional recognition of negative outcomes of episiotomy/rraphy [2,3].

Loss of sexual hormones after an iatrogenic menopause is associated with early onset and more distressing sexual disorders: loss of desire, arousal difficulties, and dyspareunia are increasingly reported with increasing years after the menopause [4,5,9,11,12,31,32] (see Chapter 27).

In the elderly, unaddressed urinary or fecal incontinence, and/or genital prolapse may occur with FSD [7,31,33,34]. The ongoing multipharmacologic treatments, because of the multiple pathologic conditions typical of the aging process, may contribute to FSD, but their potential negative effects on sexuality remain unaddressed unless the patient specifically mentions them.

Key point

The healthcare providers who interact with the woman during her life span may reduce *predisposing* factors to FSD through their early diagnosis (see Chapter 20). They may also consult about FSD while addressing acute and chronic diseases—diabetes, multiple sclerosis, coronary heart disease (CHD), chronic immunologic diseases such as lupus erythematosus or cancer—that may secondarily affect sexuality. Awareness of the importance of a satisfactory sexual life should encourage clinicians to address this issue with every patient, without assuming that chronic diseases per se excludes the need, the desire, or the possibility of a rewarding sexual life [5,8,9,11,12,17–20,35].

Iatrogenic Factors Precipitating Female Sexual Disorder

Clinicians may actively precipitate—or worsen preexisting unrecognized FSD—in their daily practice. This negative effect may be due to the known—but not completely avoidable—side effects of necessary medical and surgical treatment, or to mistakes, negligence, and overall malpractice.

Pharmacologic effects

Drug-induced sexual disorders have special characteristics: the effect dissipates with drug discontinuation or dose reduction; it is not explained by the ongoing disease or environmental stress; the onset tends to coincide with drug initiation or dose increase (although a delayed onset is possible); it is generalized, i.e. tends to be present in all sexual situations and reappears with the reintroduction of the drug [1]. Drugs more frequently associated with FSD are listed in Table 26.1. As a note, it should be remembered that some drugs—such as sexual hormones, in hormone therapy (see Chapters 20 and 27), hypoprolactinemic drugs, dopaminergic drugs, bupropion, or vasoactive drugs, to mention a few—may have a positive effect on women's sexuality [1,5,32,34].

Among the drugs most widely used, a negative sexual impact is more frequently reported with:
• *Antidepressants*: Selective serotonin reuptake inhibitors (SSRIs) are associated with loss of desire and central arousal and a specific inhibiting effect on orgasm, which increases with increasing doses [1,36].
• *Hormonal contraception*: Biologic, psychosexual, and relational factors interact in modulating the final effect of hormonal contraceptives on women's sexual response [1,6,37–39]. From the biologic point of view, sexual desire may be reduced by: the inhibition of the ovulatory peak of testosterone; the increase of liver production of sex hormone binding globulin (SHBG), which reduces the free fraction of plasmatic testosterone; the specific anti-androgenic effect of progestins such as cyproterone acetate, drospirenone or norgestimate and norelgestromine; the inhibiting effect, through a negative feedback, of vaginal dryness and dyspareunia, more frequent with "ultra light" pills, containing 15 μg ethinyl estradiol [6,37–39]. A *positive motivation* to control fertility and avoid unwanted pregnancy, and satisfaction with a rewarding cosmetic results obtained with anti-androgenic hormonal contraceptive combinations (to treat acne, hypertrichosis, or hirsutism) may nevertheless move the overall perception toward a neutral effect on sexual desire, or even a favourable one [38].
• *Chemotherapy* has a complex effect: in pre-pubertal or fertile women it may cause permanent ovarian damage, with respectively, primary hypergonadotropic amenorrhea or premature menopause [5,9,11]. This prolonged deprivation of sexual hormones, especially in women with hormone-dependent cancers, where hormone therapy is currently contraindicated, may negatively affect the whole sexual response; the younger the woman, the worse the effect, both for the impact on menopause and the impossibility of reaching critical life-goals, such as having children, unless through ovodonation, where it is legal and feasible [5,9,11,34].

• *Hormonotherapy*: Estrogen receptor-positive breast cancer has been treated with tamoxifen for almost three decades. Although reasonably well tolerated and used worldwide, this drug may specifically affect sexual function. A recent study indicates that during tamoxifen therapy the most frequent complaints were hot flushes (85%), disturbed sleep (55%), vaginal dryness and/or dyspareunia (47%), decreased sexual desire (44%), and musculoskeletal symptoms (43%) [11]. Disturbed sleep correlated with hot flushes ($p < 0.0005$) and concentration problems ($p < 0.05$). Decreased sexual interest correlated with vaginal dryness ($p < 0.0005$) and/or dyspareunia ($p < 0.0005$). After discontinuation of tamoxifen, symptoms decreased significantly [11]. More recent treatments with aromatase inhibitors such as anastrozole, which inhibit the conversion of androgens to estrogens, may also have a negative impact on sexual response.

Negative outcomes of surgery
In oncology
Surgical interventions more likely to be causally associated with FSD are those indicated in the treatment of different cancers.

Breast cancer (BC)
Breast cancer (BC) is the most frequent cancer in women, affecting 8 to 10 women in 100. Diagnosis and treatment may modify the woman's body image and sexuality [8,9]. Cancer-dependent, woman-dependent and context-dependent factors interact in contributing to the individual outcome [5,8,9].

Iatrogenic factors specifically relate to *outcomes of breast surgery* and *lymphadenectomy* [8]. Mastectomy patients had significantly ($p < 0.01$) lower body image, role, and sexual functioning scores, and their lives were, overall, more disrupted than breast-conserving therapy patients [40]. Importantly, body image, sexual functioning, and lifestyle disruptions *did not* improve over time [40]. Breast-conserving therapy, when oncologically appropriate, should be encouraged in all age groups. Body image issues and coping with change in appearance should be addressed in patient interventions.

However, Kenny *et al.* [41] suggest that, because of the need for adjuvant therapies, women treated by

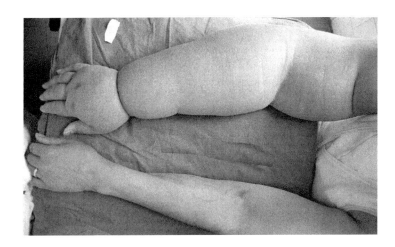

Fig. 26.1 Lymphedema in the dominant arm. Courtesy Dr Carlo Farina.

breast conservation have *better body image but worse physical function*, the latter being greater in younger patients. Negative physical and sexual symptoms may be secondary to premature iatrogenic menopause, to local sensory side effects of radiotherapy and a lack of adequate nerve-sparing techniques to maintain the sensory perception of nipple and areola [8]. An otherwise excellent cosmetic reconstruction is too frequently "silent" from the tactile and erotic point of view.

A second major iatrogenic problem, in BC surgery, is lymphedema [8,42]. The surgical removal of axillary nodes may disrupt and impair the lymphatic drainage from the arm. The arm becomes swollen and painful, causing deformity, discomfort, and disability [8,42]. Lymphedema affects the visual, tactile, pain-related, and proprioceptive dimensions of body image, more so when it pertains to the dominant arm (Fig. 26.1). When severe, it may impair body image even more than breast surgery per se. The incidence of lymphedema ranges from 6% up to 62.5% [8,40–42]. Disfigured body image and self-perception may affect the inner sense of femininity, leading to depression and avoidant coping strategies.

Gynecologic cancers
Cervical carcinoma may require radical surgery and radiotherapy [5,9,43]. Radical surgery may shorten the vagina, thus reducing its "habitability," which may be further reduced by radiotherapy, unless early

psychosexual rehabilitation is started [43]. Vaginal dryness and dyspareunia are the most frequent complaints related to vaginal shortening, while loss of desire and central arousal may be related to the concomitant oophorectomy and cancer-related problems. Concomitant bladder symptoms, if the nerve-sparing technique has not been made or has not been adequate, may further negatively impact on sexual outcomes [9,43].

Vulvar cancer requires a variably mutilating surgery. Poor techniques and infections may worsen the overall sexual outcome [44].

Colon and anal cancer
Colostomy is one of the more psychologic threatened "side effects" of anal surgery. It may affect body image, self-confidence, and self-esteem, through the feeling of shame, unworthiness, and inadequacy it may convey. Avoidance of sexual intimacy and sexual problems are reported in 40% of patients after colostomy [45].

Other cancers
Body image, self-perception, self-confidence and overall sexuality may be affected by the negative cosmetic outcomes of any type of oncologic surgery. The most vulnerable area is the face. Surgery requiring arm or limb amputation or causing asymmetry may also contribute to inhibition in sexual relationships. It is believed that the younger the patient the higher

the probability of a disrupting outcome. However, data are scant. More research is needed to define predictors of worse sexual outcomes and identify intervention for the subset of patients at higher risk of negative sexual adjustments.

In gynaecology

Bilateral oophorectomy

Bilateral oophorectomy (BO) is the most frequent iatrogenic surgery for benign reasons affecting women's sexuality. It causes surgical menopause and the associated androgen insufficiency syndrome (AIS) (see Chapters 21 and 27) [4,5]. Current recommendations suggest maintaining the ovaries, while performing a hysterectomy, unless a specific ovarian pathology indicates their removal.

Hysterectomy

Controversy on outcomes of hysterectomy persists [46]. Most studies suggest an improvement of women's sexuality after a total hysterectomy (i.e. leaving the ovaries on site). The benefit could be due to the relief from menometrorrhagia and break-through bleeding, and the associated anemia and dysmenorrhea [46].

Colporrhaphy

A Medline search from 1966 to 2004 and a manual search of conference proceedings of the International Continence Society and International Urogynaecological Association from 2001 to 2004 were carried out. The success rates for anterior colporrhaphy vary widely from 37% to 100%. Abdominal sacrocolpopexy combined with paravaginal repair significantly reduced the risk for further cystocele surgery compared to anterior colporrhaphy and sacrospinous colpopexy. The abdominal and vaginal paravaginal repair have success rates between 76% and 100%; however, no randomized trials have been performed. Different anatomical outcomes have to be tempered against complications including mesh erosions, infections, and dyspareunia [47].

Negative outcomes of radiotherapy

Radiotherapy may specifically damage sexuality through two major mechanisms [5,8,9,11]. Total body radiotherapy, associated with bone marrow transplant, may be associated with sexual disorders because of associated premature menopause, with the cohort of climacteric symptoms [5]. The negative impact on sexuality may be worsened by asthenia and fatigue, due to the primary neoplastic disease and the need for immunosuppressants, when inadequate host–donor compatibility leading to graft-versus-host reaction requires chronic immunomodulatory treatment [5].

Pelvic radiotherapy—for anal, cervical or bladder cancers—may specifically damage vaginal habitability, causing retraction, vascular damage, loss of lubrication, vaginal dryness, and dyspareunia [9,12,43].

In obstetrics

Abortion

Termination of pregnancy (TOP) may have long-term negative effects on women's sexuality. A total of 103 women who underwent an induced abortion by vacuum aspiration were interviewed 1–3 weeks before surgery and 6 months later. The data analysis report symptoms of fatigue (39%), feelings of guilt (35%), sadness (34%), and anxiety (29%). Of the total, 31% presented with at least one sexual disorder, 18% a decrease in sexual desire, 17% orgasmic disorders, 12% vaginal dryness, and 11% dyspareunia. These sexual disorders were correlated with anxiety and symptoms of depression following TOP. Six months after TOP, 57% of the women reported no change in their sexual satisfaction, 17% were "more satisfied," and 7% "less satisfied." Lessening of sexual satisfaction after TOP was correlated with diminished partner satisfaction ($p < 0.00001$), fatigue ($p < 0.0009$), feelings of guilt ($p < 0.01$), low frequency of sexual relations ($p < 0.01$), and anxiety over sexual relations ($p < 0.02$) [10].

Episiotomy

Lack of professional recognition of dyspareunia and other sexual symptoms associated with episiotomy/rraphy and vaginal dryness in lactating women is indicated as a persisting problem in current obstetric practice [2,3,34] (see Chapter 25). Up to 48% of women report vaginal dryness and dyspareunia, which persists in one-third to one-half of women one year after delivery [2]. Sexual disorders in the postpartum could be easily addressed by appropriate history taking, rehabilitation of the pelvic floor, self-massage, lubricants, and topical vaginal estrogen treatment when vaginal dryness and dyspareunia are complaints [2,3,34] (see Chapter 25).

Delivery with pelvic floor damage
On reviewing the available evidence, it appears that there are sufficient grounds to assume that vaginal delivery (or even the attempt at vaginal delivery) can cause damage to the pudendal nerve, the inferior aspects of the levator ani muscle, and fascial pelvic organ supports [48]. Risk factors for such damage have been defined and variously include operative vaginal delivery, a long second stage, and macrosomia. It is much less clear, however, whether such trauma is clinically relevant, and how important it is in the etiology of pelvic floor morbidity later in life [48].

Fecal incontinence has a female-to-male preponderance of 8:1, consistent with childbirth as the principal causative factor, although most symptomatic women do not seek medical advice until after menopause. Similarly, urinary stress incontinence is an almost exclusively female phenomenon. Obstetric injury may take the form of direct muscular damage to the anal sphincter, as occurs during a third-degree tear, and/or may be the result of cumulative damage to the pudendal nerves. Mechanical, neural, and endocrine factors may all play a causative role in fecal incontinence [49]. Both fecal and urinary incontinence may deeply affect women's sexual function and sexual relationship. Early rehabilitation of the pelvic floor may reduce the impact of childbirth-related urinary and fecal co-morbidities and associated sexual disorders in mild-moderate cases [3,34].

Iatrogenic Factors Maintaining Female Sexual Disorder

Not asking about and listening to a patient's report or complaint concerning her sexuality is the first maintenance factor of FSD. The belief that FSD is substantially psychogenic or context-dependent may induce the diagnostic omission of their potential biologic etiology. This thinking dichotomy—maintaining that male sexual disorders are mainly biologically rooted,

while female sexual disorders are psychogenically driven—is partly responsible for the two-speed progress in sexual disorders research and approval of effective drugs.

Biologic neglect is also responsible for the lack of recognition of the pathophysiology of many FSDs. This deprives women of the appropriate diagnosis and treatment of their complaint.

Sometimes the medical or surgical intervention is credited to be fully responsible for the FSD complaint, while it simply increased the woman's or couple awareness of a pre-existing problem. FSD can be caused or precipitated by medical malpractice, due to negligence, inexperience, or carelessness. The reader is referred to the specific texts of legal medicine.

Key point
The practical recommendation—to increase the positive curing and caring impact factor of the clinician and to avoid unpleasant and costly legal actions—is always to ask about sexuality and potential FSD, and report the information in the medical record, *before* any medical prescription or surgical intervention.

Post-traumatic Female Sexual Disorder

Traumas may affect FSD through multiple mechanisms. For the sake of conciseness the analysis will be limited to spinal cord injury and female genital mutilation.

Spinal cord injury
The biologic effect of a spinal cord injury (SCI) on women's sexuality depends on the level of the lesion and its severity. In women with complete upper motoneuron injuries affecting the sacral segments, the ability for reflex, but not psychogenic, lubrication, may be maintained [17–20]. In women with incomplete upper motoneuron injuries affecting the sacral segment, the ability for both reflex and reflexogenic lubrication is maintained [20]. Women with higher ability to perceive a combination of light touch and pinprick sensation in the T11–L2 dermatomes seem also to have a greater likelihood of experiencing psychogenic lubrication [17] (see Chapter 24).

The psychologic impact of SCI may contribute to sexual disorders through depression, reduced self-esteem and self-confidence, and body image concerns. Physical and emotional/motivational factors may contribute to impair SCI women's sexuality, with a spectrum of outcomes further modulated by personal and context-dependent factors (age at trauma, pre-existent satisfying couple relationship, quality of partner's and family's support, access to qualified rehabilitative care) [17].

Peer-reviewed literature has reported that women's motivation and desire for sexual activities seems to decrease after SCI [17–20]. However, in a qualitative study of women with complete spinal cord injury, Whipple *et al.* demonstrated a trajectory from cognitive genital dissociation, to sexual disenfranchisement, to sexual recovery. Higher percentages of women with SCI complained of generalized hypoactive sexual desire disorder, with a parallel decrease in self-masturbation, in comparison to controls. The reported preferred sexual activities are touching, kissing, and hugging [17,18]. The erotic expression seems therefore more focused on tender intimacy than on explicit sexual activity.

The ability to experience orgasm is less likely (17%) if women have a complete lower motoneuron injury affecting the sacral segments than if they have any other level of injury. Overall, data suggest that only 55% of SCI women are able to experience orgasm after injury, a percentage significantly lower in comparison to controls ($p < 0.001$) [18]. New data concerning orgasm in women with SCI is reported in Chapter 24.

Female genital mutilation

The wording "female genital cutting" (FGC) or "female genital mutilation" (FGM) describes a cultural custom aimed at modifying the female genitalia through an invasive intervention [21–24]. FGC and FGM are used interchangeably. Practiced mostly in Islamic countries, it is *not* an Islamic practice but a cultural practice. The proponents of FGM believe that: (1) the practice reinforces a woman's place in the society; (2) it establishes eligibility to marriage; (3) it initiates a girl into womanhood; (4) female genitals are ugly, unhygienic and in need of cleaning; (5) the practice safeguards virginity; (6) it protects fertil-

Table 26.2 Classification of female genital cutting or female genital mutilation.

Type 1	Excision of the prepuce and/or partial clitoridectomy ("sunna")
Type 2	Removal of the shaft of the clitoris and partial or total excision of the labia minora
Type 3	Clitoridectomy, excision of labia minora and majora ("pharaonic" FGM); infibulation is the reapproximation of the cut ends
Type 4	Refers to any other form of genital manipulation, for example, burning, pricking or piercing

Source: World Health Organization (1999) [24].

ity; (7) it enhances a partner's sexual pleasure [22]. The cutting can be performed at different ages, from birth to the pre-pubertal years. Different instruments may be used, with different degree of invasiveness and sepsis/asepsis, with a spectrum of short-term and long-term side effects, medical and sexual [21–24]. FGC includes a spectrum of surgical excisions from partial to complete clitoridectomy, including the removal of the labia minora and/or majora, scarifying the remnants, and even inserting a matchstick to maintain a sufficient opening for urination. The four types of FGM are summarized in Table 26.2 [24].

Associated complications can be either immediate or delayed. Their severity further contributes to the sexual disorders potentially associated with FGM. At the time of the procedure, medical complications include hemorrhage, shock, infection, urinary retention, septicemia, and even death. Severe pain, because of lack of anesthesia (except for the interventions more recently practiced by physicians in medical facilities) can contribute to emotional and physical shock. Delayed medical complications include hematocolpos, menstrual disorders, vaginal stenosis, infertility, which is reported as high as 30% when type 3 FGM is performed, urethral stenosis, recurrent bladder infections, and inability to void appropriately [22,24]. Obstetric complications include prolonged labour and fistula formation between the vagina and the bladder because of the prolonged labour secondary to the altered birth canal.

Late-appearing scars include inclusions, vulvar cysts and abscesses, and colloid formation. The impact of FGM on women's sexuality encompasses a spectrum of outcomes. Women who suffered from early and/or late complications are more likely to report a negative impact on their sexuality; the more invasive the FMG, the higher the probability of serious consequences. A research study with 250 Egyptian women who underwent type 3 FGM showed statisticially significant complaints of dysmenorrhea (80.5%), vaginal dryness during intercourse (48.5%), lack of sexual desire (45%), less frequency of sexual desire per week (28%), less initiative during sex (11%), being less pleased by sex (49%), being less orgasmic (39%), less frequency of orgasm (25%), and having difficulty experiencing orgasm (60.5%), compared with uncircumcised women [50]. However, other psychosexual problems, such as loss of interest in sex-play and dyspareunia, did not reach statistical significance. The study suggests that circumcision has a negative impact on a woman's psychosexual life [50]. Other studies report that dyspareunia is the most frequently reported FSD. It affects from 35% to 45% of women who underwent FGM; the wider the excision (type 3), the higher the probability of adverse outcomes. However, research on women who *did not* complain of early or late adverse events reported higher sexual desire, arousal, coital orgasm, and satisfaction than uncut controls. Meaning of the procedure, the perception of a higher personal value and of a better body image because of it, and the sense of a stronger social approval may modulate the psychosexual impact of the genital cutting (see the excellent review by Obermeyer [21]). Further research is needed to define the subset of women who may need sexual help after FGM. The proposal of "alternative rites" to FMG, aimed at maintaining the ritual social meaning while avoiding any physical cutting, is one of the current most credited approaches to prevent this high-risk and invasive practice.

Conclusion

Iatrogenic factors are increasingly recognized as predisposing, precipitating, and/or maintaining co-factors of FSD. Further research is needed to quantify the extent of this causality, the role of confounders, the preventive measures that should be encouraged to reduce iatrogenic FSD, and the legal implications of a claim of damaged sexuality. Clinicians should be encouraged to train in sexual medicine and include at least the basics of sexual history taking in their clinical practice, to reduce the iatrogenic contributors of FSD. Referral to a specialist in this area is also important.

References

1 Seagraves R, Balloon R. *Sexual Pharmacology: Fast Facts*. New York: WW Norton & Co, 2003.

2 Glazier CMA. Sexual function after childbirth: women's experiences, persistent morbidity and lack of professional recognition. *Brit J Obst Gynaecol* 1997;**104**:330–335.

3 Basle K, Schuster B. Pregnancy, childbirth and pelvic floor damage. In: Bouncier AP, McGuire EJ, Abrams P, eds. *Pelvic Floor Disorders*. Philadelphia, PA: Elsevier Saunders, 2004, pp. 33–42.

4 Dennerstein L, Koochaki P, Barton I, Graziottin A. Hypoactive sexual desire disorder in menopausal women: a survey of western European women. *J Sex Med* 2006;**3**:212–22.

5 Graziottin A, Basson R. Sexual dysfunction in women with premature menopause. *Menopause* 2004;**11**:766–777.

6 Graziottin A. Sexual pain disorders in adolescents. In: *Proceedings of the 12th World Congress of Human Reproduction*, International Academy of Human Reproduction. Venice, March 10–13, 2005. Roma: CIC edizioni internazionali, 2005, pp. 434–449.

7 Wesselmann U, Burnett AL, Heinberg LJ. The urogenital and rectal pain syndromes. *Pain* 1997;**73**:269–294.

8 Graziottin A. Breast cancer and its effects on women's self-image and sexual function. In: Goldstein I, Meston C, Davis S, Traish A, eds. *Women's Sexual Function and Dysfunction: Study, Diagnosis and Treatment*. London: Taylor & Francis, 2006, pp. 276–281.

9 Krychman ML, Amsterdam A, Carter J. Cancer, sexuality and sexual expression. In: Goldstein I, Meston C, Davis S, Traish A, eds. *Women's Sexual Function and Dysfunction: Study, Diagnosis and Treatment*. London: Taylor & Francis, 2006, pp. 636–643.

10 Bianchi-Demicheli F, Perrin E, Ludicke F, *et al.* Termination of pregnancy and women's sexuality. *Gynaecol Obst Invest* 2002;**53**(1):48–53.

11 Merits MJ, Beckerman I, de Varies EG, van der Zee AG, *et al.* Tamoxifen effects on subjective and psychosexual well being, in a randomized breast cancer study comparing high-dose and standard dose chemotherapy. *Br J Cancer* 2002;**86**(10):1546–1550.

12 Frumovitz M, Sun CC, Schover LR, *et al.* Quality of life and sexual functioning in cervical cancer survivors. *J Clin Oncol.* 2005;**23**(30):7428–7436.

13 Gabbard GO, Anderson C. Professional boundaries in the physician–patient relationship. *JAMA* 1995;**273**: 1445–1449.

14 Plait S. Understanding and managing professional–client boundaries. In: Levine SB, Alto SE, Risen CB, eds. *Handbook of Clinical Sexuality for Mental Health Professionals.* New York: Brunner Routledge, 2003, pp. 407–424.

15 Saloni A, Zanni G, Nappi RE, *et al.* Sexual dysfunction is common in women with lower urinary tract symptoms and urinary incontinence: results of a cross sectional study. *Eur Urol* 2004;**45**:642–648.

16 Layman EO, Paik A, Rosen RC. Sexual dysfunction in the United States: prevalence and predictors. *JAMA* 1999;**281**:537–544.

17 Sipski ML, Alexander CJ. Spinal cord injury. In: Goldstein I, Meston C, Davis S, Traish A, eds. *Women's Sexual Function and Dysfunction: Study, Diagnosis and Treatment.* London: Taylor & Francis, 2006, pp. 644–649.

18 Ferreira-Velasco ME, Barca-Buyo A, de la Barrera SS, *et al.* Sexual issues in a sample of women with spinal cord injury. *Spinal Cord* 2005;**43**(1)51–55.

19 Whipple B, Gerdes CA, Komisaruk BR. Sexual response to self-stimulation in women with complete spinal cord injury. *J Sex Res* 1996;**33**:231–240.

20 Sipski ML, Alexander CJ, Rosen RC. Physiologic parameters associated with psychogenic sexual arousal in women with incomplete spinal cord injury. *Arch Phys Med Rehabil* 1997;**78**:305–313.

21 Obermeyer CM. The consequences of female circumcision for health and sexuality: an update on the evidence. *Cult Health Sex* 2005;**7**(5):443–461.

22 Fourcroy JL. Sexuality and genital cutting. In: Goldstein I, Meston C, Davis S, Traish A, eds. *Women's Sexual Function and Dysfunction: Study, Diagnosis and Treatment.* London: Taylor & Francis, 2006, pp. 666–673.

23 Obermeyer CM. Female genital surgeries: the known, the unknown and the unknowable. *Med Anthropol Q* 1999;**13**:79–106.

24 World Health Organization (WHO). FGM: report of a World Health Organization Technical Working Group. Geneva: World Health Organization, 1996.

25 Reline AH. Sexual abuse. In: Goldstein I, Meston C, Davis S, Traish A, eds. *Women's Sexual Function and Dys-*

function: *Study, Diagnosis and Treatment.* London: Taylor & Francis, 2006, pp. 98–104.

26 Edwards L, Mason M, Phillips M. Childhood sexual and physical abuse: incidence in patients with vulvodynia. *J Reprod Med* 1997;**42**:135–139.

27 Graziottin A, Bottanelli M, Bertolasi L. Vaginismus: a clinical and neurophysiological study. In: Graziottin A. (guest ed.) "Female Sexual Dysfunction: Clinical Approach." *Urodinamica* 2004;**14**(2):117–121 (available at www.alessandragraziottin.it).

28 Harlow BL, Stewart EG. A population-based assessment of chronic unexplained vulvar pain: have we underestimated the prevalence of vulvodynia? *J Am Med Women's Assoc* 2003;**58**(2):82–88.

29 Harlow BL, Wise LA, Stewart EG. Prevalence and predictors of chronic lower genital tract discomfort. *Am J Obstet Gynecol* 2001;**185**:545–550.

30 Blake DR, Fletcher K, Joshi N, Emans SJ. Identification of symptoms that indicate a pelvic examination is necessary to exclude PID in adolescent women. *J Pediatr Adolesc Gynecol* 2003;**16**(1):25–30.

31 Graziottin A. Female sexual dysfunction. In: Bo K, Berghmans B, van Kampen M, Morkved S, eds. *Evidence Based Physiotherapy For The Pelvic Floor: Bridging Research and Clinical Practice.* Oxford: Elsevier, 2006 (in press).

32 Dennerstein L, Lehert P, Burger H. The relative effects of hormones and relationship factors on sexual function of women through the natural menopausal transition. *Fertil Steril* 2005;**84**:174–180.

33 Shafik A. The role of the levator ani muscle in evacuation, sexual performance and pelvic floor disorders. *Int Urogynecol J* 2000;**11**:361–376.

34 Graziottin A. Treatment of sexual dysfunction. In: Bo K, Berghmans B, van Kampen M, Morkved S, eds. *Evidence Based Physiotherapy for the Pelvic Floor: Bridging Research and Clinical Practice.* Oxford: Elsevier, 2006 (in press).

35 Salonia A, Briganti A, Rigatti P, Montorsi F. Medical conditions associated with female sexual dysfunctions. In: Goldstein I, Meston C, Davis S, Traish A, eds. *Women's Sexual Function and Dysfunction: Study, Diagnosis and Treatment.* London: Taylor & Francis, 2006, pp. 263–275.

36 Hensley PL, Nurnberg HG. Depression. In: Goldstein I, Meston C, Davis S, Traish A, eds. *Women's Sexual Function and Dysfunction: Study, Diagnosis and Treatment.* London: Taylor & Francis, 2006, pp. 619–626.

37 Caruso S, Agnello C, Intelisano G. *et al.* Sexual behaviour of women taking low-dose oral contraceptive containing 15 micrograms ethynlestradiol/60 micrograms gestodene. *Contraception* 2004;**69**:237–240.

38 Caruso S, Agnello C, Intelisano G, *et al.* Prospective study on sexual behaviour of women using 30 μg ethynilestradiol and 3 mg drospirenone oral contraception. *Contraception* 2005;**72**:19–23.

39 Davis AR, Castanet PM. Oral contraceptives and sexuality. In: Goldstein I, Meston C, Davis S, Traish A, eds. *Women's Sexual Function and Dysfunction: Study, Diagnosis and Treatment*. London: Taylor & Francis, 2006, pp. 290–296.

40 Engel J, Kerr J, Schlesinger-Raab A, *et al.* Quality of life following breast-conserving therapy or mastectomy: results of a 5-year prospective study. *Breast J* 2004; **10**(3):223–233.

41 Kenny P, King MT, Shiell A, *et al.* Early stage breast cancer: costs and quality of life one year after treatment by mastectomy or conservative surgery and radiation therapy. *Breast* 2000;**9**(1):37–44.

42 Runowicz CD. Lymphedema: patients and provider education: current status and future trends. *Cancer* 1998;**83**(12):2874–2876.

43 Graziottin A. Sexual function in women with gynecologic cancer: a review. *Ital J Gynaecol Obst* 2001;**2**:61–68.

44 Janda M, Obermair A, Cella D, *et al.* Vulvar cancer patients' quality of life: a qualitative assessment. *Int J Gynecol Cancer* 2004;**14**(5):875–881.

45 Nugent KP, Daniel P, Stewart B, *et al.* Quality of life in stoma patients. *Dis Colon Rectum* 1999;**42**(12):1569–1574.

46 Bradford A, Meston CC. Hysterectomy and alternative therapies. In: Goldstein I, Meston C, Davis S, Traish A, eds. *Women's Sexual Function and Dysfunction: Study, Diagnosis and Treatment*. London: Taylor & Francis, 2006, pp. 658–665.

47 Maher C, Baessler K. Surgical management of anterior vaginal wall prolapse: an evidence based literature review. *Int Urogynecol J Pelvic Floor Dysfunction* 2005;**16**(2): 132–138.

48 Dietz HP, Wilson PD. Childbirth and pelvic floor trauma. *Best Pract Res Clin Obst Gynaecol* 2005;**19**(6):913–924.

49 Fitzpatrick M, O'Hertily C. The effects of labour and delivery on the pelvic floor. *Best Pract Res Clin Obstet Gynaecol* 2001;**15**(1):63–79. Review.

50 el-Defrawi MH, Lofty G, Dandash KF, *et al.* Female genital mutilation and its psychosexual impact. *J Sex Marital Ther* 2001;**27**(5):465–473.

51 Jones KP, Kingsberg S, Whipple B. Association of Reproductive Health Professionals (ARHP) *Clinical Proceedings: Women's Sexual Health in Midlife and Beyond*, May 2005.

CHAPTER 27

Hormonal Therapy after Menopause

Alessandra Graziottin

Introduction

Menopause is characterized by the exhaustion of the ovarian production of oocytes, estrogens, and progesterone, with consequent permanent amenorrhea, anovulation, and sterility. The ovarian production of testosterone is gradually reduced from the twenties onwards, but is maintained across natural menopause [1,2]. It is completely lost in surgical menopause (bilateral oophorectomy) (Table 27.1).

The loss of sexual hormones has a widespread effect on all systems and organs, as virtually all cells of the female body have receptors for sexual hormones [3]. This loss accelerates the negative multisystemic effects of aging, with a further detrimental effect. Menopause is characterized by symptoms and signs of sexual hormone loss, with a spectrum of variability and severity, according to: age at menopause (the younger the woman the higher the vulnerability) [4,5]; its etiology (spontaneous or iatrogenic, from benign or malignant conditions) [4,5]; the genetic inheritance of the organ vulnerability to this loss, the woman's general health status and lifestyle [2,5], and the quality of medical care [5]. Predisposing, precipitating, and maintaining factors—biologic and psychosocial—specifically contribute to the pathophysiology of female sexual disorders during the menopausal transition [6]. Symptoms and signs of menopause can be attenuated by the possibility, availability, and feasibility of hormone replacement therapy (HRT) [6–10], now under further study [10–14].

Even the wording of HRT has been questioned [11,13,14]. Following the Women's Health Initiative (WHI) report [9], the National Institute of Health (NIH) suggested that a combination of estrogen and progestogen is not a physiologic replacement. The US Food and Drug Administration (FDA) has recommended the use of the term HT (hormone therapy) as a more correct description of this treatment, an indication completely accepted by the North American Menopause Society position statement (October 2004) [11]. The ongoing international debate has now accepted HT as a comprehensive term, while maintaining HRT for the symptomatic woman [10,12,14], up to five years after the menopause. The acronyms currently used in the literature to describe different hormonal treatments are summarized in Table 27.2. However, for ease of reading, the comprehensive term HT will be used, unless specific words are needed.

Current Controversy on Hormonal Therapy

Epidemiologic studies indicate that current key predictors of HT use are: *age at menopause* (the younger the woman, the higher the probability she will require and be prescribed HT); *type of menopause* (surgical menopause is three times more likely to be hormonally treated); and *education and socioeconomic level* (women better educated and with higher socioeconomic background are more likely to require and use HT) (reviewed in [5]).

Up to 75% of women with a premature, early, or natural menopause may complain of one or more impairing menopausal symptoms, affecting their quality of life, which may be alleviated or cured with appropriate HT [10–14,18–24].

Unfortunately, the Women's Health Initiative (WHI) publication [9] and the following data analysis [15,16] led to concerns, fear, and distrust toward

Table 27.1 Typical premenopausal and postmenopausal serum steroid hormone concentrations.

	Typical serum level, pg/ml		
Steroid hormone	Reproductive age	Natural menopause	Iatrogenic menopause
Estradiol	100–150	10–15	10
Testosterone	400	290	110
Androstenedione	1,900	1,000	700
DHEA	5,000	2,000	1,800
DHEAS	3,000,000	1,000,000	1,000,000

DHEA, dehydroepiandrosterone; DHEAS, dehydroepiandrosterone sulfate.

Adapted from Lobo (1999) [2].

Table 27.2 Terminology for peri- and postmenopausal therapy*.

ET:	Estrogen therapy
EPT:	Combined estrogen and progestogen therapy
Progestogen:	Encompassing both progesterone and progestin
Systemic ET/EPT:	Preparations of ET or EPT that have a systemic, not solely vaginal, effect
Local ET:	Preparations of ET that have a predominantly vaginal, not systemic, effect
HT:	Hormone therapy (encompassing both ET and EPT) in *asymptomatic* women such as those in RCT (late therapy)
HRT:	Hormone replacement therapy, which includes administration of hormones to *symptomatic* estrogen-deficient women, in the late perimenopause or early postmenopause, such as those in observational studies
CC-EPT:	Continuous combined estrogen-progestogen therapy (daily administration of both estrogen and progestogen)
CS-EPT:	Continuous sequential estrogen-progestogen therapy (estrogen daily, with progestogen added on a set sequence)

* Adapted from Sturdee & MacLennan (2003) [13], the North American Menopause Society Position statement [11], the European Menopause and Andropause Society position statement [12], and the International Menopause Society (IMS) Hormone Replacement Therapy: practical recommendations [14].

HRT, in women and in physicians [5]. WHI data exacerbated the worries previously raised by the Heart and Estrogen/Progestin Replacement Study (HERS I) [7] and HERS II [8]. The Million Women Study (MWS) [17], in spite of its lower level of evidence (II-2) compared to the WHI (I) and HERS I and HRS II (I), further increased concerns by the extensive negative media coverage it generated. Weaknesses and strength of the WHI have been discussed in previous papers [5,11–12,14,18,24,37]. Critical data emerging from the WHI are discussed under the paragraphs "Indications for HT" and "Risks of HT."

Fear was triggered by the inappropriate media reading of odds ratios. A key practical recommendation, when discussing risk and benefit with patients, is to distinguish absolute risk/benefit from relative risk/benefit, which is expressed as a percentage increase or decrease in absolute risk. This means, for example, that the reported 26% increase in the relative risk of breast cancer in the WHI is actually an absolute excess of four breast cancers for 1000 women treated for five years, or *less than one excess case per 1000 women per year of treatment* [14]. The latter simple figures should be used. In recognition of this communication and risk perception problem, the Council for International Organizations of Medical Sciences (CIOMS) task force released its report in 1998, providing a risk categorization to assist healthcare professionals and the public when interpreting risks (discussed in [11]). In this context, risks are considered as follows:

* <1/1000 = rare
* <1/10,000 = very rare

The meanings of absolute risks of HT are reviewed in detail in recent position papers [10–12].

Reactions to the findings of the randomized controlled trials (RCTs) on the impact of HT on women's health have caused a significant drop in medical prescriptions. They have dramatically illustrated the uncertainty and the emotional vulnerability of the medical profession regarding the usefulness and even the safety of HT [5]. Authoritative position statements [10–12] and practical recommendations and guidelines [14,18–20] aimed at helping clinicians by clarifying the contradictory evidence emerging from the previous observational data vs the most recent RCTs, HERS I, HERS II, and WHI, have been published. Their conclusions and the most relevant published data will be the base of the present chapter, aimed at helping the clinician in his/her daily practice with the increasing population of postmenopausal women. Indeed, the negative domino effect of a symptomatic menopause may negatively affect the sexual well-being of the woman and the couple, unless appropriately treated (see the review of RCT on HT and sexuality by Alexander *et al.* [21], the review of observational studies on menopause and sexuality by Dennerstein *et al.* [22], the comprehensive clinical approach to FSD and HT discussed by both Graziottin and Basson [4]—focused on premature menopause and sexuality, and

by Graziottin [23]—focused on natural menopause and senium).

Clinical Approach to Hormonal Therapy

HT consists of an estrogen (estradiol or equine conjugated estrogens) combined with a progestogen, in non-hysterectomized women. Progestogens are given either cyclically or continuously with the estrogen, to protect the endometrium from hyperplasia. They are not indicated in hysterectomized women. Different routes of administration are used: oral, transdermal, subcutaneous, intranasal, and vaginal. Because of the lack of the first-pass effect on the liver, the non-oral route of administration may be preferable in women with hypertriglyceridemia, migraine headache, or even increased risk of venous thrombosis [14]. Progestogens can be administered through an intrauterine device (IUD). Over 50 types and combinations of HT are available [24].

Initiation of treatment

As a general principle, HT should be initiated when menopausal symptoms occur [10–12,14,18]. In the perimenopause, treatment will be tailored according to the type of symptoms. HT includes:

* progestogens during the second half of the cycle, if menstrual disturbances are the main symptom;
* HT, if vasomotor symptoms have begun even in presence of sporadic menstrual periods, or if cycle regulation is needed;
* hormonal contraceptives (oral, preferably low-dose, patches or vaginal ring), if contraception is required.

The majority of metabolic changes, including bone resorption, start during the perimenopause.

Dose recommendation and hormone choice
Estrogens

The dose of estrogen should be the lowest needed to relieve symptoms effectively. Recommended starting doses include:

* 0.5–1 mg 17 β-estradiol
* 0.3–0.45 mg conjugated equine estrogens
* 25–37.5 μg transdermal (patch) estradiol

- 0.5 mg estradiol gel
- 150 µg intranasal estradiol.

Symptoms should be reassessed after 8–12 weeks of treatment and the dose adjusted if necessary [14]. In about 10% of patients, especially women with premature ovarian failure (POF) or early iatrogenic menopause, a higher dose may be required [10–12,14,18].

Progestogens

Three major classes of progestogens are currently available, according to their origin from 17-OH-progesterone, 19-nortestosterone, 17-alpha-spironolactone (reviewed in [6]). They may interact with five different receptors: progestinic, estrogenic, androgenic, glucocorticoid, and mineralocorticoid, with agonist, antagonist, or neutral effect [6]. Their metabolic, endocrine, and sexual action can therefore be very different from one progestogen to another. This is the major reason why some negative data emerging from RCTs, such as WHI, using the specific progestogen, medroxyprogesterone acetate (MPA), with a high mineralocorticoid affinity and therefore a negative vascular profile, *should not* be generalized to the whole class of progestogens [6,14,18]. The choice of progestogens (progesterone or synthetic progestins) should be tailored according to the patient's therapeutic needs (androgenic, anti-androgenic, neutral) and metabolic risk profile [6]. The dose and schedule should be adjusted to: the dose of estrogens, to guarantee the endometrial protection; to the regimen preferred (continuous combined versus sequential) and to the route of administration (oral, transdermal, subcutaneous, vaginal, or intrauterine [progestogen releasing intrauterine device]).

Other hormonal options for the treatment of menopausal symptoms
Androgens

RCTs indicate the positive effect of androgens, namely testosterone, on different domains of female sexual function (reviewed in [21,22]). The use of androgens locally for vulvar dystrophy and clitoral insensitivity is often overlooked, but is a very efficacious treatment for genital sexual dysfunction [14]. Dehydroepiandrosterone (DHEA) administration is able to improve the quality of life in elderly patients. It also determines an estrogen-like restoration of β-endorphin basal and stimulated level, indicating a modulation of the neuroendocrine function. In addition, the positive effect on Kuppermann score (which quantifies the severity of menopausal symptoms), with no changes on endometrial thickness, suggests that DHEA administration in the postmenopause may be considered as a possible real replacement treatment [20]. However, no androgenic treatment for the menopause has yet been approved at the time of writing (November 2005).

Tibolone

This molecule is a derivative of norethynodrel, a progestogen with androgenic activity. It has been defined as a selective tissue estrogenic activity regulator (STEAR). Tibolone is a prodrug that rapidly converts after intake, in the intestinal tract and liver, to various metabolites that are systemically active as progestogen, androgen, or estrogen. It has different actions on different target organs, which provide an overall favorable risk–benefit profile [14,19,23,26]. Clinically, tibolone treats menopausal symptoms, including hot flushes and vaginal dryness, as effectively as estrogen therapy (ET), and, most importantly, improves sexual response, while having a positive effect on bone [14,19]. Widely used across the world, it is not approved in the USA at the time of writing (November 2005).

Duration of treatment

The duration of treatment is based on the indication and the persistence of symptoms. Guidelines and position statement [10–12,14,18] recommend that:
- the appropriate indication, dose and type of HT should be re-evaluated annually;
- the need for continuing treatment to relieve menopausal symptoms can be determined only by temporarily discontinuing the therapy. In general, this can be considered after 2–3 years. If symptoms do not recur, HT does not need to be reinstated;
- long-term therapy, usually topical, i.e. vaginal, may be required for ongoing relief from the symptom of urogenital atrophy (see also Chapters 23 and 25).

Monitoring treatment

Pretreatment clinical assessment should include history and physical examination, with measurement of weight and blood pressure. The history should be directed, in particular, to potential indications and contraindications (see below). Menopausal symptoms, menstrual and *sexual* history, co-morbidity between urogenital and sexual disorders [4,23], personal and or family history of osteoporotic fracture, venous thromboembolism, breast cancer, cardiovascular disease, and Alzheimer disease should be evaluated and reported in the medical record [12,14,18]. The clinical examination should include a complete breast and gynecologic examination [12]. It should pay special attention to vulvovaginal trophism, including the measurement of vaginal pH, the pelvic floor tonus, which may indicate specific non-hormonal—besides topical hormonal—treatment to address urogenital and sexual co-morbidities [25,26], and the presence of painful vulvar, mid-vaginal, and deep painful points (see also Chapter 25) [4,23,25]. Patients should be re-evaluated annually. Additional investigations should be guided by this evaluation [14].

Additional instrumental assessments

- *Mammography*: frequency according to local national guidelines. When mammographic density is present, to avoid diagnostic difficulties, discontinuation of HT for 2–4 weeks before mammography can be considered.
- *Vaginal ultrasound and/or endometrial biopsy*: if indicated by abnormal vaginal bleeding.
- *Bone mineral density measurement* based on national guidelines [10–12,14,18].

Indications for and Benefits of Hormonal Therapy

Menopausal symptoms and quality of life

Menopause-related decline in estradiol has been linked to a decline in sexual interest, enjoyment, arousal, and orgasm in observational studies [23] and has been found in RCTs to have positive effects on a number of domains of sexual function (see the review of RCTs by Alexander *et al.* [21]). The direction of causality is that decline in estradiol increases

vasomotor symptoms, which affect mood, and which then affects sexual response.

Autonomic disturbances such as hot flushes, sweating, insomnia, and palpitations can be relieved by HT [2,4–6,10–12,14,18,26]. Other symptoms such as fatigue, irritability, nervousness, and depressed mood may be improved [2,4–6, 10–12,14,18]. Sexual symptoms, when caused by a domino negative effect consensual to the menopausal autonomic disruption, and loss of genital trophism, may be improved as well. In this way, the quality of life can be maintained. Progestogens, according to their structure and metabolic and endocrine profile [6,14,18], can potentiate or oppose the action of estrogens. Every systemic ET/estrogen-progestogen therapy (EPT) product is government-approved for this indication [11].

Premature menopause

Women undergoing premature menopause (PM) (either premature ovarian failure (POF) or iatrogenic) are exposed to the dramatic long-term consequences of deprivation of sexual hormones; the earlier the menopause, the worse the impact on general health and sexual well-being [4]. This neglected group of patients is increasing. Table 27.3 outlines the various etiologies underlying PM, including genetic, autoimmune, those associated with chronic disease, as well as iatrogenic, in the context of benign or malignant disease (reviewed in [4]). Spontaneous ovarian failure affects on average 1% of women under 40 years of age [27], although percentages as high as 7.1% have been recently reported [28]. The Study of Women Across the Nation (SWAN) [27] indicates that POF was reported by 1.1% of women. By ethnicity, 1.0% of Caucasian, 1.4% of African American, 1.4% of Hispanic, 0.5% of Chinese, and 0.1% of Japanese women experienced POF. The differences in frequency across ethnic groups were statistically significant ($p = 0.01$). Lifestyle-related sociocultural factors may be important contributors to age at menopause, as well as modulators of its impact on sexual well-being.

Iatrogenic menopause, for benign and malignant conditions, affects 3.4–4.5% of women under 40 [4,29,30] and up to 15% between 40 and 45 years of age. The five-year survival for all malignancies in

Table 27.3 Factors affecting sexual outcome after premature menopause.

---

1 Etiological factors
- POF vs. PM associated with chronic disease
- iatrogenic: benign vs. malignant
- debility from associated medical conditions
- severity of the residual chronic pelvic pain & deep dyspareunia in endometriosis
- type of cancer, stage and prognosis, conservative vs. radical surgery
- cancer hormone-dependence (breast cancer and genital adenocarcinomata)
- adjuvant chemo/radiotherapy/bone marrow transplant.

2 Factors associated with life stage
- more complex negative effects on sexuality in younger women
- teenage PM interrupts psychosexual maturity
- fulfilment of life goals prior to diagnosis

3 Factors personal to the woman
- coping strategies
- premenopausal sexual experiences and quality
- premorbid personality and psychiatric status
- previous erotic self-perception, sexual self-confidence
- education, social and professional role

4 Contextual factors
- family dynamics (attachment vs. autonomy, in peripubertal children and adolescents)
- couple's dynamics and marital status
- support network (family, friends, colleagues, self-help groups)
- quality of medical and psychosexual care
- ethnicity and sociocultural issues

POF, premature ovarian failure; PM, premature menopause. Adapted from Graziottin & Basson (2004) [4].

childhood and adolescence is 72% (up to 90% for some cancers) [31–33], with an increasing number of survivors facing the challenges of adulthood deprived of their gonadal hormones, unless an appropriate HT for dosage, type and *length of treatment* is prescribed. Premature menopause is associated with an accelerated risk of osteoporosis, and probably coronary heart disease (CHD) [12,14,18] and Alzheimer disease. Distressing sexual disorders are more frequently reported in women with PM [4,34], particularly after bilateral oophorectomy. A recently published randomized placebo-controlled trial was conducted in surgically menopausal women (aged 24–70) who developed stressful hypoactive sexual desire disorder [35]. Treatment with 300 μg/day testosterone patches on estrogen-repleted women increased sexual desire and frequency of satisfying sexual activity, and were well tolerated [35]. However, this treatment has not been approved at this time.

In PM women, the risk of breast cancer after HT corresponds to the risk found in premenopausal women of similar age who have not suffered an iatrogenic or premature menopause. Consensus therefore exists on the recommendation that women who have undergone PM (unless associated with hormone-dependent cancer, such as breast cancer or genital adenocarcinomata) should be offered HT, *at least until the average age of menopause* (51 years) [10–12,14,18].

Urogenital and sexual symptoms

Atrophic changes in the urogenital tract and their consequences (for example, vaginal dryness, dyspareunia, urinary frequency and urgency, postcoital cystitis) are improved by ET. When prescribed *solely* for the treatment of such symptoms, topical low-dose vaginal products are the treatment of choice [4–6,10,12,14,18]. ET may well address the urogenital co-morbidity [35] that increases with increasing age, unless appropriate ET is prescribed. Long-term treatment is often required as symptoms can recur on cessation of therapy. Every systemic and local ET/EPT product is government-approved for this indication [11].

Osteoporosis

Necessary but not sufficient measures in the prevention and treatment of postmenopausal osteoporosis include regular weight-bearing exercise, cessation of smoking, adequate calcium intake, and insuring normal levels of vitamin D. Estrogens prevent postmenopausal bone loss and reduce fracture risk (as shown both in observational studies and in RCT) [8,9], reviewed in [19].

Some progestogens (19-nortestosterone derivatives) potentiate the action of estrogens. Low-dose HT prevents the loss of spinal and hip bone mass both in recently postmenopausal women and in elderly patients. Standard dose HT lowers the risk of spine, hip, and forearm fractures [10–12,14,18,19]. HT may be an initial option for osteoporosis prevention and for fracture risk reduction in the asymptomatic woman at significantly increased fracture risk. Such treatment could be the first step of a long-term program, which may subsequently involve the use of selective estrogen receptor modulators (SERMs), and/or bisphosphonates and teriparatide, when indicated [10–12,14,18,19].

Colon cancer

EPT reduces the risk of colorectal cancer. Both previous observational data and the EPT part of the WHI trial show a significant reduced risk. It is unknown how long the effect of combined HT persists after treatment is stopped or how HT affects mortality from colorectal cancer. The reduction of risk has not been shown with ET [12].

Diabetes

HT may decrease the risk of developing type 2 diabetes by increasing insulin sensitivity. The EPT part of the WHI study [9] as well as HERS [7,8] demonstrated a significant decreased risk of developing diabetes in hormone-treated women [12].

Other benefits

HT can slow the typical thinning of the skin and the mucosal atrophy that occurs after menopause. Lacrimal and salivary secretion are modulated by sexual hormones. Eye dryness and mouth dryness, increasingly complained of after the menopause, can be attenuated by HT. The positive impact of skin appearance and trophism can greatly improve personal confidence and feeling of well-being [4,14,23].

Table 27.4 summarizes the latest recommendations of the European Menopause and Andropause Society, EMAS [12].

Risks of Hormonal Therapy

Breast cancer

Breast cancer risk probably increases with EPT use beyond five years [11]. In absolute terms, this increased risk is small in the WHI, being four to six ad-

ditional invasive cancers per 10,000 women who use it for five or more years, and of possible statistical significance [11]. *There is no mortality difference between users and non-users.* Women in the estrogen-only (CEE) arm of the WHI demonstrated no increased risk of breast cancer after an average of 6.8 years of use. There was a non-significant trend toward *reduction* of breast cancer in women overall, with this trend strongest in women under age 60 (seven fewer breast cancers per 10,000 women) [11,12]. Specific subgroups may be affected in different ways [11,12]. To place the above in perspective, the increased risk of diagnosis of breast cancer with HT is similar to the increased risk of it with such factors as an early menarche (before age 11 years), a late first pregnancy (over 35), nulliparity, and moderate alcohol consumption (>20 g/day). *The increased risk attributed to HT is much less than that associated with obesity* [36]. Due to the risk of recurrence, HT should not be prescribed to women with previous breast cancer (grade B recommendation) [12].

Endometrial cancer

In women with an intact uterus, unopposed ET causes a dose- and duration-dependent increase in the risk of endometrial hyperplasia and cancer. *Estrogen should therefore be combined with progestogen therapy* (grade A recommendation). Endometrial protection is currently the only menopause-related indication for progestogen use [10–12,14,18,36]. No increased risk of endometrial cancer has been found with continuous combined regimens.

Ovarian cancer

Observational studies and the WHI indicate that EPT may be associated with a slightly, albeit significant, risk of epithelial ovarian cancer after long-term use (>10 years) [12]. However, with continuous combined therapy this risk does not seem apparent.

Venous thromboembolism

HT should not be prescribed to women with a previous episode of deep venous thromboembolism (DVT) (grade A recommendation). HT increases risk of DVT three-fold with the highest risk occurring in the first year of use. The overall risk in menopausal women age 50–59 is of the order of 3–4 in 10,000 per

Table 27.4 EMAS* 2005 position statement on peri- and postmenopausal hormonal therapy, with grade of recommendation.

Positive statements

- Lifestyle management, with emphasis on exercise, dietary intake, and cessation of smoking is recommended, to increase the quality of life and reduce the risk of cardiovascular disease, osteoporotic fractures, and also breast cancer (grade A clinical recommendation)
- Systemic ET or EPT alleviates moderate and severe climacteric symptoms, especially vasomotor symptoms (grade A recommendation). No alternative treatment exists with similar effect.
- HRT can beneficially affect quality of life in women with climacteric symptoms (grade A-B clinical recommendations). The effect is independent of the route of administration
- An overall beneficial risk-benefit ratio of HRT in women with an early (<45 years) natural or iatrogenic menopause is documented (grade A-B recommendation). In particular, the risk of breast cancer corresponds to the risk found in premenopausal women of similar age, who have not suffered an iatrogenic or premature menopause
- ET and EPT reduce the risk of both spine and hip as well as other osteoporotic fractures. HRT is an effective method of preventing fracture in all age groups of women who are most susceptible (grade A recommendation). HRT may be the best option in young women or menopausally symptomatic women. Alternatives to HRT use are available and may generally be preferable for the long-term prevention and treatment of osteoporosis in elderly women
- HRT decreases the risk of developing type 2 diabetes (Grade A-B recommendation)

Risks and controversies

- HT should *not* be used as prevention against CHD (grade A clinical recommendation). Results from both the secondary prevention HERS and the EPT of the WHI study show that EPT does not confer cardiac protection and may increase the early risk of CHD. However, the information from the ET WHI study indicates no harmful effect of ET on the CHD rate
- HT should *not* be used as prevention against Alzheimer disease (grade A clinical recommendation). HT does not improve *established* brain damage
- HRT is associated with an increased risk of breast cancer. The magnitude of the excess relative risk is greater when estrogen is combined with progestogen, sequentially or continuously. The absolute excess risk corresponds to 1–2 cases per 100 women among the age groups of 50 to 70 years

---

CHD, coronary heart disease; EPT, combined estrogen and progestogen therapy; ET, estrogen therapy; HERS, Heart and Estrogen/Progestin Replacement Study; HRT, hormone replacement therapy; HT, hormone therapy; WHI, Women's Health Initiative.
* EMAS: European Menopause and Andropause Society, which has 21 affiliated National Menopause Societies.
Adapted from Skouby and the EMAS Writing Group: *Sven O. Skouby (President), David Barlow, Martina Dören, Göran Samsioe, Anne Gompel, Amos Pines, Farook Al-Azzawi, Alessandra Graziottin, Decebal Hudita, Erdogan Ertüngealp, Joaquin Calaf-Alsina, Serge Rozenberg, and John C. Stevenson* [12]. With acknowledgments to: Sven S. Skouby, President of the European Society of Menopause and Andropause (EMAS), and Marco Gambacciani, Member of the Board of the International Menopause Society (IMS), for their constructive comments.

year. The absolute rate increase is impacted by body mass index (BMI) and genetic predisposition.

The absolute risk of pulmonary embolism (PE) based on data from all trials implies that in 1000 women 50–59 years of age, taking HT for five years there would be an additional two cases [12]. According to CIOMS criteria, this is a rare event [11]. Transdermal estradiol could be different in that the metabolic impact on thrombophylia is different according to the route of administration, being higher with oral continuous combined (CC).

Stroke

HT should not be prescribed to women with previous stroke (grade A recommendation) [12]. The WHI trial evidence that both ET and ERT increase the risk of stroke, with an excess risk of eight more strokes per year for every 10,000 women on HT. When separating by stroke subtypes, ERT was associated with an increased risk of ischemic stroke only. In women 50–59 years of age, five years use of HT would yield one additional case of stroke per 1000 women [12], a rare event according to CIOMS criteria [11].

Gallbladder

The WHI confirmed the observation of HERS that HT increases the risk of gallbladder disease. As gallbladder disease increases with aging and with obesity, HT users may have a silent pre-existing disease [24].

Controversial Risk/Benefit Issues and "Window of Opportunity"

Based on observational studies [38,39], prevention of CHD and of Alzheimer disease were considered an indication for HT. The recent RCTs (WHI, HERS I, and HERS II) questioned this indication. Accurate revision of data per cohort of age suggest that *HT prescribed soon after the menopause may have a favorable protective effect on all vessels*, when treated women are still relatively healthy. HT may precipitate adverse vascular events when prescribed later in life, when vascular atherosclerotic damage has already been established. Similar mechanisms seem to be valid for the brain.

The concept of *"window of opportunity"* [14] suggests therefore that *timing of HT* may be critical in modulating positive or adverse effects. In particular:
• HT may have a positive cardiovascular effect when prescribed during and after the menopausal transition [14].
• HT should *not* be used as prevention against CHD (grade A clinical recommendation). Results from both the secondary prevention HERS and the EPT of the WHI study show that EPT does not confer cardiac protection and may increase the early risk of CHD. However, the information from the ET WHI study indicates no harmful effect of ET on the rate of CHD. The concept of "window of opportunity" or "therapeutic window" may help to understand the contradictory data between early observational data and the HERS and WHI trial [14].
• HT should *not* be used as a prevention against Alzheimer disease (grade A clinical recommendation). HT does not improve *established* brain damage. The WHI found a two-fold risk of dementia (possibly of thrombotic origin), significant in women only over the age of 75. Deterioration of cognitive functions in the WHI was found in women over age 65, especially in those with lower cognitive function at the initiation of treatment. However, the cohort analysis, indicating a cognitive benefit for women on HRT soon after the menopause, suggests that the concept of "therapeutic window" may apply to brain health as well.

Contraindications

According to regulatory authorities, contraindications can be summarized as follows [36]:
• Current, past or suspected breast cancer
• Known or suspected estrogen-dependent genital malignant tumors (e.g. adenocarcinoma of the endometrium, ovary, and cervix)
• Undiagnosed genital bleeding
• Untreated endometrial hyperplasia
• Previous idiopathic or current venous thromboembolism (deep venous thrombosis, pulmonary thromboembolism)
• Active or recent arterial disease (e.g. angina, myocardial infarction)
• Untreated hypertension
• Active liver disease (hepatitis)
• Porphyria cutanea tarda (an absolute contraindication)
• Known hypersensitivity to the active substances or to any of the excipients.

Therapeutic Options and Alternatives

When HT is not tolerated, or is contraindicated, a number of alternative therapies can be considered [14,37,40,41]:
• Phytoestrogen-rich herbal extracts may improve menopausal symptoms, although such improvement may be similar to that seen with placebo. The plausibility of this effect is based on the affinity of phytoestrogens for the estrogen beta receptors. The total picture produced by conscientious review of the studies is bleak overall, but there seems to be good reason to pursue the possibilities inherent in soy protein with phytoestrogens in populations of women who endogenously produce equol [40]. However, the phytoestrogen's action is currently being investigated with contradictory findings. No conclusions on their specific role, efficacy dose, side effects, and

contraindications can be determined at the time of writing (November 2005) [14,37,40,41].

• Phyoestrogens may slow the rate of bone loss, but fracture risk reduction has not been demonstrated [14,19,37].

• Alpha-adrenergic agonists, such as clonidine, are moderately effective in relieving hot flushes.

• High doses of progestogens (5–10 mg norethisterone acetate (NETA), 20–40 mg MPA or megestrol acetate/day) effectively reduce hot flushes. Long-term safety on the breast has not been demonstrated [14,19].

• Neuroactive drugs, e.g. selective serotonin receptor inhibitors (SSRIs), are able to relieve vasomotor symptoms with moderate efficacy and may be tried for short periods when HT is contraindicated or not desired [42].

• Recent reports, including a RCT in 420 breast cancer patients [43], suggest that gabapentin, an antiseizure medication, reduces hot flushes.

• Bisphosphonates can be used to treat osteoporosis, especially in older postmenopausal women with a history of osteoporotic fracture [14,19,37].

• Selective estrogen receptor modulators (SERMs), such as raloxifene, are licensed for the prevention and treatment of spinal osteoporosis in postmenopausal women. They have not been shown to reduce hip fracture risk. In early postmenopausal women, SERMs are not able to reduce the vasomotor symptoms and may make them worse [14,44]. Preliminary evidence suggests that they may reduce breast cancer risk.

Conclusions

Healthy lifestyle, with emphasis on exercise, dietary intake, and cessation of smoking, is recommended, to increase the quality of life and reduce the risk of cardiovascular disease, osteoporotic fractures, and also breast cancer, before and after menopause.

With the current level of evidence, HT should only be prescribed when it is clearly indicated, primarily *for symptom relief*. In this context, there is no effective alternative to estrogen or estrogen-progestogen treatment. HT has a specific role in women with premature menopause, and should be considered until the age of natural menopause (51 years). It has numerous beneficial effects, if prescribed soon after the menopause, when the "window of opportunity" potentiates its beneficial impact on likely healthy organs and tissue. HT involves some additional risks of venous thromboembolic disease, stroke, and breast cancer after long-term therapy. The incidence of these risks is evaluated as rare or very rare, according to CIOMS criteria. The need to continue with treatment and the indications for HT should be reviewed regularly when used in the long term. Constant updating is required in the rapidly evolving field of menopausal management.

References

1 Burger HG, Dudley EC, Hopper JL, *et al.* Prospectively measured levels of serum follicle-stimulating hormone, estradiol, and the dimeric inhibins during the menopausal transition in a population-based cohort of women. *J Clin Endocrinol Metab* 1999;**84**:4025–4030.

2 Lobo RA. *Treatment of the Postmenopausal Woman: Basic and Clinical Aspects*. Philadelphia, PA: Lippincott Williams & Wilkins, 1999.

3 Gronemeyer H, Gustafsson JA, Laudet V. Principles for modulation of the nuclear receptor superfamily. *Nature* 2004;**3**:950–964.

4 Graziottin A, Basson R. Sexual dysfunction in women with premature menopause. *Menopause* 2004;**11**(6 Pt 2):766–777.

5 Graziottin A. The woman patient after WHI. *Maturitas* 2005;**51**(1):29–37.

6 Graziottin A, Leiblum SR. Biological and psychosocial pathophysiology of female sexual dysfunction during the menopausal transition. *J Sex Med* 2005;suppl 3: 133–145.

7 Hsia J, Simon JA, Lin F, *et al.* Peripheral arterial disease in randomized trial of estrogen with progestin in women with coronary heart disease: the Heart and Estrogen/progestin Replacement Study (HERS I). *Circulation* 2000;**102**:2228–2232.

8 Grady D, Herrington D, Bittner V, *et al.* for the HERS Research Group. Cardiovascular disease outcomes during 6.8 years of hormone therapy: Heart and Estrogen/progestin Replacement Study follow-up (HERS II). *JAMA* 2002;**288**:49–57.

9 Writing Group for the Women's Health Initiative Investigators. Risk and benefits of estrogens plus progestins in healthy postmenopausal women: principal results from the Women's Health Initiative randomized controlled trial. *JAMA* 2002;**288**:321–333.

10 Writing Group of the International Menopause Society Executive Committee. Guidelines for the hormone treatment of women in the menopausal transition and beyond. *Climacteric* 2004;**7**:8–11.

11 The North American Menopause Society Position statement. Recommendations for estrogen and progestogen use in peri and postmenopausal women: October 2004. *Menopause* 2004;**11**(6):589–600.

12 Skouby SO and the EMAS Writing Group (David Barlow, Martina Dören, Göran Samsioe, Anne Gompel, Amos Pines, Farook Al-Azzawi, Alessandra Graziottin, Decebal Hudita, Erdogan Ertüngealp, Joaquin Calaf-Alsina, Serge Rozenberg and John C. Stevenson). Climacteric medicine: European Menopause and Andropause Society (EMAS) Position statements on postmenopausal hormonal therapy. *Maturitas* 2004; **48**:19–25.

13 Sturdee DW, MacLennan A. HT or HRT, that is the question? (editorial) *Climacteric* 2003;**6**:1.

14 Burger H, and the IMS Writing group. Practical recommendations for hormone replacement therapy in the peri and post menopause. *Climacteric* 2004;**7**:1–7.

15 Chlebowsky RT, Hendrix SL, Langer RD, *et al.* for the Women's Health Initiative Investigators. Influence of estrogens plus progestin on breast cancer and mammography in healthy postmenopausal women: the Women's Health Initiative randomized trial. *JAMA* 2003;**289**:3243–3253.

16 Manson JE, Hsia J, Johnson KC, *et al.* for the Women's Health Initiative Investigators. Estrogens plus progestin and the risk of coronary heart disease. *N Engl J Med* 2003;**349**:523–534.

17 Million Women Study Collaborators. Breast cancer and hormone replacement study. *Lancet* 2003;**362**:419–427.

18 Naftolin F, Schneider HPG, Sturdee DW, and The Writing Group of the IMS Executive Committee.Guidelines for the hormone treatment of women in the menopausal transition and beyond: Position statement by the Executive Committee of the International Menopause Society. *Maturitas* 2004;**48**:27–31.

19 Genazzani AR, Gambacciani M, Schneider HPG, Christiansen C. Controversial issues in climacteric medicine IV. Postmenopausal osteoporosis: therapeutic options. *Climacteric* 2005;**8**:99–109.

20 Genazzani AR, Gambacciani M, Simoncini, Schneider HPG. Controversial issues in climacteric medicine. Series 3rd Pisa workshops "HRT in Climacteric and aging brain." *Maturitas* 2003;**46**:7–26.

21 Alexander JL, Kotz K, Dennerstein L, Kutner SJ, Whallen K, Notelovitz M. The effects of menopausal hormone therapies on female sexual functioning: review of double-blind randomized controlled trials. *Menopause* 2004;**11**(4):749–765.

22 Dennerstein L, Alexander JL, Kotz K. The menopause and sexual functioning: a review of the population-based studies. *Annu Rev Sex Res* 2003;**14**:64–82.

23 Graziottin A. Sexuality in postmenopause and senium. In: Lauritzen C, Studd J, eds. *Current Management of the Menopause.* London: Martin Dunitz, 2004, pp. 185–203.

24 Rees M. Unravelling the confusion about HRT in women. *J Mens Health Gend* 2005;**2**(3):287–291.

25 Graziottin A. Treatment of sexual dysfunction. In: Bo K, Berghmans B, van Kampen M, Morkved S, eds. *Evidence Based Physiotherapy for the Pelvic Floor: Bridging Research and Clinical Practice.* Oxford: Elsevier, 2005.

26 Donati Sarti C, Chiantera A, Graziottin A, Ognisanti F, Sidoli C, Mincigrucci M, Parazzini F, Gruppo di Studio I per AOGOI. Hormone therapy and sleep quality in women around menopause. *Menopause* 2005;**12**(5): 545–551.

27 Luborsky JL, Meyer P, Sowers MF, Gold EB, Santoro N. Premature menopause in a multiethnic population study of the menopause transition. *Hum Reprod* 2003;**8**(1):199–206.

28 Adamopoulos DA, Karamertzanis MD, Thomopoulos A, Pappa A, Koukkou E, Nicopoulou SC. Age at menopause and prevalence of its different types in contemporary Greek women. *Menopause* 2002;**9**(6): 443–448.

29 Anasti JN. Premature ovarian failure: an update. *Fertil Steril* 1998;**70**:1–15.

30 Laml T, Schultz-Lobmeyr I, Obruca A, *et al.* Premature ovarian failure: etiology and prospects. *Gynecol Endocrinol* 2000;**14**:292–302.

31 Rauck A, Green DM, Yasui Y, Mertens A, Robinson LL. Marriage in the survivors of childhood cancer: a preliminary study description from the Childhood Cancer Survivor Study *Med Pediatr Oncol* 1999;**33**:60–63.

32 Larsen EC, Muller J, Schmiegelow K, Rechnitzer C, Andersen AN. Reduced ovarian function in long term survivors of radiation- and chemotherapy-treated childhood cancer. *J Clin Endocrinol Metab* 2003;**88**: 5307–5314.

33 Thomson AB, Critchley HOD, Kelnar CJH, Wallace WHB. Late reproductive sequelae following treatment of childhood cancer and options for fertility preservation. *Bailliere's Best Pract Res Clin Endocrinol Metab* 2002;**6**(2):311–334.

34 Dennerstein L, Koochaki PE, Barton I, Graziottin A. Hypoactive sexual desire disorder in menopausal

women: a survey of Western European women. *J Sex Med* 2006;**3**:212–22.

35 Braunstein GD, Sundwall DA, Katz M, Shifren JL, Buster JE, Simon JA, *et al.* Safety and efficacy of a testosterone patch for the treatment of hypoactive sexual desire disorder in surgically menopausal women. *Arch Intern Med* 2005;**165**: 1582–1589.

36 Simunic V, Banovic I, Ciglar S, Jeren L, Pavicic Baldani D, Sprem M. Local estrogen treatment in patients with urogenital symptoms. *Int J Gynecol Obstet* 2003;**82**: 187–197.

37 IMS Writing Group. Hormone Replacement Therapy—practical recommendations—meeting report. *Climacteric* 2004;**7**(suppl) I:11–35.

38 GrodsteinF, Manson JE, Colditz GA, Willett WC, Speizer FE, Stampfer MI. A prospective, observational study of postmenopausal hormone therapy and primary prevention of cardiovascular disease. *Ann Intern Med* 2000;**133**:933–941.

39 Grodstein F, Stampfer MI, Manson JE, *et al.* Postmenopausal estrogen and progestin use and the risk of cardiovascular disease. *N Engl J Med* 1996;**335**:453–461.

40 Speroff L. Alternative therapies for postmenopausal women. *Int J Fertil Womens Med* 2005;**50**(3):101–114.

41 Haimov-Kochman R, Hochner-Celnikier D. Hot flashes revisited: pharmacological and herbal options for hot flashes management. What does the evidence tell us? *Acta Obstet Gynecol Scand* 2005;**84**(10):972–979. Review.

42 Nagata H, Nozaki M, Nakano K. Short-term combinational therapy of low-dose estrogen with selective serotonin re-uptake inhibitor (fluvoxamine) for oophorectomized women with hot flashes and depressive tendencies. *J Obstet Gynaecol Res* 2005;**31**(2): 107–114.

43 Pandya KJ, Morrow GR, Roscoe JA, *et al.* Gabapentin for hot flashes in 420 women with breast cancer: a randomised double-blind placebo-controlled trial. *Lancet* 2005;**366**(9488):818–824.

44 Martino S, Disch D, Dowsett SA, *et al.* Safety assessment of raloxifene over eight years in a clinical trial setting. *Curr Med Res Opin* 2005;**21**(9):1441–1452.

Female Sexual Disorders: Future Trends and Conclusions

Alessandra Graziottin, Beverly Whipple, Lorraine Dennerstein, Jeanne L Alexander, Linda Banner, and Annamaria Giraldi

Historically, recognition and treatment of the biological basis of female sexual health issues mirrored the recognition and treatment of female urologic disorders [1]. Both were poorly understood, and therefore, under diagnosed and under treated.

On a positive note, urologists have been the specialists who recently took the lead in the revolutionary understanding of the biologic basis of FSD. The contribution of key urologists, including Raz, McGuire and Kursh, began a new era [2,3]. Women's anatomy, and specifically the role of the pelvic floor, was reconsidered, with increasing attention to the physiologic role of sexual hormones in the bladder, genitals and in sexual response [4,7].

Research on neurobiologic bases of women's sexual response added further visibility to the physical basis of their sexual function or disorders, with a multidisciplinary involvement [8–11]. Parallel research on hormonal, vascular, psychosexual and contextual factors is contributing to give meaning to the complexity of women's sexual function and disorders [4–17].

Urologists deserve as well to be credited for a tremendous educational effort, aimed at involving a larger audience of clinicians in this biologically based medical perspective. The first International Consensus Conference on FSD was convened in October 1998, in Boston, under the auspices and sponsorship of the American Foundation for Urologic Diseases (AFUD) [18]. In 2003, under the same AFUD' sponsorship, the Consensus Conference was further updated [19].

Since then, research on the biologic pathophysiology of FSD has had a renaissance. Similarities and differences between men's and women's sexual function and disorders have undergone intense scrutiny [1–3,7–8,11–14,15–18,20]. A significant research commitment to investigate the biologic basis of FSD is ongoing. However, so far (December 2005) no specific pharmacologic treatment has been specifically approved for FSD. The gap between the different research speeds between the two genders has not yet been filled.

The International Society for Sexual Medicine (ISSM), with a prominent urologic component, is to be acknowledged for a tremendous educational effort in sexual medicine, for men first, and now also for women. This book witnesses the increasing attention dedicated to the biologic basis of FSD, and to the educational effort to translate a huge dataset into a meaningful clinical practice.

The FSD sub-committee wishes to express gratitude to ISSM for hosting this section, and for promoting awareness of women's rights to be counseled on their sexual concerns and appropriately treated for their sexual problems with a balanced approach between medical and psychosexual/contextual co-factors.

The future of FSD is challenging and exciting, in the research, in the educational and in the clinical arena. The commitment is huge, the effort demanding, the reward (emotional, ethical and human) is increasing. But it requires integrated, multidisciplinary work, witnessed in the various scientific and clinical backgrounds of different specialists and health care providers working with passion in the FSD field.

References

1 Kellogg-Spat S, Whitmore K. Role of the female urologist/urogynecologist. In: Goldstein I, Meston C, Davis S, Traish A, eds. *Women's Sexual Function and Dysfunction: Study, Diagnosis and Treatment*. Taylor and Francis: Abingdon, UK, 2006, pp. 708–714.

2 Raz S. *Female Urology*. WB Saunders, Philadelphia, 1983.

3 Kursh ED, McGuire EJ. *Female Urology*, JB Lippincott, Philadelphia, 1994.

4 Basle K, Schuster B. Pregnancy, childbirth and pelvic floor damage. In: Bourcier AP, McGuire EJ, Arams P. *Pelvic Floor Disorders*. Elsevier Saunders: Philadelphia, 2004, pp. 33–42.

5 Bourcier AP, McGuire EJ, Arams P. *Pelvic Floor Disorders*. Elsevier Saunders: Philadelphia, 2004.

6 Graziottin A. Treatment of sexual dysfunction. In: Bo K, Berghmans B, van Kampen M, Morkved S, eds. *Evidence Based Physiotherapy for the Pelvic Floor. Bridging Research and Clinical Practice*, Elsevier: Oxford, UK, 2005.

7 Bancroft J. Biological factors in human sexuality. *J Sex Res* 2002;**39**:15–21.

8 Pfaus J, Everitt B. The Psychopharmacology of Sexual Behaviour. In: Bloom FE, Kupfer D, eds. *Psychopharmacology*. Raven Press: New York, 1995, chapt. 65, pp. 743–758.

9 Komisaruk B, Whipple B. Brain activity imaging during sexual response in women with spinal cord injury. In: Hyde J, ed. *Biological Substrates of Human Sexuality*. American Psychological Association: Washington, DC, 2005, pp. 109–146.

10 Meston CM, Frohlich PF. The neurobiology of sexual function. *Arch Gen Psychiatry* 2000;**57**:1012–30.

11 Graziottin A. Libido: the biologic scenario. *Maturitas* 2000;**34**(suppl 1):S9–16.

12 Dennerstein L, Hayes R. The Impact of Aging on Sexual Function and Sexual Dysfunction in Women: A Review of Population-Based Studies. *J Sex Med* 2005;**2**: 317–330.

13 Dennerstein L, Randolph J, Taffe J, Dudley E, Burger H. Hormones, mood, sexuality, and the menopausal transition. *Fertil Steril* 2002;**77**(suppl 4):S42–8.

14 Goldstein I, Berman JR. Vasculogenic female sexual dysfunction: vaginal engorgement and clitoral erectile insufficiency syndromes. *Int J Impot Res* 1998;**10** (suppl 2):S84–90; discussion S98–101.

15 Bancroft J, Loftus J, Long JS. Distress about sex: A national survey of women in heterosexual relationships. *Arch Sex Behav* 2003;**32**(3):193–204.

16 Klausmann D. Sexual motivation and the duration of the relationship. *Arch Sex Behav* 2002;**31**:275–287.

17 Liu C. Does quality of marital sex decline with duration? *Arch Sex Behav*, 2003;**32**(1):55–60.

18 Basson R, Bertian J, Burnett A, Derogatis L, Ferguson D, Fourcroy J, Goldstein I, Graziottin A. *et al.* Report of the International Consensus Development Conference on Female Sexual Dysfunction: Definitions and Classifications. *J Urol* 2000;**163**:888–93.

19 Basson R, Leiblum S, Brotto L, Derogatis L, Fourcroy J, Fugl-Meyer K, Graziottin A, Heiman JR, Laan E, Meston C, Schover L, van Lankveld J, Schultz WW. Definitions of women's sexual dysfunction reconsidered: advocating expansion and revision. *J Psychosom Obstet Gynaecol* 2003;**24**:221–9.

20 Graziottin A. Similarities and differences between male and female sexual dysfunctions. In Kandeel F, Lue T, Pryor J, Swerdloff R, eds. *Male Sexual Dysfunction: Pathophysiology and Treatment*. New York, Marcel Dekker, 2006 (in press).

CHAPTER 28

Cardiovascular Issues in Male and Female Sexual Dysfunction

Graham Jackson and Adolph Hutter

Cardiovascular Response to Physical and Sexual Activity in Men and Women

When advising cardiac patients about sexual activity it is important to individualize the advice. We have a statistical framework to support our recommendations but each person being advised will have, as well as a general cardiac condition (e.g. being post-myocardial infarction), varying degrees of effort restriction, determined by, for example, the size of the infarction. In addition, each person will have personal issues regarding safety of sex, treatment of erectile dysfunction (ED), and their confidence in returning to normal activities including sex. As we advise on sex we need to remember that the problems may have preceded the cardiac event, with important relationship issues as a consequence.

Cardiovascular Response to Physical and Sexual Activity in Men and Women

Several studies have been performed using ambulatory electrocardiogram (ECG) and blood pressure (BP) monitoring, comparing the heart rate, ECG, and BP response to sexual activity with other normal daily activities [1]. The energy requirement during sexual intercourse is not excessive for couples in a longstanding relationship. The average peak heart rate is 110–130 beats per minute and the peak systolic BP is 150–180 mmHg, resulting in a rate pressure product of 16,000–22,000. Expressed as a multiple of the metabolic equivalent (MET) of energy expenditure expanded in the resting state (MET = 1), sexual intercourse is associated with a work load of 2–3 METs before orgasm and 3–4 METs during orgasm. Younger couples, who are not usually the individuals we advise, may be more vigorous in their

activity, expending 5–6 METs. The average duration of sexual intercourse is 5–15 minutes. Therefore, sexual intercourse is not an extreme or sustained cardiovascular stress for patients in a longstanding relationship who are comfortable with each other. Casual sexual intercourse, which must be separated from extramarital sexual intercourse with a longstanding "other partner," may involve a greater cardiac workload because of lack of familiarity and age mismatch (usually an older man with a younger woman), with different activities and expectations [2].

The incidence of ED increases with age as does the prevalence of coronary artery disease (CAD) [2,3]. The heart rate response to exercise decreases with age and the presence of heart rate lowering antiischemic drugs such as the beta blockers. The elderly remain sexually active with no evidence of increased cardiovascular risk from sexual activity or treatment with sildenafil, providing the relationship is longstanding [38]. While sildenafil does not have any adverse effect on exercise-induced arrhythmias, cardiopulmonary responses during activity, or QT intervals on the ECG, by facilitating sexual activity sildenafil may encourage elderly patients to seek a more challenging casual younger partner [30]. Elevated catecholamine levels may result and adversely affect myocardial oxygen demand or overcome the protective action of beta blockers (which work on the basis of competition) and thereby increase the potential for an ischemic event.

By using our knowledge of MET equivalents in the clinical setting we can advise on sexual safety by comparing sexual intercourse to other activities. Some of the daily activities and MET equivalents are shown in Table 28.1.

Table 28.1 MET equivalents as a guide to relating daily activity to sexual activity.

Daily activity	METs
Sexual intercourse with established partner	
lower range (normal)	2–3
lower range (orgasm)	3–4
upper range (vigorous activity)	5–6
Lifting and carrying objects (9–20 kg)	4–5
Walking one mile in 20 minutes on the level	3–4
Golf	4–5
Gardening (digging)	3–5
Do-it-yourself, wallpapering, and so on	4–5
Light housework, e.g. ironing, polishing	2–4
Heavy housework, e.g. making beds, scrubbing floors, cleaning windows	3–6

Table 28.2 Relative risk of MI during the two hours after sexual activity: physically fit equals sexually fit.

Patient type	Relative risk
All patients	2.5 (1.7–3.7)
Men	2.7 (1.8–4.0)
Women	1.3 (0.3–5.2)
Previous MI	2.9 (1.3–6.5)
Sedentary life	3.0 (2.0–4.5)
Physically active	1.2 (0.4–3.7)

Source: [6].

Exercise Testing

Using METs, sexual intercourse is equivalent to 3–4 minutes of the standard Bruce treadmill protocol. Where doubts exist about the safety of sexual intercourse, an exercise test can help guide decision making. If a person can manage at least four minutes on the treadmill without significant symptoms, ECG evidence of ischemia, a fall in systolic BP, or dangerous arrhythmias, it will be safe to advise on sexual activity [2,3]. Drory et al. [4,5] studied 88 men with CAD (off therapy) using ambulatory ECGs and bicycle exercise tests. On ambulatory ECGs one-third of the men had ischemia during sexual intercourse and all of them had ischemia on the bicycle exercise ECG. All patients without ischemia on the exercise test (n = 34) also had no ECG changes during sexual intercourse. All ischemic episodes during sexual intercourse were associated with an increasing heart rate, identifying a potentially important therapeutic role for heart rate lowering drugs (β-adrenoreceptor antagonists, verapamil, diltiazem).

If a patient is unable to perform an exercise test because of mobility problems, a pharmacologic stress test should be utilized (e.g. dobutamine stress echocardiography—an infusion of dobutamine accelerates the heart rate with the patient supine; the 12-lead ECG records evidence of ischemia and the echocardiogram ischemic-induced left ventricular wall motion abnormalities).

A man who cannot achieve 3–4 METs should be further evaluated by angiography if appropriate [2].

Advice on METs in the clinical setting and relating this advice to sexual intercourse should also include advice to avoiding stress, a heavy meal, or excess alcohol consumption prior to sexual intercourse.

Positions

As long as the couple are not stressed by the sexual position they use, there is no evidence of increased cardiac stress to a man or woman. Man on top, woman on top, side to side, oral sex, and masturbation are cardiologically equivalent. In homosexual relationships, other than casual, anal intercourse is not associated with increased cardiac stress provided proper lubrication is used and amyl nitrate ("poppers") are not used in the presence of a phosphodiesterase type-5 (PDE-5) inhibitor.

Cardiac Risk

There is only a small myocardial infarction risk associated with sex. The relative risk of a myocardial infarction (MI) during the two hours following sex is shown in Table 28.2.

The baseline absolute risk of an MI during normal daily life is low—one chance in a million per hour for

Risk factors

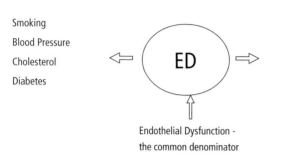

Coronary heart disease

Smoking
Blood Pressure
Cholesterol
Diabetes

ED

Endothelial Dysfunction -
the common denominator

Erectile dysfunction

Smoking

Blood Pressure

Cholesterol

Diabetes

Fig. 28.1 Risk factors for erectile dysfunction (ED) and coronary heart disease; endothelial dysfunction (ED) = erectile dysfunction (ED). Source [8].

a healthy adult, and 10 chances in a million per hour for a patient with documented cardiac disease. Therefore, during the two hours following sex, the risk increases to 2.5 in a million for a healthy adult and 25 in a million for a patient with documented cardiac disease; but, importantly, there is no risk increase in those who are physically active.

A similar study from Sweden has reported identical findings [7]. If we take a baseline annual rate of 1% for a 50-year-old man, as a result of weekly sexual activity, the risk of an MI increases to 1.01% in those without a history of a previous MI and to 1.1% in those with a previous history.

Coital sudden death is very rare. In three large studies, sex activity-related death was 0.6% in Japan, 0.18% in Frankfurt, and 1.7% in Berlin. Extramarital sex was responsible for 75%, 75%, and 77% respectively, and the victims were men in 82%, 94%, and 93% of cases, respectively [1]. An older man with a younger woman was the commonest scenario.

Vasculogenic Erectile Dysfunction

Vascular diseases are the most common cause of ED, with endothelial dysfunction now recognized as the common denominator (Fig. 28.1).

ED and CAD share the same risk factors, which explains the endothelial link (age, hyperlipidemia, hypertension, diabetes, smoking, inactivity, obesity, and depression). However, before attributing ED to a purely vascular cause it is important to evaluate the patient thoroughly as other factors may be contributing to the problem or occasionally be the cause. As men age, there may be co-morbid conditions that need to be addressed (endocrine, cellular, neural, or iatrogenic, e.g. drug therapy), and organic ED will have psychologic consequences needing counseling and support.

A large number of drugs, whether prescribed or recreational, can affect sexual function [2]. These drugs include:
• Cardiovascular drugs: thiazide diuretics, β-adrenoceptor antagonists, calcium channel antagonists, centrally acting agents (e.g. methyldopa, clonidine, reserpine, ganglion blockers), digoxin, lipid-lowering agents, angiotensin-converting enzyme (ACE) inhibitors.
• Recreational drugs, such as alcohol (ethanol), marijuana, amphetamines, cocaine, anabolic steroids, heroin (diamorphine).
• Psychotropic drugs: major tranquillizers, anxiolytics and hypnotics, tricyclic antidepressants, selective serotonin reuptake inhibitors.
• Endocrine drugs: anti-adrogens, estrogens, gonadotropin-releasing hormone analogs.
• Others: cimetidine, ranitidine, metoclopramide, carbamazepine.
The negative impact may be on erections, ejaculation, or sex drive. There is little evidence that changing cardiovascular drug therapy will restore erectile function, suggesting that it is the underlying disease

process that is more important. However, if there is a strong temporal relationship between the commencement of treatment and the onset of ED (2–4 weeks) it is logical to change therapy if it is safe to do so. Antihypertensive agents, especially thiazide diuretics, are the most frequently incriminated and a switch to angiotensin II receptor antagonists or α-adrenoceptor antagonists should be considered [9]. Where drugs are prognostically important, such as β-adrenoceptor antagonists after myocardial infarction, the decision to discontinue therapy should be approached with caution and only undertaken after considering overall risks [3].

The role of statins, either in improving endothelial function and thereby ED or causing ED due to a drug adverse effect, remains unclear [41]. There is overwhelming evidence that statins are prognostically important drugs that also reduce cardiovascular morbidity. They are therefore universally prescribed in cardiovascular patients. Until the exact relationship is clarified, that will need to take into account drug interactions due to frequent co-prescribing, men should be warned of the potential for an adverse ED effect. A switch from a lipophilic statin such as simvastatin to a hydrophilic statin (pravastatin, fluvastatin) may resolve drug-induced ED and allow for the cardiovascular statin benefits to continue [42].

Erectile Dysfunction and Cardiovascular Disease

The Massachusetts Male Aging Study [10] was a random sample, cross-sectional, observational study of 1709 healthy men aged 40–70 years to assess the impact of aging on a wide range of health-related issues. A total of 52% of respondents reported some degree of ED (17% mild, 25% moderate, 10% complete) with the prevalence increasing with age. Cardiovascular disease was significantly associated with ED. The incidence was doubled in patients with hypertension, tripled in diabetic patients, and in those with established coronary disease it was quadrupled. Cigarette smoking increased the prevalence two-fold for all of these conditions and a positive relationship was found for reduced high-density lipoprotein-cholesterol and ED.

The association between hyperlipidemia and ED

has been studied in apparently healthy men who complained of ED [11]. Over 60% had hyperlipidemia and 90% of these had evidence of penile arterial disease using doppler ultrasound studies. Diabetes is commonly associated with ED with a prevalence of 50% (range 27–70% depending on age and disease severity). The onset of ED usually occurs within the first 10 years of diagnosis of diabetes [12].

Men aged over 50 years with established CAD have an ED incidence of 40% and in those post-myocardial infarction or post-vascular surgery the incidence ranges from 39% to 64%, depending on diagnostic criteria [13].

Erectile Dysfunction as a Marker of Vascular Disease

As ED and vascular disease share the same risk factors, the possibility arises that ED in otherwise asymptomatic men may be a marker of silent vascular disease, especially CAD [14]. This has now been established to be the case and represents an important new means of identifying those at risk of vascular disease.

Pritzker [15] studied 50 asymptomatic men (other than ED) aged 40–60 years who had cardiovascular risk factors (multiple in 80%). Exercise ECG was abnormal in 28 men and subsequent coronary angiography in 20 men identified severe CAD in six, moderate two-vessel disease in seven, and significant single-vessel CAD in a further seven men. In a study of 132 men attending day case angiography, 65% had experienced ED before their CAD diagnosis had been made [16]. ED also correlates with the severity of CAD with single-vessel disease patients having less difficulty in obtaining an erection [17].

The smaller penile arteries (diameter 1–2 mm) suffer obstruction earlier from plaque burden than the larger coronary (3–4 mm), carotid (5–7 mm), or iliofemoral (6–8 mm) arteries, hence ED may be symptomatic before a coronary event [18]. Addressing cardiovascular risk early after the presentation of ED and aggressive intervention to reduce risk may have long-term symptomatic and prognostic cardiac benefits [19]. Most acute coronary syndromes follow from asymptomatic lipid-rich plaques rupturing

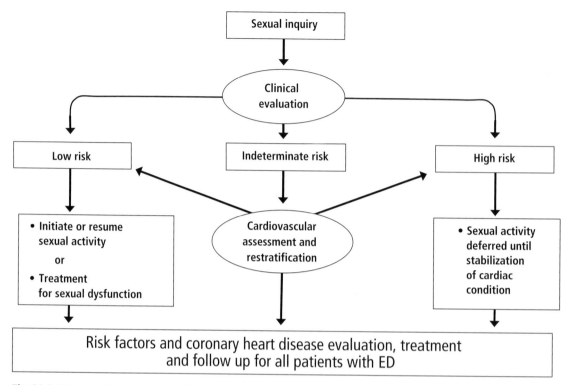

Fig. 28.2 Princeton II evaluation algorithm.

and ED may therefore be a marker for reducing the risk of this happening [22].

Billups and colleagues have developed a risk assessment and management algorithm for primary care patients with ED, with the aim of facilitating the early diagnosis, intervention, and prevention of cardiovascular disease [21].

Any asymptomatic man who presents with ED that does not have an obvious cause (e.g. trauma) should be screened for vascular disease and have blood glucose, lipids, and blood pressure measurements. Ideally, all at-risk patients should undergo an elective exercise ECG to facilitate risk stratification [22].

Treating Erectile Dysfunction in Patients at Cardiovascular Risk

Recognizing the need for advice on management of ED, two consensus panels (UK and American) have produced similar guidelines dividing cardiovascular risk into three practical categories with management recommendations [2,3]. The Princeton consensus guidelines have recently been updated (Table 28.3).

It is recommended that all men with ED should undergo a full medical assessment (Fig. 28.2). Baseline physical activity needs to be established and cardiovascular risk graded low, intermediate, or high. Most patients with low or intermediate cardiac risk can have their ED managed in the outpatient or primary care setting.

There is no evidence that treating ED in patients with cardiovascular disease increases cardiac risk; however, this is with the proviso that the patient is properly assessed and the couple or individual (self-stimulation may be the only form of sexual activity) are appropriately counseled. Oral drug therapy is the most widely used because of its acceptability and effectiveness, but all therapies have a place in management. The philosophy is to always be positive during

Table 28.3 Risk from sexual activity in cardiovascular diseases: Second Princeton Consensus Conference.

Low risk: typically implied by the ability to perform exercise of modest intensity without symptoms
Asymptomatic and <3 major risk factors (excluding gender)
Major CVD risk factors include age, male gender, hypertension, diabetes mellitus, cigarette smoking, dyslipidemia, sedentary lifestyle, and family history of premature CAD
Controlled hypertension
Beta-blockers and thiazide diuretics may predispose to ED
Mild, stable angina pectoris
Noninvasive evaluation recommended
Anti-anginal drug regimen may require modification
Post-revascularization and without significant residual ischemia
ETT may be beneficial to assess risk
Post-MI (>6–8 weeks), but asymptomatic and without ETT-induced ischemia, or post-revascularization
If post-revascularization or no ETT-induced ischemia, intercourse may be resumed 3–4 weeks post MI
Mild valvular disease
May include select patients with mild aortic stenosis
LVD (NYHA class I)
Most patients are low risk

Intermediate or indeterminate risk: evaluate to reclassify as high or low risk
Asymptomatic and ≥3 CAD risk factors (excluding gender)
Increased risk for acute MI and death
ETT may be appropriate, particularly in sedentary patients
Moderate, stable angina pectoris
ETT may clarify risk
MI >2 weeks but <6 weeks
Increased risk of ischemia, reinfarction, and malignant arrhythmias
ETT may clarify risk
LVD/CHF (NYHA class II)
Moderate risk of increased symptoms
Cardiovascular evaluation and rehabilitation may permit reclassification as low risk
Noncardiac atherosclerotic sequelae (peripheral arterial disease, history of stroke, or transient ischemic attacks)
Increased risk of MI
Cardiologic evaluation should be considered

High risk: defer resumption of sexual activity until cardiologic assessment and treatment
Unstable or refractory angina
Increased risk of MI
Uncontrolled hypertension
Increased risk of acute cardiac and vascular events (i.e. stroke)
CHF (NYHA class III, IV)
Increased risk of cardiac decompensation
Recent MI (<2 weeks)
Increased risk of reinfarction, cardiac rupture, or arrhythmias, but impact of complete revascularization on risk is unknown
High-risk arrhythmias
Rarely, malignant arrhythmias during sexual activity may cause sudden death
Risk is decreased by an implanted defibrillator or pacemaker
Obstructive hypertrophic cardiomyopathies
Cardiovascular risks of sexual activity are poorly defined
Cardiologic evaluation (i.e. exercise stress testing and echocardiography) may guide patient management
Moderate to severe valve disease
Use vasoactive drugs with caution

CAD, coronary artery disease; CHF, congestive heart failure; CV, cardiovascular; CVA, cerebrovascular accident; ED, erectile dysfunction; ETT, exercise tolerance test; LVD, left ventricular dysfunction; MI, myocardial infarction; NYHA = New York Heart Association.

Adapted from Kostis *et al.* (2005) [3].

what, for many men and their partners, is an uncertain time.

Phosphodiesterase inhibitors

To say that sildenafil has transformed the management of ED would be a substantial understatement. Its mechanism of action by blocking degradation of cGMP by phosphodiesterase-5 (PDE-5) promotes blood flow into the penis and the restoration of erectile function. Vardenafil and tadalafil have been added to this family of drugs [23,24]. Because their mechanism of action is the same, there is no reason to assume there will be any significant differences in ED effectiveness, but their half-life may be of cardiac clinical importance.

Hemodynamically, PDE-5 inhibitors have mild nitrate-like actions (sildenafil was originally intended to be a drug for stable angina) [25]. As PDE-5 is present in smooth muscle cells throughout the vasculature and the NO/cGMP pathway is involved in the regulation of BP, PDE-5 inhibitors have a modest hypotensive action. In healthy men a single dose of 100 mg sildenafil transiently lowered BP by an average of 10/7 mmHg, with a return to baseline after six hours. There was no effect on heart rate [25]. As NO is an important neurotransmitter throughout the vasculature and is involved in the regulation of vascular smooth muscle relaxation, a synergistic and clinically important interaction with oral or sublingual nitrates can occur and a profound fall in BP can result. The mechanism involves the combination of nitrates increasing cGMP formation by activating guanylate cyclase and PDE-5 inhibition—decreasing cGMP breakdown by inhibiting PDE-5. The concomitant administration of PDE-5 inhibitors and nitrates is a contraindication to their use and this recommendation also extends to other NO donors, such as nicorandil. Clinical guidelines regarding timing of sublingual nitrate use post PDE-5 inhibitor are 24 hours for sildenafil and vardenafil [3]. Tadalafil, with its long half-life, did not react with nitrates at 48 hours after use [26]. Oral nitrates are not prognostically important drugs and they can therefore be discontinued and, if needed, alternative agents substituted [27]. After oral nitrate cessation, and provided there has been no clinical deterioration, PDE-5 inhibitors can be used safely. It is recommended

that the time interval prior to PDE-5 inhibitor use is five half-lives, which equals five days for the most popular once-daily oral nitrate agents.

Sildenafil

Sildenafil is the first oral treatment for ED and the most extensively evaluated [28]. Overall success rates in patients with cardiovascular disease of 80% or greater have been recorded with no evidence of tolerance. Patients with diabetes with or without additional risk factors, with their more complex and extensive pathophysiology, have an average success rate of 60%. In randomized trials to date, open-label or outpatient monitoring studies, the use of sildenafil is not associated with any excess risk of myocardial infarction, stroke, or mortality [29,30]. In patients with stable angina pectoris there is no evidence of an ischemic effect due to coronary steal, and in one large, double-blind, placebo-controlled, exercise study sildenafil 100 mg increased exercise time and diminished ischemia [31]. A study of the hemodynamic effects in men with severe CAD identified no adverse cardiovascular effects and a potentially beneficial effect on coronary blood flow reserve [32]. Studies in patients with and without diabetes have demonstrated improved endothelial function acutely and after long-term oral dose administration, which may have implications beyond the treatment of ED [25]. Sildenafil has also been shown to attenuate the activation of platelet IIb/IIIa receptor activity [33]. Hypertensive patients on mono- or multiple therapy have experienced no increase in adverse events with the exception of doxazosin, a non-selective α-adrenoceptor antagonist. Occasional postural effects have occurred with sildenafil when taken within four hours of doxazosin 4 mg; an advisory to avoid this time interval is now in place. Sildenafil has also been proven effective in heart failure patients who were deemed suitable for ED therapy [34]. The incidence of ED in heart failure patients is 80%, making this finding of major clinical importance. On average, the sildenafil dose is 50 mg with 25 mg advised initially in those over 80 years of age because of delayed excretion. Sildenafil 100 mg is invariably needed in patients with diabetes. An empty stomach and avoiding alcohol or cigarette smoking facilitates the effect. Sildenafil

100 mg has no additional adverse cardiac effects above the 50 mg dose and should be routinely prescribed if the 50 mg dose is not effective after four attempts.

Sildenafil's short half-life makes it the drug of choice in patients with the more severe cardiovascular disease, allowing early use of support therapy if an adverse clinical event occurs.

Tadalafil

Tadalafil has also been extensively evaluated in patients with cardiovascular disease and has a similar safety and efficacy profile to sildenafil [35]. Studies have shown no adverse effects on cardiac contraction, ventricular repolarization, or ischemic threshold. A similar hypotensive effect has been recorded with a dose of doxazosin of 8 mg, so caution is needed. As hypotension does not occur in the supine position, and as tadalafil has a long half-life, it is suggested that tadalafil is taken in the morning and doxazosin in the evening. There is no interaction of tadalafil with the selective α-adrenoceptor antagonist tamsulosin which can, therefore, be prescribed as an alternative to doxazosin for benign prostate hypertrophy [36].

Because of its long half-life, tadalafil may not be the first choice for patients with more complex cardiovascular disease. However, as 80% of patients with cardiovascular disease stratify into low risk it is an alternative for the majority.

Vardenafil

Since vardenafil has a very similar chemical structure to sildenafil, it is not surprising that it has a similar clinical profile. One study has reported no impairment of exercise ability in stable CAD patients receiving vardenafil 20 mg [37]. Similar clinical efficiency for all three agents has been observed in patients with diabetes.

Other therapies

When oral agents are not effective, intracavernous injection therapy, transurethral alprostadil, or a vacuum pump are alternatives requiring specialized referral and advice [2,3]. There is no evidence of increased cardiovascular risk from using any of these therapeutic options. If surgical intervention with general anesthetic is being anticipated, a full cardiologic risk evaluation is recommended.

Androgens

The use of testosterone replacement therapy for the treatment of hypogonadism and ED may assist PDE5 inhibitors if they have failed to be effective [39]. Testosterone levels within the normal range have neutral or potentially beneficial effects on the cardiovascular system [40]. Androgen replacement therapy should be offered to men with CAD and hypogonadism if symptomatically appropriate [3]. The absence of long-term studies needs to be addressed in terms of possible preventive properties on the vascular wall, reduction in low-density lipoprotein levels and the reduction of insulin resistance in contrast to the increase in hematocrit and risk of exacerbating prostate cancer [3,40].

Female Sexual Dysfunction and Cardiovascular Disease

Women share the same cardiovascular risk factors as men and CAD is as common in women as men [43]. The guidelines for assessing cardiovascular risks from the second Princeton Consensus are applicable to women as well as men. In treating ED, care should be taken to evaluate the cardiovascular condition (if present) of his partner as both will have similar cardiovascular responses to exercise. Female sexual disorder (see Chapters 19–27) has not been evaluated as a potential risk factor or marker for asymptomatic vascular disease in a large study but it has been reported to occur frequently enough in the female population to be a consideration in those with and without symptomatic vascular disease. For example, in 1987, Riley *et al.* reported on the prevalence of sexual dysfunction in hypertensive men and women [44]. This was a questionnaire-based study including 178 women which identified significantly more women with arousal difficulties than men with ED ($p < 0.0001$). Of particular interest, arousal dysfunction was not age-related and there was no difference between treated and untreated women—that is, it was not drug-induced. Burchardt *et al.* [45] reported on 67 hypertensive women (mean age 60.4 years), identifying untreated sexual dysfunction in 42.6%

of the 81.3% who had a sexual partner, and in the report by Duncan *et al.* [46], hypertensive women had more difficulty in achieving lubrication and orgasm than healthy controls. A small study of 30 women with angina pectoris suggested sexual dysfunction was common (nine, 30%) with seven (23%) experiencing problems before developing cardiac symptoms [47]. Larger studies are needed before conclusions can be made but it is clear that FSD needs to be queried as part of cardiovascular management.

Drug therapy of FSD should take into account potential cardiovascular adverse effects of the therapy itself and the cardiovascular risk of facilitating sexual activity. In addition, we need more information on the possibility that cardiac drug therapy may lead to FSD.

Conclusion

ED is common in patients with cardiovascular disease and should be routinely enquired about. The cardiac risk of sexual activity in patients with cardiovascular disease is minimal in properly assessed patients. The restoration of a sexual relationship is a possibility for the majority of patients with cardiovascular disease and ED using oral PDE5 inhibitors, which have an excellent safety profile (avoiding nitrate use). ED is a marker for cardiovascular disease as well as its consequence; therefore, its identification (in the asymptomatic male) provides the opportunity to address other cardiovascular risk factors and detect silent but significant vascular pathology. FSD is common and CAD is as common in women as men. Women should therefore receive the same cardiovascular risk and therapeutic advice as men. Though at present we do not know if FSD is a marker for silent vascular disease, we need to be alert to this possibility.

References

1 Drory Y. Sexual activity and cardiovascular risk. *Eur Heart J* 2002;**4**(suppl H):H13–18.
2 Jackson G, Betteridge J, Dean J, *et al.* A systematic approach to erectile dysfunction in the cardiovascular patient: a consensus statement: update 2002. *Int J Clin Pract* 2002;**56**:633–671.

3 Kostis JB, Jackson G, Rosen R, *et al.* Sexual dysfunction and cardiac risk (the Second Princeton Consensus Conference). *Am J Cardiol* 2005;**96**:313–321.
4 Drory Y, Fisman EZ, Shapira Y, *et al.* Ventricular arrhythmias during sexual activity in patients with coronary artery disease. *Chest* 1996;**109**:922–924.
5 Drory Y, Shapira I, Fisman EZ, *et al.* Myocardial ischaemia during sexual activity in patients with coronary artery disease. *Am J Cardiol* 1995;**75**:835–837.
6 Müller JE, Mittleman A, MacLure M, *et al.* Determinants of myocardial infarction onset study investigators. Triggering myocardial infarction by sexual activity: low absolute risk and prevention by regular physical exercise. *JAMA* 1996;**275**:1405–1409.
7 Müller J, Ahlbom A, Hulting J, *et al.* Sexual activity as a trigger of myocardial infarction: a case cross-over analysis in the Stockholm Heart Epidemiology Programme (SHEEP). *Heart* 2001;**86**:387–390.
8 Solomon H, Man JW, Jackson G. Erectile dysfunction and the cardiovascular patient: endothelial dysfunction is the common denominator. *Heart* 2004;**89**:251–254.
9 Jackson G. Erectile dysfunction and hypertension. *Int J Clin Pract* 2002;**56**:491–492.
10 Feldman HA, Goldstein I, Hatzichristou DG, *et al.* Impotence and its medical and psychological correlates: results of the Massachusetts Male Aging Study. *J Urol* 1994;**151**:54–61.
11 Kaiser DR, Billups K, Mason C, *et al.* Impaired brachial artery endothelium-dependent and -independent vasodilation in men with erectile dysfunction and no other clinical cardiovascular disease. *J Am Coll Cardiol* 2004;**43**(2):179–184.
12 Snow KJ. Erectile dysfunction in patients with diabetes mellitus: advances in treatment with phosphodiesterase Type 5 inhibitors. *Br J Diabetes Vasc Dis* 2002;**2**:282–287.
13 Bortolotti A, Parazzini F, Colli E, *et al.* The epidemiology of erectile dysfunction and its risk factors. *Int J Androl* 1997;**20**:323–334.
14 Kirby M, Jackson G, Betteridge J, *et al.* Is erectile dysfunction a marker for cardiovascular disease? *Int J Clin Pract* 2001;**55**:614–618.
15 Pritzker M. The penile stress test: a window to the heart of the man? [abstract] *Circulation* 1999;**100**: 3751.
16 Solomon H, Man JW, Wierzbicki AS, *et al.* Relation of erectile dysfunction to angiographic coronary artery disease. *Am J Cardiol* 2003;**91**:230–231.
17 Greenstein A, Chen J, Miller H, *et al.* Does severity of ischaemic coronary disease correlate with erectile function? *Int J Impot Res* 1997;**9**:123–126.

18 Montorsi P, Montorsi F, Schulman CC. Is erectile dysfunction the 'Tip of the Iceberg' of a systemic vascular disorder? *Eur Urol* 2003;**44**:352–354.

19 Kirby M, Jackson G, Simonsen U. Endothelial dysfunction links erectile dysfunction to heart disease? *Int J Clin Pract* 2005;**59**:225–229.

20 Montorsi F, Briganti I, Salonia A, *et al.* Erectile dysfunction prevalence, time of onset and association with risk factors in 300 consecutive patients with acute chest pain and angiographically documented coronary artery disease. *Eur Urol* 2003;**44**:360–365.

21 Billups KL, Bank AJ, Padma-Nathan H, *et al.* Erectile dysfunction is a marker for cardiovascular disease: results of the Minority Health Institute Expert Advisory Panel. *J Sex Med* 2005;**2**:40–52.

22 Solomon H, Man J, Wierzbicki AS, *et al.* Erectile dysfunction: cardiovascular risk and the role of the cardiologist. *Int J Clin Pract* 2003;**57**:96–99.

23 Brock GB, McMahon CG, Chen KK, *et al.* Efficiency and safety of tadalafil for the treatment of erectile dysfunction: results of integrated analysis. *J Urol* 2002;**168**: 1332–1336.

24 Porst H, Rosen R, Padma-Nathan H, *et al.* Efficacy and tolerability of vardenafil, a new selective phosphodiesterase type 5 inhibitor, in patients with erectile dysfunction: the first at home clinical trial. *Int J Impot Res* 2001;**13**:192–199.

25 Gillies HC, Roblin D, Jackson G. Coronary and systemic haemodynamic effects of sildenafil citrate: from basic science to clinical studies in patients with cardiovascular disease. *Int J Cardiol* 2002;**86**:131–141.

26 Kloner RA, Hutter AM, Emmick JT, *et al.* Time course of the interaction between tadalafil and nitrates. *J Am Coll Cardiol* 2004;**42**:1855–1860.

27 Jackson G, Martin E, McGing E, Cooper A. Successful withdrawal of oral long-acting nitrates to facilitate phosphodiesterase type 5 inhibitor use in stable coronary disease patients with erectile dysfunction. *J Sex Med* 2005;**2**:513–516.

28 Padma-Nathan H, ed. Sildenafil citrate (Viagra) and erectile dysfunction: a comprehensive four year update on efficacy, safety, and management approaches. *Urology* 2002;**60**(2B):1–90.

29 Mittleman MA, MacClure M, Glasser DB. Evaluation of acute risk for myocardial infarction in men treated with sildenafil citrate. *Am J Cardiol* 2005;**96**:443–446.

30 Jackson G, Gillies H, Osterloh I. Past, present and future: a 7-year update of Viagra (sildenafil citrate). *Int J Clin Pract* 2005;**59**:680–691.

31 Fox KM, Thadani U, Ma PTS, *et al.* Sildenafil citrate does not reduce exercise tolerance in men with erectile dysfunction and chronic stable angina. *Eur Heart J* 2003;**24**:2206–2212.

32 Herrman HC, Chang G, Klugherz BD, *et al.* Haemodynamic effects of sildenafil in men with severe coronary artery disease. *N Engl J Med* 2000;**342**:1662–1666.

33 Halcox JPJ, Nour KRA, Zalos G, *et al.* The effect of sildenafil on human vascular function, platelet activation and myocardial ischaemia. *J Am Coll Cardiol* 2002;**40**: 1232–1240.

34 Katz SD. Potential role of type 5 phosphodiesterase inhibition in the treatment of congestive heart failure. *Congest Heart Fail* 2003;**9**:9–15.

35 Jackson G, Kloner RA, Costigan TM, *et al.* Update on clinical trials of tadalafil demonstrates no increased risk of cardiovascular adverse events. *J Sex Med* 2004;**1**: 161–167.

36 Kloner RA, Jackson G, Emmick JT, *et al.* Interaction between phosphodiesterase 5 inhibitor, tadalafil, and two alpha blockers, doxazosin and tamsulosin, in healthy normotensive men. *J Urol* 2004;**172**:1935–1940.

37 Thadani U, Smith W, Nash S, *et al.* The effect of vardenafil, a potent and highly selective phosphodiesterase-5 inhibitor for the treatment of erectile dysfunction, on the cardiovascular response to exercise in patients with coronary artery disease. *J Am Coll Cardiol* 2002;**40**: 2006–2012.

38 Wagner G, Montorsi F, Auerbach S, Collins M. Sildenafil citrate (Viagra) improves erectile function in elderly patients with erectile dysfunction: a subgroup analysis. *J Geront* 2001;**50A**:M113–119.

39 Shabsigh R, Kaufman JM, Steidle C, Padma-Nathan H. Randomised study of testosterone gel as adjunctive therapy to sildenafil in hypogonadal men with erectile dysfunction who do not respond to sildenafil alone. *J Urol* 2004;**172**:658–663.

40 Muller M, Van Der Schouw YT, Thijssen JHH, Grobbee DE. Endogenous sex hormones and cardiovascular disease in men. *J Clin Endocrinol Metab* 2003;**88**:5076–5086.

41 Bruckert E, Giral P, Heshmati HM, Turpin G. Men treated with hypolipidaemic drugs complain more frequently of erectile dysfunction. *J Clin Pharm Ther* 1996;**21**:89–94.

42 Jackson G. Simvastatin and impotence. *Brit Med J* 1997;**351**:31.

43 Wenger NK, Collins P, eds. *Women and Heart Disease*. London: Taylor & Francis, 2005.

44 Riley AJ, Steiner JA, Cooper R, McPherson CK. The prevalence of sexual dysfunction in male and female

hypertensive patients. *J Sex Marital Ther* 1987;**2**:131–138.

45 Burchardt M, Burchardt T, Anastasiadis AG, *et al.* Sexual dysfunction is common and overlooked in female patients with hypertension. *Sex Marital Ther* 2002;**28**:17–26.

46 Duncan LE, Lewis C, Smith CE, *et al.* Sex, drugs and hypertension: a methodological approach for studying a sensitive subject. *Int J Impot Res* 2001;**13**:31–40.

47 Salonia A, Briganti A, Montorsi P. Sexual dysfunction in women with coronary artery disease. *Int J Impot Res* 2002;**14**(suppl 4):S80.

Index